# MicroRNAs: Novel Biomarkers and Therapeutic Targets for Human Cancers

# MicroRNAs: Novel Biomarkers and Therapeutic Targets for Human Cancers

Special Issue Editors

**Takahiro Ochiya**
**Ryou-u Takahashi**

MDPI • Basel • Beijing • Wuhan • Barcelona • Belgrade

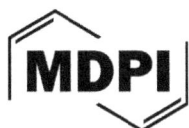

MDPI

*Special Issue Editors*

Takahiro Ochiya
Tokyo Medical University,
National Cancer Center Research Institute
Japan

Ryou-u Takahashi
Hiroshima University,
National Cancer Center Research Institute
Japan

*Editorial Office*
MDPI
St. Alban-Anlage 66
Basel, Switzerland

This is a reprint of articles from the Special Issue published online in the open access journal *Journal of Clinical Medicine* (ISSN 2077-0383) from 2015 to 2016 (available at: http://www.mdpi.com/journal/jcm/special_issues/MicroRNAs-Cancers)

For citation purposes, cite each article independently as indicated on the article page online and as indicated below:

LastName, A.A.; LastName, B.B.; LastName, C.C. Article Title. *Journal Name* **Year**, *Article Number*, Page Range.

ISBN 978-3-03897-252-5 (Pbk)
ISBN 978-3-03897-253-2 (PDF)

# Contents

# About the Special Issue Editors

**Takahiro Ochiya** is Chief of the Division of Molecular and Cellular Medicine at the National Cancer Center Research Institute, Tokyo. He is also appointed as an invited professor at Waseda University (since 2004) and Tokyo Institute of Technology (since 2008). After he earned a Ph.D. in 1988 from Osaka University, he completed a postdoctoral fellowship at La Jolla Cancer Research (Burnham Institute for Medical Research), CA, USA. Dr. Ochiya's lab focuses the development of novel animal models, methods, and strategies to study cancer development and metastasis. In particular, his current focus is on the development of novel diagnostic strategies and treatments for cancer patients.

**Ryou-u Takahashi** is an associate professor of the Department of Cellular and Molecular Biology at the School of Pharmaceutical Sciences, Hiroshima University, Japan. After he earned a Ph.D. in 2008 from the Tokyo Institute of Technology, he then completed a postdoctoral fellowship and worked as a staff scientist at the National Cancer Center Research Institute. His current focus is on siRNA- and microRNA-based therapies against cancer stem cells.

# Preface to "MicroRNAs: Novel Biomarkers and Therapeutic Targets for Human Cancers"

We are pleased to present to you MDPI Press Review: This Special Issue is a collection of research and review articles from the *Journal of Clinical Medic*ine in order to provide readers with the latest information and developments of microRNA-based diagnostic markers and therapeutics. Articles were selected and reviewed by invited experts who specialize in the field of cancer research and RNA biology. This issue covers a wide range of topics from basic research to clinical study.

**Takahiro Ochiya, Ryou-u Takahashi**
*Special Issue Editors*

Journal of
*Clinical Medicine*

MDPI

*Communication*

# Preliminary Analysis of the Expression of Selected Proangiogenic and Antioxidant Genes and MicroRNAs in Patients with Non-Muscle-Invasive Bladder Cancer

Magdalena Kozakowska [1,†], Barbara Dobrowolska-Glazar [2,3,†], Krzysztof Okoń [4], Alicja Józkowicz [1], Zygmunt Dobrowolski [3,5,‡] and Józef Dulak [1,6,*,‡]

1   Department of Medical Biotechnology, Faculty of Biochemistry, Biophysics and Biotechnology, Jagiellonian University, 30-387 Krakow, Poland; m.kozakowska@uj.edu.pl (M.K.); alicja.jozkowicz@uj.edu.pl (A.J.)
2   Department of Pediatric Urology, Jagiellonian University Medical College, 30-688 Krakow, Poland; bdobrowolska@o2.pl
3   Department and Clinic of Urology, Jagiellonian University Medical College, 31-530 Krakow, Poland; zdobrowol@su.krakow.pl
4   Department of Pathomorphology, Jagiellonian University Medical College, 31-531 Krakow, Poland; k.okon@uj.edu.pl
5   Department of Urology, University of Rzeszow, 35-959 Rzeszow, Poland
6   Malopolska Centre of Biotechnology, Jagiellonian University, 30-387 Krakow, Poland
*   Correspondence: jozef.dulak@uj.edu.pl; Tel.: +48-12-664-63-75; Fax: +48-12-664-69-18
†   These authors contributed equally to the work.
‡   These authors contributed equally as senior authors to the work.

Academic Editors: Takahiro Ochiya and Ryou-u Takahashi
Received: 5 November 2015; Accepted: 14 February 2016; Published: 25 February 2016

**Abstract:** Heme oxygenase-1 (HO-1) is an enzyme contributing to the development and progression of different cancer types. HO-1 plays a role in pathological angiogenesis in bladder cancer and contributes to the resistance of this cancer to therapy. It also regulates the expression of microRNAs in *rhabdomyosarcoma* and non-small cell lung cancer. The expression of HO-1 may be regulated by hypoxia inducible factors (HIFs) and Nrf2 transcription factor. The expression of HO-1 has not so far been examined in relation to Nrf2, HIF-1$\alpha$, and potential mediators of angiogenesis in human bladder cancer. We measured the concentration of proinflammatory and proangiogenic cytokines and the expression of cytoprotective and proangiogenic mRNAs and miRNAs in healthy subjects and patients with bladder cancer. HO-1 expression was upregulated together with HIF-1$\alpha$, HIF-2$\alpha$, and Nrf2 in bladder cancer in comparison to healthy tissue. VEGF was elevated both at mRNA and protein level in the tumor and in sera, respectively. Additionally, IL-6 and IL-8 were increased in sera of patients affected with urothelial bladder cancer. Moreover, miR-155 was downregulated whereas miR-200c was elevated in cancer biopsies in comparison to healthy tissue. The results indicate that the increased expression of HO-1 in bladder cancer is paralleled by changes in the expression of other potentially interacting genes, like Nrf2, HIF-1$\alpha$, HIF-2$\alpha$, IL-6, IL-8, and VEGF. Further studies are necessary to also elucidate the potential links with miR-155 and miR-200c.

**Keywords:** bladder cancer; urothelial cancer; heme oxygenase-1; hypoxia inducible factor; Nrf2; miR-155; miR-200c; VEGF; angiogenesis

## 1. Introduction

Bladder cancer (*urothelial cancer*) is the 7th most common cancer in men and 17th in women, and is more frequent in well-developed regions, where 60% of all incidents occur. Non-muscle-invasive bladder cancer is characterized by a high rate of recurrence—despite the total resection of the tumor it reappears in 75% of patients. The five-year survival rate is around 57% [1,2]. The major cause of development of bladder cancer is long-term exposure to environmental risk factors. The primary culprits are smoking, chemical compounds binding DNA (like aromatic amines), or arsenic (the metabolism of which is associated with the generation of reactive oxygen species) [2]. Recent data indicate the role of oxidative stress in the progression of bladder cancer [3].

Among transcription factors affected by oxidative stress, and which are altered in bladder cancer, are hypoxia inducible factors (HIF-1$\alpha$, HIF-2$\alpha$), and Nrf2 transcription factor [3]. In response to oxidative stress, Nrf2 binds to promoters of genes encoding antioxidative enzymes [4]. It is believed to be a mediator of action of chemopreventive compounds [5–8], and it also contributes to resistance to cisplatin [9] and photodynamic therapy [10]. HIF-1$\alpha$ and HIF-2$\alpha$, which regulate cellular redox homeostasis, are factors inducing angiogenesis and inflammatory reaction [11,12]. They are correlated with increasing invasiveness, macrophage infiltration, and angiogenesis in bladder cancer [13–15]. Among the direct mediators of HIFs in bladder cancer, vascular endothelial growth factor (VEGF) is usually listed [13,15–17]. Its expression correlates with enhanced angiogenesis, proliferation, and metastatic potential in urothelial tumors [18–20]. However, since clinical trials based on VEGF-targeted anti-angiogenic therapies of bladder cancer have not given satisfactory results [21], there is a need to search for other mediators of both pro-angiogenic and anti-cytotoxic effects of HIFs and Nrf2.

Heme oxygenase-1 (HO-1) is a heme-degrading enzyme of known pro-angiogenic and cytoprotective effects, the expression of which may be induced by both Nrf2 and HIF-1$\alpha$ [22]. Moreover, HO-1 has a potent impact on the development of different types of cancer [23]. In recent years, an increasing body of evidence points to the role of HO-1 in pathological angiogenesis in bladder cancer [24] and in some cases in the resistance of this cancer to chemo- and radiotherapy [10,25,26]. However, only a few of the studies analyzed clinical material from patients affected by bladder cancer, confirming a positive correlation of HO-1 level with the proliferation of cancer cells, VEGF-induced angiogenesis, and, finally, the malignant behavior of the cancer [24,27–29], whereas none of them involved comparison to the healthy tissue. Furthermore, the expression of HO-1 was never assessed together with Nrf2 in the clinical samples and only one study showed the analysis of HO-1 with HIF-1$\alpha$ and HIF-2$\alpha$ in urothelial tumors, suggesting the correlation between their expressions [24].

HO-1 is known to potently regulate the expression of miRNAs in muscle myoblasts and rhabdomyosarcoma [30–32]. The expression of miRNAs is also changed in bladder cancer, which may be a diagnostic parameter [33,34]. Changes in miR-200c are suggested to be associated with the pathogenesis of bladder cancer and to affect the efficacy of therapeutic treatment [35,36]. Similar tendencies were demonstrated for other types of cancer [37,38], but the current data for bladder cancer are ambiguous and show either an induction of miR-200c expression [39–41] or an inhibition [33,42–45]. On the other hand, miR-133b [46–48] and miR-133a [39,46,49–52], shown by us to be strongly affected by HO-1 [30], are also downregulated in bladder cancer.

The aim of this study was to analyze the level of proinflammatory and proangiogenic cytokines in the sera and determine the expression of genes associated with cytoprotection and angiogenesis as well as selected miRNAs in clinical samples collected from patients subjected to diagnostic and control cystoscopy.

## 2. Experimental Section

### 2.1. Patient Samples

Patients with known bladder cancer in stages Ta, Tis, or T1 and patients with suspected bladder cancer were recruited ($N$ = 21; age 51–80, mean age = 67; five females and 16 males). Two hours prior to the TURBT (transurethral resection of the bladder tumor) procedure, patients underwent bladder instillation with 50 mL of 8 mM solution of HAL (hexyl aminolevulinate) hydrochloride in phosphate buffered saline (Hexvix, Photocure) through a Foley catheter. After the HAL solution was evacuated, the bladder was inspected by white light cystoscopy. Lesions or suspicious areas were classified and mapped onto a bladder chart in blue. The bladder was then inspected by HAL fluorescence cystoscopy. Lesions or suspicious areas were classified and mapped onto the bladder chart in red. Fluorescence cystoscopy was a supplementary but not substitutional procedure. The diameter of the lesions or suspicious areas were 0.2–2 cm, while the majority did not exceed 1 cm. Biopsies (0.1–0.3 cm diameter) were taken from all mapped areas. Test materials were collected for histopathological analysis and some of them were used for the isolation of RNA. Among 27 samples collected for mRNA and miRNA analysis, papillary urothelial neoplasm of low malignant potential, according to the International Society of Urological Pathology guidelines [53], was diagnosed in two cases, low-grade urothelial carcinoma in 13, and high-grade urothelial carcinoma in one (out of the initial group of 21 patients, bladder cancer was diagnosed in $N = 16$ cases; age 51–80, mean age 67; five females and 11 males). Eleven samples for mRNA and miRNA analysis were histologically assessed as unaltered, healthy tissue—$N = 11$, age 57–74, mean age 67; two females and nine males. Those 11 samples were derived from patients finally diagnosed as healthy ($N = 5$, age 58–73, mean age 69; 5 males) and 6 samples of healthy tissue were also found among patients who had bladder cancer confirmed in another area.

Serum was collected for the analysis of cytokines from all patients subjected to cystoscopy (16 patients with subsequently diagnosed bladder cancer and five assessed histopathologically as healthy) as well as from additional healthy, voluntary, age-matched controls (the total number of healthy controls included for the measurement of cytokine: $N = 9$, age 51–73, mean age = 65; three females and six males).

The research was completed in September 2012; it complied with the Declaration of Helsinki and was approved by the Local Bioethical Commission (agreement No. KBET/197/B/2012). Patients provided written informed consent for the study.

### 2.2. RNA Isolation and qRT-PCR

RNA isolation followed by reverse transcription and quantitative PCR for genes and miRNA were performed with standard procedures, described elsewhere [30]. Primers used in qRT-PCR are presented in Tables 1 and 2.

**Table 1.** Sequences of starters for genes.

| Gene | | Sequence of Starters |
|------|--|----------------------|
| EF2 | forward | 5′-GAC ATC ACC AAG GGT GTG CAG-3′ |
|  | reverse | 5′-TCA GCA CAC TGG CAT AGA GGC-3′ |
| HO-1 | forward | 5′-GTG GAG MCG CTT YAC RTA GYG C-3′ |
|  | reverse | 5′-CTT TCA GAA GGG YCA GGT GWC C-3′ |
| VEGF | forward | 5′-ATG CGG ATC AAA CCT CAC CAA GGC-3′ |
|  | reverse | 5′-TTA ACT CAA GCT GCC TCG CCT TGC-3′ |
| Nrf2 | forward | 5′-GGG GTA AGA ATA AAG TGG CTG CTC-3′ |
|  | reverse | 5′-ACA TTG CCA TCT CTT GTT TGC TG-3′ |
| HIF-1$\alpha$ | forward | 5′-TGC TTG GTG CTG ATT TGT GA-3′ |
|  | reverse | 5′-GGT CAG ATG ATC AGA GTC CA-3′ |
| HIF-2$\alpha$ | forward | 5′-TCC GAG CAG TGG AGT CAT TCA-3′ |
|  | reverse | 5′-GTC CAA ATG TGC CGT GTG AAA-3′ |

**Table 2.** Sequences of starters for miRNA.

| miRNA | Sequence Of Specific Starters |
|-------|-------------------------------|
| U6 | 5′-CGC AAG GAT GAC ACG CAA ATT C-3′ |
| miRNA-133a | 5′-TTG GTC CCC TTC AAC CAG CTG T-3′ |
| miRNA-155 | 5′-TTA ATG CTA ATT GTG ATA GGG GT-3′ |
| miRNA-200c | 5′-TAA TAC TGC CGG GTA ATG ATG GA-3′ |

### 2.3. Luminex Analysis of Cytokine and Growth Factor Concentrations in Plasma

Concentrations of interferon-γ (IFN-γ), interleukin (IL)-1β, IL-6, IL-8, IL-10, IL-12, IL-17, monocyte chemoattractant protein-1 (MCP-1), tumor necrosis factor-α (TNFα), and VEGF in plasma were evaluated using Milliplex FlexMap 3D (Millipore, Billerica, MA, USA) according to the vendor's protocol.

### 2.4. Statistical Analysis

The normal distribution of data was checked using the D'Agostino–Pearson test. Statistical significance was assessed using the Student's t-test or Welch's Mann–Whitney $U$-test, and accepted at $p < 0.05$. Correlation was analyzed using Spearman's rank correlation.

## 3. Results

### 3.1. Level of Cytokine in the Sera

The analysis of cytokine levels was performed in the sera of patients with diagnosed bladder cancer ($N = 16$) and aged-matched healthy controls ($N = 9$). IL-6 was significantly increased in the material collected from patients affected by bladder cancer, whereas TNFα showed a tendency to be induced ($p = 0.08$) (Figure 1). Proangiogenic VEGF and IL-8 were both significantly increased in urological patients (Figure 1), whereas IFNγ, IL-1β, MCP-1, IL-10, IL-12, and IL-17 were unchanged (data not shown).

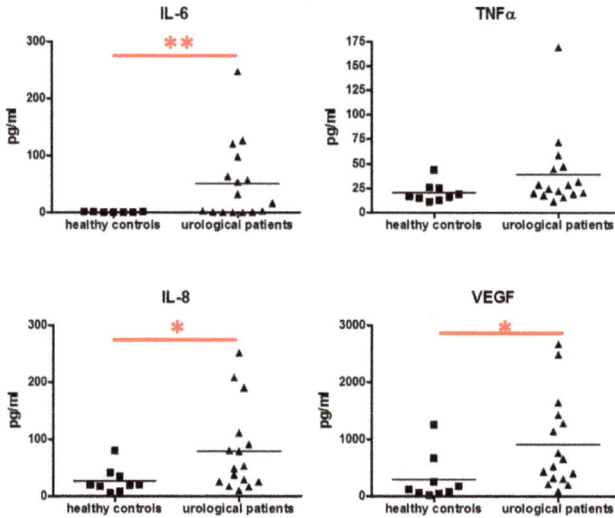

**Figure 1.** Concentrations of cytokines in the serum of patients with diagnosed bladder cancer and in healthy controls. Luminex, $N = 9$–16; each dot represents one individual, line represents a mean; * $p < 0.05$; ** $p < 0.01$.

## 3.2. Expression of Proangiogenic and Cytoprotective Genes in Tumor Samples

The analysis of gene expressions at mRNA level revealed that Nrf2 (a transcription factor and regulator of the expression of proteins that are a second line of cell defense against oxidative stress), and its downstream target HO-1, were upregulated in samples of bladder cancer ($N = 16$) in comparison to healthy tissue ($N = 11$) (Figure 2). Similarly, factors regulated by hypoxia (HIF-1$\alpha$ and HIF-2$\alpha$) and their target VEGF were upregulated in bladder cancer samples (Figure 2).

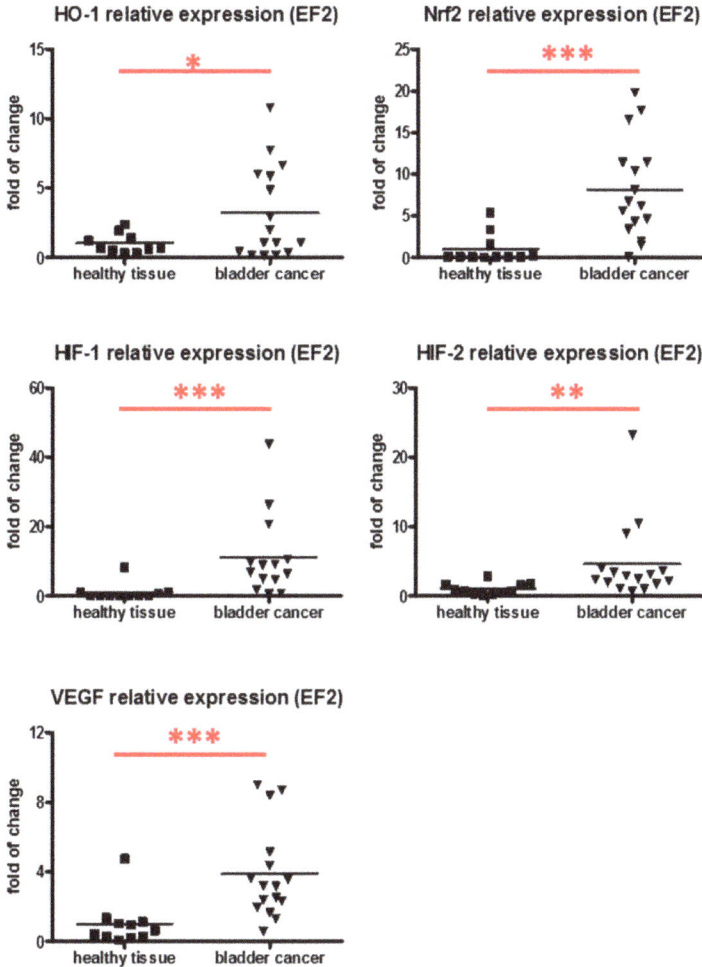

**Figure 2.** Gene expression at mRNA level in samples of bladder cancer and in healthy tissue. qRT-PCR, $N = 11$–16; each dot represents one individual, line represents a mean; $^* p < 0.05$; $^{**} p < 0.01$; $^{***} p < 0.001$.

## 3.3. Analysis of miRNA Expression in Cancer Samples

Analysis of miRNAs showed that the level of miR-200c is significantly induced in samples of bladder cancer, whereas miR-155 is downregulated. No changes were observed in the case of miR-133a (Figure 3).

**miR-133a relative expression (U6)**

**miR-155 relative expression (U6)**

**miR-200c relative expression (U6)**

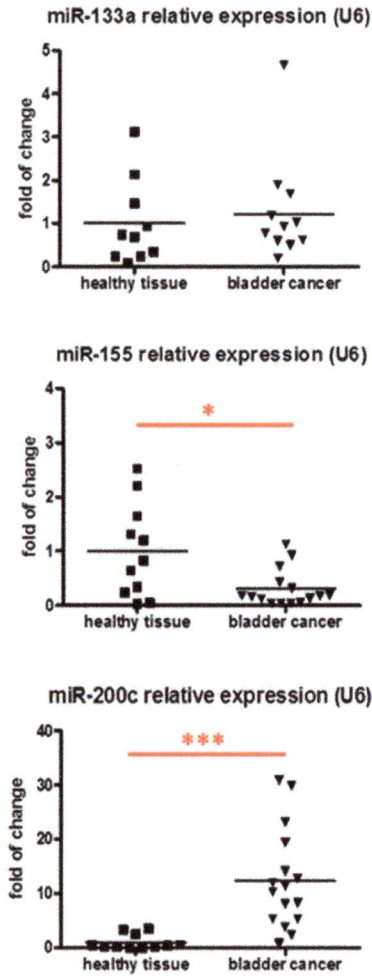

**Figure 3.** The expression of selected miRNAs in samples of bladder cancer and in healthy tissue. qRT-PCR, $N$ = 11–16; each dot represents one individual, line represents a mean; * $p < 0.05$; *** $p < 0.001$.

Spearman's rank correlation coefficient was used to determine the correlation between miRNAs and the expression of genes analyzed. MiR-200c was found to positively correlate to VEGF expression in bladder cancer (Table 3).

**Table 3.** Spearman's rank correlation of tested miRNA/mRNA; * $p < 0.05$.

|  | HO-1 | Nrf2 | VEGF | HIF1 | HIF2 |
|---|---|---|---|---|---|
| miR-133a | −0.329 | −0.347 | 0.161 | 0.063 | 0.109 |
| miR-155 | 0.194 | −0.151 | −0.009 | 0.411 | −0.385 |
| miR-200c | 0.259 | 0.406 | 0.606 * | 0.365 | 0.424 |

## 4. Discussion

Our results confirm previous data showing the increased production of proinflammatory and proangiogenic cytokines in patients affected by bladder cancer, and suggesting their diagnostic importance [20,54–56].

Upregulation of IL-6 was detected in the sera and urine of bladder cancer patients [56,57], as well as in tumors [58,59]. IL-6 was correlated with higher clinical stage, higher recurrence rate, and reduced survival of patients with bladder cancer [58]. TNFα was also detected in the sera and in peripheral blood mononuclear cells of patients with bladder cancer, although no correlation with tumor stages was shown [59,60]. Our results confirm a significantly enhanced level of IL-6 and only a tendency toward such an induction in the case of TNFα.

IL-8 was shown to induce both angiogenesis and tumorigenecity, and in this way it can enhance the metastatic potential of bladder cancer [18–20,55,61]. A similar relationship was demonstrated for VEGF expression, which enhances angiogenesis, proliferation, and metastatic potential in urothelial tumors [18–20]. Accordingly, we observed the induction of IL-8 (at protein level in sera) and VEGF (at protein level in sera and at mRNA level in the specimen of urothelial bladder cancer).

The upregulation of VEGF correlates to HIF-1α expression. We have also showed for the first time the elevated expression of both Nrf2 and HO-1 in urothelial bladder cancer. However, both Nrf2 and HIFs transcription factors are mostly regulated at protein stability [12,62], though its mRNA increase also indicates possible protein upregulation. It is therefore possible that Nrf2, a known inducer of HO-1 expression in different tissues [22], is also responsible for elevating HO-1 expression in bladder cancer. This supports previous *in vitro* data suggesting that Nrf2 may be associated with the enhanced expression of HO-1 in bladder cancer cells [10], which in turn enhances pathological angiogenesis in tumors and the viability of cells during therapy [10,24–26].

The mechanism of proangiogenic, and especially cytoprotective properties of HO-1 in bladder cancer is not well understood. It is associated with increased VEGF, HIF-1α, and HIF-2α [24]. Taking into account that HO-1 also potentiates the expression of other proangiogenic factors [22,63], and that our results show increased IL-8 in the sera of bladder cancer patients, the involvement of other mediators is also possible. HO-1 regulates the cell cycle via the modulation of soluble guanylyl cyclase activity, p38-signalling pathway, or PI3K pathway, which are activated by one of the heme degradation end products, carbon monoxide (CO) [22]. It is therefore possible that these mechanisms might also play a role in bladder cancer. Moreover, in other studies the HO-1 level was shown to correlate with the expression of cyclooxygenase-2 (COX-2) both *in vivo* (in samples of bladder cancer patients [28]) and *in vitro* (in bladder cancer cell lines cultured in hypoxic conditions [24]). COX-2 is a factor associated with carcinogenesis and higher pathological stages of bladder cancer [64]. It requires further analysis to examine the possible link between HO-1 and COX-2 in bladder cancer.

Furthermore, HO-1 is a potent regulator of miRNAs [30], inhibiting among others miR-133a, miR-133b, and miR-1 [30]. The importance of these miRNAs has been suggested in bladder cancer [46–52,65,66]. However, our analysis does not show the changes in the expression of miR-133a.

In turn, we have observed a decreased expression of miR-155, which was previously shown to be increased in the urine of the patients affected by urothelial bladder cancer [33]. Accordingly, the results showed that miR-155 is upregulated in urothelial tumors and associated with poor survival [67] as well as with the induction of the proliferation of bladder cancer cell line *in vitro* [68]. These results seem contradictory to those presented here; however, it must be noted that the sequence of primers used in that study [67] did not cover the mature miR-155-5p, which is detected in our analysis. MiR-155 was shown to target HIF-1α in murine and human cells [69,70]; therefore, its downregulation may be responsible for the upregulation of HIF-1α observed here in bladder cancer cells. Although miR-155 was demonstrated to target HO-1 in rodent models [71,72] it must be noted that in human cells it upregulates HO-1 expression by targeting Bach1—a repressor of HO-1 transcription [73]. Further studies are necessary to determine if there is any direct link between miR-155 and HO-1 in bladder cancer.

Finally, we have also demonstrated the increased expression of miR-200c in specimens of bladder cancer in comparison to healthy controls, which supports previous data showing an upregulation of this miRNA in bladder cancer [39–41]. As miR-200c has so far been shown to target HO-1 and is associated with HO-1 decreased expression in other tissues and cancer types [74,75], we did not expect that it could be a mediator of HO-1 upregulation or action in bladder cancer. On the other hand, miR-200c was positively correlated with VEGF expression in samples of bladder cancer. Similarly, miR-200c overexpression was shown to induce VEGF expression in non-small cell lung cancer [76], although opposite results suggesting that miR-200c directly targets VEGF expression were also obtained for different cancer types [38,77,78]. Therefore it seems that the relationship between miR-200c and VEGF depends on cell type.

In conclusion, we have shown here for the first time that the expression of both HO-1 and Nrf2 is elevated in specimens of bladder cancer. Additionally, HIF-1$\alpha$ and HIF-2$\alpha$ are upregulated at the mRNA level in urothelial bladder cancer and correlate with elevated VEGF expression in tumors and with its increased concentration in the plasma of patients affected by bladder cancer in comparison to healthy controls. The elevated level of proinflammatory and proangiogenic cytokines was also observed in the sera of patients with bladder cancer. Among the miRNAs analyzed, upregulation of miR-200c and downregulation of miR-155 were observed, which may be responsible for the induction of HIF-1$\alpha$ mRNA. The expression of both HO-1 and Nrf2 is increased in bladder cancer compared to healthy tissue.

Further studies with increased number of patients, and the functional assays for the potential targets of microRNAs and transcription factors are necessary to validate the results described here.

**Acknowledgments:** This research was conducted in the scope of the MiR-TANGO International Associated Laboratory (LIA) created by the Jagiellonian University (Department of Medical Biotechnology) and the CNRS, France (Centre de Biophysique Moleculaire, Orléans). The Faculty of Biochemistry, Biophysics, and Biotechnology of Jagiellonian University is a partner of the Leading National Research Centre (KNOW) supported by the Ministry of Science and Higher Education.

**Author Contributions:** M.K. collected samples, performed the experiments and wrote the paper; B.D.G collected samples, performed the experiments, and contributed to writing the paper; K.O. performed the histopathological analysis; A.J. contributed to the analysis of data; Z.D. conceived and designed the experiments; J.D. conceived and designed the experiments and contributed to writing the paper.

**Conflicts of Interest:** The authors declare no conflict of interest.

# References

1. Ferlay, J.; Soerjomataram, I.; Dikshit, R.; Eser, S.; Mathers, C.; Rebelo, M.; Parkin, D.M.; Forman, D.; Bray, F. Cancer incidence and mortality worldwide: Sources, methods and major patterns in globocan 2012. *Int. J. Cancer* **2015**, *136*, E359–E386. [CrossRef] [PubMed]

2. Wein, A.J. *Cambell-Walsh Urology*, 10th ed.; Elsevier Saunders: Philadelphia, PA, USA, 2012.

3. Sawicka, E.; Lisowska, A.; Kowal, P.; Dlugosz, A. The role of oxidative stress in bladder cancer. *Postepy Hig. Med. Dosw.* **2015**, *69*, 744–752. [CrossRef] [PubMed]

4. Florczyk, U.; Loboda, A.; Stachurska, A.; Jozkowicz, A.; Dulak, J. Role of Nrf2 transcription factor in cellular response to oxidative stress. *Postepy Biochem.* **2010**, *56*, 147–155. [PubMed]

5. Iida, K.; Itoh, K.; Kumagai, Y.; Oyasu, R.; Hattori, K.; Kawai, K.; Shimazui, T.; Akaza, H.; Yamamoto, M. Nrf2 is essential for the chemopreventive efficacy of oltipraz against urinary bladder carcinogenesis. *Cancer Res.* **2004**, *64*, 6424–6431. [CrossRef] [PubMed]

6. Iida, K.; Itoh, K.; Maher, J.M.; Kumagai, Y.; Oyasu, R.; Mori, Y.; Shimazui, T.; Akaza, H.; Yamamoto, M. Nrf2 and p53 cooperatively protect against bbn-induced urinary bladder carcinogenesis. *Carcinogenesis* **2007**, *28*, 2398–2403. [CrossRef] [PubMed]

7. Paonessa, J.D.; Ding, Y.; Randall, K.L.; Munday, R.; Argoti, D.; Vouros, P.; Zhang, Y. Identification of an unintended consequence of Nrf2-directed cytoprotection against a key tobacco carcinogen plus a counteracting chemopreventive intervention. *Cancer Res.* **2011**, *71*, 3904–3911. [CrossRef] [PubMed]

8.  Paonessa, J.D.; Munday, C.M.; Mhawech-Fauceglia, P.; Munday, R.; Zhang, Y. 5,6-dihydrocyclopenta[*c*][1,2]-dithiole-3(4*H*)-thione is a promising cancer chemopreventive agent in the urinary bladder. *Chem. Biol. Interact.* **2009**, *180*, 119–126. [CrossRef] [PubMed]

9.  Hayden, A.; Douglas, J.; Sommerlad, M.; Andrews, L.; Gould, K.; Hussain, S.; Thomas, G.J.; Packham, G.; Crabb, S.J. The Nrf2 transcription factor contributes to resistance to cisplatin in bladder cancer. *Urol. Oncol.* **2014**, *32*, 806–814. [CrossRef] [PubMed]

10. Kocanova, S.; Buytaert, E.; Matroule, J.Y.; Piette, J.; Golab, J.; de Witte, P.; Agostinis, P. Induction of heme-oxygenase 1 requires the p38$^{MAPK}$ and PI3K pathways and suppresses apoptotic cell death following hypericin-mediated photodynamic therapy. *Apoptosis* **2007**, *12*, 731–741. [CrossRef] [PubMed]

11. Loboda, A.; Jozkowicz, A.; Dulak, J. HIF-1 *versus* HIF-2—Is one more important than the other? *Vasc. Pharmacol.* **2012**, *56*, 245–251. [CrossRef] [PubMed]

12. Loboda, A.; Jozkowicz, A.; Dulak, J. HIF-1 and HIF-2 transcription factors–similar but not identical. *Mol. Cells* **2010**, *29*, 435–442. [CrossRef] [PubMed]

13. Theodoropoulos, V.E.; Lazaris, A.; Sofras, F.; Gerzelis, I.; Tsoukala, V.; Ghikonti, I.; Manikas, K.; Kastriotis, I. Hypoxia-inducible factor 1 alpha expression correlates with angiogenesis and unfavorable prognosis in bladder cancer. *Eur. Urol.* **2004**, *46*, 200–208. [CrossRef] [PubMed]

14. Ioachim, E.; Michael, M.; Salmas, M.; Michael, M.M.; Stavropoulos, N.E.; Malamou-Mitsi, V. Hypoxia-inducible factors HIF-1α and HIF-2α expression in bladder cancer and their associations with other angiogenesis-related proteins. *Urol. Int.* **2006**, *77*, 255–263. [CrossRef] [PubMed]

15. Chai, C.Y.; Chen, W.T.; Hung, W.C.; Kang, W.Y.; Huang, Y.C.; Su, Y.C.; Yang, C.H. Hypoxia-inducible factor-1 alpha expression correlates with focal macrophage infiltration, angiogenesis and unfavourable prognosis in urothelial carcinoma. *J. Clin. Pathol.* **2008**, *61*, 658–664. [CrossRef] [PubMed]

16. Deniz, H.; Karakok, M.; Yagci, F.; Guldur, M.E. Evaluation of relationship between HIF-1α immunoreactivity and stage, grade, angiogenic profile and proliferative index in bladder urothelial carcinomas. *Int. Urol. Nephrol.* **2010**, *42*, 103–107. [CrossRef] [PubMed]

17. Jones, A.; Fujiyama, C.; Blanche, C.; Moore, J.W.; Fuggle, S.; Cranston, D.; Bicknell, R.; Harris, A.L. Relation of vascular endothelial growth factor production to expression and regulation of hypoxia-inducible factor-1 alpha and hypoxia-inducible factor-2 alpha in human bladder tumors and cell lines. *Clin. Cancer Res.* **2001**, *7*, 1263–1272. [PubMed]

18. Inoue, K.; Slaton, J.W.; Karashima, T.; Yoshikawa, C.; Shuin, T.; Sweeney, P.; Millikan, R.; Dinney, C.P. The prognostic value of angiogenesis factor expression for predicting recurrence and metastasis of bladder cancer after neoadjuvant chemotherapy and radical cystectomy. *Clin. Cancer Res.* **2000**, *6*, 4866–4873. [PubMed]

19. Kopparapu, P.K.; Boorjian, S.A.; Robinson, B.D.; Downes, M.; Gudas, L.J.; Mongan, N.P.; Persson, J.L. Expression of VEGF and its receptors VEGFR1/VEGFR2 is associated with invasiveness of bladder cancer. *Anticancer Res.* **2013**, *33*, 2381–2390. [PubMed]

20. Nakanishi, R.; Oka, N.; Nakatsuji, H.; Koizumi, T.; Sakaki, M.; Takahashi, M.; Fukumori, T.; Kanayama, H.O. Effect of vascular endothelial growth factor and its receptor inhibitor on proliferation and invasion in bladder cancer. *Urol. Int.* **2009**, *83*, 98–106. [CrossRef] [PubMed]

21. Mazzola, C.R.; Chin, J. Targeting the VEGF pathway in metastatic bladder cancer. *Expert Opin. Investig. Drugs* **2015**, *24*, 913–927. [CrossRef] [PubMed]

22. Loboda, A.; Jazwa, A.; Grochot-Przeczek, A.; Rutkowski, A.J.; Cisowski, J.; Agarwal, A.; Jozkowicz, A.; Dulak, J. Heme oxygenase-1 and the vascular bed: From molecular mechanisms to therapeutic opportunities. *Antioxid. Redox Signal.* **2008**, *10*, 1767–1812. [CrossRef] [PubMed]

23. Was, H.; Dulak, J.; Jozkowicz, A. Heme oxygenase-1 in tumor biology and therapy. *Curr. Drug Targets* **2010**, *11*, 1551–1570. [CrossRef] [PubMed]

24. Miyake, M.; Fujimoto, K.; Anai, S.; Ohnishi, S.; Kuwada, M.; Nakai, Y.; Inoue, T.; Matsumura, Y.; Tomioka, A.; Ikeda, T.; *et al.* Heme oxygenase-1 promotes angiogenesis in urothelial carcinoma of the urinary bladder. *Oncol. Rep.* **2011**, *25*, 653–660. [CrossRef] [PubMed]

25. Miyake, M.; Fujimoto, K.; Anai, S.; Ohnishi, S.; Nakai, Y.; Inoue, T.; Matsumura, Y.; Tomioka, A.; Ikeda, T.; Okajima, E.; *et al.* Inhibition of heme oxygenase-1 enhances the cytotoxic effect of gemcitabine in urothelial cancer cells. *Anticancer Res.* **2010**, *30*, 2145–2152. [PubMed]

26. Miyake, M.; Ishii, M.; Kawashima, K.; Kodama, T.; Sugano, K.; Fujimoto, K.; Hirao, Y. Sirna-mediated knockdown of the heme synthesis and degradation pathways: Modulation of treatment effect of 5-aminolevulinic acid-based photodynamic therapy in urothelial cancer cell lines. *Photochem. Photobiol.* **2009**, *85*, 1020–1027. [CrossRef] [PubMed]

27. Miyake, M.; Fujimoto, K.; Anai, S.; Ohnishi, S.; Nakai, Y.; Inoue, T.; Matsumura, Y.; Tomioka, A.; Ikeda, T.; Tanaka, N.; *et al.* Clinical significance of heme oxygenase-1 expression in non-muscle-invasive bladder cancer. *Urol. Int.* **2010**, *85*, 355–363. [CrossRef] [PubMed]

28. Miyata, Y.; Kanda, S.; Mitsunari, K.; Asai, A.; Sakai, H. Heme oxygenase-1 expression is associated with tumor aggressiveness and outcomes in patients with bladder cancer: A correlation with smoking intensity. *Transl. Res. J. Lab. Clin. Med.* **2014**, *164*, 468–476. [CrossRef] [PubMed]

29. Kim, J.H.; Park, J. Prognostic significance of heme oxygenase-1, S100 calcium-binding protein A4, and syndecan-1 expression in primary non-muscle-invasive bladder cancer. *Hum. Pathol.* **2014**, *45*, 1830–1838. [CrossRef] [PubMed]

30. Kozakowska, M.; Ciesla, M.; Stefanska, A.; Skrzypek, K.; Was, H.; Jazwa, A.; Grochot-Przeczek, A.; Kotlinowski, J.; Szymula, A.; Bartelik, A.; *et al.* Heme oxygenase-1 inhibits myoblast differentiation by targeting myomirs. *Antioxid. Redox Signal.* **2012**, *16*, 113–127. [CrossRef] [PubMed]

31. Skrzypek, K.; Tertil, M.; Golda, S.; Ciesla, M.; Weglarczyk, K.; Collet, G.; Guichard, A.; Kozakowska, M.; Boczkowski, J.; Was, H.; *et al.* Interplay between heme oxygenase-1 and miR-378 affects non-small cell lung carcinoma growth, vascularization, and metastasis. *Antioxid. Redox Signal.* **2013**, *19*, 644–660. [CrossRef] [PubMed]

32. Tertil, M.; Golda, S.; Skrzypek, K.; Florczyk, U.; Weglarczyk, K.; Kotlinowski, J.; Maleszewska, M.; Czauderna, S.; Pichon, C.; Kieda, C.; *et al.* Nrf2-heme oxygenase-1 axis in mucoepidermoid carcinoma of the lung: Antitumoral effects associated with down-regulation of matrix metalloproteinases. *Free Radic. Biol. Med.* **2015**, *89*, 147–157. [CrossRef] [PubMed]

33. Wang, G.; Chan, E.S.; Kwan, B.C.; Li, P.K.; Yip, S.K.; Szeto, C.C.; Ng, C.F. Expression of microRNAs in the urine of patients with bladder cancer. *Clin. Genitourin. Cancer* **2012**, *10*, 106–113. [CrossRef] [PubMed]

34. Schaefer, A.; Stephan, C.; Busch, J.; Yousef, G.M.; Jung, K. Diagnostic, prognostic and therapeutic implications of microRNAs in urologic tumors. *Nat. Rev.* **2010**, *7*, 286–297. [CrossRef] [PubMed]

35. Adam, L.; Zhong, M.; Choi, W.; Qi, W.; Nicoloso, M.; Arora, A.; Calin, G.; Wang, H.; Siefker-Radtke, A.; McConkey, D.; *et al.* miR-200 expression regulates epithelial-to-mesenchymal transition in bladder cancer cells and reverses resistance to epidermal growth factor receptor therapy. *Clin. Cancer Res.* **2009**, *15*, 5060–5072. [CrossRef] [PubMed]

36. Zhou, H.; Tang, K.; Xiao, H.; Zeng, J.; Guan, W.; Guo, X.; Xu, H.; Ye, Z. A panel of eight-miRNA signature as a potential biomarker for predicting survival in bladder cancer. *J. Exp. Clin. Cancer Res. CR* **2015**, *34*, 53. [CrossRef] [PubMed]

37. Gravgaard, K.H.; Lyng, M.B.; Laenkholm, A.V.; Sokilde, R.; Nielsen, B.S.; Litman, T.; Ditzel, H.J. The miRNA-200 family and miRNA-9 exhibit differential expression in primary *versus* corresponding metastatic tissue in breast cancer. *Breast Cancer Res. Treat.* **2012**, *134*, 207–217. [CrossRef] [PubMed]

38. Panda, H.; Pelakh, L.; Chuang, T.D.; Luo, X.; Bukulmez, O.; Chegini, N. Endometrial miR-200c is altered during transformation into cancerous states and targets the expression of ZEBs, VEGFA, FLT1, IKKβ, KLF9, and FBLN5. *Reprod. Sci.* **2012**, *19*, 786–796. [CrossRef] [PubMed]

39. Han, Y.; Chen, J.; Zhao, X.; Liang, C.; Wang, Y.; Sun, L.; Jiang, Z.; Zhang, Z.; Yang, R.; Chen, J.; *et al.* MicroRNA expression signatures of bladder cancer revealed by deep sequencing. *PLoS ONE* **2011**, *6*, e18286. [CrossRef] [PubMed]

40. Li, X.; Chen, J.; Hu, X.; Huang, Y.; Li, Z.; Zhou, L.; Tian, Z.; Ma, H.; Wu, Z.; Chen, M.; *et al.* Comparative mrna and microRNA expression profiling of three genitourinary cancers reveals common hallmarks and cancer-specific molecular events. *PLoS ONE* **2011**, *6*, e22570. [CrossRef] [PubMed]

41. Mahdavinezhad, A.; Mousavi-Bahar, S.H.; Poorolajal, J.; Yadegarazari, R.; Jafari, M.; Shabab, N.; Saidijam, M. Evaluation of miR-141, miR-200c, miR-30b expression and clinicopathological features of bladder cancer. *Int. J. Mol. Cell. Med.* **2015**, *4*, 32–39. [PubMed]

42. Wszolek, M.F.; Rieger-Christ, K.M.; Kenney, P.A.; Gould, J.J.; Silva Neto, B.; Lavoie, A.K.; Logvinenko, T.; Libertino, J.A.; Summerhayes, I.C. A microRNA expression profile defining the invasive bladder tumor phenotype. *Urol. Oncol.* **2011**, *29*, 794–801. [CrossRef] [PubMed]

43. Wiklund, E.D.; Bramsen, J.B.; Hulf, T.; Dyrskjot, L.; Ramanathan, R.; Hansen, T.B.; Villadsen, S.B.; Gao, S.; Ostenfeld, M.S.; Borre, M.; *et al.* Coordinated epigenetic repression of the miR-200 family and miR-205 in invasive bladder cancer. *Int. J. Cancer* **2011**, *128*, 1327–1334. [CrossRef] [PubMed]

44. Liu, L.; Qiu, M.; Tan, G.; Liang, Z.; Qin, Y.; Chen, L.; Chen, H.; Liu, J. miR-200c inhibits invasion, migration and proliferation of bladder cancer cells through down-regulation of BMI-1 and E2F3. *J. Transl. Med.* **2014**, *12*, 305. [CrossRef] [PubMed]

45. Xie, P.; Xu, F.; Cheng, W.; Gao, J.; Zhang, Z.; Ge, J.; Wei, Z.; Xu, X.; Liu, Y. Infiltration related miRNAs in bladder urothelial carcinoma. *J. Huazhong Univ. Sci. Technol.* **2012**, *32*, 576–580. [CrossRef] [PubMed]

46. Song, T.; Xia, W.; Shao, N.; Zhang, X.; Wang, C.; Wu, Y.; Dong, J.; Cai, W.; Li, H. Differential miRNA expression profiles in bladder urothelial carcinomas. *Asian Pac. J. Cancer Prev.* **2011**, *11*, 905–911.

47. Ichimi, T.; Enokida, H.; Okuno, Y.; Kunimoto, R.; Chiyomaru, T.; Kawamoto, K.; Kawahara, K.; Toki, K.; Kawakami, K.; Nishiyama, K.; *et al.* Identification of novel microRNA targets based on microRNA signatures in bladder cancer. *Int. J. Cancer* **2009**, *125*, 345–352. [CrossRef] [PubMed]

48. Catto, J.W.; Miah, S.; Owen, H.C.; Bryant, H.; Myers, K.; Dudziec, E.; Larre, S.; Milo, M.; Rehman, I.; Rosario, D.J.; *et al.* Distinct microRNA alterations characterize high- and low-grade bladder cancer. *Cancer Res.* **2009**, *69*, 8472–8481. [CrossRef] [PubMed]

49. Yoshino, H.; Chiyomaru, T.; Enokida, H.; Kawakami, K.; Tatarano, S.; Nishiyama, K.; Nohata, N.; Seki, N.; Nakagawa, M. The tumour-suppressive function of miR-1 and miR-133a targeting taglun2 in bladder cancer. *Br. J. Cancer* **2011**, *104*, 808–818. [CrossRef] [PubMed]

50. Chiyomaru, T.; Enokida, H.; Kawakami, K.; Tatarano, S.; Uchida, Y.; Kawahara, K.; Nishiyama, K.; Seki, N.; Nakagawa, M. Functional role of LASP1 in cell viability and its regulation by microRNAs in bladder cancer. *Urol. Oncol.* **2012**, *30*, 434–443. [CrossRef] [PubMed]

51. Chiyomaru, T.; Enokida, H.; Tatarano, S.; Kawahara, K.; Uchida, Y.; Nishiyama, K.; Fujimura, L.; Kikkawa, N.; Seki, N.; Nakagawa, M. miR-145 and miR-133a function as tumour suppressors and directly regulate fscn1 expression in bladder cancer. *Br. J. Cancer* **2010**, *102*, 883–891. [CrossRef] [PubMed]

52. Uchida, Y.; Chiyomaru, T.; Enokida, H.; Kawakami, K.; Tatarano, S.; Kawahara, K.; Nishiyama, K.; Seki, N.; Nakagawa, M. miR-133a induces apoptosis through direct regulation of GSTP1 in bladder cancer cell lines. *Urol. Oncol.* **2011**, *31*, 115–123. [CrossRef] [PubMed]

53. Epstein, J.I.; Amin, M.B.; Reuter, V.R.; Mostofi, F.K. The world health organization/international society of urological pathology consensus classification of urothelial (transitional cell) neoplasms of the urinary bladder. Bladder consensus conference committee. *Am. J. Surg. Pathol.* **1998**, *22*, 1435–1448. [CrossRef] [PubMed]

54. Beecken, W.D.; Engl, T.; Hofmann, J.; Jonas, D.; Blaheta, R. Clinical relevance of serum angiogenic activity in patients with transitional cell carcinoma of the bladder. *J. Cell. Mol. Med.* **2005**, *9*, 655–661. [CrossRef] [PubMed]

55. Mahmoud, M.A.; Ali, M.H.; Hassoba, H.M.; Elhadidy, G.S. Serum interleukin-8 and insulin like growth factor-1 in egyptian bladder cancer patients. *Cancer Biomark.* **2010**, *6*, 105–110. [PubMed]

56. Seguchi, T.; Yokokawa, K.; Sugao, H.; Nakano, E.; Sonoda, T.; Okuyama, A. Interleukin-6 activity in urine and serum in patients with bladder carcinoma. *J. Urol.* **1992**, *148*, 791–794. [PubMed]

57. Kovacs, E. Investigation of interleukin-6 (il-6), soluble IL-6 receptor (sIL-6r) and soluble gp130 (sgp130) in sera of cancer patients. *Biomed. Pharmacother.* **2001**, *55*, 391–396. [CrossRef]

58. Chen, M.F.; Lin, P.Y.; Wu, C.F.; Chen, W.C.; Wu, C.T. Il-6 expression regulates tumorigenicity and correlates with prognosis in bladder cancer. *PLoS ONE* **2013**, *8*, e61901. [CrossRef] [PubMed]

59. Agarwal, A.; Verma, S.; Burra, U.; Murthy, N.S.; Mohanty, N.K.; Saxena, S. Flow cytometric analysis of Th1 and Th2 cytokines in pbmcs as a parameter of immunological dysfunction in patients of superficial transitional cell carcinoma of bladder. *Cancer Immunol. Immunother. CII* **2006**, *55*, 734–743. [CrossRef] [PubMed]

60. Salman, T.; el-Ahmady, O.; el-Shafee, M.; Omar, S.; Salman, I. The clinical value of cathepsin-D and TNF-alpha in bladder cancer patients. *Anticancer Res.* **1997**, *17*, 3087–3090. [PubMed]

61. Chikazawa, M.; Inoue, K.; Fukata, S.; Karashima, T.; Shuin, T. Expression of angiogenesis-related genes regulates different steps in the process of tumor growth and metastasis in human urothelial cell carcinoma of the urinary bladder. *Pathobiology* **2008**, *75*, 335–345. [CrossRef] [PubMed]

62. Ma, Q. Role of Nrf2 in oxidative stress and toxicity. *Annu. Rev. Pharmacol. Toxicol.* **2013**, *53*, 401–426. [CrossRef] [PubMed]

63. Deshane, J.; Chen, S.; Caballero, S.; Grochot-Przeczek, A.; Was, H.; Li Calzi, S.; Lach, R.; Hock, T.D.; Chen, B.; Hill-Kapturczak, N.; *et al.* Stromal cell-derived factor 1 promotes angiogenesis via a heme oxygenase 1-dependent mechanism. *J. Exp. Med.* **2007**, *204*, 605–618. [CrossRef] [PubMed]

64. Zhu, Z.; Shen, Z.; Xu, C. Inflammatory pathways as promising targets to increase chemotherapy response in bladder cancer. *Med. Inflamm.* **2012**, *2012*, 528690. [CrossRef] [PubMed]

65. Yoshino, H.; Enokida, H.; Chiyomaru, T.; Tatarano, S.; Hidaka, H.; Yamasaki, T.; Gotannda, T.; Tachiwada, T.; Nohata, N.; Yamane, T.; *et al.* Tumor suppressive microRNA-1 mediated novel apoptosis pathways through direct inhibition of splicing factor serine/arginine-rich 9 (SRSF9/SRp30c) in bladder cancer. *Biochem. Biophys. Res. Commun.* **2012**, *417*, 588–593. [CrossRef] [PubMed]

66. Wang, T.; Yuan, J.; Feng, N.; Li, Y.; Lin, Z.; Jiang, Z.; Gui, Y. Hsa-miR-1 downregulates long non-coding rna urothelial cancer associated 1 in bladder cancer. *Tumour Biol.* **2014**, *35*, 10075–10084. [CrossRef] [PubMed]

67. Wang, H.; Men, C.P. Correlation of increased expression of microRNA-155 in bladder cancer and prognosis. *Lab. Med.* **2015**, *46*, 118–122. [CrossRef] [PubMed]

68. Peng, Y.; Dong, W.; Lin, T.X.; Zhong, G.Z.; Liao, B.; Wang, B.; Gu, P.; Huang, L.; Xie, Y.; Lu, F.D.; *et al.* MicroRNA-155 promotes bladder cancer growth by repressing the tumor suppressor DMTF1. *Oncotarget* **2015**, *6*, 16043–16058. [CrossRef] [PubMed]

69. Hu, R.; Zhang, Y.; Yang, X.; Yan, J.; Sun, Y.; Chen, Z.; Jiang, H. Isoflurane attenuates LPS-induced acute lung injury by targeting miR-155-HIF1-alpha. *Front. Biosci.* **2015**, *20*, 139–156.

70. Bruning, U.; Cerone, L.; Neufeld, Z.; Fitzpatrick, S.F.; Cheong, A.; Scholz, C.C.; Simpson, D.A.; Leonard, M.O.; Tambuwala, M.M.; Cummins, E.P.; *et al.* Microrna-155 promotes resolution of hypoxia-inducible factor 1α activity during prolonged hypoxia. *Mol. Cell. Biol.* **2011**, *31*, 4087–4096. [CrossRef] [PubMed]

71. Zhang, J.; Braun, M.Y. Protoporphyrin treatment modulates susceptibility to experimental autoimmune encephalomyelitis in miR-155-deficient mice. *PLoS ONE* **2015**, *10*, e0145237. [CrossRef] [PubMed]

72. Zhang, J.; Vandevenne, P.; Hamdi, H.; Van Puyvelde, M.; Zucchi, A.; Bettonville, M.; Weatherly, K.; Braun, M.Y. Micro-RNA-155-mediated control of heme oxygenase 1 (HO-1) is required for restoring adaptively tolerant cd4+ T-cell function in rodents. *Eur. J. Immunol.* **2015**, *45*, 829–842. [CrossRef] [PubMed]

73. Pulkkinen, K.H.; Yla-Herttuala, S.; Levonen, A.L. Heme oxygenase 1 is induced by miR-155 via reduced bach1 translation in endothelial cells. *Free Radic. Biol. Med.* **2011**, *51*, 2124–2131. [CrossRef] [PubMed]

74. Stachurska, A.; Ciesla, M.; Kozakowska, M.; Wolffram, S.; Boesch-Saadatmandi, C.; Rimbach, G.; Jozkowicz, A.; Dulak, J.; Loboda, A. Cross-talk between microRNAs, nuclear factor E2-related factor 2, and heme oxygenase-1 in ochratoxin a-induced toxic effects in renal proximal tubular epithelial cells. *Mol. Nutr. Food Res.* **2013**, *57*, 504–515. [CrossRef] [PubMed]

75. Gao, C.; Peng, F.H.; Peng, L.K. miR-200c sensitizes clear-cell renal cell carcinoma cells to sorafenib and imatinib by targeting heme oxygenase-1. *Neoplasma* **2014**, *61*, 680–689. [CrossRef] [PubMed]

76. Tejero, R.; Navarro, A.; Campayo, M.; Vinolas, N.; Marrades, R.M.; Cordeiro, A.; Ruiz-Martinez, M.; Santasusagna, S.; Molins, L.; Ramirez, J.; *et al.* miR-141 and miR-200c as markers of overall survival in early stage non-small cell lung cancer adenocarcinoma. *PLoS ONE* **2014**, *9*, e101899. [CrossRef] [PubMed]

77. Chuang, T.D.; Panda, H.; Luo, X.; Chegini, N. miR-200c is aberrantly expressed in leiomyomas in an ethnic-dependent manner and targets ZEBs, VEGFA, TIMP2, and FBLN5. *Endocr. Relat. Cancer* **2012**, *19*, 541–556. [CrossRef] [PubMed]

78. Erturk, E.; Cecener, G.; Tezcan, G.; Egeli, U.; Tunca, B.; Gokgoz, S.; Tolunay, S.; Tasdelen, I. Brca mutations cause reduction in miR-200c expression in triple negative breast cancer. *Gene* **2015**, *556*, 163–169. [CrossRef] [PubMed]

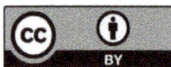

Journal of
*Clinical Medicine*

MDPI

*Article*

# Enhanced Efficacy of Doxorubicin by microRNA-499-Mediated Improvement of Tumor Blood Flow

Ayaka Okamoto [1], Tomohiro Asai [1], Sho Ryu [1], Hidenori Ando [1], Noriyuki Maeda [2], Takehisa Dewa [3] and Naoto Oku [1,*]

[1]   Department of Medical Biochemistry, University of Shizuoka School of Pharmaceutical Sciences, 52-1 Yada, Suruga-ku, Shizuoka 422-8526, Japan; s14803@u-shizuoka-ken.ac.jp (A.O.); asai@u-shizuoka-ken.ac.jp (T.A.); rorange0805@gmail.com (S.R.); h.ando@tokushima-u.ac.jp (H.A.)
[2]   Nippon Fine Chemical Co. Ltd., 5-1-1 Umei, Takasago, Hyogo 676-0074, Japan; n-maeda@nipponseika.com
[3]   Department of Life and Materials Engineering, Nagoya Institute of Technology, Gokiso-cho, Showa-ku, Nagoya 466-8555, Japan; takedewa@nitech.ac.jp
*   Correspondence: oku@u-shizuoka-ken.ac.jp; Tel.: +81-54-264-5701; Fax: +81-54-264-5705

Academic Editors: Takahiro Ochiya and Ryou-u Takahashi
Received: 30 November 2015; Accepted: 14 January 2016; Published: 19 January 2016

**Abstract:** Genetic therapy using microRNA-499 (miR-499) was combined with chemotherapy for the advanced treatment of cancer. Our previous study showed that miR-499 suppressed tumor growth through the inhibition of vascular endothelial growth factor (VEGF) production and subsequent angiogenesis. In the present study, we focused on blood flow in tumors treated with miR499, since some angiogenic vessels are known to lack blood flow. Tetraethylenepentamine-based polycation liposomes (TEPA-PCL) were prepared and modified with Ala-Pro-Arg-Pro-Gly peptide (APRPG) for targeted delivery of miR-499 (APRPG-miR-499) to angiogenic vessels and tumor cells. The tumor blood flow was significantly improved, so-called normalized, after systemic administration of APRPG-miR-499 to Colon 26 NL-17 carcinoma–bearing mice. In addition, the accumulation of doxorubicin (DOX) in the tumors was increased by pre-treatment with APRPG-miR-499. Moreover, the combination therapy of APRPG-miR-499 and DOX resulted in significant suppression of the tumors. Taken together, our present data indicate that miR-499 delivered with APRPG-modified-TEPA-PCL normalized tumor vessels, resulting in enhancement of intratumoral accumulation of DOX. Our findings suggest that APRPG-miR-499 may be a therapeutic, or a combination therapeutic, candidate for cancer treatment.

**Keywords:** microRNA; miR-499; cancer therapy; gene delivery; liposomes; tumor blood perfusion

## 1. Introduction

miR-499 is one of the miRNAs that regulate the expression of several genes, especially under hypoxia/ischemia conditions such as those found in cancer, myocardial infarction, and so on [1]. It is known that miR-499 is involved in particular signaling pathways including Wnt signaling and calcineurin pathways [1,2]. It has also been reported that the Wnt signaling pathway is involved in carcinogenesis and cell differentiation, and the calcineurin pathway in cancer cell growth. Additionally, both of these signaling pathways induce angiogenesis [3,4]. It is well established that the calcineurin catalytic subunit $\alpha$ isoform (CnA$\alpha$) is involved in the promotion of angiogenesis following activation of the transcriptional factor nuclear factor of activated T cells (NFAT). It is known that hypoxia-inducible factor 1-$\alpha$ (HIF1-$\alpha$) is regulated by the calcineurin-NFAT pathway. HIF1-$\alpha$ causes vascular endothelial growth factor (VEGF) secretion from cells, resulting in promotion of angiogenesis. In addition, in some kinds of tumors, the Wnt signaling pathway also regulates the production of VEGF. Since miR-499 inhibits the Wnt and calcineurin signaling pathways through the suppression of target genes that construct these pathways, it has been expected that miR-499 might be a good candidate for cancer treatment (Scheme 1). Indeed, we showed earlier that miR-499 suppresses the growth of tumor cells and the capillary tube formation of human umbilical vein endothelial cells (HUVECs) *in vitro* [5].

A miRNA delivery system is necessary for application of miRNAs to cancer therapy. Previously, we developed a small RNA delivery system using tetraethylenepentamine-based polycation liposomes (TEPA-PCL) [6–8] and demonstrated that miR-499/TEPA-PCL reduces the secretion of VEGF and the production of other pro-angiogenic factors, e.g., CnAα and frizzled family receptor 8 (FZD8), in Colon 26 NL-17 mouse carcinoma cells [5]. For systemic administration and tumor targeting, we modified the Ala-Pro-Arg-Pro-Gly (APRPG) peptide on the surface of miR-499/TEPA-PCL (APRPG-miR-499) and showed that APRPG-miR-499 significantly suppresses tumor growth through silencing of target genes in Colon 26 NL-17-carcinoma–grafted mice [5]. Since it is shown that miR-499 could be a potential predictive biomarker in patients with lung cancer treated with chemotherapy [9], elucidation of miR-499 activity *in vivo* is of considerable interest.

In general, tumors construct angiogenic vessels to secure a supply route from blood to obtain oxygen and nutrients [10,11]. Since the production of tumor vessels is rapid, these vessels are immature and leaky, and are chaotically constructed, resulting in loops or dead-end conformations. These factors lead to intratumoral hypertension, which causes difficulty in delivery of anti-cancer drugs into the tumors [12]. Since these vessels do not extend to all parts of the tumors, some regions in the tumor tissue become severely hypoxic. Fewer blood vessels mean not only poor delivery of anti-cancer drugs, but also a hypoxic environment. Such an environment works negatively when the anti-cancer drug has been administered as follows: Tumors metabolize the nutrients anaerobically in hypoxia, resulting in the accumulation of lactic acid in the tumor tissue, which causes acidosis. In this case, the efficacy of basic anti-cancer drugs such as doxorubicin and paclitaxel is decreased dramatically. Therefore, the normalization of tumor blood vessels is a meaningful goal in cancer therapy. Inhibition of angiogenesis ameliorates blood perfusion in the tumor due to the decrease of defective tumor vessels without blood flow. Anti-cancer drugs that extend deeply into the tumors via improved blood flow are expected to show potent cytotoxic effects. Recent studies showed that the combination therapy of anti-angiogenic agents and anti-cancer drugs is effective for the treatment of cancer [13–17]. Such therapy is based on the concept of vascular normalization, *i.e.*, the tumor vessels temporally show the function similarly to normal vessels [18–20]. In fact, Avastin®, an anti-VEGF antibody, which has been used as an anti-angiogenic agent in combination therapies with anti-cancer drugs, causes the extension of progression-free survival in the clinical setting [21].

In the present study, we focused on the anti-angiogenic effect of miR-499. We developed APRPG-miR-499 as a partner of DOX for combination therapy and examined its therapeutic effects in tumor-grafted mice.

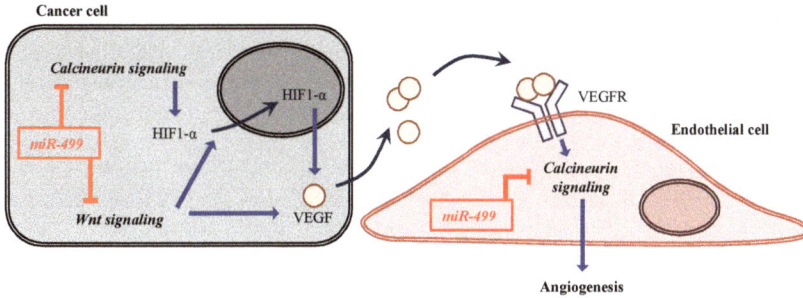

**Scheme 1.** Associations of signaling pathways and miR-499. The blue arrows indicate upregulation. The red symbols mean inhibition.

## 2. Experimental Section

### 2.1. Preparation of Tetraethylenepentamine-Based Polycation Liposomes (TEPA-PCL) and Lipoplex

Cholesterol-conjugated miR-499 (miR-499-C) and cholesterol-conjugated control miRNA (miCont-C) were purchased from Hokkaido System Science (Hokkaido, Japan). The 3′ end of the passenger strand of miRNAs was modified with cholesterol as previously reported [7,8]. miR-499 was composed of miR-499-5p and miR-499-3p. The sequences of the strands were as follows: miR-499-5p: 5′-UUAAGACUUGCAGUGAUGUUU-3′, miR-499-3p: 5′-AACAU CACAGCAAGUCUGUGCU-3′. Dicetyl phosphate-tetraethylenepentamine (DCP-TEPA) was synthesized as described earlier [6]. Cholesterol, dipalmitoylphosphatidylcholine (DPPC), dioleoylphosphatidylethanolamine (DOPE), and Ala-Pro-Arg-Pro-Gly (APRPG)-grafted polyethylene glycol (6000)-distearoylphosphatidylethanolamine (APRPG-PEG-DSPE) were synthesized by Nippon Fine Chemical (Hyogo, Japan).

TEPA-PCL was prepared as described previously [6]. DOPE, cholesterol, DPPC, and DCP-TEPA (4:4:3:1 as a molar ratio) were mixed and lyophilized overnight. Then the lipid was hydrated with diethylpyrocarbonate (DEPC)-treated water. These liposomes were extruded 10 times through a polycarbonate membrane filter with a pore size of 100 nm (Nuclepore, Maidstone, UK). To form miR-499-C/TEPA-PCL lipoplexes, we mixed miR-499-C with TEPA-PCL in DEPC-treated water at a ratio of the nitrogen moiety derived from TEPA-PCL to the phosphorus from miR-499-C (N/P ratio) of 18 and incubated this mixture for 20 min at room temperature. In order to apply them to systemic administration, miR-499-C/TEPA-PCL were modified with APRPG-PEG-DSPE. APRPG-PEG-DSPE at a ratio of 10% of total lipids was incubated with miR-499-C/TEPA-PCL at 50 °C for 20 min to obtain APRPG-modified miR-499-C/TEPA-PCL lipoplex (APRPG-miR-499). Cholesterol-conjugated non-targeting miRNA (miCont-C) instead of miR-499-C was used to prepare APRPG-modified miCont-C/TEPA-PCL lipoplex (APRPG-miCont). The particle size and ζ-potential of APRPG-miR-499 diluted with 10 mM phosphate buffer were measured with a Zetasizer Nano ZS (Malvern, Worcestershire, UK).

### 2.2. Cell Culture

Colon 26 NL-17 mouse carcinoma cells were established by Yamori (Japanese Foundation for Cancer Research, Tokyo, Japan) and were kindly provided by Nakajima (SBI Pharmaceuticals, Tokyo, Japan). The cells were cultured in DMEM/Ham's F-12 medium (Wako, Osaka, Japan), which was supplemented with 10% fetal bovine serum (FBS, AusGeneX, Oxenford, Australia), 100-units/mL penicillin G (MP Biomedicals, Irvine, CA, USA), and 100-µg/mL streptomycin (MP Biomedicals), in a $CO_2$ incubator.

## 2.3. Experimental Animals

BALB/c mice (male, five weeks old) were purchased from Japan SLC (Shizuoka, Japan). The animals were cared for according to the Animal Facility Guidelines of the University of Shizuoka. All animal experiments were approved by the Animal and Ethics Committee of the University of Shizuoka on september 18, 2013 (Approved No. 136048).

For preparation of tumor-bearing mice, Colon 26 NL-17 cells ($1 \times 10^6$ cells/mouse) were implanted subcutaneously into the left posterior flank of BALB/c mice. Lipoplex samples were administered via a tail vein at selected times after the implantation, as described in each experiment.

## 2.4. Evaluation of Tumor Blood Flow

APRPG-miR-499 or APRPG-miCont (2 mg/kg as miRNA) lipoplexes were intravenously injected into the tumor-bearing mice seven days after the implantation. The mice were injected Biotynylated Lycopersicon esculentum (tomato) Lectin (Vector laboratories, Inc., Burlingame, CA, USA) four days after administration of APRPG-miRNAs in order to stain the vessels with blood perfusion. Ten minutes later, the mice were fixed by reflux flow with 1% paraformaldehyde. The tumors were excised and embedded in Tissue-Tek® O.C.T. Compound (Sakura Finetek Japan, Tokyo, Japan). Frozen tumor sections of 10 μm thickness were prepared with a Microm HM 505 E Cryostat (Micro-edge Instruments, Tokyo, Japan) and mounted on MAS-coated slides (Matsunami Glass, Osaka, Japan). After having been fixed with acetone and blocked with 3% bovine serum albumin in phosphate-buffered saline (PBS), these tumor sections were incubated with streptavidin-Alexa Fluor® 594 conjugate (Life Technologies, Gaithersburg, MD, USA) for 1 h in a humid chamber, and then with anti-mouse CD31 (PECAM-1) antibody labeled with FITC (eBioscience, San Diego, CA, USA) for 1 h. The fluorescence of Alexa Fluor® 594-labeled Lycopersicon esculentum Lectin and FITC-labeled CD31 was observed by confocal laser-scanning microscopy (LSM 510 META, Carl Zeiss, Oberkochen, Germany). To obtain the percentage of vessels with blood flow, we divided the co-localized area of Alexa Fluor® 594 (blood flow area) and FITC (total vessels) by the FITC-positive area (total vessels).

## 2.5. Accumulation of Doxorubicin in the Tumor

APRPG-miR-499 or APRPG-miCont (2 mg/kg as miRNA) lipoplexes were intravenously injected into the tumor-bearing mice seven days after the implantation. Four days later, the mice were intravenously injected with DOX at a dose of 10 mg/kg. The tumors were refluxed with PBS and excised 3 h after the injection. After the tumors had been homogenized in 0.3 M HCl in 70% ethanol by use of a ShakeMan 2 (Biomedical Science, Tokyo, Japan), the fluorescence of DOX (excitation wavelength (Ex.): 470 nm, emission wavelength (Em.): 590 nm) were measured with Infinite M200 (TECAN, Männedorf, Switzerland).

## 2.6. Therapeutic Experiment

For investigation of APRPG-miR-499 mono-therapy, tumor-bearing mice were prepared and injected with APRPG-miR-499 (2 mg/kg as miR-499) intravenously on the day when the tumor size had reached 50 mm³. The tumor size and body weight of each mouse were monitored daily from day four after the injection. Tumor volume was calculated from the following formula: $0.4 \times a \times b^2$ (a; largest diameter, b; smallest diameter). On the other hand, for the combination therapy, the tumor-bearing mice were administered APRPG-miR-499 or APRPG-miCont (2 mg/kg as miRNAs) intravenously as described above. Then, at four days after the injection, the mice were injected intravenously with DOX at a dose of 5 mg/kg. The tumor size and body weight were monitored as mentioned above.

## 2.7. Statistical Analysis

The statistical differences in more than three groups were evaluated by analysis of variance (ANOVA) with the Tukey *post-hoc* test, whereas those in two groups were determined by using Student's *t* test.

## 3. Results and Discussion

### 3.1. Amelioration of Incomplete Blood Flow in Tumors Treated with miR-499

Physicochemical properties of APRPG-miR-499 were as follows: particle size, 163 ± 13 nm; $\zeta$-potential, −0.30 ± 0.46 mV. Because the complexes of miR-499 and TEPA-PCL (lipoplexes) themselves had a strong positive charge (*ca.* +45 mV), we modified the surface of the lipoplexes with PEG6000 in order to mask the charge and prolong their blood circulation. Our previous study revealed that APRPG-modified TEPA-PCL accumulates in tumor tissues after intravenous injection and becomes associated with tumor endothelial cells owing to the potent affinity of APRPG for VEGF receptor 1 (VEGFR 1) on the endothelial cells [5]. Therefore, it would be expected that APRPG-modified TEPA-PCL would enable miR-499 to arrive at the tumor tissues and to become internalized effectively in the target cells. By confocal microscopic observation at four days after the administration of miR-499 to mice, we found that the tumor vessels had much more blood flow compared with the APRPG-miCont–injected group (Figure 1A). Quantitative analysis showed that the tumor vessels that had been treated with APRPG-miR-499 had blood flow about 1.5 times higher than that of the other groups, although the number of blood vessels was not significantly different between APRPG-miR-499 and APRPG-miCont (Figure 1B). The proportion of vessels with blood perfusion was about 60% in the APRPG-miCont–treated group; however, more than 90% of the vessels had blood flow after the APRPG-miR-499 treatment, indicating that miR-499 might have affected the improvement of tumor blood vessels. Previously we reported that miR-499 inhibits the capillary tube networks *in vitro* [5]. We consider that miR-499 regulated the balance of pro-angiogenic factors and anti-angiogenic ones by inhibiting VEGF secretion.

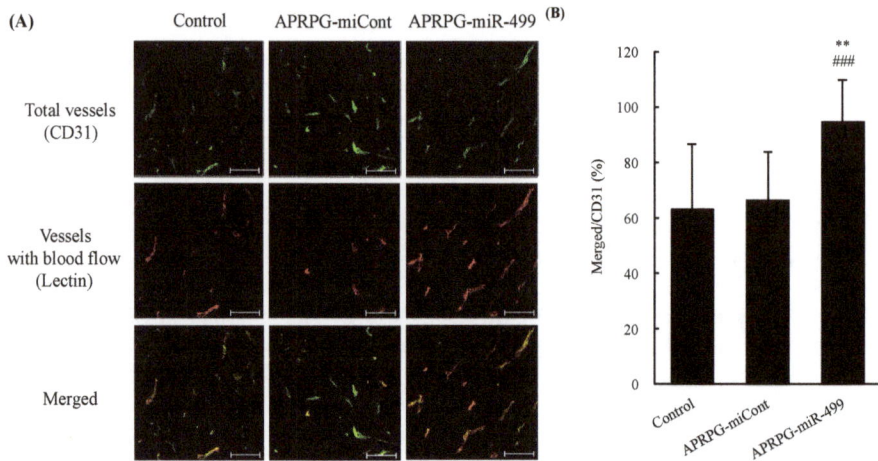

**Figure 1.** miR-499-mediated improvement of blood flow in tumor blood vessels. Colon 26 NL-17 cells were subcutaneously implanted into the left posterior flank of BALB/c mice. APRPG-miR-499 or APRPG-miCont (2 mg/kg as miRNA) were administered intravenously seven days after the implantation. Perfused vessels were labeled by intravenous injection of biotin-conjugated Lycopersicon esculentum Lectin at 96 h after the lipoplex injection. The tumor vessels were fixed by reflux flow with 1% paraformaldehyde. After the solid tumors had been dissected, 10-µm frozen sections were prepared. CD31 of the vasculature was immunostained with FITC. Biotin-conjugated Lycopersicon esculentum Lectin was labeled with Streptavidin-Alexa Fluor® 594. Green indicates vasculature, red indicates vessels with blood flow. Yellow color indicates areas of double-stained vessels. (**A**) Confocal images are shown. Scale bars indicate 100 µm; (**B**) Percent lectin$^+$CD31$^+$ double-positive area/total CD31$^+$ area was determined to assess perfusion efficiency of the tumor vasculature. Data are presented as percent ratio of merged area/CD31$^+$ area. Asterisks indicate significant differences (** $p < 0.01$ *vs.* control, ### $p < 0.001$ *vs.* APRPG-miCont).

### 3.2. Improvement of Doxorubicin (DOX) Accumulation in Tumors Treated with miR-499

The accumulation of DOX in the tumors four days after its administration to the tumor-bearing mice was determined by measuring the fluorescence of DOX. The results showed that more DOX accumulated in the tumor tissue in the miR-499-treated mice than in the other groups (Figure 2). Since the tumor blood vessels treated with miR-499 had the blood perfusion as mentioned, a high amount of DOX was carried to the tumor tissue with blood perfusion. In general, it is known that tumor vessels are defective and leaky because of rapid angiogenesis [12]. Additionally, lymphatic dysfunction in tumors causes intratumoral hypertension, resulting in less accumulation of an anti-cancer drug in the deeper part of the tumor. The inhibition of VEGF production results in the regression of incomplete tumor blood vessels and drives the improvement of the vessels [13–15]. The normalization of tumor vessels leads to reduced stromal pressure, which increases the amount of anti-cancer drugs delivered to the tumors [22,23]. Our findings suggest that miR-499 could enhance the accumulation of DOX in the tumors due to the development of a favorable environment for drug delivery via VEGF regulation.

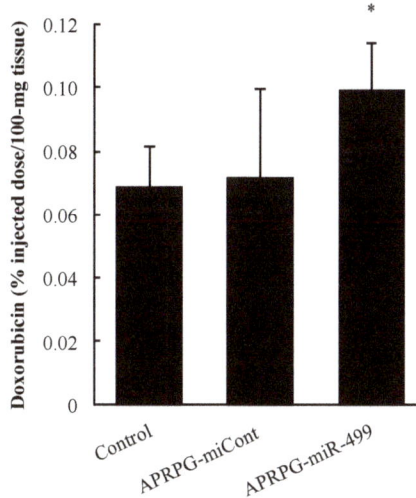

**Figure 2.** Improvement of DOX accumulation in tumors treated with miR-499. Colon 26 NL-17 cells were subcutaneously implanted into the left posterior flank of BALB/c mice. APRPG-miR-499 or APRPG-miCont were administered intravenously seven days after implantation. Four days after the lipoplex injection, DOX was administered intravenously. Three hours after DOX injection, tumor tissues were excised. The tumors were homogenized with ShakeMan2 and then centrifuged. DOX accumulation was quantified by measuring the fluorescence of DOX (Ex. 470 nm, Em. 590 nm). Asterisks indicate significant differences (* $p < 0.05$).

### 3.3. Combination Therapy with miR-499 and DOX

For the therapeutic experiment, tumor-bearing mice were intravenously administered APRPG-miR-499 and/or DOX. Although APRPG-miR-499 did not inhibit the tumor growth with a single injection at a dose of 2 mg/kg as miR-499 (Figure 3A), it did enhance the antitumor effect of DOX (Figure 3B). These data suggest that APRPG-miR-499 contributed to the normalization of blood flow in the tumor vessels, allowing DOX to accumulate in the tumor tissue and resulting in an enhanced antitumor effect of DOX. Previously, we reported that APRPG-miR-499 monotherapy caused a significant inhibition of tumor growth when given twice to mice bearing smaller tumors at a dose of 2 mg/kg/day as miR-499 [5]. These data indicate that a low dose of miR-499 mainly improved blood flow due to the normalization of incomplete tumor blood vessels, and a high dose mainly reduced blood vessels themselves due to the suppression of angiogenesis, resulting in the inhibition of tumor growth. Also, importantly, there was no weight loss in any group after the injection (Figure 3C,D). Considering the clinical application of anti-cancer drugs, it is meaningful that a smaller amount of DOX would be enough for the treatment of cancer. We expect that combination therapy of miR-499 and DOX would enable patients to have reduced side effects and to maintain their quality of life at a high level. These results suggest that miR-499 could be a good candidate for increasing the efficacy of anti-cancer drugs. Taken together, our data indicate that miR-499 enhanced the effect of an anti-cancer drug, DOX, possibly through vascular normalization, suggesting that combination therapy with miR-499 and anti-cancer drugs can be a potential therapeutic strategy.

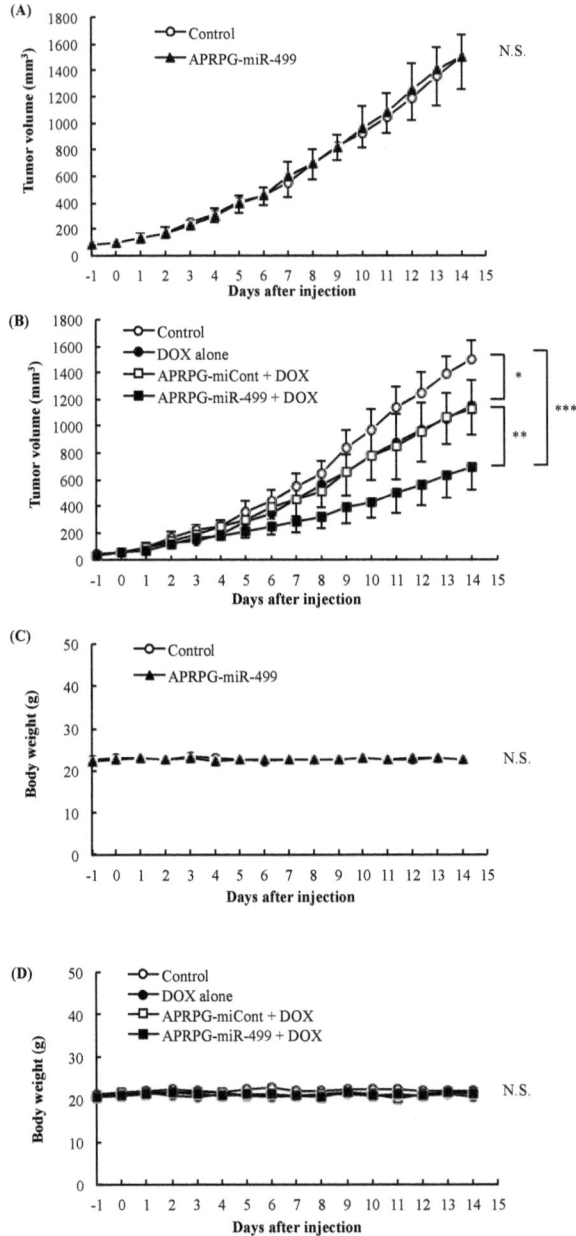

**Figure 3.** Combination therapy with miR-499 and DOX. Colon 26 NL-17 cells were subcutaneously implanted into the left posterior flank of BALB/c mice. APRPG-miR-499 was administered intravenously when the tumor volume had reached 50 mm³. In the case of combination therapy, DOX (5 mg/kg) was intravenously injected via a tail vein at four days after the lipoplex injection. The tumor size (**A,B**); and body weight (**C,D**) of each mouse were monitored daily from one day before lipoplex injection. Asterisks indicate significant differences (* $p < 0.05$, ** $p < 0.01$, *** $p < 0.001$). N.S. means no significant difference.

## 4. Conclusions

In the present study, we found that the tumor blood flow was increased significantly after the administration of APRPG-miR-499. In addition, the accumulation of DOX in the tumor tissue was also increased after the treatment with APRPG-miR-499. Furthermore, the tumor growth was suppressed significantly with DOX and miR-499 combination therapy compared with DOX monotherapy. Our findings provide a novel strategy for cancer therapy and contribute to the development of genetic drugs and/or therapeutic modalities based on RNA interference.

**Acknowledgments:** This research was supported by a grant-in-aid for scientific research from the Japan Society for the Promotion of Science.

**Author Contributions:** Tomohiro Asai and Naoto Oku designed the research; Tomohiro Asai, Hidenori Ando, Sho Ryu, and Naoto Oku designed the experiments; Takehisa Dewa synthesized the DCP-TEPA; Noriyuki Maeda did the DOPE, cholesterol, DPPC, and APRPG-PEG-DSPE; Sho Ryu, Ayaka Okamoto, and Hidenori Ando performed the *in vivo* assay with supervision from Naoto Oku. Ayaka Okamoto, Sho Ryu, Tomohiro Asai and Naoto Oku wrote the manuscript. All authors discussed the results and commented on the manuscript.

**Conflicts of Interest:** The authors declare no conflict of interest.

## References

1. Wilson, K.D.; Hu, S.; Venkatasubrahmanyam, S.; Fu, J.-D.; Sun, N.; Abilez, O.J.; Baugh, J.J.A.; Jia, F.; Ghosh, Z.; Li, R.A.; *et al.* Dynamic microRNA expression programs during cardiac differentiation of human embryonic stem cells: Role for miR-499. *Circ. Cardiovasc. Genet.* **2010**, *3*, 426–435. [CrossRef] [PubMed]
2. Zhang, L.L.; Liu, J.J.; Liu, F.; Liu, W.H.; Wang, Y.S.; Zhu, B.; Yu, B. MiR-499 induces cardiac differentiation of rat mesenchymal stem cells through Wnt/β-catenin signaling pathway. *Biochem. Biophys. Res. Commun.* **2012**, *420*, 875–881. [CrossRef] [PubMed]
3. Drzewiecka, A.W.; Ratajewski, M.; Wagner, W.; Dastych, J. HIF-1α is up-regulated in activated mast cells by a process that involves calcineurin and NFAT. *J. Immunol.* **2008**, *181*, 1665–1672. [CrossRef]
4. Zhang, X.; Gaspard, J.P.; Chung, D.C. Regulation of vascular endothelial growth factor by the Wnt and K-ras pathways in colonic neoplasia. *Cancer Res.* **2001**, *61*, 6050–6054. [PubMed]
5. Ando, H.; Asai, T.; Koide, H.; Okamoto, A.; Maeda, N.; Tomita, K.; Dewa, T.; Minamino, T.; Oku, N. Advanced cancer therapy by integrative antitumor actions via systemic administration of miR-499. *J. Control Release* **2014**, *181*, 32–39. [CrossRef] [PubMed]
6. Asai, T.; Matsushita, S.; Kenjo, E.; Tsuzuku, T.; Yonenaga, N.; Koide, H.; Hatanaka, K.; Dewa, T.; Nango, M.; Maeda, N.; *et al.* Dicetyl phosphate-tetraethylenepentamine-based liposomes for systemic siRNA delivery. *Bioconj. Chem.* **2011**, *22*, 429–435. [CrossRef] [PubMed]
7. Ando, H.; Okamoto, A.; Yokota, M.; Shimizu, K.; Asai, T.; Dewa, T.; Oku, N. Development of a miR-92a delivery system for anti-angiogenesis-based cancer therapy. *J. Gene Med.* **2013**, *15*, 20–27. [CrossRef] [PubMed]
8. Ando, H.; Okamoto, A.; Yokota, M.; Asai, T.; Dewa, T.; Oku, N. Polycation liposomes as a vector for potential intracellular delivery of microRNA. *J. Gene Med.* **2013**, *15*, 375–383. [CrossRef] [PubMed]
9. Qiu, F.; Yang, L.; Ling, X.; Yang, R.; Yang, X.; Zhang, L.; Fang, W.; Xie, C.; Huang, D.; Zhou, Y.; *et al.* Sequence variation in mature microRNA-499 confers unfavorable prognosis of lung cancer patients treated with platinum-based chemotherapy. *Clin. Cancer Res.* **2015**, *21*, 1602–1163. [CrossRef] [PubMed]
10. Folkman, J. Tumor angiogenesis: Therapeutic implications. *N. Engl. J. Med.* **1971**, *285*, 1182–1186. [PubMed]
11. Folkman, J.; Klagsbrun, M. Angiogenic factors. *Science* **1987**, *235*, 442–447. [CrossRef] [PubMed]
12. Jain, R.K. Barriers to drug delivery in solid tumors. *Sci. Am.* **1994**, *271*, 58–65. [CrossRef] [PubMed]
13. Wildiers, H.; Guetens, G.; Boeck, G.D.; Verbeken, E.; Landuyt, B.; Landuyt, W.; de Bruijn, E.A.; van Oosterom, A.T. Effect of antivascular endothelial growth factor treatment on the intratumoral uptake of CPT-11. *Br. J. Cancer* **2003**, *88*, 1979–1986. [CrossRef] [PubMed]
14. Fukumura, D.; Jain, R.K. Tumor microvasculature and microenvironment: Targets for anti-angiogenesis and normalization. *Microvasc. Res.* **2007**, *74*, 72–84. [CrossRef] [PubMed]

15. Tong, R.T.; Boucher, Y.; Kozin, S.V.; Winkler, F.; Hicklin, D.J.; Jain, R.K. Vascular normalization by vascular endothelial growth factor receptor 2 blockade induces a pressure gradient across the vasculature and improves drug penetration in tumors. *Cancer Res.* **2004**, *64*, 3731–3736. [CrossRef] [PubMed]
16. Saranadasa, M.; Wang, E.S. Vascular endothelial growth factor inhibition: Conflicting roles in tumor growth. *Cytokine* **2011**, *53*, 115–129. [CrossRef] [PubMed]
17. Klement, G.; Huang, P.; Mayer, B.; Green, S.K.; Man, S.; Bohlen, P.; Hicklin, D.; Kerbel, R.S. Differences in therapeutic indexes of combination metronomic chemotherapy and an anti-VEGFR-2 antibody in multidrug-resistant human breast cancer xenografts. *Clin. Cancer Res.* **2002**, *8*, 221–232. [PubMed]
18. Jain, R.K. Normalization of tumor vasculature: An emerging concept in antiangiogenic therapy. *Science* **2005**, *307*, 58–62. [CrossRef] [PubMed]
19. Lin, M.I.; Sessa, W.C. Antiangiogenic therapy: Creating a unique "window" of opportunity. *Cancer Cell* **2004**, *6*, 529–531. [CrossRef] [PubMed]
20. Winkler, F.; Kozin, S.V.; Tong, R.T.; Chae, S.S.; Booth, M.F.; Garkavtsev, I.; Xu, L.; Hicklin, D.J.; Fukumura, D.; di Tomaso, E.; *et al.* Kinetics of vascular normalization by VEGFR2 blockade governs brain tumor response to radiation: Role of oxygenation, angiopoietin-1, and matrix metalloproteinases. *Cancer Cell* **2004**, *6*, 553–563. [CrossRef] [PubMed]
21. Hurwitz, H.; Fehrenbacher, L.; Novotny, W.; Cartwright, T.; Hainsworth, J.; Heim, W.; Berlin, J.; Baron, A.; Griffing, S.; Holmgren, E.; *et al.* Bevacizumab plus irinotecan, fluorouracil, and leucovorin for metastatic colorectal cancer. *N. Engl. J. Med.* **2004**, *350*, 2335–2342. [CrossRef] [PubMed]
22. Huang, G.; Chen, L. Recombinant human endostatin improves anti-tumor efficacy of paclitaxel by normalizing tumor vasculature in Lewis lung carcinoma. *J. Cancer Res. Clin. Oncol.* **2010**, *136*, 1201–1211. [CrossRef] [PubMed]
23. Datta, M.; Via, L.E.; Kamoun, W.S.; Liu, C.; Chen, W.; Seano, G.; Weiner, D.M.; Schimel, D.; England, K.; Martin, J.D.; *et al.* Anti-vascular endothelial growth factor treatment normalizes tuberculosis granuloma vasculature and improves small molecule delivery. *Proc. Natl. Acad. Sci. USA* **2015**, *112*, 1827–1832. [CrossRef] [PubMed]

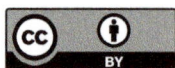

Journal of
*Clinical Medicine*

MDPI

*Article*

# Detection of Exosomal miRNAs in the Plasma of Melanoma Patients

Susan R. Pfeffer [1,†], Kenneth F. Grossmann [2,†], Pamela B. Cassidy [3], Chuan He Yang [1], Meiyun Fan [1], Levy Kopelovich [4], Sancy A. Leachman [3] and Lawrence M. Pfeffer [1,*]

[1]   Department of Pathology and Laboratory Medicine, Center for Cancer Research,
      University of Tennessee Health Science Center, 19 South Manassas Street, Memphis, TN 38163, USA;
      spfeffer@uthsc.edu (S.R.P.); cyang@uthsc.edu (C.H.Y.); mfan2@uthsc.edu (M.F.)
[2]   Department of Oncology, University of Utah, Salt Lake City, UT 84112, USA;
      kenneth.grossmann@hci.utah.edu
[3]   Department of Dermatology, Oregon Health & Science University, Portland, OR 97239, USA;
      cassidyp@ohsu.edu (P.B.C.); leachmas@ohsu.edu (S.A.L.)
[4]   Department of Medicine, Weill Cornell College of Medicine, New York, NY 10065, USA;
      kopelovichl@gmail.com
*     Correspondence: LPFEFFER@UTHSC.EDU; Tel.: +1-901-448-7855; Fax: +1-901-448-3910
†     These authors contributed equally to this work.

Academic Editors: Takahiro Ochiya and Ryou-u Takahashi
Received: 3 August 2015; Accepted: 4 December 2015; Published: 17 December 2015

**Abstract:** MicroRNAs (miRNAs) are a class of 22–25 nucleotide RNAs that control gene expression at the post-transcriptional level. MiRNAs have potential as cancer biomarkers. Melanoma is a highly aggressive form of skin cancer accounting for almost 4% of cancers among men and women, and ~80% of skin cancer-related deaths in the US. In the present study we analyzed plasma-derived exosomal miRNAs from clinically affected and unaffected familial melanoma patients (CDKN2A/p16 gene carriers) and compared them with affected (nonfamilial melanoma) and unaffected control subjects in order to identify novel risk biomarkers for melanoma. Intact miRNAs can be isolated from the circulation because of their presence in exosomes. A number of differentially regulated miRNAs identified by NanoString human V2 miRNA array were validated by quantitative PCR. Significantly, miR-17, miR-19a, miR-21, miR-126, and miR-149 were expressed at higher levels in patients with metastatic sporadic melanoma as compared with familial melanoma patients or unaffected control subjects. Surprisingly, no substantial differences in miRNA expression were detected between familial melanoma patients (all inclusive) and unaffected control subjects. The miRNAs differentially expressed in the different patient cohorts, especially in patients with metastatic melanoma, may play important roles in tumor progression and metastasis, and may be used as predictive biomarkers to monitor remission as well as relapse following therapeutic intervention.

**Keywords:** miRNAs; melanoma; exosomes; metastasis

## 1. Introduction

MicroRNAs (miRNAs) are an abundant class of small RNAs that control gene expression at the post-transcriptional level through degradation or repression of mRNA translation [1]. MiRNAs are able to regulate the expression of multiple targets by binding to the 3′-untranslated regions of genes. Emerging evidence suggests that miRNAs are involved in critical biological processes, including development, differentiation, apoptosis, proliferation and antiviral defense [2]. Most importantly, aberrant expression of miRNAs appears to be causatively linked to the pathogenesis of cancer [3]. Thus, miRNAs have potential as risk biomarkers, particularly following therapeutic intervention.

Exosomes are small (30–100 nm) extracellular vesicles that are produced by a wide variety of cell types, including tumor cells [4]. Although exosomes were originally considered to be cellular waste products, recent studies have demonstrated that they promote intercellular communication and immunoregulatory processes by shuttling proteins, lipids, and miRNAs between cells [5,6]. Moreover, intact miRNAs can be isolated from the circulation in significant quantities despite the presence of high levels of RNase activity because of their presence in exosomes [7,8]. The remarkable stability of circulating exosomal miRNAs makes them candidates to monitor disease progression in a variety of cancers.

Skin cancer is the most common human cancer. The incidence of melanoma, the most lethal skin cancer, is one of the few cancers in the U.S. that continues to rise [9]. Melanoma is a highly aggressive form of skin cancer that accounts for almost 5% of cancers among men and women, and ~80% of skin cancer-related deaths in the US. The clustering of several melanomas within a single family, several independent primary melanomas in a single individual, and co-incidence of several melanomas and other cancers such as pancreatic cancer in the same family are all associated with inheritance of germline mutations in a high-penetrance melanoma susceptibility gene [10]. The most common high-penetrance melanoma predisposition gene is cyclin-dependent kinase inhibitor 2A, which encodes two independent predisposition genes, CDKN2A/p16 and CDKN2A/ARF. CDKN2A mutations occur in approximately 20%–40% of melanoma-prone families worldwide [11,12]. Variable rates of mutation have been found in sporadic melanomas, in some studies being as high as 50% in primary lesions [13]. The CDKN2A gene locus generates two proteins through alternate reading frames: p16$^{INK4a}$ and p14$^{arf}$. The p16$^{INK4a}$ protein binds to CDK4 and CDK6, inhibiting their ability to phosphorylate the retinoblastoma protein. The p14$^{arf}$ protein stabilizes the tumor suppressor protein p53. Collectively, these CDKN2A gene products are potent tumor suppressors that play distinct but critical roles in cell cycle progression and apoptosis [14]. Heterozygous loss of p16$^{INK4a}$ function is sufficient to confer a 67% lifetime risk of melanoma [15].

According to the National Cancer Institute, in 2015 an estimated 76,100 new melanoma cases will be diagnosed and 9710 deaths will occur in the US. Identifying early biomarkers for melanoma would enable discovery of potential targets and presumably agents for early intervention in persons at risk of developing melanoma. A noninvasive screening tool to identify patients with a predisposition to melanoma is presently lacking. Whole blood holds several advantages as a biomarker specimen, most notably because sampling and processing is much simpler than that of skin. In this regard it holds significant potential as a point-of-care test, which would be attractive in determining an ideal cancer-screening tool.

We previously showed that gene expression profiles are altered in phenotypically normal skin fibroblasts from familial melanoma families with distinct CDKN2A/p16 mutations (DKN2A:c.377T>A (p.V126D) and CDKN2A:c.259G>T (p.R87P)) when compared to skin fibroblasts from normal controls [16]. Furthermore, UV-irradiation of skin fibroblasts from such familial melanoma cohorts resulted in specific alterations in the expression of genes that regulate cell cycle and DNA damage response, and similar alterations in gene expression were also observed in melanoma lesions. In the present study, we investigated whether exosomal-derived miRNAs in the plasma from both clinically symptomatic and asymptomatic familial (CDKN2A:c.377T>A (p.V126D)) and sporadic melanoma patients, including unaffected family members, may be used as prognostic biomarkers to identify individuals at high risk of developing melanoma. However, this proof of principle experiment did not identify miRNAs specifically dysregulated in plasma-derived exosomes from familial melanoma patients. Nonetheless, several miRNAs were differentially expressed in patients with metastatic disease, not only in melanoma tumor tissue but also in plasma-derived exosomes. This result substantiates the finding of miRNA dysregulation in metastatic melanoma [17–19]. These findings form the basis for future studies on their applicability as diagnostic and prognostic biomarkers in melanoma.

## 2. Results

*2.1. Characterization of miRNA Expression in Plasma-Derived Exosomes from Patients with a Predisposition to Melanoma and Patients with Metastatic Melanoma*

We performed miRNA profiling on RNA prepared from plasma-derived exosomes from four specific patient cohorts. The general patient information is shown in Table 1. Cohort A comprised 8 clinically affected individuals from a single large family, who carried a CDKN2A/p16 (CDKN2A:c.377T>A (p.V126D)) mutation but were free of disease at the time of blood draw. Cohort B comprised 5 individuals from the same family as in Cohort A with CDKN2A/p16 mutations, but with no history of melanoma at the time of this study. Cohort C comprised 13 spouse controls in the same kindred as A and B above, and Cohort D consisted of 10 non-related metastatic melanoma patients with currently active disease. We hypothesized that genetically predisposed individuals such as those who carried a CDKN2A/p16 mutation might share the expression profile with individuals having sporadic metastatic melanoma.

**Table 1.** General patient information.

| Cohort | Age | Gender | p16 Mutation Status | Melanoma Diagnosis |
|--------|-----|--------|---------------------|--------------------|
| A1 | 37 | M | 377T>A (p.V126D) | N |
| A2 | 40 | M | 377T>A (p.V126D) | N |
| A3 | 37 | M | 377T>A (p.V126D)) | N |
| A4 | 46 | M | 377T>A (p.V126D) | N |
| A5 | 64 | F | 377T>A (p.V126D) | N |
| B1 | 86 | M | 377T>A (p.V126D) | Y |
| B2 | 56 | M | 377T>A (p.V126D) | Y |
| B3 | 83 | M | 377T>A (p.V126D) | Y |
| B4 | 66 | F | 377T>A (p.V126D) | Y |
| B5 | 50 | M | 377T>A (p.V126D) | Y |
| B6 | 39 | F | 377T>A (p.V126D) | Y |
| B7 | 42 | F | 377T>A (p.V126D) | Y |
| B8 | 52 | F | 377T>A (p.V126D) | Y |
| C1 | 68 | M | negative | N |
| C2 | 40 | F | negative | N |
| C3 | 41 | M | negative | N |
| C4 | 46 | M | negative | N |
| C5 | 45 | F | negative | N |
| C6 | 36 | M | negative | N |
| C7 | 58 | M | negative | N |
| C8 | 63 | M | negative | N |
| C9 | 88 | M | negative | N |
| C10 | 34 | F | negative | N |
| C11 | 36 | F | negative | N |
| C12 | 40 | F | negative | N |
| C13 | 68 | F | negative | N |
| D1 | 50 | M | Not tested | met mel |
| D2 | 48 | F | Not tested | met mel |
| D3 | 38 | M | Not tested | met mel |
| D4 | 55 | M | Not tested | met mel |
| D5 | 34 | M | Not tested | met mel |
| D6 | 81 | M | Not tested | met mel |
| D7 | 82 | F | Not tested | met mel |
| D8 | 40 | M | Not tested | met mel |
| D9 | 40 | M | Not tested | met mel |
| D10 | 55 | M | Not tested | met mel |

In brief, the miRNA expression data from the 36 samples was analyzed with nSolver software to identify alterations in miRNA expression. Among the ~700 human miRNAs examined, 75 miRNAs were detected in plasma-derived exosomes from more than half of the patients. The 50 miRNAs that showed highest total reads (most abundant) in the exosomes of the 36 patient samples were then subjected to unsupervised hierarchal clustering with the expression heat maps of the individual patient samples shown in Figure 1. The twenty most variable miRNAs among all samples were then further validated by qPCR analysis to examine their differential expression within the four patient cohorts described in Table 1. These miRNAs included let-7b, let-7g, miR-17, miR-19a, miR-19b, miR-20b, miR-21, miR-23a, miR-29a, miR-92a, miR-125b, miR-126, miR-128, miR-137, miR-148a, miR-149, miR-199a, miR-221, miR-222 and miR-423 (Table 2).

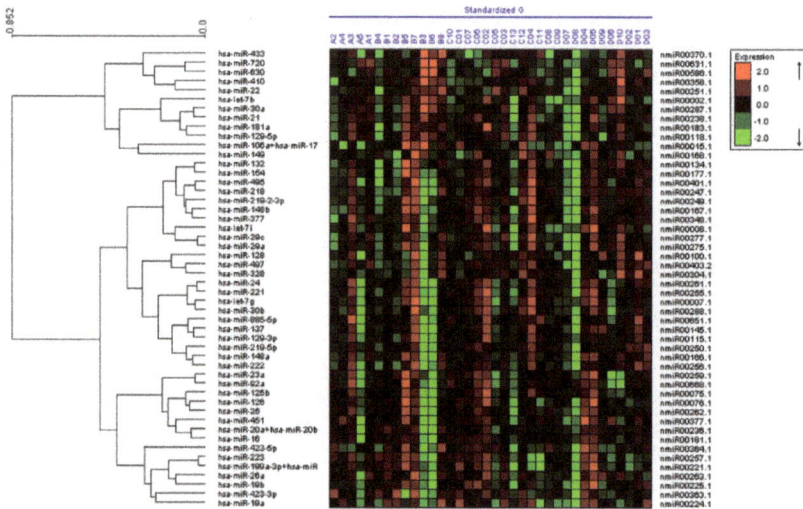

**Figure 1.** Characterization of miRNA expression in plasma-derived exosomes from individuals with a genetic predisposition to melanoma (all inclusive), spouse controls and patients with sporadic metastatic melanoma. RNA was prepared from plasma-derived exosomes from the patient cohorts listed in Table 1, and miRNA expression profiling was conducted on the nCounter Analysis System using the human V1 miRNA assay kit.

**Table 2.** Primers used for miRNA expression.

| | |
|---|---|
| hsa-let-7b | TGAGGTAGTAGGTTGTGTGGTT |
| hsa-let-7g-5p | TGAGGTAGTAGTTTGTACAGTT |
| hsa-miR-125b | TCCCTGAGACCCTAACTTGTGA |
| hsa-miR-126 | TCGTACCGTGAGTAATAATGCG |
| hsa-miR-128 | TCACAGTGAACCGGTCTCTTT |
| hsa-miR-137 | TTATTGCTTAAGAATACGCGTAG |
| hsa-miR-148a | AAAGTTCTGAGACACTCCGACT |
| hsa-miR-149 | TCTGGCTCCGTGTCTTCACTCCC |
| hsa-miR-17 | CAAAGTGCTTACAGTGCAGGTAG |
| hsa-miR-199a-5p | CCCAGTGTTCAGACTACCTGTTC |
| hsa-miR-19a | TGTGCAAATCTATGCAAAACTGA |
| hsa-miR-19b | TGTGCAAATCCATGCAAAACTGA |
| hsa-miR-20b | TAAAGTGCTTATAGTGCAGGTAG |
| hsa-miR-21 | TAGCTTATCAGACTGATGTTGA |
| hsa-miR-221 | AGCTACATTGTCTGCTGGGTTTC |
| hsa-miR-222 | AGCTACATCTGGCTACTGGGT |
| hsa-miR-23a | ATCACATTGCCAGGGATTTCC |
| hsa-miR-29a | TAGCACCATCTGAAATCGGTTA |
| hsa-miR-423-5p | TGAGGGGCAGAGAGCGAGACTTT |
| hsa-miR-92a | TATTGCACTTGTCCCGGCCTGT |

## 2.2. Detection of Circulating miRNA in Plasma-Derived Exosomes

Since there are no known control or house-keeping microRNAs in exosomes, we adopted the strategy of using spiked-in *C. elegans* miRNAs directly into Qiazol prior to RNA extraction as normalizing controls [20]. To determine whether our miRNA assays by qPCR were within the linear range of detection, a reference standard Cel-39 was spiked into Qiazol at 0.05 fmol/mL and 0.0005 fmol/mL prior to RNA extraction, and the expression of miR-21, miR-92b and miR-126 in plasma-derived exosomes was determined. These assays demonstrated the appropriate miRNA expression levels relative to the known quantity of spiked-in Cel39, demonstrating that our qPCR assay conditions for miRNAs were within the linear range.

We then examined the expression of circulating miRNAs by qPCR using the RNAs derived from the original cohort, plus an additional 3 metastatic melanoma patient samples. Thus, we analyzed miRNA expression in 13 individuals with metastatic melanoma, 13 control volunteers, 5 individuals with the p16 mutation (CDKN2A:c.377T>A (p.V126D)) but with no clinical evidence of melanoma incidence, and 8 individuals with the p16 mutation with melanoma. We subjected the qPCR data on the circulating miRNAs to statistical analysis as shown in Tables 3–5 and presented as "box plots" in Figures 2 and 3. In Table 3 we compared the expression levels of these miRNAs between individuals with the CDKN2A:c.377T>A (p.V126D) mutation to those of normal volunteers, and found that there were no statistically significant differences between expression of any of the 20 exosomal miRNAs measured. In Table 4 and Figure 2 we show the comparison in miRNA expression between individuals with the p16 mutation (CDKN2A:c.377T>A (p.V126D)) that had no evidence of melanoma *versus* those individuals that had a history of melanoma. Most interestingly, expression of miR-125b was 1.5-fold higher in those individuals with the p16 mutation (CDKN2A:c.377T>A (p.V126D)) that had no evidence of melanoma as compared to individuals with this mutation that had a history of melanoma (*p* value of 0.025). In Table 5 and Figure 3 we show the comparison in miRNA expression between control individuals and patients with metastatic melanoma. Most interestingly, miR-17, miR-19a, miR-21, miR-126 and miR-149 were expressed at 1.8-fold, 2.3-fold, 1.7-fold, 2.8-fold and 3.9-fold higher levels, respectively, in patients with metastatic melanoma (*p* values of 0.044, 0.015, 0.038, 0.040 and 0.021, respectively).

**Table 3.** MiRNA expression in plasma-derived exosomes from p16 mutation carriers.

| MiRNA | Control | p16 Carriers | *p* Value |
|---|---|---|---|
| hsa-let-7b | $0.118 \pm 0.001$ | $0.104 \pm 0.012$ | 0.217 |
| hsa-let-7g | $0.056 \pm 0.007$ | $0.051 \pm 0.011$ | 0.350 |
| hsa-miR-125b | $1.319 \pm 0.125$ | $1.251 \pm 0.150$ | 0.368 |
| hsa-miR-126 | $0.113 \pm 0.019$ | $0.127 \pm 0.018$ | 0.425 |
| hsa-miR-128 | $2.034 \pm 0.210$ | $1.826 \pm 0.206$ | 0.242 |
| hsa-miR-137 | $0.052 \pm 0.005$ | $0.045 \pm 0.006$ | 0.252 |
| hsa-miR-148a | $0.094 \pm 0.011$ | $0.083 \pm 0.008$ | 0.224 |
| hsa-miR-149 | $0.024 \pm 0.004$ | $0.028 \pm 0.006$ | 0.310 |
| hsa-miR-17 | $0.101 \pm 0.17$ | $0.097 \pm 0.013$ | 0.418 |
| hsa-miR-199a | $0.017 \pm 0.004$ | $0.016 \pm 0.010$ | 0.451 |
| hsa-miR-19a | $0.421 \pm 0.067$ | $0.409 \pm 0.053$ | 0.446 |
| hsa-miR-19b | $0.558 \pm 0.090$ | $0.543 \pm 0.077$ | 0.450 |
| hsa-miR-20b | $0.123 \pm 0.020$ | $0.107 \pm 0.012$ | 0.273 |
| hsa-miR-21 | $0.775 \pm 0.074$ | $0.789 \pm 0.054$ | 0.441 |
| hsa-miR-221 | $0.335 \pm 0.030$ | $0.311 \pm 0.023$ | 0.273 |
| hsa-miR-222 | $0.589 \pm 0.062$ | $0.519 \pm 0.062$ | 0.182 |
| hsa-miR-23a | $0.520 \pm 0.095$ | $0.473 \pm 0.072$ | 0.350 |
| hsa-miR-29a | $0.625 \pm 0.054$ | $0.593 \pm 0.044$ | 0.323 |
| hsa-miR-423-3p | $0.088 \pm 0.014$ | $0.078 \pm 0.006$ | 0.264 |
| hsa-miR-92a | $0.341 \pm 0.053$ | $0.306 \pm 0.034$ | 0.292 |

**Table 4.** MiRNA expression in plasma-derived exosomes from p16 mutation carriers with or without melanoma.

| MiRNA | p16 No Melanoma | p16 with Melanoma | *p* Value |
|---|---|---|---|
| hsa-let-7b | 0.119 ± 0.017 | 0.094 ± 0.016 | 0.162 |
| hsa-let-7g | 0.048 ± 0.007 | 0.052 ± 0.018 | 0.422 |
| hsa-miR-125b | 1.571 ± 0.081 | 1.052 ± 0.214 | 0.025 |
| hsa-miR-126 | 0.140 ± 0.007 | 0.120 ± 0.030 | 0.274 |
| hsa-miR-128 | 1.908 ± 0.223 | 1.774 ± 0.315 | 0.368 |
| hsa-miR-137 | 0.036 ± 0.004 | 0.051 ± 0.009 | 0.103 |
| hsa-miR-148a | 0.089 ± 0.004 | 0.079 ± 0.013 | 0.256 |
| hsa-miR-149 | 0.021 ± 0.002 | 0.032 ± 0.010 | 0.172 |
| hsa-miR-17 | 0.111 ± 0.012 | 0.088 ± 0.021 | 0.187 |
| hsa-miR-199a | 0.020 ± 0.006 | 0.013 ± 0.002 | 0.183 |
| hsa-miR-19a | 0.404 ± 0.037 | 0.411 ± 0.087 | 0.471 |
| hsa-miR-19b | 0.485 ± 0.053 | 0.579 ± 0.123 | 0.252 |
| hsa-miR-20b | 0.121 ± 0.016 | 0.099 ± 0.018 | 0.191 |
| hsa-miR-21 | 0.757 ± 0.046 | 0.809 ± 0.085 | 0.301 |
| hsa-miR-221 | 0.354 ± 0.029 | 0.285 ± 0.031 | 0.068 |
| hsa-miR-222 | 0.577 ± 0.046 | 0.483 ± 0.061 | 0.125 |
| hsa-miR-23a | 0.542 ± 0.069 | 0.430 ± 0.110 | 0.205 |
| hsa-miR-29a | 0.544 ± 0.061 | 0.623 ± 0.061 | 0.193 |
| hsa-miR-423-3p | 0.094 ± 0.012 | 0.068 ± 0.005 | 0.063 |
| hsa-miR-92a | 0.382 ± 0.075 | 0.258 ± 0.018 | 0.088 |

**Table 5.** MiRNA expression in plasma-derived exosomes from patients with metastatic melanoma.

| MiRNA | Control | Metastatic Melanoma | *p* Value |
|---|---|---|---|
| hsa-let-7b | 0.118 ± 0.001 | 0.192 ± 0.066 | 0.146 |
| hsa-let-7g | 0.056 ± 0.007 | 0.065 ± 0.027 | 0.378 |
| hsa-miR-125b | 1.319 ± 0.125 | 1.219 ± 0.468 | 0.420 |
| hsa-miR-126 | 0.113 ± 0.019 | 0.320 ± 0.096 | 0.040 |
| hsa-miR-128 | 2.034 ± 0.210 | 1.420 ± 0.322 | 0.063 |
| hsa-miR-137 | 0.052 ± 0.005 | 0.102 ± 0.030 | 0.067 |
| hsa-miR-148a | 0.094 ± 0.011 | 0.126 ± 0.028 | 0.150 |
| hsa-miR-149 | 0.024 ± 0.004 | 0.094 ± 0.030 | 0.021 |
| hsa-miR-17 | 0.101 ± 0.17 | 0.181 ± 0.040 | 0.044 |
| hsa-miR-199a | 0.017 ± 0.004 | 0.028 ± 0.006 | 0.084 |
| hsa-miR-19a | 0.421 ± 0.067 | 0.986 ± 0.222 | 0.015 |
| hsa-miR-19b | 0.558 ± 0.090 | 1.203 ± 0.290 | 0.259 |
| hsa-miR-20b | 0.123 ± 0.020 | 0.202 ± 0.046 | 0.071 |
| hsa-miR-21 | 0.775 ± 0.074 | 1.305 ± 0.268 | 0.038 |
| hsa-miR-221 | 0.335 ± 0.030 | 0.390 ± 0.085 | 0.279 |
| hsa-miR-222 | 0.589 ± 0.062 | 0.680 ± 0.123 | 0.258 |
| hsa-miR-23a | 0.520 ± 0.095 | 0.773 ± 0.208 | 0.142 |
| hsa-miR-29a | 0.625 ± 0.054 | 0.795 ± 0.150 | 0.154 |
| hsa-miR-423-3p | 0.088 ± 0.014 | 0.082 ± 0.010 | 0.369 |
| hsa-miR-92a | 0.341 ± 0.053 | 0.267 ± 0.036 | 0.133 |

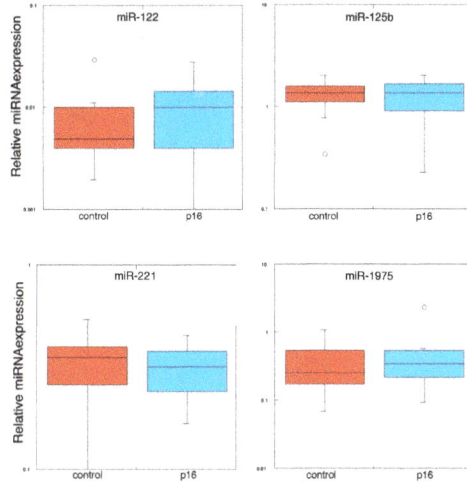

**Figure 2.** MiRNA expression in plasma-derived exosomes from individuals with the p16 mutation and normal volunteers. RNA was prepared from plasma-derived exosomes from individuals with the p16 mutation (CDKN2A:c.377T>A (p.V126D)) and normal volunteers. MiRNA expression was determined by qPCR ($n = 3$) and normalized to the spiked-in levels of Cel39.

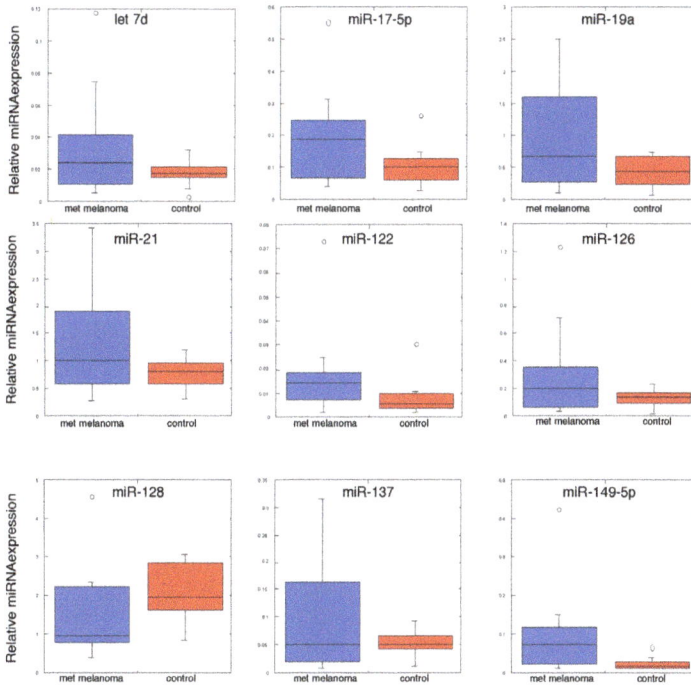

**Figure 3.** MiRNA expression in plasma-derived exosomes from individuals with metastatic melanoma and normal volunteers. RNA was prepared from plasma-derived exosomes from individuals with metastatic melanoma and normal volunteers. MiRNA expression was determined by qPCR ($n = 3$) and normalized to the spiked-in levels of Cel39.

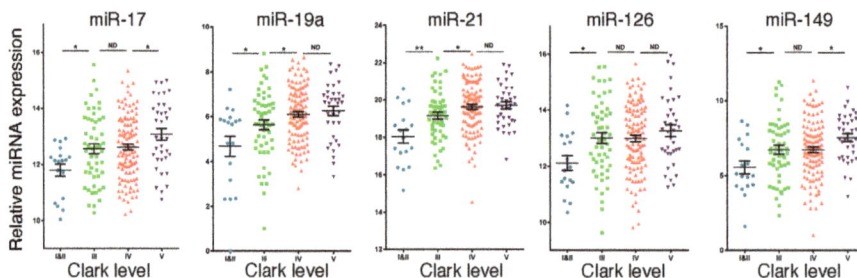

**Figure 4.** High expression of miR-17, miR-19a, miR-21, miR-126 and miR-149 is associated with melanoma tumor grade. Expression of miR-17, miR-19a, miR-21, miR-126 and miR-149 in the TCGA database for 216 independent melanoma patient samples according to Clark level (Level 1 is the least aggressive and Level V is the most aggressive).

### 2.3. Expression of Potential miRNA Biomarkers in Melanoma

Based on the results from the above studies, we then sought to determine whether miRNAs, which were differentially expressed in plasma exosomes derived from patients with metastatic melanoma, were also differentially expressed in melanoma tumor tissue. Therefore, we examined the TCGA database for miRNA expression in 216 melanoma specimens, which were classified according to Clark level (level I/II is minimally invasive cancer and level V is the most highly invasive form). As shown in Figure 4, low expression of miR-17, miR-19a, miR-21, miR-126 and miR-149 was found in thinner melanoma (Clark level I/II) and high expression was found in thicker melanoma (Clark level III, IV and V). These results provide additional evidence that these exosomal miRNAs are associated with the occurrence of melanoma *in situ*. Such melanoma samples include the tumor cells as well as the cells in tumor microenvironment that coordinately regulate tumorigenesis.

### 2.4. The Potential Biological Functions of the miRNAs Upregulated in Metastatic Melanoma

To investigate the potential biological functions of the miRNAs upregulated in metastatic melanoma, the target sites of miR-17-5p, miR-19a-3p, miR-149-5p, miR-21 and miR-126-3p were mapped to the 3-UTRs of a panel of genes that have been previously found to be associated with melanoma progression [21–23]. Forty genes associated with melanoma progression were found to be putative targets of these miRNAs (Table 6). To gain insights into the biological pathways that these putative miRNA targets may affect, we performed gene set enrichment analysis using the Molecular Signatures Database v5.0 [24], which is a computational method used to identify over-represented gene sets with defined biological meanings [25]. As shown in Figure 5, the most significantly enriched gene sets contain genes downregulated by ultraviolet (UV) irradiation (*i.e.*, genes included in the ENK_UV_RESPONSE_EPIDERMIS_DN and ENK_UV_RESPONSE_KERATINOCYTE_DN gene sets), targeted by the tumor protein p53 (TP53)/retinoblastoma protein (RB1) (*i.e.*, genes included in the MARTINEZ_RB1_AND_TP53_TARGETS_UP, MARTINEZ_RB1_TARGETS_UP and MARTINEZ_TP53_TARGETS_UP gene sets) and genes related to the tumor growth factor-beta (TGFB)/SMAD pathways (*i.e.*, genes included in the PANGAS_TUMOR_SUPPRESSION_BY_SMAD1 _AND_SMAD5_UP gene set).

**Table 6.** Putative targets of miRNAs upregulated in metastatic melanoma.

| Genes | | miR-17 | miR-19a | miR-149 | miR-21 |
|---|---|---|---|---|---|
| ADD3 | adducin 3 (gamma) | | | y | |
| ARL4C | ADP-ribosylation factor-like 4C | y | | | |
| BCL11A | B-cell CLL/lymphoma 11A (zinc finger protein) | | y | | y |
| BCL11B | B-cell CLL/lymphoma 11B (zinc finger protein) | y | | | y |
| CD34 | CD34 molecule | | | y | |
| CDS1 | CDP-diacylglycerol synthase (phosphatidate cytidylyltransferase) 1 | | y | | |
| CXCL12 | chemokine (C-X-C motif) ligand 12 (stromal cell-derived factor 1) | | y | | |
| CYBB | cytochrome b-245, beta polypeptide | y | | | |
| DSC3 | desmocollin 3 | | | y | |
| EREG | epiregulin | y | y | | |
| ESR1 | estrogen receptor 1 | y | y | | |
| FAT2 | FAT tumor suppressor homolog 2 | y | | | |
| FBLN1 | fibulin 1 | y | | y | |
| GJA1 | gap junction protein, alpha 1, 43 kDa | y | y | | |
| GRHL2 | grainyhead-like 2 (Drosophila) | y | | | |
| HLF | hepatic leukemia factor | y | y | | |
| ID2 | inhibitor of DNA binding 2, dominant negative helix-loop-helix protein | | y | | |
| LRIG1 | leucine-rich repeats and immunoglobulin-like domains 1 | y | y | | |
| LRRK1 | leucine-rich repeat kinase 1 | | y | | |
| LTB4R | leukotriene B4 receptor | | | y | |
| MACF1 | microtubule-actin crosslinking factor 1 | | y | | |
| MBNL1 | muscleblind-like (Drosophila) | y | y | | y |
| MGEA5 | meningioma expressed antigen 5 (hyaluronidase) | y | | | |
| MPZL2 | myelin protein zero-like 2 | y | | | |
| NFATC3 | nuclear factor of activated T-cells, cytoplasmic, calcineurin-dependent 3 | | | y | |
| NLRP3 | NLR family, pyrin domain containing 3 | y | | | |
| NMT2 | N-myristoyltransferase 2 | | y | | |
| NTRK2 | neurotrophic tyrosine kinase, receptor, type 2 | y | | y | |
| PAIP2B | poly(A) binding protein interacting protein 2B | | | y | y |
| PTGER3 | prostaglandin E receptor 3 (subtype EP3) | y | | | |
| PTGS1 | prostaglandin-endoperoxide synthase 1 (prostaglandin G/H synthase and cyclooxygenase) | y | | | |
| RAPGEFL1 | Rap guanine nucleotide exchange factor (GEF)-like 1 | y | y | | |
| RORA | RAR-related orphan receptor A | y | y | y | |
| RTN1 | reticulon 1 | | y | | |
| TCF4 | transcription factor 4 | y | | | |
| TMEM45A | transmembrane protein 45A | | y | | |
| TNFRSF25 | tumor necrosis factor receptor superfamily, member 25 | | | y | |
| TP63 | tumor protein p63 | y | | y | |
| TXNIP | thioredoxin interacting protein | y | | | |
| ZFP36L2 | zinc finger protein 36, C3H type-like 2 | | | | y |

No binding sites of miR-126 were found in the 3′-UTRs of the genes associated with melanoma progression.

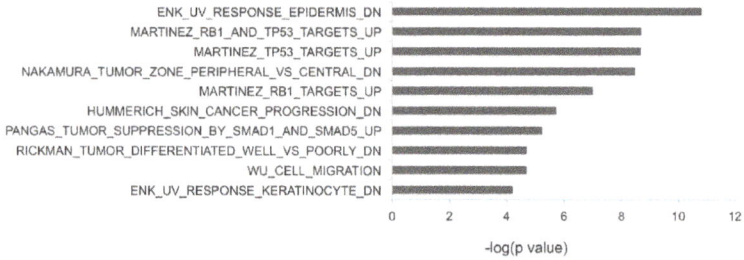

**Figure 5.** Enriched gene sets of putative targets of miRNAs upregulated in metastatic melanoma. The conserved target sites of miR-17-5p, miR-19a-3p, miR-149-5p, miR-21 and miR-126-3p were mapped to the 3-UTRs of a panel of genes that have been associated with melanoma progression according to TargetScan V6.2. Gene set enrichment analysis of putative miRNA targets was conducted by using the Molecular Signatures Database v5.0.

## 3. Discussion

To date, over 1800 human miRNAs have been identified, and miRNAs are predicted to control over 60% of all human genes [2,26]. MiRNAs regulate a wide variety of cellular processes, including cancer. The miRNAs differentially expressed in patients with metastatic melanoma may play important roles in tumor progression and metastasis, as well as be explored as diagnostic biomarkers. Exosomal miRNAs may transfer or shuttle signals between cancer cells and normal cells, and may contribute to malignant transformation. Differentially-expressed exosomal miRNA has now been demonstrated for many forms of cancer [27], and a recent study has shown that a panel of 5 miRNAs can be used to estimate risk of recurrence in stage II melanoma patients [28]. The measurement of tumor-derived miRNAs in serum or plasma may be an important approach to cancer detection [20]. In a previous study, higher levels of circulating miR-221 were found in serum samples of malignant melanoma patients as compared to healthy volunteers [29].

In the present study, we investigated miRNA signatures of plasma-derived exosomes from familial and sporadic melanoma patients and unaffected family members. Several miRNAs were differentially expressed in plasma-derived exosomes, which may form the basis for future studies on their applicability as predisposition biomarkers and potential chemoprevention targets. An important aspect of our studies was the finding that miR-17, miR-19a, miR-21, miR-126 and miR-149 were expressed at higher levels in plasma-derived exosomes from patients with metastatic melanoma. Many of these miRNAs have been associated with various cancers, and in some cases with melanoma specifically. For example, using a high-throughput approach, miR-17 was identified as a potential oncogenic miRNA in melanoma [30]. Previous studies demonstrated that miR-17 is highly expressed in leukemia and lung cancer, and it promotes cell proliferation by targeting p21 [31,32] as well as PTEN and RB [33,34]. Also, increased expression of miR-19a leads to increased melanoma invasiveness [35]. MiR-19a is an important member of the oncogenic miR-17-92 cluster. MiR-19a is upregulated in acute myeloid leukemia, colorectal cancer and gastric cancer, and is believed to act through promoting tumor growth and metastasis [36,37]. MiR-21 is frequently upregulated in human tumor cells where it appears to play an important role in the oncogenic process through its association with increased proliferation, low apoptosis, high invasion and metastatic potential [38–44]. However, miR-21 is also upregulated in the inflammatory response, which also may play an important role in tumor progression as well as in tumor elimination (reviewed in [45]). We recently found that IFN upregulated miR-21 expression in both melanoma and prostate cancer cells, which diminished their apoptotic sensitivity [46,47]. In contrast, knockdown (KD) of miR-21 expression enhanced apoptotic sensitivity to IFN as well as to several chemotherapeutic agents. Consistent with these findings, miR-21 inhibition in human melanoma cells increases expression of the PTEN target gene, leading to suppression of AKT phosphorylation and subsequently increased Bax/Bcl-2 ratio [48]. Most interestingly, using mouse B16 melanoma, we found that while the parent cell line exclusively formed large tumors in the lungs of tail-vein injected mice, miR-21 KD cells formed only small lung tumors [47], and mice injected with miR-21 KD cells exhibited markedly prolonged animal survival. Elevated miR-126 expression has been observed in normal melanocytes and primary melanoma cell lines, while it was reportedly reduced in metastatic melanoma [49]. Overexpression of miR-126 was found to enhance melanogenesis. MiR-149 is upregulated in melanoma cells and is expressed in response to p53 activation [50]. However, miR-149 provides a mechanism to bypass the induction of apoptosis by p53 activation by directly targeting glycogen synthetase-3α and thereby stabilizing MCL-1.

Consistent with the reported function of these miRNAs in regulating cell proliferation and metastatic potential, target site mapping to genes associated with melanoma progression suggests that miR-17-5p, miR-19a-3p, miR-149-5p and miR-21 play a role in modulating cell response to TP53/RB1 activation and TGFβ/SMAD signaling pathways. Since these pathways play an important role in regulating the G1/S checkpoint of normal melanocytes and are major regulators of melanocyte transformation [51,52], the upregulation of miRNAs controlling TP53/RB1 activation and TGFβ/SMAD signaling pathways may contribute to G1/S checkpoint abnormalities that are frequently observed during melanoma progression. Since these signaling pathways are critical to the malignant process, further studies will be needed to define the roles of these pathways directly in melanoma cells themselves and in the stromal cells surrounding the tumor.

Although we hypothesized that genetically predisposed familial melanoma patients with/without evidence of disease might share their miRNA expression profile with sporadic metastatic melanoma patients, no major differences between p16 mutation (CDKN2A:c.377T>A (p.V126D)) gene carriers and normal controls were detected. There are several possible explanations for our inability to discern miRNAs that are risk biomarkers in cohorts of familial melanoma. These possibilities include: (1) differences in miRNA profiles of the cohorts in our p16 families are too small to be detected with the sample size available in this work (although relative to the uniqueness of the cohort, the number of samples used in this study is large); (2) the miRNA profile of an affected p16 mutation carrier (CDKN2A:c.377T>A (p.V126D)) is not significantly different from a carrier that has not had a melanoma or from a normal control; (3) other p16 mutations such as the CDKN2A:c.259G>T (p.R87P) mutation [16,53] may more closely share the miRNA pattern associated with the pattern observed in plasma-derived exosomes from sporadic malignant melanoma patients; and (4) the metastatic patients may have had circulating tumor cells which contributed and further amplified the differences seen in exosomes, and tumor exosomes are different from those that might be associated with genetic predisposition to melanoma. Our findings are consistent with the occurrence of miRNA dysregulation in metastatic melanoma. Therefore, this technology might be better suited for detecting recurrent metastatic melanoma following therapeutic intervention.

Taken together, our results show that we have been able to identify several circulating miRNAs that are up-regulated in plasma-derived exosomes from patients with sporadic metastatic melanoma. While the increased expression of these unique miRNAs in the plasma-derived exosomes may be due, in part, to the occurrence of tumor cells in the circulation, these circulating miRNAs have prognostic potential in patients with metastatic melanoma. Future studies should be directed at discerning the role of these individual miRNAs in melanoma progression and metastasis, particularly in response to therapy.

## 4. Materials and Methods

### 4.1. Plasma

Archived citrate-treated plasma samples from 8 individuals with CDKN2A/p16 mutations with a history of melanoma, 5 individuals with CDKN2A/p16 mutations with no history of melanoma, 13 spouse controls and 10 patients with metastatic melanoma were obtained from the Huntsman

Cancer Institute of the University of Utah. All subjects gave their informed consent for inclusion before they participated in the study. The study was conducted in accordance with the Declaration of Helsinki, and the protocol was approved by the Ethics Committee of the University of Utah (7916-00). General clinical patient information is shown in Table 1.

### 4.2. Preparation of Plasma-Derived Exosomes and Isolation of RNA

Following a protocol previously established in our group [8], citrate-treated plasma was incubated at 37 °C for 15 min with Thromboplastin-D to remove clotting factors, and centrifuged (8000× $g$ for 15 min at 22 °C). The resultant supernatant (1.2 mL) was mixed by inversion with 140 µL of ExoQuick solution (System Biosciences, Mountain View, CA, USA) overnight at 4 °C. The ExoQuick/plasma mixture was centrifuged (1500× $g$ for 15 min at 22 °C), and the exosomal pellet was washed twice with PBS. The exosomal pellet was resuspended in 700 µL of Qiazol (containing 0.05 fmol/mL of Cel39 for miRNA normalization) and incubated for 5 min at 22 °C. The RNA was extracted by addition of 140 µL of chloroform by incubating for 5 min at RT. After centrifugation at 12,000× $g$ for 15 min at 4 °C, 280 µL of the upper aqueous phase was transferred to a new tube, mixed with 420 µL of 100% ethanol and loaded on a miRNeasy MinElute spin column. After centrifugation at 8000× $g$ for 15 s at 22 °C, the column was washed three times with RNeasy buffer RWT followed by centrifugation. The RNA was concentrated to a final volume of 20 µL with RNase-free water with an Amicon Ultra YM-3 filter by centrifugation at 14,000× $g$ at 22 °C for 45 min.

### 4.3. miRNA Expression Profiling

Microarray analysis on RNA prepared from plasma-derived exosomes was performed using the human V1 miRNA assay kit (NanoString Technologies, Seattle, WA, USA) that contains ~700 human miRNAs. The integrity and quantity of the RNA was assessed using the Agilent 2100 Bioanalyzer and RNA 6000 Pico Kit (Agilent Technologies, Santa Clara, CA, USA). In brief, total RNA was mixed with pairs of capture and reporter probes, hybridized on the nCounter Prep Station, and purified complexes were quantified on the nCounter digital analyzer. To account for differences in hybridization and purification, data were normalized to the average counts for all control spikes in each sample and analyzed with nSolver software.

### 4.4. miRNA Expression Using SYBR Green Real Time PCR

PolyA-tailed total RNA was prepared from plasma-derived exosomes using (polyA) polymerase (NEB; Ipswich, MA, USA) at 37 °C for 1 h as previously described [46]. The final reaction mixture was extracted with phenol/chloroform, precipitated with isopropanol, redissolved in diethylpyrocarbonate (DEPC)-treated water, and was reverse-transcribed into first-strand cDNA using Superscript III transcriptase (Invitrogen) with the oligo-dT adapter primer 5′GCGAGCACAGAATTAATACGACTCACTATAGGTTTTTTTTTTTTTVN3′. For PCR, 40 ng of cDNA was used as a template in each reaction. The reverse primer was from the adapter sequence: 5′GCGAGCACAGAATTAATACGACTCAC3′ and the forward primers were specific to miRNA mature sequences (shown in Table 2). The SYBR Green-based real-time PCR was performed to quantify miRNA expression, and Cel39 was used to normalize miRNA expression. The expression data was normalized to the expression of the spiked in C. elegans miRNA (Cel39) as a normalizing control as previously described [20].

### 4.5. TCGA Data Query

To examine the relationship between miR-17, miR-19a, miR-21, miR-126 and miR-149 expression in human cancer specimens from cutaneous melanoma, we queried the TCGA data portal [54] for all samples with Level 3 miRNA expression data available, as well as the accompanying clinical data. The data set was filtered for samples having expression data for these selected miRNAs and clinical data, yielding a final set of 216 melanoma independent patient samples.

## 4.6. Statistical Analysis

At least two independent PCR experiments were performed in triplicate, and data are presented as means ± sd. ANOVA and post-hoc least significant difference analysis or Student *t* tests were performed using Graphpad InStat 3 software, with *p*-values < 0.05 considered statistically significant.

**Acknowledgments:** This work was supported by National Cancer Institute HHSN261200433000C and by funds from the Muirhead Chair Endowment at the University of Tennessee Health Science Center. We thank John F. Quackenbush for his assistance in preparing plasma-derived exosomes and in the initial miRNA analysis.

**Author Contributions:** Kenneth F. Grossmann, Levy Kopelovich, Sancy A. Leachman and Lawrence M. Pfeffer conceived and designed the experiments; Susan R. Pfeffer and Chuan He Yang performed the experiments; Susan R. Pfeffer, Kenneth F. Grossmann, Meiyun Fan, Pamela B. Cassidy, Chuan He Yang, Sancy A. Leachman and Lawrence M. Pfeffer analyzed the data; Chuan He Yang, Kenneth F. Grossmann, Meiyun Fan, Pamela B. Cassidy, Sancy A. Leachman and Lawrence M. Pfeffer contributed reagents/materials/analysis tools; Susan R. Pfeffer, Levy Kopelovich, Sancy A. Leachman and Lawrence M. Pfeffer wrote the paper.

## References

1. Vasudevan, S.; Tong, Y.; Steitz, J.A. Switching from repression to activation: MicroRNAs can up-regulate translation. *Science* **2007**, *318*, 1931–1934. [CrossRef] [PubMed]
2. Bartel, D.P. MicroRNAs: Genomics, biogenesis, mechanism, and function. *Cell* **2004**, *116*, 281–297. [CrossRef]
3. Cho, W.C. Oncomirs: The discovery and progress of microRNAs in cancers. *Mol. Cancer* **2007**, *6*, 60. [CrossRef] [PubMed]
4. Rabinowits, G.; Gercel-Taylor, C.; Day, J.M.; Taylor, D.D.; Kloecker, G.H. Exosomal microRNA: A diagnostic marker for lung cancer. *Clin. Lung Cancer* **2009**, *10*, 42–46. [CrossRef] [PubMed]
5. Thery, C.; Ostrowski, M.; Segura, E. Membrane vesicles as conveyors of immune responses. *Nat. Rev. Immunol.* **2009**, *9*, 581–593. [CrossRef] [PubMed]
6. Pegtel, D.M.; Cosmopoulos, K.; Thorley-Lawson, D.A.; van Eijndhoven, M.A.; Hopmans, E.S.; Lindenberg, J.L.; de Gruijl, T.D.; Wurdinger, T.; Middeldorp, J.M. Functional delivery of viral miRNAs via exosomes. *Proc. Natl. Acad. Sci. USA* **2010**, *107*, 6328–6333. [CrossRef] [PubMed]
7. Kottel, R.H.; Hoch, S.O.; Parsons, R.G.; Hoch, J.A. Serum ribonuclease activity in cancer patients. *Br. J. Cancer* **1978**, *38*, 280–286. [CrossRef] [PubMed]
8. Quackenbush, J.F.; Cassidy, P.B.; Pfeffer, L.M.; Boucher, K.M.; Hawkes, J.E.; Pfeffer, S.R.; Kopelovich, L.; Leachman, S.A. Isolation of circulating microRNAs from microvesicles found in human plasma. *Methods Mol. Biol.* **2014**, *1102*, 641–653. [PubMed]
9. Siegel, R.; Naishadham, D.; Jemal, A. Cancer statistics, 2012. *CA Cancer J. Clin.* **2012**, *62*, 10–29. [CrossRef] [PubMed]
10. Aoude, L.G.; Wadt, K.A.; Pritchard, A.L.; Hayward, N.K. Genetics of familial melanoma: 20 years after CDKN2A. *Pigment Cell Melanoma Res.* **2015**, *28*, 148–160. [CrossRef] [PubMed]
11. Eliason, M.J.; Larson, A.A.; Florell, S.R.; Zone, J.J.; Cannon-Albright, L.A.; Samlowski, W.E.; Leachman, S.A. Population-based prevalence of CDKN2A mutations in Utah melanoma families. *J. Investig. Dermatol.* **2006**, *126*, 660–666. [CrossRef] [PubMed]
12. Goldstein, A.M.; Chan, M.; Harland, M.; Hayward, N.K.; Demenais, F.; Bishop, D.T.; Azizi, E.; Bergman, W.; Bianchi-Scarra, G.; Bruno, W.; *et al.* Features associated with germline CDKN2A mutations: A genomel study of melanoma-prone families from three continents. *J. Med. Genet.* **2007**, *44*, 99–106. [CrossRef] [PubMed]
13. Hodis, E.; Watson, I.R.; Kryukov, G.V.; Arold, S.T.; Imielinski, M.; Theurillat, J.P.; Nickerson, E.; Auclair, D.; Li, L.; Place, C.; *et al.* A landscape of driver mutations in melanoma. *Cell* **2012**, *150*, 251–263. [CrossRef] [PubMed]
14. Stott, F.J.; Bates, S.; James, M.C.; McConnell, B.B.; Starborg, M.; Brookes, S.; Palmero, I.; Ryan, K.; Hara, E.; Vousden, K.H.; *et al.* The alternative product from the human CDKN2A locus, p14(ARF), participates in a regulatory feedback loop with p53 and MDM2. *EMBO J.* **1998**, *17*, 5001–5014. [CrossRef] [PubMed]

15. Bishop, D.T.; Demenais, F.; Goldstein, A.M.; Bergman, W.; Bishop, J.N.; de Paillerets, B.; Chompret, A.; Ghiorzo, P.; Gruis, N.; Hansson, J.; *et al.* Geographical variation in the penetrance of CDKN2A mutations for melanoma. *J. Natl. Cancer Inst.* **2002**, *94*, 894–903. [CrossRef] [PubMed]

16. Fan, M.; Pfeffer, S.R.; Lynch, H.T.; Cassidy, P.; Leachman, S.; Pfeffer, L.M.; Kopelovich, L. Altered transcriptome signature of phenotypically normal skin fibroblasts heterozygous for CDKN2A in familial melanoma: Relevance to early intervention. *Oncotarget* **2013**, *4*, 128–141. [CrossRef] [PubMed]

17. Caramuta, S.; Egyhazi, S.; Rodolfo, M.; Witten, D.; Hansson, J.; Larsson, C.; Lui, W.O. MicroRNA expression profiles associated with mutational status and survival in malignant melanoma. *J. Investig. Dermatol.* **2010**, *130*, 2062–2070. [CrossRef] [PubMed]

18. Glud, M.; Klausen, M.; Gniadecki, R.; Rossing, M.; Hastrup, N.; Nielsen, F.C.; Drzewiecki, K.T. MicroRNA expression in melanocytic nevi: The usefulness of formalin-fixed, paraffin-embedded material for miRNA microarray profiling. *J. Investig. Dermatol.* **2009**, *129*, 1219–1224. [CrossRef] [PubMed]

19. Segura, M.F.; Belitskaya-Levy, I.; Rose, A.E.; Zakrzewski, J.; Gaziel, A.; Hanniford, D.; Darvishian, F.; Berman, R.S.; Shapiro, R.L.; Pavlick, A.C.; *et al.* Melanoma microRNA signature predicts post-recurrence survival. *Clin. Cancer Res.* **2010**, *16*, 1577–1586. [CrossRef] [PubMed]

20. Mitchell, P.S.; Parkin, R.K.; Kroh, E.M.; Fritz, B.R.; Wyman, S.K.; Pogosova-Agadjanyan, E.L.; Peterson, A.; Noteboom, J.; O'Briant, K.C.; Allen, A.; *et al.* Circulating microRNAs as stable blood-based markers for cancer detection. *Proc. Natl. Acad. Sci USA* **2008**, *105*, 10513–10518. [CrossRef] [PubMed]

21. Talantov, D.; Mazumder, A.; Yu, J.X.; Briggs, T.; Jiang, Y.; Backus, J.; Atkins, D.; Wang, Y. Novel genes associated with malignant melanoma but not benign melanocytic lesions. *Clin. Cancer Res.* **2005**, *11*, 7234–7242. [CrossRef] [PubMed]

22. Smith, A.P.; Hoek, K.; Becker, D. Whole-genome expression profiling of the melanoma progression pathway reveals marked molecular differences between nevi/melanoma *in situ* and advanced-stage melanomas. *Cancer Biol. Ther.* **2005**, *4*, 1018–1029. [CrossRef] [PubMed]

23. Jaeger, J.; Koczan, D.; Thiesen, H.J.; Ibrahim, S.M.; Gross, G.; Spang, R.; Kunz, M. Gene expression signatures for tumor progression, tumor subtype, and tumor thickness in laser-microdissected melanoma tissues. *Clin. Cancer Res.* **2007**, *13*, 806–815. [CrossRef] [PubMed]

24. Molecular Signatures Database v5.0. Available online: http://software.broadinstitute.org/gsea/index.jsp (accessed on 30 June 2015).

25. Subramanian, A.; Tamayo, P.; Mootha, V.K.; Mukherjee, S.; Ebert, B.L.; Gillette, M.A.; Paulovich, A.; Pomeroy, S.L.; Golub, T.R.; Lander, E.S.; *et al.* Gene set enrichment analysis: A knowledge-based approach for interpreting genome-wide expression profiles. *Proc. Natl. Acad. Sci. USA* **2005**, *102*, 15545–15550. [CrossRef] [PubMed]

26. Lim, L.P.; Lau, N.C.; Garrett-Engele, P.; Grimson, A.; Schelter, J.M.; Castle, J.; Bartel, D.P.; Linsley, P.S.; Johnson, J.M. Microarray analysis shows that some microRNAs downregulate large numbers of target mRNAs. *Nature* **2005**, *433*, 769–773. [CrossRef] [PubMed]

27. Reid, G.; Kirschner, M.B.; van Zandwijk, N. Circulating microRNAs: Association with disease and potential use as biomarkers. *Crit. Rev. Oncol. Hematol.* **2011**, *80*, 193–208. [CrossRef] [PubMed]

28. Friedman, E.B.; Shang, S.; de Miera, E.; Fog, J.U.; Teilum, M.W.; Ma, M.W.; Berman, R.S.; Shapiro, R.L.; Pavlick, A.C.; Hernando, E.; *et al.* Serum microRNAs as biomarkers for recurrence in melanoma. *J. Trans. Med.* **2012**, *10*, 155. [CrossRef] [PubMed]

29. Kanemaru, H.; Fukushima, S.; Yamashita, J.; Honda, N.; Oyama, R.; Kakimoto, A.; Masuguchi, S.; Ishihara, T.; Inoue, Y.; Jinnin, M.; *et al.* The circulating microRNA-221 level in patients with malignant melanoma as a new tumor marker. *J. Dermatol. Sci.* **2011**, *61*, 187–193. [CrossRef] [PubMed]

30. Greenberg, E.; Hershkovitz, L.; Itzhaki, O.; Hajdu, S.; Nemlich, Y.; Ortenberg, R.; Gefen, N.; Edry, L.; Modai, S.; Keisari, Y.; *et al.* Regulation of cancer aggressive features in melanoma cells by microRNAs. *PLoS ONE* **2011**, *6*, e18936. [CrossRef] [PubMed]

31. Wong, P.; Iwasaki, M.; Somervaille, T.C.; Ficara, F.; Carico, C.; Arnold, C.; Chen, C.Z.; Cleary, M.L. The miR-17-92 microRNA polycistron regulates MLL leukemia stem cell potential by modulating p21 expression. *Cancer Res.* **2010**, *70*, 3833–3842. [CrossRef] [PubMed]

32. Rao, E.; Jiang, C.; Ji, M.; Huang, X.; Iqbal, J.; Lenz, G.; Wright, G.; Staudt, L.M.; Zhao, Y.; McKeithan, T.W.; *et al.* The miRNA-17 approximately 92 cluster mediates chemoresistance and enhances tumor growth in mantle cell lymphoma via pi3k/akt pathway activation. *Leukemia* **2012**, *26*, 1064–1072. [CrossRef] [PubMed]

33. Hayashita, Y.; Osada, H.; Tatematsu, Y.; Yamada, H.; Yanagisawa, K.; Tomida, S.; Yatabe, Y.; Kawahara, K.; Sekido, Y.; Takahashi, T. A polycistronic microRNA cluster, miR-17-92, is overexpressed in human lung cancers and enhances cell proliferation. *Cancer Res.* **2005**, *65*, 9628–9632. [CrossRef] [PubMed]

34. Ebi, H.; Sato, T.; Sugito, N.; Hosono, Y.; Yatabe, Y.; Matsuyama, Y.; Yamaguchi, T.; Osada, H.; Suzuki, M.; Takahashi, T. Counterbalance between rb inactivation and miR-17-92 overexpression in reactive oxygen species and DNA damage induction in lung cancers. *Oncogene* **2009**, *28*, 3371–3379. [CrossRef] [PubMed]

35. Levy, C.; Khaled, M.; Iliopoulos, D.; Janas, M.M.; Schubert, S.; Pinner, S.; Chen, P.H.; Li, S.; Fletcher, A.L.; Yokoyama, S.; *et al.* Intronic miR-211 assumes the tumor suppressive function of its host gene in melanoma. *Mol. Cell* **2010**, *40*, 841–849. [CrossRef] [PubMed]

36. Wu, Q.; Yang, Z.; An, Y.; Hu, H.; Yin, J.; Zhang, P.; Nie, Y.; Wu, K.; Shi, Y.; Fan, D. MiR-19a/b modulate the metastasis of gastric cancer cells by targeting the tumour suppressor MXD1. *Cell Death Dis.* **2014**, *5*, e1144. [CrossRef] [PubMed]

37. Lepore, I.; Dell'Aversana, C.; Pilyugin, M.; Conte, M.; Nebbioso, A.; de Bellis, F.; Tambaro, F.P.; Izzo, T.; Garcia-Manero, G.; Ferrara, F.; *et al.* HDAC inhibitors repress BARD1 isoform expression in acute myeloid leukemia cells via activation of miR-19a and/or b. *PLoS ONE* **2013**, *8*, e83018. [CrossRef] [PubMed]

38. Si, M.L.; Zhu, S.; Wu, H.; Lu, Z.; Wu, F.; Mo, Y.Y. MiR-21-mediated tumor growth. *Oncogene* **2007**, *26*, 2799–2803. [CrossRef] [PubMed]

39. Volinia, S.; Calin, G.A.; Liu, C.G.; Ambs, S.; Cimmino, A.; Petrocca, F.; Visone, R.; Iorio, M.; Roldo, C.; Ferracin, M.; *et al.* A microRNA expression signature of human solid tumors defines cancer gene targets. *Proc. Natl. Acad. Sci. USA* **2006**, *103*, 2257–2261. [CrossRef] [PubMed]

40. Folini, M.; Gandellini, P.; Longoni, N.; Profumo, V.; Callari, M.; Pennati, M.; Colecchia, M.; Supino, R.; Veneroni, S.; Salvioni, R.; *et al.* miR-21: An oncomir on strike in prostate cancer. *Mol. Cancer* **2010**, *9*, 12. [CrossRef] [PubMed]

41. Loffler, D.; Brocke-Heidrich, K.; Pfeifer, G.; Stocsits, C.; Hackermuller, J.; Kretzschmar, A.K.; Burger, R.; Gramatzki, M.; Blumert, C.; Bauer, K.; *et al.* Interleukin-6 dependent survival of multiple myeloma cells involves the stat3-mediated induction of microRNA-21 through a highly conserved enhancer. *Blood* **2007**, *110*, 1330–1333. [CrossRef] [PubMed]

42. Chan, J.A.; Krichevsky, A.M.; Kosik, K.S. MicroRNA-21 is an antiapoptotic factor in human glioblastoma cells. *Cancer Res.* **2005**, *65*, 6029–6033. [CrossRef] [PubMed]

43. Zhu, S.; Wu, H.; Wu, F.; Nie, D.; Sheng, S.; Mo, Y.Y. MicroRNA-21 targets tumor suppressor genes in invasion and metastasis. *Cell Res.* **2008**, *18*, 350–359. [CrossRef] [PubMed]

44. Wang, P.; Zou, F.; Zhang, X.; Li, H.; Dulak, A.; Tomko, R.J., Jr.; Lazo, J.S.; Wang, Z.; Zhang, L.; Yu, J. MicroRNA-21 negatively regulates Cdc25A and cell cycle progression in colon cancer cells. *Cancer Res.* **2009**, *69*, 8157–8165. [CrossRef] [PubMed]

45. Sheedy, F.J. Turning 21: Induction of miR-21 as a key switch in the inflammatory response. *Front. Immunol.* **2015**, *6*, 19. [CrossRef] [PubMed]

46. Yang, C.H.; Yue, J.; Fan, M.; Pfeffer, L.M. IFN induces miR-21 through a signal transducer and activator of transcription 3-dependent pathway as a suppressive negative feedback on IFN-induced apoptosis. *Cancer Res.* **2010**, *70*, 8108–8116. [CrossRef] [PubMed]

47. Yang, C.H.; Yue, J.; Pfeffer, S.R.; Handorf, C.R.; Pfeffer, L.M. MicroRNA miR-21 regulates the metastatic behavior of b16 melanoma cells. *J. Biol. Chem.* **2011**, *286*, 39172–39178. [CrossRef] [PubMed]

48. Jiang, L.; Lv, X.; Li, J.; Li, J.; Li, X.; Li, W.; Li, Y. The status of microRNA-21 expression and its clinical significance in human cutaneous malignant melanoma. *Acta Histochem.* **2012**, *114*, 582–588. [CrossRef] [PubMed]

49. Felli, N.; Felicetti, F.; Lustri, A.M.; Errico, M.C.; Bottero, L.; Cannistraci, A.; de Feo, A.; Petrini, M.; Pedini, F.; Biffoni, M.; *et al.* miR-126&126* restored expressions play a tumor suppressor role by directly regulating ADAM9 and MMP7 in melanoma. *PLoS ONE* **2013**, *8*, e56824. [CrossRef] [PubMed]

50. Jin, L.; Hu, W.L.; Jiang, C.C.; Wang, J.X.; Han, C.C.; Chu, P.; Zhang, L.J.; Thorne, R.F.; Wilmott, J.; Scolyer, R.A.; *et al.* MicroRNA-149*, a p53-responsive microRNA, functions as an oncogenic regulator in human melanoma. *Proc. Natl. Acad. Sci. USA* **2011**, *108*, 15840–15845. [CrossRef] [PubMed]

51. Sauroja, I.; Smeds, J.; Vlaykova, T.; Kumar, R.; Talve, L.; Hahka-Kemppinen, M.; Punnonen, K.; Jansen, C.T.; Hemminki, K.; Pyrhonen, S. Analysis of G(1)/S checkpoint regulators in metastatic melanoma. *Genes Chromosomes Cancer* **2000**, *28*, 404–414. [CrossRef]

52. Perrot, C.Y.; Javelaud, D.; Mauviel, A. Insights into the transforming growth factor-beta signaling pathway in cutaneous melanoma. *Ann. Dermatol.* **2013**, *25*, 135–144. [CrossRef] [PubMed]
53. Lynch, H.T.; Fusaro, R.M.; Lynch, J.F.; Brand, R. Pancreatic cancer and the fammm syndrome. *Fam. Cancer* **2008**, *7*, 103–112. [CrossRef] [PubMed]
54. TCGA Data Portal. Available online: https://tcga-data.nci.nih.gov/tcga/tcgaHome2.jsp (accessed on 23 July 2015).

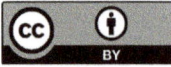

Journal of
*Clinical Medicine*

MDPI

*Article*

# MicroRNA Library-Based Functional Screening Identified Androgen-Sensitive miR-216a as a Player in Bicalutamide Resistance in Prostate Cancer

Toshiaki Miyazaki [1], Kazuhiro Ikeda [1], Wataru Sato [1], Kuniko Horie-Inoue [1], Koji Okamoto [2] and Satoshi Inoue [1,3,4,]*

[1] Division of Gene Regulation and Signal Transduction, Research Center for Genomic Medicine, Saitama Medical University, 1397-1 Yamane, Hidaka-shi, Saitama 350-1241, Japan; tmiyaza@saitama-med.ac.jp (T.M.); ikeda@saitama-med.ac.jp (K.I.); wsatou@saitama-med.ac.jp (W.S.); khorie07@saitama-med.ac.jp (K.H.-I.)

[2] Division of Cancer Differentiation, National Cancer Center Research Institute, 5-1-1 Tsukiji, Chuo-ku, Tokyo 104-0045, Japan; kojokamo@ncc.go.jp

[3] Department of Geriatric Medicine, Graduate School of Medicine, The University of Tokyo, 7-3-1 Hongo, Bunkyo-ku, Tokyo 113-8655, Japan

[4] Department of Anti-Aging Medicine, Graduate School of Medicine, The University of Tokyo, 7-3-1 Hongo, Bunkyo-ku, Tokyo 113-8655, Japan

* Author to whom correspondence should be addressed; sinoue07@saitama-med.ac.jp or INOUE-GER@h.u-tokyo.ac.jp; Tel.: +81-42-984-4606; Fax: +81-42-984-4541.

Academic Editors: Takahiro Ochiya and Ryou-u Takahashi

Received: 30 June 2015; Accepted: 10 October 2015; Published: 20 October 2015

**Abstract:** Prostate cancer is a major hormone-dependent tumor affecting men, and is often treated by hormone therapy at the primary stages. Despite its initial efficiency, the disease eventually acquires resistance, resulting in the recurrence of castration-resistant prostate cancer. Recent studies suggest that dysregulation of microRNA (miRNA) function is one of the mechanisms underlying hormone therapy resistance. Identification of critical miRNAs involved in endocrine resistance will therefore be important for developing therapeutic targets for prostate cancer. In the present study, we performed an miRNA library screening to identify anti-androgen bicalutamide resistance-related miRNAs in prostate cancer LNCaP cells. Cells were infected with a lentiviral miRNA library and subsequently maintained in media containing either bicalutamide or vehicle for a month. Microarray analysis determined the amounts of individual miRNA precursors and identified 2 retained miRNAs after one-month bicalutamide treatment. Of these, we further characterized miR-216a, because its function in prostate cancer remains unknown. miR-216a could be induced by dihydrotestosterone in LNCaP cells and ectopic expression of miR-216a inhibited bicalutamide-mediated growth suppression of LNCaP cells. Furthermore, a microarray dataset revealed that the expression levels of miR-216a were significantly higher in clinical prostate cancer than in benign samples. These results suggest that functional screening using an miRNA expression library could be useful for identifying novel miRNAs that contribute to bicalutamide resistance in prostate cancer.

**Keywords:** microRNA; hormone therapy resistance; androgen; prostate cancer

## 1. Introduction

Prostate cancer is the second most common cancer among men worldwide and the incidence of prostate cancer has been increasing in Japan. Because the growth of prostate cancer is primarily regulated by androgen signaling, androgen deprivation therapy is often performed as prostate cancer treatment. The hormone therapy is initially effective for inhibiting the growth of prostate cancer by suppressing androgen receptor (AR) activity. Nevertheless, patients eventually acquire resistance to

*J. Clin. Med.* **2015**, *4*, 1853–1865

hormonal therapy during long-term treatment, and develop an advanced form of the disease, termed castration-resistant prostate cancer (CRPC) [1–3]. Patients with CRPC have a poor prognosis and account for the majority of deaths due to the disease.

Interestingly, recent studies have shown that AR signaling regulates prostate cancer growth even under the condition of androgen deprivation in CRPC. CRPC is commonly associated with increased AR signaling due to AR overexpression, AR mutation, transcription cofactor activation, AR phosphorylation, and other processes [4–8]. Indeed, overexpression of AR mRNA or protein is found in most cases of CRPC [6–8]. These findings suggest that AR plays a critical role in the development and progression of prostate cancer at both primary and CRPC stages [9–13]. However, the precise molecular mechanisms underlying the resistance to endocrine therapy and recurrence in CRPC remain to be studied, in terms of its key regulators and signaling events. As one of the new transcriptional regulators involved in cancer biology, the dysregulation of microRNAs (miRNAs) has been paid attention to various disease states including tumor progression, metastasis, and angiogenesis [14–16]. miRNAs function as transcriptional modulators by binding to complementary sequences in the 3'-untranslated region of their target mRNAs [17].

In the present study, we performed lentiviral miRNA library screening to identify novel miRNAs modulating the response to the anti-androgen bicalutamide in human prostate cancer LNCaP cells. By comparing the integrated miRNAs in the genomes of cells treated with bicalutamide and vehicle for one-month, two retained miRNAs were selected based on the fold change values of array signal intensities (by >5-fold). We focused on miR-216a, one of the retained miRNAs in the bicalutamide-treated cells, and examined its effect on the growth of LNCaP cells. Overexpression of miR-216a inhibited bicalutamide-mediated growth suppression of LNCaP cells. We found that miR-216a was overexpressed in long-term androgen-deprived bicalutamide-resistant LNCaP (LTAD-BicR) cells compared with parental LNCaP cells. Moreover, clinical prostate cancer samples showed higher levels of miR-216a expression than benign samples. These results show that miRNA library-based functional screening is useful for identification of novel miRNAs that are critical for bicalutamide responses in prostate cancer. These miRNAs could be applied for the development of alternative options for the diagnosis and treatment of prostate cancer.

## 2. Results

### 2.1. Screening for miRNAs Affecting Bicalutamide Responses in Prostate Cancer LNCaP Cells

To identify miRNAs involved in the bicalutamide responses in LNCaP cells, we performed functional screening with a lentiviral library comprising 445 miRNA precursors. LNCaP cells were infected with the library at different multiplicities of infection, and cell populations showing 30%–40% infection efficiency were selected, screened, and continuously cultured for one month in the presence of 1 or 10 μM bicalutamide or vehicle (Figure 1A). At the end of the cultivation period, genomic DNA was extracted from the surviving cells. The miRNAs that had integrated into the genome were amplified by PCR, using specific primers against the common sequences that flanked each miRNA, and then quantified by custom-made microarrays using the two-color of Cy-3 and Cy-5 fluorescent probe hybridization system. The array signal plots comparing the 2 control samples were linearly distributed along a diagonal line (Figure 1B), indicating that the biological duplicates exhibited high reproducibility. In contrast, plots comparing the bicalutamide-treated samples with the control samples were widely distributed. The upper left- or lower right-positioned plots separated by the diagonal line corresponding to the ectopic miRNAs that were retained or dropped out after one-month bicalutamide treatment, respectively (Figure 1C, 10 μM bicalutamide Sample 1 *versus* Control 1; Figure 1D, 1 μM bicalutamide Sample 2 *versus* Control 2; Figure 1E, 1 μM bicalutamide Sample 3 *versus* Control 3). Based on fold changes and *p* values (>5-fold at a threshold of *p* < 0.01), we identified two retained miRNAs that were upregulated in bicalutamide-treated cells (Table 1). The distribution of the retained miRNAs can be visualized by volcano plotting using averaged values for fold change and inverse $p$ value as $x$- and $y$-axes, respectively (Figure 2).

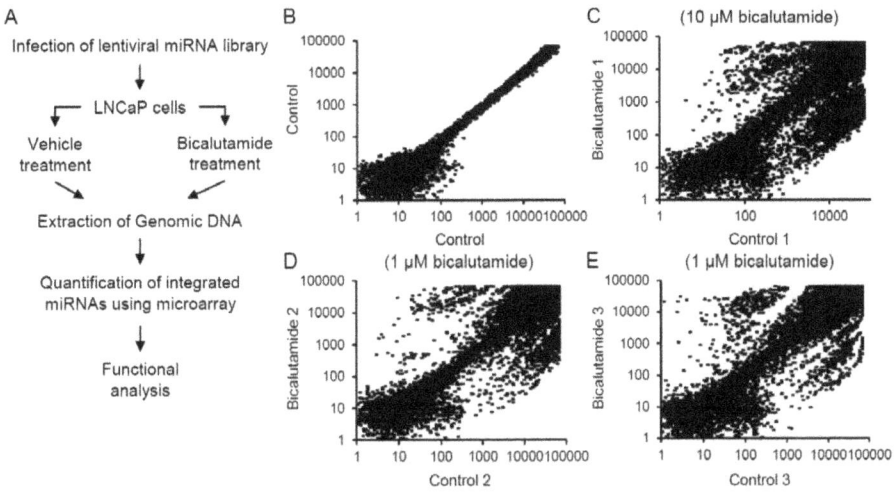

**Figure 1.** Screening of miRNAs associated with bicalutamide responses in LNCaP cells. (**A**) Schematic representation of screening procedure using a lentiviral miRNA library to identify mediators of the bicalutamide responses in human prostate cancer LNCaP cells. In brief, cells were infected with a lentiviral miRNA library and further cultured in regular media containing normal FBS with or without anti-androgen bicalutamide. Amounts of miRNAs integrated in the genomic DNAs of surviving cells were quantified by microarray; (**B**) Validation of miRNA screening reproducibility using two controls experiment is shown; (**C–E**) Scatter plots of array signal intensities for individual miRNAs for three groups of bicalutamide-treated and vehicle-treated samples ((**C**) 10 µM bicalutamide Sample 1 *versus* Control 1; (**D**) 1 µM bicalutamide Sample 2 *versus* Control 2; (**E**) 1 µM bicalutamide Sample 3 *versus* Control 3).

**Table 1.** Retained miRNAs after bicalutamide treatment.

| miRNA | Control [a] | Bicalutamide [b] | Bicalutamide/Control | $p$ Value |
|---|---|---|---|---|
| miR-345 | 4737.4 ± 4127.3 | 32086.3 ± 4257.2 | 6.77 | 0.0013 |
| miR-216a | 7534.2 ± 7345.9 | 40038.2 ± 8824 | 5.31 | 0.0087 |

[a] Averaged signal intensity of miRNA in the vehicle-treated control cells was quantified by microarray. The results are shown as mean ± S.D. [b] Averaged signal intensity of miRNA in the bicalutamide-treated cells was quantified by microarray. The results are shown as mean ± S.D.

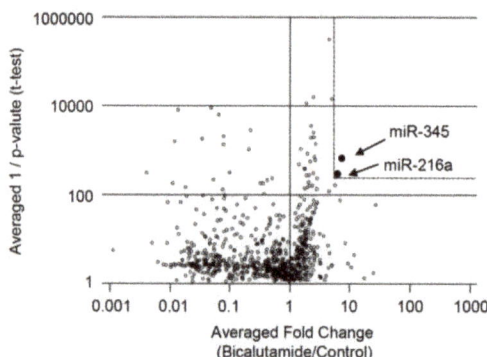

**Figure 2.** Volcano plot shows comparative analysis of miRNA microarray of the averaged three groups of the bicalutamide-treated cells and vehicle-treated cells. Volcano plot of microarray data generated by clustering based on probes that were retained (fold change >5; $p < 0.01$) in the averaged three groups of the bicalutamide-treated cells compared to vehicle-treated cells (Control). Closed circles represent selected miRNAs in this study.

## 2.2. miR-216a is Androgen-inducible and Overexpression of miR-216a Inhibits Bicalutamide-dependent Suppression of LNCaP Cell Growth

Alteration of miRNA expression may account for the change of bicalutamide resistance or sensitivity in LNCaP cells by modulating their target gene expression. Overexpressed miRNAs in cancers that promote oncogenesis are known as oncomiRs, whereas underexpressed miRNAs act as tumor suppressor miRs [18,19]. In this study, we focused on the retained miRNAs that could silence the expression of tumor suppressor genes. One of the retained miRNAs was miR-345, which has been reported to be associated with drug resistance and markers in cancers including breast and colorectal cancers [20,21]. miR-216a was further investigated because miR-216a is a candidate miRNA regulated by the androgen pathway [22]. We examined endogenous miR-216a expression in LNCaP cells and showed that the miRNA is upregulated by 5α-dihydrotestosterone (DHT) (10 nM) treatment (Figure 3A). To examine whether the miR-216a modulates bicalutamide resistance, LNCaP cells were infected with recombinant lentivirus that expresses the miR-216a precursor and subjected to the cell viability assay using 2-(2-methoxy-4-nitrophenyl)-3-(4-nitrophenyl)-5-(2,4-disulfophenyl)-2H-tetrazolium (WST-8). WST-8 assay revealed that ectopic miR-216a expression blunted the bicalutamide-mediated suppression of LNCaP cell growth, whereas bicalutamide treatment significantly repressed the growth of LNCaP cells infected with a control miRNA (miR-Control) (Figure 3B). Lentiviral transduction of miR-216a precursor elicited substantial ectopic expression of the mature miRNA in the cells at Day 7, as shown by qPCR (Figure 3C).

## 2.3. miR-216a is Upregulated in Bicalutamide-resistant LNCaP Cells and Clinical Prostate Cancer Samples

To determine the endogenous expression levels of the miR-216a, we generated bicalutamide-resistant cells, LTAD-BicR by long-term culture (>3 months) of LNCaP with bicalutamide and phenol red-free medium. Small RNA sequencing using RNAs prepared from LTAD-BicR and parental LNCaP cells showed that the expression levels of miR-216a were significantly upregulated in LTAD-BicR cells, as compared to parental cells (Figure 3D). We next examined the expression levels of miR-216a in clinical samples based on the miRNA sequencing dataset (#SDS144) retrieved from The Cancer Genome Atlas (TCGA) (Figure 3E). We found that the miR-216a expression levels were significantly higher in prostate cancers with Gleason score 8 and 9 compared to normal prostate tissues ($p < 0.05$), and also significantly higher in prostate cancers with Gleason score 8 and 9 compared to those with Gleason score 6 and 7 ($p < 0.05$). Taken together, studies on cultured cancer cells and clinical samples suggest that endogenous miR-216a expression associates with endocrine resistance and progression of prostate cancer.

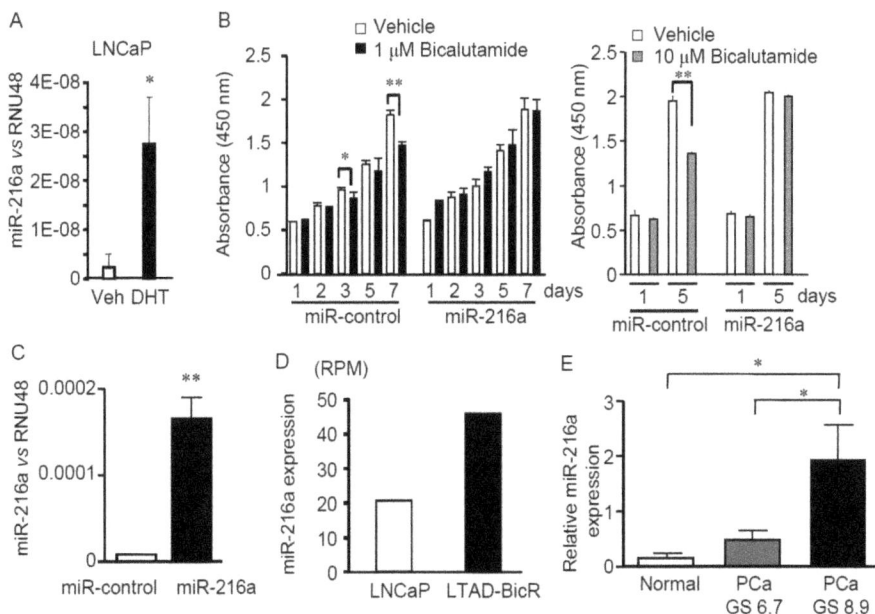

**Figure 3.** Overexpression of miR-216a inhibited bicalutamide-dependent suppression of LNCaP cell growth and upregulation of miR-216a in bicalutamide-resistant LNCaP cells and clinical prostate cancer samples. (**A**) Endogenous miR-216a expression is androgen-inducible in LNCaP cells. Cells maintained in hormone-deprived medium (phenol red-free medium with charcoal stripped FBS) were treated with 5α-dihydrotestosterone (DHT) (10 nM) or vehicle for 48 h and relative expression of mature miR-216a was determined by normalization to RNU48 expression evaluated by qPCR. Statistical analysis was performed using Student's *t*-test. *, $p < 0.05$; (**B**) Overexpression of miR-216a inhibits bicalutamide-dependent suppression of LNCaP cell growth. Cells were infected with miR-216a precursor or miR-control, and then treated with 1 µM bicalutamide or vehicle in regular media with normal FBS. Cell proliferation was examined using WST-8 at indicated time points. The absorbance was read on a microplate reader at a wavelength of 450 nm. The results are shown as mean values ± S.D. ($n$ = 4). Statistical analysis was performed using Student's *t*-test. * $p < 0.05$; ** $p < 0.01$; (**C**) Relative expression of mature miR-216a on Day 7 after lentiviral transduction of miR-216a or miR-control was determined by normalization to RNU48 expression evaluated by qPCR. **, $p < 0.01$. Cells were cultured in regular media with normal FBS; (**D**) Small RNA sequencing using RNAs from LNCaP and LTAD-BicR cells shows that miR-216a expression was significantly upregulated in bicalutamide-resistant LTAD-BicR cells as compared to parental LNCaP cells. LNCaP and LTAD-BicR cells were maintained in regular media with normal FBS and phenol red-free media with charcoal-stripped FBS, respectively. The miRNA expression is quantified in terms of RPM (Reads Per Million) value, which is normalized against total reads in the sample; (**E**) Increased expression levels of miR-216a in advanced prostate cancer samples (Gleason score 8 and 9) compared with normal prostate samples or with lower-grade prostate cancer samples (Gleason score 6 and 7), based on an miRNA sequencing SDS144 dataset in The Cancer Genome Atlas. Relative miR-216a expression levels were calculated from original log2 values in the dataset. Normal prostate tissues, $n$ = 4; prostate cancers with Gleason score 6 and 7, $n$ = 23; and prostate cancers with Gleason score 8 and 9, $n$ = 8. *, $p < 0.05$.

## 3. Discussion

In the present study, we performed a functional screening using a lentiviral miRNA library to identify miRNAs associated with acquired resistance for endocrine therapy in prostate cancer. LNCaP cells infected with the miRNA library were treated with bicalutamide or vehicle for one month, and then the profiles of the genome-integrated miRNAs were compared. We identified two retained miRNAs in the bicalutamide-treated cells compared with the control cells. These miRNAs might be involved in the modulation of bicalutamide resistance in LNCaP cells. We focused on one of the upregulated miRNAs, miR-216a, and found that this miRNA is androgen-inducible. Then, we demonstrated that the overexpression of miR-216a significantly inhibited the bicalutamide-mediated growth suppression of LNCaP cells. We used 1 μM bicalutamide because it was shown that μM order of bicalutamide is a sufficient concentration for repressing the growth of LNCaP cells [23]. Our study showed that miR-216a expression increased in bicalutamide-resistant LNCaP cells, and an miRNA-seq dataset from TCGA also revealed the upregulation of miR-216a in clinical prostate cancer samples at advanced disease stages.

miR-216a is reported as an miRNA that is regulated by the androgen pathway at early stages of hepatocarcinogenesis. Consistently, we showed that miR-216a is an androgen-inducible miRNA as determined by our qPCR analysis. It is also notable that several androgen-dependent AR binding sites are located in the upstream genomic region of miR-216a as shown in the ChIP-on-chip data for prostate cancer [24]. Among them, the nearest AR binding site is located at ~6 kb upstream region of miR-216a and the sequence of the binding site contains at least five consensus androgen response elements analyzed by the JASPER open-access database of transcription factor binding profiles [25]. Thus, miR-216a could be an androgen target miRNA in prostate cancer cells. In addition, miR-216a targets tumor suppressor in lung cancer-1 (*TSLC1*), which modulates cell cycle progression, cell proliferation, and apoptosis [22]. Upregulation of miR-216a has been also reported in diabetic glomerular mesangial cells and this miRNA, together with miR-217, targets PTEN and activates AKT, leading to glomerular mesangial cell survival and hypertrophy [26]. In our screening of miR-216a target genes using several predicting programs (TargetScan, DIANA-microT, miRDB, and miRTarBase), we found that this miRNA could targets PTEN and TGFBR2. As loss of PTEN and TGFBR2 from prostate has been shown to result in castration-resistant cancer with metastases [27], we assume that miR-216a would play a critical role in the modulation of AR signaling and development of endocrine resistance. Future studies are required to clarify the precise role of miR-216a in prostate cancer.

We also identified miR-345 as another retained miRNA. miR-345 was found to be differentially expressed between breast cancer MCF-7 cells and the derivative cisplatin-resistant cells. In this report, miR-345 was demonstrated to target the multidrug resistance-associated protein 1 (MRP1) and suggested to be responsible for development of resistance to anticancer drugs [20]. In addition, miR-345 level in whole blood was a prognostic biomarker for overall survival and progression-free survival of patients with metastatic colorectal cancer treated with cetuximab and irinotecan [21]. These observations suggest that miR-345 may modulate drug resistance and could serve as a prognostic marker in cancers. Thus, miR-345 might be also involved in prostate cancer.

We recently reported of an miRNA library screen to identify miRNAs modulating tamoxifen responses in human breast cancer MCF-7 cells. By comparing miRNA expression in cells treated with 4-hydroxytamoxifen (OHT) to that in vehicle-treated cells, we successfully identified miR-574-3p as a modulating factor for tamoxifen response in breast cancer [28]. Indeed, miR-574-3p has been reported as a tumor suppressor in prostate, bladder, and gastric cancers [29–31]. The present study was also designed to identify miRNAs associated with anti-hormone resistance. We speculate that the results of these studies can provide new information regarding miRNAs that play critical roles in the development of hormone therapy resistance.

In summary, we showed that functional screening based on lentiviral miRNA library is useful for identifying miRNAs involved in bicalutamide resistance in prostate cancer cells. This approach could provide new targets for the diagnosis and treatment of advanced prostate cancer.

## 4. Materials and Methods

### 4.1. Screening of Lentiviral miRNA Library and Microarray Analysis

Experimental concepts of our screen method were based on previous literature [32]. Briefly, a human miRNA precursor lentivirus library that was consisted of a pool of 445 human miRNA precursor clones coexpressing GFP was purchased from System Biosciences (Mountain View, CA, USA). The library was infected to LNCaP cells with at different multiplicities of infection together with 5 mg/mL polybrene. Transduction efficiency was evaluated by GFP expression 48 h after infection using FACS Calibur (Becton Dickinson, CA, USA).

To avoid the possibility of multiple infections, we selected cell populations with 30 to 40% infection efficiency. Cells were continuously cultured in RPMI medium containing 1 or 10 μM bicalutamide or vehicle for 4 weeks. During the culture period, medium was replaced every 2 to 3 days. Then, miRNA precursors integrated into the surviving cells were amplified by PCR using specific primers against the sequences in the lentivirus vector (forward primer: 5'-GCCTGGAGACGCCATCCACGCTG-3'; reverse primer: 5'-GATGTGCGCTCTGCCCACTGAC-3'), in order to amplify miRNA precursor sequences. PCR products from bicalutamide-treated and vehicle-treated LNCaP cells were labeled with Cy-3 or Cy-5, respectively, using the Genome DNA Enzymatic Labeling Kit (Agilent Technologies, Santa Clara, CA, USA) and then subjected to microarray hybridization (Oligo cDGH/ChIP-on-ChIP Hybridization Kit, Agilent Technologies). Agilent Feature Extractor software was used to scan microarray images and to normalize signal intensities. A volcano plot was generated by clustering based on probes. Signals (fold change >5; $p < 0.01$) in the averaged 3 groups of the bicalutamide-treated LNCaP cells compared to vehicle-treated cells were selected as candidate miRNAs potentially involved in the bicalutamide resistance.

### 4.2. Cell Culture and Transduction of miRNA Precursors by Lentiviral Vector

LNCaP prostate cancer cells were purchased from the American Type Culture Collection (Manassas, VA, USA). LNCaP cells were cultured in RPMI supplemented with 10% fetal bovine serum, penicillin (50 U/mL), and streptomycin (50 μg/mL) at 37 °C in a humidified atmosphere containing 5% $CO_2$. Long-term androgen-deprived bicalutamide-treated cells (LTAD-BicR cells) were established from LNCaP cells by long-term (>3 months) treatment with 1 μM bicalutamide in phenol-red free RPMI supplemented with 10% charcoal-dextran-treated fetal bovine serum, penicillin (50 U/mL), and streptomycin (50 μg/mL) at 37 °C in a humidified atmosphere containing 5% $CO_2$. Transduction of miR-216a precursor or control miRNA (Pre-miR™ miRNA Precursor, Life Technologies, CA, USA) into LNCaP cells were carried out by generating virus-containing supernatants as previously reported [32]. Briefly, lentivirus plasmids were co-transfected with pLP1, pLP2, and pLP/VSVG (Invitrogen) into 293FT cells (Invitrogen), and virus containing supernatants were prepared according to manufacturer's instructions. For infection, cells were incubated with virus-containing supernatants in the presence of 6 mg/mL polybrene.

### 4.3. RNA Extraction and High-throughput Sequencing

Total RNAs were isolated from LNCaP and LTAD-BicR cells using the ISOGEN reagent (Nippon Gene, Toyama, Japan) in accordance with the manufacturer's instruction. Small RNA cDNA library was generated from the total RNAs and high-throughput sequencing was performed using an Illumina GAIIx sequencer (Illumina, San Diego, CA, USA) [33]. Mapping of small RNA reads were performed on human genomes (NCBI35 assembly). In quantitative PCR (qPCR) experiments, miRNA levels in LNCaP cells were determined by StepOne Real-time PCR System (Applied Biosystems) using TaqMan microRNA assays (Applied Biosystems, CA, USA). Results from three independent experiments were normalized to the expression of endogenous RNU48. 5α-Dihydrotestosterone (DHT) (Nacalai Tesque, Kyoto, Japan) treatment was performed at 10 nM concentration for 48 h.

*J. Clin. Med.* **2015**, *4*, 1853–1865

*4.4. Cell Growth Assay*

The effects of bicalutamide or miRNAs on cell viability were determined by the WST-8 assay using the Cell Count Reagent SF (NACALAI TESQUE, Kyoto, Japan). LNCaP cells were lentivirally transduced with miR-216a or miR-control and were seeded into 96-well plates at a density of 5000 or 3000 cells per well, and 10 μL of WST-8 solution was added to each well at the indicated time points (24, 48, 72, 120 or 168 h) after transfection. Cells were further incubated for 3 h at 37 °C in a 5% $CO_2$ incubator. The absorbance was measured at 450 nm with Multiscan FC Microplate Photometer (Thermo Fisher Scientific, MA, USA). The results were shown as mean ± S.D. ($n = 4$). Statistical analysis was carried out using Student's *t*-test. *, $p < 0.05$; **, $p < 0.01$.

**Acknowledgments:** The authors thank RIKEN Omics Science Center for sequencing our samples. This work was supported in part by Grants of the Cell Innovation Program, P-DIRECT and "Support Project of Strategic Research Center in Private Universities" from the MEXT, Japan; the Ministry of Health, Labor, and Welfare; the JSPS; the Advanced research for medical products Mining Program of the NIBIO; and the Takeda Science Foundation.

**Author Contributions:** Toshiaki Miyazaki, Kazuhiro Ikeda, and Satoshi Inoue conceived and designed the experiments; Toshiaki Miyazaki, Kazuhiro Ikeda, and Wataru Sato performed the experiments and analyzed the data; Koji Okamoto contributed to reagents/materials/analysis tools; Toshiaki Miyazaki, Kazuhiro Ikeda, Kuniko Horie-Inoue, and Satoshi Inoue wrote the manuscript; and all authors reviewed the manuscript.

**Conflicts of Interest:** The authors declare no conflict of interest.

# References

1.  Debes, J.D.; Tindall, D.J. Mechanism of androgen-refractory prostate cancer. *N. Engl. J. Med.* **2004**, *351*, 1488–1490. [PubMed]
2.  Antonarakis, E.S.; Carducci, M.A.; Eisenberger, M.A. Novel targeted therapeutics for metastatic castration-resistant prostate cancer. *Cancer Lett.* **2010**, *291*, 1–13. [CrossRef] [PubMed]
3.  Chen, Y.; Sawyers, C.L.; Scher, H.I. Targeting the androgen receptor pathway in prostate cancer. *Curr. Opin. Pharmacol.* **2008**, *8*, 440–448. [CrossRef] [PubMed]
4.  Mostaghel, E.A.; Page, S.T.; Lin, D.W.; Fazli, L.; Coleman, I.M.; True, L.D.; Knudsen, B.; Hess, D.L.; Nelson, C.C.; Matsumoto, A.M.; *et al.* Intraprostatic androgens and androgen-regulated gene expression persist after testosterone suppression: Therapeutic implications for castration-resistant prostate cancer. *Cancer Res.* **2007**, *67*, 5033–5041. [CrossRef] [PubMed]
5.  Balk, S.P.; Knudsen, K.E. AR, the cell cycle, and prostate cancer. *Nucl. Recept. Signal.* **2008**, *6*, e001. [CrossRef] [PubMed]
6.  Chen, C.D.; Welsbie, D.S.; Tran, C.; Baek, S.H.; Chen, R.; Vessella, R.; Rosenfeld, M.G.; Sawyers, C.L. Molecular determinants of resistance to antiandrogen therapy. *Nat. Med.* **2004**, *10*, 33–39. [CrossRef] [PubMed]
7.  Feldman, B.J.; Feldman, D. The development of androgen-independent prostate cancer. *Nat. Rev. Cancer* **2001**, *1*, 34–45. [CrossRef] [PubMed]
8.  Gregory, C.W.; He, B.; Johnson, R.T.; Ford, O.H.; Mohler, J.L.; French, F.S.; Wilson, E.M. A mechanism for androgen receptor-mediated prostate cancer recurrence after androgen deprivation therapy. *Cancer Res.* **2001**, *61*, 4315–4319. [PubMed]
9.  Vis, A.N.; Schröder, F.H. Key targets of hormonal treatment of prostate cancer. Part 1: The androgen receptor and steroidogenic pathways. *BJU Int.* **2009**, *104*, 438–448. [CrossRef] [PubMed]
10. Hååg, P.; Bektic, J.; Bartsch, G.; Klocker, H.; Eder, I.E. Androgen receptor down regulation by small interference RNA induces cell growth inhibition in androgen sensitive as well as in androgen independent prostate cancer cells. *J. Steroid Biochem. Mol. Biol.* **2005**, *96*, 251–258. [CrossRef] [PubMed]
11. Yuan, X.; Li, T.; Wang, H.; Zhang, T.; Barua, M.; Borgesi, R.A.; Bubley, G.J.; Lu, M.L.; Balk, S.P. Androgen receptor remains critical for cell-cycle progression in androgen-independent CWR22 prostate cancer cells. *Am. J. Pathol.* **2006**, *169*, 682–696. [CrossRef] [PubMed]
12. Compagno, D.; Merle, C.; Morin, A.; Gilbert, C.; Mathieu, J.R.; Mauduit, C.; Benahmed, M.; Cabon, F. SIRNA-directed *in vivo* silencing of androgen receptor inhibits the growth of castration-resistant prostate carcinomas. *PLoS ONE* **2007**, *2*, e1006. [CrossRef] [PubMed]

13. Gregory, C.W.; Johnson, R.T., Jr.; Mohler, J.L.; French, F.S.; Wilson, E.M. Androgen receptor stabilization in recurrent prostate cancer is associated with hypersensitivity to low androgen. *Cancer Res.* **2001**, *61*, 2892–2898. [PubMed]

14. Iorio, M.V.; Croce, C.M. MicroRNA dysregulation in cancer: Diagnostics, monitoring and therapeutics. A comprehensive review. *EMBO Mol. Med.* **2012**, *4*, 143–159. [CrossRef] [PubMed]

15. Croce, C.M. Causes and consequences of microRNA dysregulation in cancer. *Nat. Rev. Genet.* **2009**, *10*, 704–714. [CrossRef] [PubMed]

16. Dykxhoorn, D.M. MicroRNAs and metastasis: little RNAs go a long way. *Cancer Res.* **2010**, *70*, 6401–6406. [CrossRef] [PubMed]

17. Bartel, D.P. MicroRNAs: Target recognition and regulatory functions. *Cell* **2009**, *136*, 215–233. [CrossRef] [PubMed]

18. Zhang, B.; Pan, X.; Cobb, G.P.; Anderson, T.A. microRNAs as oncogenes and tumor suppressors. *Dev. Biol.* **2007**, *302*, 1–12. [CrossRef] [PubMed]

19. Hata, A.; Lieberman, J. Dysregulation of microRNA biogenesis and gene silencing in cancer. *Sci. Signal.* **2015**, *8*, re3. [CrossRef] [PubMed]

20. Pogribny, I.P.; Filkowski, J.N.; Tryndyak, V.P.; Golubov, A.; Shpyleva, S.I.; Kovalchuk, O. Alterations of microRNAs and their targets are associated with acquired resistance of MCF-7 breast cancer cells to cisplatin. *Int. J. Cancer* **2010**, *127*, 1785–1794. [CrossRef] [PubMed]

21. Schou, J.V.; Rossi, S.; Jensen, B.V.; Nielsen, D.L.; Pfeiffer, P.; Høgdall, E.; Yilmaz, M.; Tejpar, S.; Delorenzi, M.; Kruhøffer, M.; Johansen, J.S. miR-345 in metastatic colorectal cancer: a non-invasive biomarker for clinical outcome in non-KRAS mutant patients treated with 3rd line cetuximab and irinotecan. *PLoS ONE* **2014**, *9*, e99886. [CrossRef] [PubMed]

22. Chen, P.J.; Yeh, S.H.; Liu, W.H.; Lin, C.C.; Huang, H.C.; Chen, C.L.; Chen, D.S.; Chen, P.J. Androgen pathway stimulates microRNA-216a transcription to suppress the tumor suppressor in lung cancer-1 gene in early hepatocarcinogenesis. *Hepatology* **2012**, *56*, 632–643. [CrossRef] [PubMed]

23. Pignatta, S.; Arienti, C.; Zoli, W.; Di Donato, M.; Castoria, G.; Gabucci, E.; Casadio, V.; Falconi, M.; De Giorgi, U.; Silvestrini, R.; *et al.* Prolonged exposure to (*R*)-bicalutamide generates a LNCaP subclone with alteration of mitochondrial genome. *Mol. Cell Endocrinol.* **2014**, *382*, 314–324. [CrossRef] [PubMed]

24. Wang, Q.; Li, W.; Liu, X.S.; Carroll, J.S.; Jänne, O.A.; Keeton, E.K.; Chinnaiyan, A.M.; Pienta, K.J.; Brown, M. A hierarchical network of transcription factors governs androgen receptor-dependent prostate cancer growth. *Mol. Cell* **2007**, *27*, 380–392. [CrossRef] [PubMed]

25. Mathelier, A.; Zhao, X.; Zhang, A.W.; Parcy, F.; Worsley-Hunt, R.; Arenillas, D.J.; Buchman, S.; Chen, C.Y.; Chou, A.; Ienasescu, H.; *et al.* JASPAR 2014: an extensively expanded and updated open-access database of transcription factor binding profiles. *Nucleic Acids Res.* **2014**, *42*, D142–D147. [CrossRef] [PubMed]

26. Kato, M.; Putta, S.; Wang, M.; Yuan, H.; Lanting, L.; Nair, I.; Gunn, A.; Nakagawa, Y.; Shimano, H.; Todorov, I.; *et al.* TGF-beta activates Akt kinase through a microRNA-dependent amplifying circuit targeting PTEN. *Nat. Cell. Biol.* **2009**, *11*, 881–889. [CrossRef] [PubMed]

27. Bjerke, G.A.; Yang, C.S.; Frierson, H.F.; Paschal, B.M.; Wotton, D. Activation of Akt signaling in prostate induces a TGFβ-mediated restraint on cancer progression and metastasis. *Oncogene* **2014**, *33*, 3660–3667. [CrossRef] [PubMed]

28. Ujihira, T.; Ikeda, K.; Suzuki, T.; Yamaga, R.; Sato, W.; Horie-Inoue, K.; Shigekawa, T.; Osaki, A.; Saeki, T.; Okamoto, K.; *et al.* MicroRNA-574-3p, identified by microRNA library-based functional screening, modulates tamoxifen response in breast cancer. *Sci. Rep.* **2015**, *5*, 7641. [CrossRef] [PubMed]

29. Chiyomaru, T.; Yamamura, S.; Fukuhara, S.; Hidaka, H.; Majid, S.; Saini, S.; Arora, S.; Deng, G.; Shahryari, V.; Chang, I.; *et al.* Genistein up-regulates tumor suppressor microRNA-574-3p in prostate cancer. *PLoS ONE* **2013**, *8*, e58929. [CrossRef] [PubMed]

30. Tatarano, S.; Chiyomaru, T.; Kawakami, K.; Enokida, H.; Yoshino, H.; Hidaka, H.; Nohata, N.; Yamasaki, T.; Gotanda, T.; Tachiwada, T.; *et al.* Novel oncogenic function of mesoderm development candidate 1 and its regulation by MiR-574-3p in bladder cancer cell lines. *Int. J. Oncol.* **2012**, *40*, 951–959. [PubMed]

31. Su, Y.; Ni, Z.; Wang, G.; Cui, J.; Wei, C.; Wang, J.; Yang, Q.; Xu, Y.; Li, F. Aberrant expression of microRNAs in gastric cancer and biological significance of miR-574-3p. *Int. Immunopharmacol.* **2012**, *13*, 468–475. [CrossRef] [PubMed]

*J. Clin. Med.* **2015**, *4*, 1853–1865

32. Okamoto, K.; Ishiguro, T.; Midorikawa, Y.; Ohata, H.; Izumiya, M.; Tsuchiya, N.; Sato, A.; Sakai, H.; Nakagama, H. miR-493 induction during carcinogenesis blocks metastatic settlement of colon cancer cells in liver. *EMBO J.* **2012**, *31*, 1752–1763. [CrossRef] [PubMed]

33. Burroughs, A.M.; Kawano, M.; Ando, Y.; Daub, C.O.; Hayashizaki, Y. pre-miRNA profiles obtained through application of locked nucleic acids and deep sequencing reveals complex 5′/3′ arm variation including concomitant cleavage and polyuridylation patterns. *Nucleic Acids Res.* **2012**, *40*, 1424–1437. [CrossRef] [PubMed]

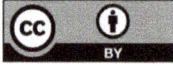

Journal of
*Clinical Medicine*

MDPI

Article

# Bioinformatic Interrogation of 5p-arm and 3p-arm Specific miRNA Expression Using TCGA Datasets

Wei-Ting Kuo [1,2], Ming-Wei Su [1,3], Yungling Leo Lee [1,3], Chien-Hsiun Chen [1], Chew-Wun Wu [4], Wen-Liang Fang [4], Kuo-Hung Huang [4] and Wen-chang Lin [1,2,*]

[1]  Institute of Biomedical Sciences, Academia Sinica, Taipei 115, Taiwan; raxkuo@hotmail.com (W.-T.K.);
     a8802137@gmail.com (M.-W.S.); leolee@ntu.edu.tw (Y.L.L.); chchen@ibms.sinica.edu.tw (C.-H.C.)
[2]  Institute of Biotechnology in Medicine, National Yang-Ming University, Taipei 112, Taiwan
[3]  Institute of Epidemiology and Preventive Medicine, National Taiwan University, Taipei 100, Taiwan
[4]  Department of Surgery, Veterans General Hospital and National Yang-Ming University, Taipei 112, Taiwan;
     chewwunwu@gmail.com (C.-W.W.); wlfang@vghtpe.gov.tw (W.-L.F.); khhuang@vghtpe.gov.tw (K.-H.H.)
*   Author to whom correspondence should be addressed; wenlin@ibms.sinica.edu.tw;
     Tel.: +886-2-2652-3967; Fax: +886-2-2782-7654.

Academic Editors: Takahiro Ochiya and Ryou-u Takahashi
Received: 23 June 2015; Accepted: 9 September 2015; Published: 15 September 2015

**Abstract:** MicroRNAs (miRNAs) play important roles in cellular functions and developmental processes. They are also implicated in oncogenesis mechanisms and could serve as potential cancer biomarkers. Using high-throughput miRNA sequencing information, expression of both the 5p-arm and 3p-arm mature miRNAs were demonstrated and generated from the single miRNA hairpin precursor. However, current miRNA annotations lack comprehensive 5p-arm/3p-arm feature annotations. Among known human mature miRNAs, only half of them are annotated with arm features. This generated ambiguous results in many miRNA-Sequencing (miRNA-Seq) studies. In this report, we have interrogated the TCGA (the Cancer Genome Atlas) miRNA expression datasets with an improved, fully annotated human 5p-arm and 3p-arm miRNA reference list. By utilizing this comprehensive miRNA arm-feature annotations, enhanced determinations and clear annotations were achieved for the miRNA isoforms (isomiRs) recognized from the sequencing reads. In the gastric cancer (STAD) dataset, as an example, 32 5p-arm/3p-arm specific miRNAs were found to be down-regulated and 24 5p-arm/3p-arm specific miRNAs were found to be up-regulated. We have further extended miRNA biomarker discoveries to additional TCGA miRNA-Seq datasets and provided extensive expression information on 5p-arm/3p-arm miRNAs across multiple cancer types. Our results identified several miRNAs that could be potential common biomarkers for human cancers.

**Keywords:** microRNA; 5p-arm; 3p-arm; bioinformatics; TCGA; biomarker

---

## 1. Introduction

Cancer is one of the most devastating human diseases [1] and there are devoted efforts to improve cancer treatments. With only limited successes in new anti-cancer drug discovery for clinical usages, it is generally recognized that early diagnosis and surgical resection are the most effective therapeutic procedures for curing human cancers. However, early discovery of cancer is not feasible for most cancer types due to the lack of useful and convenient non-invasive screening biomarkers. The current clinical serum based protein biomarkers for cancers are often unsatisfactory and lack specificity [2]. Therefore, there are substantial research efforts in many countries to identify better biomarkers for early cancer diagnosis and detection.

MicroRNAs (miRNAs) have become the emerging potential cancer biomarkers in recent years [3–6]. They are small RNA molecules, which are derived from endogenous non-protein-coding gene transcripts [7,8]. Extensive studies have implicated that miRNAs could play significant roles in tumorigenesis mechanisms and cancer malignant progression [9–12]. Intriguingly, miRNAs can be released from cancer cells into body fluids via secreting exosomes particles [6,13]. Therefore, circulating miRNAs could be utilized as novel liquid biopsy biomarkers [14–20]. In the miRNA biogenesis processes, the primary miRNA transcripts are transcribed and cleaved by the Drosha enzyme before being exported to the cytoplasm. They are further processed by the Dicer enzyme to generate the mature miRNA duplex [21–23]. Subsequently, one arm of the mature miRNA duplex is preferentially selected to form the ultimate RNA-induced silencing complex and the other arm of the duplex (miR-star) is often degraded [24]. However, with the increasing depth of Next Generation Sequencing (NGS) data, scientists have observed that both arms (strands) of the miRNA duplex could be utilized by the RNA-induced silencing complex (RISC) [25,26]. Therefore, 5p-arm and 3p-arm feature assignments would be essential to clearly distinguish the expressed miRNAs from the same pre-miRNAs during analysis. Thus, missing or incomplete arm feature annotations on human miRNAs might generate ambiguous miRNA data interpretations.

In previous report, we have established a comprehensive arm feature annotation list on almost all known human miRNAs in order to better understand the intrinsic properties of 5p-arm and 3p-arm miRNAs [27]. In this report, we have utilized such an annotated 5p-arm and 3p-arm miRNA list to further analyze the TCGA (the Cancer Genome Atlas) miRNA-Seq dataset for the interrogation of miRNAs as useful cancer biomarkers. The Cancer Genome Atlas is a comprehensive and coordinated effort to accelerate the understanding of the molecular basis of cancer through the application of various genome analysis technologies, including miRNA-Seq [28]. With the large collection of miRNA NGS data, our results demonstrated that the arm-specific miRNA expression profile would be beneficial for thorough analysis of dys-regulated miRNAs in human cancers.

## 2. Experimental Section

### 2.1. Arm Feature Assignment of Human Mature miRNAs

We downloaded all known miRNA information from miRBase release 20 (miRNA.dat, hairpin.fa and mature.fa), which contained 24,521 miRNA precursors and 30,424 mature miRNA sequences [29,30]. There were 206 species reported and we classified them using the species prefix for subsequent analysis. Among all reported miRNAs, there were only 15,398 miRNAs annotated with arm features. We assigned the arm features according to each individual species. For the human genome, there are 2578 mature miRNAs reported. To generate 5p-arm feature/3p-arm feature annotations, we adapted a mapping and classification strategy similar to those used by Zhou *et al.* [26]. In brief, the arm features of all mature miRNAs were annotated by mapping them back to the hairpin precursor sequences using the bowtie program as described [27]. The hairpin precursors were first divided into 5p-arm strand regions (37.5% of the hairpin length), loop regions (25% of the hairpin length) and 3p-arm strand regions (37.5% of the hairpin length) from their 5′-end starting positions. Assignment of the arm features was performed according to the bowtie mapping results (5p-arm or 3p-arm), and we discarded the miRNA records mapped to the loop regions. For human miRNAs, we have assigned 1297 miRNAs with 5p-arm and 1279 miRNAs with 3p-arm. Only two miRNAs were mapped to the loop region; therefore, they could not be assigned to the 5p-arm or 3p-arm. The complete human miRNA 5p-arm and 3p-arm annotation list is provided as the supplementary table. Python scripts were developed to process all data and analysis results using the Linux server (running Scientific Linux 6).

### 2.2. miRNA-Seq Datasets from TCGA

We obtained the level three miRNA-Seq data from TCGA website excluding cancer types with low numbers of tissue samples [28]. The final 13 TCGA cancer type datasets retrieved included: bladder urothelial carcinoma (BLCA), breast invasive carcinoma (BRCA), head and neck squamous cell carcinoma (HNSC), kidney chromophobe carcinoma (KICH), kidney renal clear cell carcinoma (KIRC), kidney renal papillary cell carcinoma (KIRP), liver hepatocellular carcinoma (LIHC), lung adenocarcinoma (LUAD), lung squamous cell carcinoma (LUSC), prostate adenocarcinoma (PRAD), Thyroid carcinoma (THCA), Uterine corpus endometrial carcinoma (UCEC), and stomach adenocarcinoma (STAD). In summary, we obtained 3972 tumor samples and 578 normal (adjacent tumor) samples. All datasets were processed and calculated for rpm (reads per million). We also excluded libraries with less than one million reads in subsequent miRNA expression analysis.

### 2.3. Bioinformatic Analysis with Comprehensive Arm-Feature-Annotated miRNA

In order to measure the 5p-arm and 3p-arm miRNA expression, we used the top three expression miRNA isoforms (isomiRs) from 5p-arm and 3p-arm miRNA regions to represent the expression level of 5p-arm miRNAs and 3p-arm miRNAs. For each 5p-arm miRNA or 3p-arm miRNA, we filtered out the lowly expressed miRNAs (rpm less than one). We selected only miRNAs expressed in over 50% of the TCGA libraries for comparison analysis. In the case of specifically interrogating miRNA precursor loci expression, we then combined the 5p-arm and 3p-arm expression reads and calculated their rpm values. Analysis of variance (ANOVA) was performed to identify differentially expressed miRNAs or arm-specific miRNAs using Partek Genomic Suite software (St. Louis, MO, USA).

### 3. Results and Discussion

Due to the significance of miRNAs in cancer development and progression, there are many studies interrogating the roles of miRNAs in human cancers [4,5,12,31], including the TCGA project [28]. However, detailed analysis on the specific expression of miRNA arms across different cancer types is lacking. In order to comprehensively interrogate the expression of miRNA arms, we have obtained the TCGA miRNA-Seq data in 13 different cancer types with the total of 3972 cancer tissue samples and 578 normal (adjacent tumor) tissues. As in the available TCGA miRNA-Seq dataset, we observed that opposite arm miRNAs were often neglected since TCGA pipeline used the standard miRBase annotations. Therefore, our analysis pipeline here would be helpful to assign the expression values of all possible 5p-arm and 3p-arm miRNAs in the TCGA datasets.

### 3.1. Arm Features and isomiR Quantifications

In a previous report [27], we analyzed the reported 30,424 mature miRNAs in miRBase, and there were only 15,398 miRNAs annotated with arm features. To resolve this incomplete annotation limitation, we have mapped all un-assigned mature miRNA sequences to their respective precursor miRNA sequences. For human miRNAs, there are 2578 reported mature miRNAs, and we have assigned 1297 miRNAs with 5p-arm and 1279 miRNAs with 3p-arm. Only two miRNAs were mapped to the loop region; therefore, they could not be assigned to the 5p-arm or 3p-arm. Following the arm feature annotation, additional issues to be clarified are the determination and quantification of isomiRs [32]. Typically, reported mature miRNA expressions are only annotated by matching with the known mature miRNA sequences reported (as a defined length and nucleotide sequences). However, it is often observed that length and sequence variants of the reported miRNAs could be readily seen from the NGS data (Figure 1, hsa-let-7a-1 as an example). These miRNA isoforms or variants were named isomiRs.

As reported previously, there are many mature miRNA isoforms of the same pre-miRNA gene loci that existed following the NGS reads mapping procedures [25]. This isomiR phenomenon existed in all TCGA miRNA-Seq datasets. It has been reported that isomiRs could also associate with RISC and be involved in the target mRNA silencing [26]. This would generate issues in quantification of miRNA expression, since we should not ignore the existence of isomiRs. One can certainly use the miRBase annotated mature miRNA as the only standard for quantification, but this would miss some of the un-annotated opposite arm miRNAs. Besides, in some miRNA loci, we observed that the most abundant isomiR is not necessary the one annotated by miRBase [25]. In Figure 1, as an example, the miRBase reported that hsa-let-7a-1-5p (ugagguaguagguuguauaguu; MIMAT0000062; labeled with

*J. Clin. Med.* **2015**, *4*, 1798–1814

5p) and hsa-let-7a-1-3p (cuauacaaucuacugucuuuc; MIMAT0004481; labeled with 3p) are not the most abundantly expressed isomiRs in this gastric cancer NGS dataset. Therefore, we believe that it is not practical to use just the miRBase annotated mature miRNA sequence as the sole standard expression reference for NGS data quantification. Another way of tabulating is to include all isomiRs mapped to the pre-miRNA locus to cover all the length and sequence isomiR variants in some reported analysis pipelines. However, this would include both the 5p-arm and 3p-arm mature miRNAs expressions into the same miRNA loci. This might be acceptable and utilized in earlier miRNA expression studies with only single mature miRNA arm expected and annotated. Nevertheless, this is not satisfactory with current understanding of NGS datasets with both arms of miRNAs recognized. Therefore, with the comprehensive 5p-arm and 3p-arm miRNA list, we suggested that it is better to carefully quantify the expression of 5p-arm and 3p-arm miRNAs separately.

```
hsa-let-7a-1    hg19:9:96938124-96938418:+
....UGGGAUGAGGUAGUAGGUUGUAUAGUUUUAGGGUCACACCCACCACUGGGAGAUAACUAUACAAUCUACUGUCUUUCCUA....


.......AUGAGGUAGUAGGUUGUAUAGUU.......................................................     3      0.659618
........AUGAGGUAGUAGGUUGUAUAGUUU.....................................................     9      1.978854
........AUGAGGUAGUAGGUUGUAUAGUUUU....................................................     1      0.219873
.........UGAGGUAGUAGGUUGUAUAG........................................................   192     42.215542
.........UGAGGUAGUAGGUUGUAUAGU.......................................................  4563   1003.27874
5p.....UGAGGUAGUAGGUUGUAUAGUU.........................................................  8307   1826.481809
........UGAGGUAGUAGGUUGUAUAGUUU...................................................... 16342   3593.158268
........UGAGGUAGUAGGUUGUAUAGUUUU.....................................................   203     44.634141
........UGAGGUAGUAGGUUGUAUAGUUUA.....................................................    10      2.198726
........UGAGGUAGUAGGUUGUAUAGUUUAGGG..................................................     1      0.219873
.........GAGGUAGUAGGUUGUAUAGUU.......................................................     2      0.439745
.........GAGGUAGUAGGUUGUAUAGUUU......................................................    12      2.638471
..........AGGUAGUAGGUUGUAUAGUUU......................................................     1      0.219873
...........GGUAGUAGGUUGUAUAGU........................................................     7      1.539108
...........GGUAGUAGGUUGUAUAGUU.......................................................    17      3.737834
...........GGUAGUAGGUUGUAUAGUUU......................................................    63     13.851975
...........GGUAGUAGGUUGUAUAGUUUU.....................................................     5      1.099363
............GUAGUAGGUUGUAUAGUU.......................................................     2      0.439745
............GUAGAGGUUGUAUAGUUU.......................................................    19      0.219873
.............UAGUAGGUUGUAUAGUUU......................................................     2      0.439745
.............UAGUAGGUUGUAUAGUUUUAGGG.................................................     3      0.659618
..............UAGUAGGUUGUAUAGUUUUAGGGUC..............................................     2      0.439745
..............GUAGGUUGUAUAGUUU.......................................................     3      0.659618
...................UUAGGGUCACACCCACCACUGGGAG.........................................     1      0.219873
..................................................CUAUACAAUCUACUGUCUU.................     2      0.439745
..................................................CUAUACAAUCUACUGUCUUU................     1      0.219873
3p................................................CUAUACAAUCUACUGUCUUUC...............    16      3.517962
..................................................CUAUACAAUCUACUGUCUUUCC..............    40      8.794905
..................................................CUAUACAAUCUACUGUCUUUCCU.............    33      7.255796
...................................................UAUACAAUCUACUGUCUUU................     1      0.219873
...................................................UAUACAAUCUACUGUCUUUCCU.............     1      0.219873
...................................................UAUACAAUCUACUGUCUUUCCUA............     1      0.219873
....................................................AUACAAUCUACUGUCUUUCCUA...........     1      0.219873
.....................................................UACAAUCUACUGUCUUUCCUA...........     1      0.219873

                                                                                     Read      Reads per
                                                                                     counts    million
```

**Figure 1.** Next Generation Sequencing (NGS) reads alignments of hsa-let-7a-1 miRNA isoforms (isomiRs). A small RNA NGS library from a gastric cancer cell line (AGS cells) was prepared and sequenced with Illumina Solexa platform. The NGS reads were aligned to the hsa-let-7a-1 miRNA genomic locus using Bowtie mapping program following adaptor trimming. We allowed no mismatch at the mapping procedure using standard Bowtie parameter. We trimmed the last 3′ end mismatch one by one until the mapping perfect-match reads were at least 18 nucleotides in length [25]. Here, the hsa-let-7a-1 miRNA precursor sequences and genomic coordinates are displayed on the top section. The NGS reads are aligned and their sequences, read counts and rpm (reads per million) values are displayed. The miRBase annotated hsa-let-7a-1-5p (MIMAT0000062) and hsa-let-7a-1-3p (MIMAT0004481) are marked with 5p and 3p in red, respectively.

After tabulating and ranking the expression value of each isomiRs in different miRNA arms (read counts as well as rpm value), we noted a significant pattern on the uppermost expressed isomiRs. We tabulated the expression of all isomiRs in the 5p-arm and 3p-arm miRNAs separately, and calculated the distribution percentage of each isomiR. In Figure 2, we observed that the most abundantly expressed isomiR represented around 80% of the total expression level of all isomiRs. This observation is similar in the 5p-arm miRNA group as well as in 3p-arm miRNA group, respectively. Again, the topmost expressed isomiR is not necessarilyy the one annotated by the miRBase. In addition, the highest three expressed isomiRs could cover nearly 95% of the total expression amounts. Thus, we propose using read counts or rpm values of the uppermost three isomiR expression as the expression level of the 5p-arm and 3p-arm miRNAs. This procedure would be particularly beneficial in determining the un-annotated opposite arm miRNA expression level for those miRNAs with only one single arm miRNA reported by miRBase, since there are no official defined mature miRNA sequences and lengths.

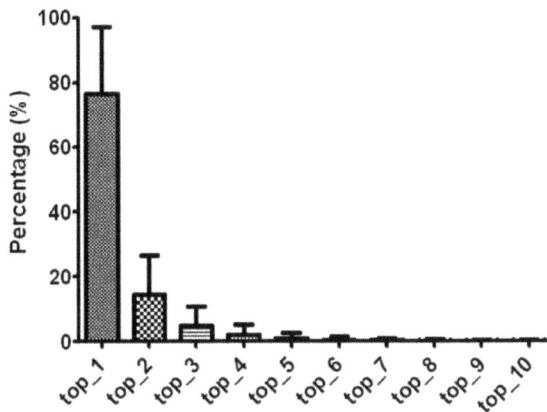

**Figure 2.** Expression level distribution of miRNA isoform (isomiR) reads. The read counts of each isomiR were tabulated and ranked by their expression percentage within each miRNA gene loci, *i.e.*, read counts of each isomiR divided by the total read counts of all isomiRs in the miRNA gene loci. The top ten expressed isomiRs percentages are displayed.

*3.2. TCGA miRNA-Seq Analysis: STAD Gastric Cancer Dataset*

We then applied this analysis pipeline for the obtained 3972 TCGA datasets. Using the gastric cancer (STAD) data as an example, there were 261 cancer samples and 38 normal samples obtained from TCGA. We used the level 3 expression data and convert the read counts and rpm values from the TCGA STAD dataset. As described earlier, TCGA initial analysis used only the miRBase annotation information; therefore, the arm feature was not well annotated. In addition, many opposite arm (lagging strand) miRNAs were not annotated at all. Following our analysis pipeline and assignment of all 5p-arm and 3p-arm miRNA expression values using the top three expressed isomiRs, we obtained a comprehensive 5p-arm and 3p-arm miRNA expression profile in STAD gastric cancers.

We first examined the miRNA gene loci (combined 5p-arm and 3p-arm miRNA together) expression profile in STAD normal samples. In Figure 3A, the utmost ten expressed miRNAs are miR-143, miR-148a, miR-21, miR-22, miR-375, miR-10a, miR-30a, miR-192, miR-99b and miR-145. In order to compare the expression pattern between 5p-arm and 3p-arm miRNAs in detail, we then analyzed the expression values of separated 5p-arm and 3p-arm miRNAs. When one further interrogated the preferential expression on the 5p-arm and 3p-arm miRNAs in details, preferential expression of single miRNA arm is noted in these highly expressed miRNAs (Figure 3b). Six miRNAs have higher expression levels in 5p-arm and 4 miRNAs have more expression in 3p-arm.

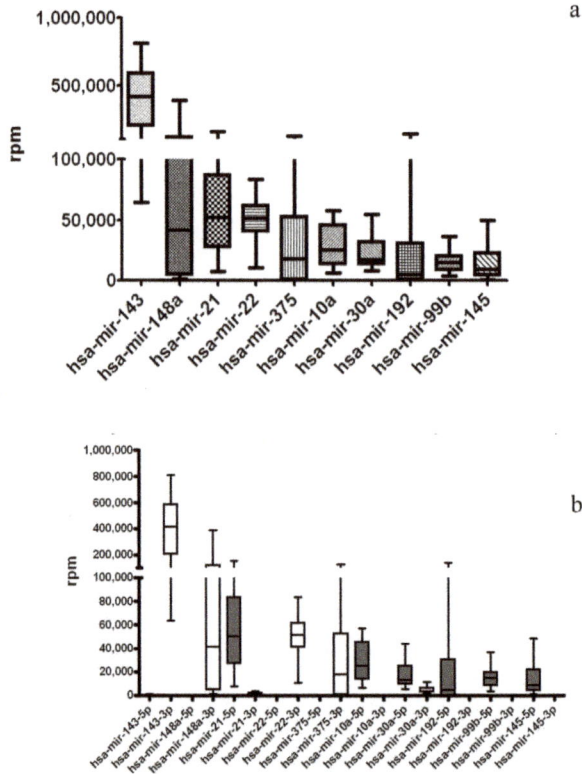

**Figure 3.** Distribution of the top ten expressed miRNAs from the TCGA (the Cancer Genome Atlas) normal gastric tissue dataset. miRNA expression data of 38 normal samples in TCGA stomach adenocarcinoma (STAD) libraries were re-analyzed using the new arm feature list. (**a**) The rpm (reads per million) values of each miRNAs were tabulated by combining the 5p-arm and 3p-arm together to represent the miRNA loci expression; (**b**) 5p-arm and 3p-arm expression levels were tabulated separately and displayed. miR-143 is the most expressed miRNA in the TCGA clinical normal samples.

Similar miRNA expression patterns were observed in the STAD cancer samples (Figure 4). The highly expressed miRNA genes (combined 5p-arm and 3p-arm together) in the STAD cancer group are: miR-21, miR-143, miR-22, miR-148a, miR-10a, miR-192, miR-375, miR-99b, let-7a-2 and miR-30a. The 5p-arm miRNA and 3p-arm miRNA expression dominance pattern is also similar in the STAD cancer samples (Figure 4b) following the examination on separated 5p-arm and 3p-arm expression levels. Finally, we observe most of highly expressed miRNAs in both the normal and cancer STAD groups, including miR-143, miR-21, miR-22, miR-148a, miR-10a, miR-192, miR-375, miR-99b and miR-30a. However, it is significant to observe the increase of expression rpm numbers of miR-21, specifically miR-21-5p. This implied the significant role of miR-21-5p in gastric cancer oncogenesis as previously reported [18,33].

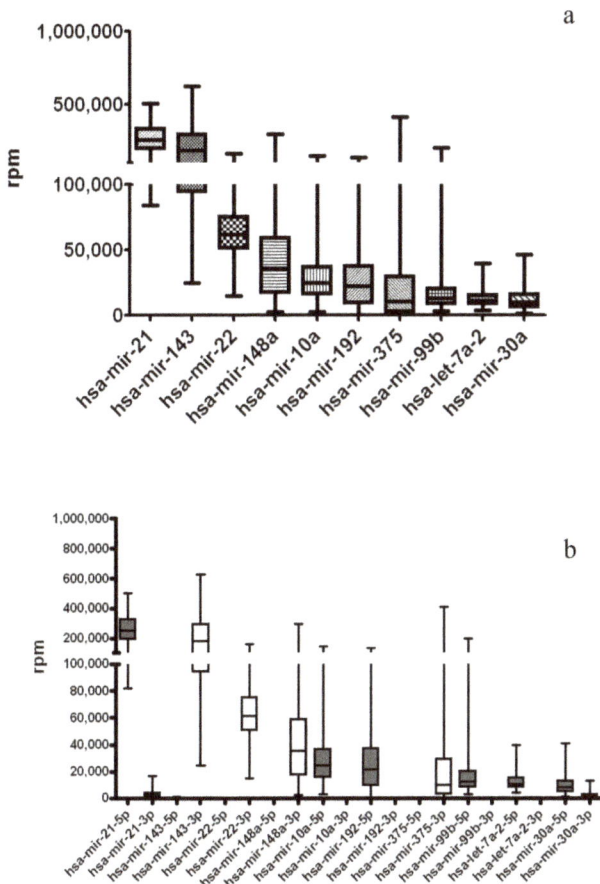

**Figure 4.** Distribution of highly expressed miRNAs in 261 gastric cancer samples from TCGA (The Cancer Genome Atlas) datasets. miRNA expression data of TCGA stomach adenocarcinoma (STAD) were retrieved and re-analyzed using the comprehensive arm feature annotated miRNA list. (**a**) The rpm values of each miRNAs were tabulated by combining the 5p-arm and 3p-arm to represent the miRNA loci expression; (**b**) 5p-arm and 3p-arm expression levels were tabulated separately and displayed. miR-21 is the most expressed miRNAs in the TCGA clinical cancer samples.

Finally, we used ANOVA analysis to identify the significantly expressed miRNAs in the TCGA STAD dataset. We filtered out the miRNAs with low expression (rpm less than one) and selected only miRNAs expressed in over 50% of the TCGA STAD sample libraries. The subsequent normalization and ANOVA analysis were performed by the Partek software package. In Figure 5a, with the selection criteria of fold-change value > 2.5 and $p$-value < 0.05, we interrogated the miRNA gene loci expression by the combined 5p-arm and 3p-arm expression values. We identified 22 down-regulated miRNAs and 18 up-regulated miRNAs from close to 300 clinical STAD samples (Table 1; overall miRNA precursor). Among these 40 miRNAs, 23 miRNAs have been reported to have significant association with human gastric cancers in a previous review paper [3]. With our new analysis pipeline, we could achieve better resolutions and coverage on the arm-specific isomiR expressions. We further interrogated the separate expression levels of 5p-arm miRNAs and 3p-arm miRNAs. In the 5p-arm and 3p-arm separated analysis group, there are 32 miRNAs down-regulated and 24 miRNAs up-regulated (Figure 5b and Table 1; separate 5p-arm and 3p-arm miRNAs). More arm-specific miRNAs were identified here in the arm separate group as expected (56 arm-specific miRNAs *vs.* 40 miRNA genes). In the up-regulated miRNAs, we found the five miRNAs have both 5p-arm and 3p-arm expression significantly increased (miR-146b, miR-200a, miR-141 miR-192 and miR-194). In the down-regulated group, there are seven miRNA pairs (miR-139, miR-29c, miR-145, miR-378, miR-30a, miR-143 and miR-144) with both the 5p-arm and 3p-arm identified as significantly dys-regulated miRNAs. Many of the miRNAs were also reported by a recent systems biology paper from TCGA in 2014 [34].

We further compare the expression pattern between 5p-arm and 3p-arm miRNAs in more detail. We selected only miRNAs expressing both 5p-arm and 3p-arm miRNAs for analysis, and there are 196 miRNAs identified from the TCGA STAD library with both the 5p-arm and 3p-arm expressed. It is noted there is a significant expression level difference between the guide strand miRNAs and passenger strand miRNAs (miRNA*) as researchers have previously noted [25,35–37]. If one investigates the 5p-arm/3p-arm expression ratios of these single arm dominant miRNAs across over 4000 TCGA samples examined here, there is no significant difference between 5p-arm expression dominance and 3p-arm expression dominance miRNA populations. Similar findings on consistency of isomiR expression profiles in different cell types were also reported by Guo *et al.* [38]. Therefore, the arm-switching events were not detected among the large numbers of TCGA data examined here. This also illustrated the advantages of our arm-feature annotation efforts to provide clearer and better miRNA analysis results systematically in large numbers of samples. The arm-switching phenomenon is mentioned previously by observing that the arm from which the dominant mature miRNA is processed can switch in different tissues or developmental periods [39]. It is believed that arm selection is governed by the asymmetrical stability of hairpins and that the determinant sequences critical to arm dominance is outside the mature miRNA duplex. Just recently, in addition to the secondary hairpin structure, it has been reported that certain primary sequence motifs are also required in hairpin recognition and processing, including the downstream SRp20-binding motif, the basal UG motif in the stem, and the apical stem GUG motif [40].

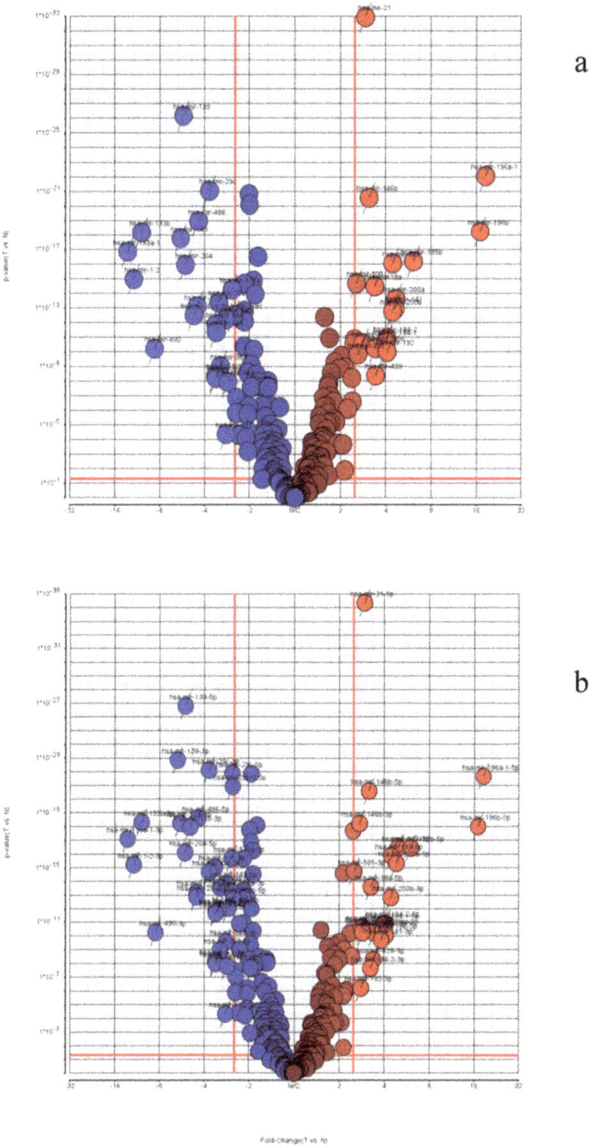

**Figure 5.** Volcano plot of combined miRNA expression and separate 5p-arm/3p-arm miRNA expression in TCGA (The Cancer Genome Atlas) gastric cancer tissues. miRNA expression data of TCGA stomach adenocarcinoma (STAD) were retrieved and re-analyzed using the comprehensive arm feature annotated miRNA list. The miRNA expression information of gastric cancer tissues is illustrated here by calculating the mean expression level from TCGA samples. Following analysis of variance (ANOVA) in the Partek software package, the volcano plot is displayed for selecting differentially expressed miRNA genes. (**a**) Precursor miRNAs gene loci expression by combining the 5p-arm and 3p-arm miRNAs together for analysis; (**b**) 5p-arm and 3p-arm miRNAs tabulated separately for their expression and analyzed.

**Table 1.** Dys-regulated miRNAs in TCGA (the Cancer Genome Atlas) STAD gastric cancer tissues.

| TCGA STAD (Stomach Adenocarcinoma) | | | |
|---|---|---|---|
| Overall miRNA Precursors | | Separate 5p-arm and 3p-arm miRNAs | |
| Down regulated | Up regulated | Down regulated | Up regulated |
| hsa-miR-139 | hsa-miR-21 | hsa-miR-139-5p | hsa-miR-21-5p |
| hsa-miR-29c | hsa-miR-196a-1 | hsa-miR-139-3p | hsa-miR-196a-1-5p |
| hsa-miR-486 | hsa-miR-146b | hsa-miR-29c-3p | hsa-miR-146b-5p |
| hsa-miR-133b | hsa-miR-196b | hsa-miR-29c-5p | hsa-miR-146b-3p |
| hsa-miR-145 | hsa-miR-135b | hsa-miR-29b-2-5p | hsa-miR-196b-5p |
| hsa-miR-133a-1 | hsa-miR-183 | hsa-miR-486-5p | hsa-miR-141-5p |
| hsa-miR-204 | hsa-miR-501 | hsa-miR-133b-3p | hsa-miR-135b-5p |
| hsa-miR-1-2 | hsa-miR-18a | hsa-miR-145-5p | hsa-miR-183-5p |
| hsa-miR-378a | hsa-miR-200a | hsa-miR-145-3p | hsa-miR-200a-5p |
| hsa-miR-30a | hsa-miR-141 | hsa-miR-133a-1-3p | hsa-miR-501-3p |
| hsa-miR-129-1 | hsa-miR-200b | hsa-miR-204-5p | hsa-miR-18a-5p |
| hsa-miR-129-2 | hsa-miR-194-2 | hsa-miR-378a-5p | hsa-miR-200b-3p |
| hsa-miR-378c | hsa-miR-194-1 | hsa-miR-1-2-3p | hsa-miR-194-2-5p |
| hsa-miR-195 | hsa-miR-182 | hsa-miR-195-3p | hsa-miR-194-1-5p |
| hsa-miR-144 | hsa-miR-200c | hsa-miR-30a-3p | hsa-miR-335-3p |
| hsa-miR-143 | hsa-miR-192 | hsa-miR-143-5p | hsa-miR-182-5p |
| hsa-miR-490 | hsa-miR-335 | hsa-miR-30a-5p | hsa-miR-200a-3p |
| hsa-miR-363 | hsa-miR-429 | hsa-miR-378a-3p | hsa-miR-200c-3p |
| hsa-miR-9-2 | | hsa-miR-129-1-5p | hsa-miR-708-5p |
| hsa-miR-9-1 | | hsa-miR-129-2-5p | hsa-miR-192-5p |
| hsa-miR-149 | | hsa-miR-378c-5p | hsa-miR-141-3p |
| hsa-miR-187 | | hsa-miR-195-5p | hsa-miR-429-3p |
| | | hsa-miR-30c-2-3p | hsa-miR-194-2-3p |
| | | hsa-miR-144-5p | hsa-miR-192-3p |
| | | hsa-miR-143-3p | |
| | | hsa-miR-490-3p | |
| | | hsa-miR-144-3p | |
| | | hsa-miR-363-3p | |
| | | hsa-miR-9-2-5p | |
| | | hsa-miR-9-1-5p | |
| | | hsa-miR-149-5p | |
| | | hsa-miR-187-3p | |

### 3.3. miRNA-Seq Analysis on Additional 12 TCGA Cancer Types

By using a comprehensive 5p-arm and 3p-arm miRNA reference list, our analysis pipeline could provide clear and comprehensive miRNA expression profiles. Since there are no systematic examinations on arm specific miRNAs, we are interested in interrogating the arm-specific miRNAs dys-regulated in different cancers. We further applied this analysis pipeline to interrogate other miRNA-Seq datasets from TCGA, especially on the 5p-arm and 3p-arm annotated miRNAs. The same criteria (fold-change value > 2.5 and *p*-value < 0.05) were applied to identify significantly dys-regulated arm-specific miRNAs (Supplementary Figures S1a to S1l). It is interesting to note that the numbers of dys-regulated miRNAs varied between different cancer types, which might be related to the diverse sample size and library qualities, since we do filter out low-expression miRNAs. Many of the miRNAs identified in each cancer type were reported in the literatures [3]. Here, we would like to inquire if any of the dys-regulated could be utilized as potential cancer biomarkers for most cancer types, which would be beneficial to serve as routine cancer screening biomarkers. We first explored arm-specific miRNAs found in all cancer types analyzed (233 miRNAs) and then examined the significance distribution of each 5p-arm and 3p-arm miRNA using hierarchical clustering (Figure 6).

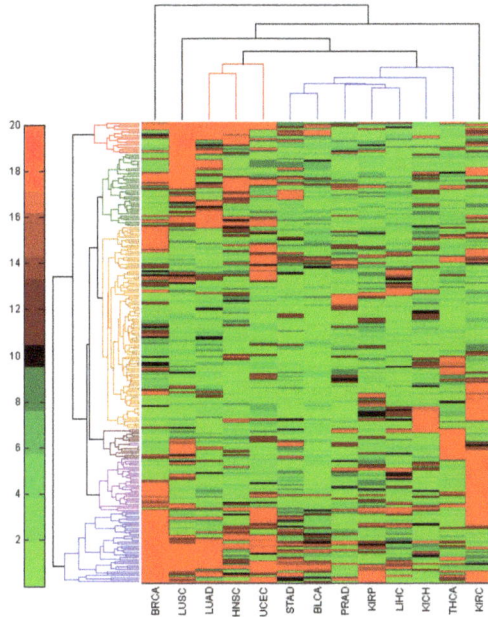

**Figure 6.** Hierarchical clustering analysis on significantly dys-regulated miRNAs in 13 TCGA (the Cancer Genome Atlas) cancer types. 233 arm-specific miRNAs were expressed in all 13 cancer types and further selected for hierarchical clustering analysis to reveal their significance in each cancer type.

Among these 233 miRNAs, there are several miRNAs seems to be important in the basic oncogenesis processes and found to be significant in multiple cancer types. They could be utilized as general cancer biomarkers [5,33,41–45]. Some of the up-regulated arm specific miRNAs include miR-182-5p, miR-183-5p, miR-21-5p, miR-141-5p, miR-1307-5p, miR-130b-3p, miR-196b-5p, miR-210-3p, miR-21-3p and miR-141-3p. The down-regulated miRNAs include miR-139-5p, miR-139-3p, miR-145-5p, miR-145-3p, miR-486-5p, and miR-1-2-3p. In some cases, we observed the few miRNAs have contradictory associations in different cancer types, which indicate multiple biological functions for some of the miRNAs, such as miR-141-5p and miR-141-3p, miR-486-5p. There are few miRNA 5p-arm and 3p-arm pairs identified in our study: miR-21-5p and miR-21-3p; miR-141-5p and miR-141-3p; miR-139-5p and miR-139-3p; miR-145-5p and miR-145-3p. The 5p-arm mature miRNA is totally different from the 3p-arm mature miRNA in terms of sequences and target spectrum, not to mention expression level. miR-139-5p has been known to be a tumor suppressor miRNA by inhibiting the metastasis pathway [46]; however, miR-139-3p has not been well studied and is often neglected, since much literature has only used miR-139. There are few studies suggested that both arms of mature miRNAs (miR-582-5p and miR-582-3p) from a single pri-miRNA locus were cooperatively involved in the modulation of critical cellular pathways in human cancer cells [47]. More studies should be conducted to carefully interrogate 5p-arm and 3p-arm miRNA functions. Therefore, our study provides better annotations and improved understanding of arm-specific miRNAs in human cancers.

## 4. Conclusions

In conclusion, with comprehensive 5p-arm and 3p-arm feature annotations, we could achieve more comprehensive and in-depth investigation on dys-regulated miRNAs in human cancers. In earlier reports, while certain miRNAs were reported with the correct arm assignment annotations, the arm

*J. Clin. Med.* **2015**, *4*, 1798–1814

annotation information was often lacking in other reports. This would generate confusion in the interpretation of data, since one would not know which arm was being referred to. Using miR-30a as an example, in some papers miR-30a-3p is a signature biomarker for breast cancer recurrence [4], and another study mentioned miR-30a-5p as a tumor-suppressive miRNA in colon cancer [48]. Nonetheless, we could encounter literature lacking clear descriptions of the miR-30a 5p-arm or miR-30a 3p-arm, which would create uncertainty and bafflement for people interested in their studies. Thus, it is beneficial to have complete, comprehensive 5p-arm/3p-arm assignment for all human miRNAs. This is especially important for NGS miRNA analysis, since more miRNA reads from both 5p-arm and 3p-arm could be observed with the increasing depth of sequencing. By utilizing the comprehensive miRNA arm-feature annotations, we could improve the miRNA expression pipeline with better and well-defined annotated miRNA expression information and provided extended expression information on opposite arms of the miRNA hairpin precursors. With the systematical interrogation of multiple cancer miRNA-Seq datasets from TCGA, we were able to apply our analysis pipeline to discover arm-specific miRNAs important in the oncogenesis processes and useful as common cancer biomarkers for different cancer types.

**Acknowledgments:** This work was supported by research grants from Academia Sinica and Ministry of Science and Technology, Taiwan.

**Author Contributions:** Wei-Ting Kuo and Ming-Wei Su performed the main experiments and data analysis. Yungling Leo Lee and Chien-Hsiun Chen helped with the statistical assessment and manuscript suggestions. Chew-Wun Wu provided the clinical information and manuscript discussion. Wen-Liang Fang and Kuo-Hung Huang provided the clinical samples. Wen-chang Lin was responsible for the experimental design and manuscript preparation. All authors contributed significantly to the drafting and critical revision of this manuscript.

**Conflicts of Interest:** The authors declare no conflict of interest.

## References

1. Hanahan, D.; Weinberg, R.A. Hallmarks of cancer: The next generation. *Cell* **2011**, *144*, 646–674. [CrossRef] [PubMed]

2. He, C.Z.; Zhang, K.H.; Li, Q.; Liu, X.H.; Hong, Y.; Lv, N.H. Combined use of AFP, CEA, CA125 and CAL9-9 improves the sensitivity for the diagnosis of gastric cancer. *BMC Gastroenterol.* **2013**, *13*. [CrossRef] [PubMed]

3. Liao, Y.L.; Tsai, K.W.; Lin, W.C. miRNAs in gastric cancer. In *Gastric Carcinoma—Molecular Aspects and Current Advances*; Lotfy, D.M., Ed.; InTech Open: Rijeka, Croatia, 2011; pp. 87–104.

4. Perez-Rivas, L.G.; Jerez, J.M.; Carmona, R.; de Luque, V.; Vicioso, L.; Claros, M.G.; Viguera, E.; Pajares, B.; Sanchez, A.; Ribelles, N.; *et al.* A microRNA signature associated with early recurrence in breast cancer. *PLoS ONE* **2014**, *9*, e91884. [CrossRef] [PubMed]

5. Tsai, K.W.; Liao, Y.L.; Wu, C.W.; Hu, L.Y.; Li, S.C.; Chan, W.C.; Ho, M.R.; Lai, C.H.; Kao, H.W.; Fang, W.L.; *et al.* Aberrant expression of miR-196a in gastric cancers and correlation with recurrence. *Genes Chromosomes Cancer* **2012**, *51*, 394–401. [CrossRef] [PubMed]

6. Kosaka, N.; Iguchi, H.; Ochiya, T. Circulating microRNA in body fluid: A new potential biomarker for cancer diagnosis and prognosis. *Cancer Sci.* **2010**, *101*, 2087–2092. [CrossRef] [PubMed]

7. Bartel, D.P. MicroRNAs: Genomics, biogenesis, mechanism, and function. *Cell* **2004**, *116*, 281–297. [CrossRef]

8. Bartel, D.P. MicroRNAs: Target recognition and regulatory functions. *Cell* **2009**, *136*, 215–233. [CrossRef] [PubMed]

9. Lujambio, A.; Lowe, S.W. The microcosmos of cancer. *Nature* **2012**, *482*, 347–355. [CrossRef] [PubMed]

10. Rosenfeld, N.; Aharonov, R.; Meiri, E.; Rosenwald, S.; Spector, Y.; Zepeniuk, M.; Benjamin, H.; Shabes, N.; Tabak, S.; Levy, A.; *et al.* MicroRNAs accurately identify cancer tissue origin. *Nat. Biotechnol.* **2008**, *26*, 462–469. [CrossRef] [PubMed]

11. Takahashi, R.U.; Miyazaki, H.; Ochiya, T. The role of microRNAs in the regulation of cancer stem cells. *Front. Genet.* **2014**, *4*. [CrossRef] [PubMed]

12. Takahashi, R.U.; Miyazaki, H.; Ochiya, T. The roles of microRNAs in breast cancer. *Cancers (Basel)* **2015**, *7*, 598–616. [CrossRef] [PubMed]

13. Kosaka, N.; Iguchi, H.; Yoshioka, Y.; Takeshita, F.; Matsuki, Y.; Ochiya, T. Secretory mechanisms and intercellular transfer of microRNAs in living cells. *J. Biol. Chem.* **2010**, *285*, 17442–17452. [CrossRef] [PubMed]

14. Schwarzenbach, H.; Nishida, N.; Calin, G.A.; Pantel, K. Clinical relevance of circulating cell-free microRNAs in cancer. *Nat. Rev. Clin. Oncol.* **2014**, *11*, 145–156. [CrossRef] [PubMed]

15. Tominaga, N.; Kosaka, N.; Ono, M.; Katsuda, T.; Yoshioka, Y.; Tamura, K.; Lotvall, J.; Nakagama, H.; Ochiya, T. Brain metastatic cancer cells release microRNA-181c-containing extracellular vesicles capable of destructing blood-brain barrier. *Nat. Commun.* **2015**, *6*. [CrossRef] [PubMed]

16. Sugimachi, K.; Matsumura, T.; Hirata, H.; Uchi, R.; Ueda, M.; Ueo, H.; Shinden, Y.; Iguchi, T.; Eguchi, H.; Shirabe, K.; *et al.* Identification of a *bona fide* microRNA biomarker in serum exosomes that predicts hepatocellular carcinoma recurrence after liver transplantation. *Br. J. Cancer* **2015**, *112*, 532–538. [CrossRef] [PubMed]

17. Matsumura, T.; Sugimachi, K.; Iinuma, H.; Takahashi, Y.; Kurashige, J.; Sawada, G.; Ueda, M.; Uchi, R.; Ueo, H.; Takano, Y.; *et al.* Exosomal microRNA in serum is a novel biomarker of recurrence in human colorectal cancer. *Br. J. Cancer* **2015**, *113*, 275–281. [CrossRef] [PubMed]

18. Kuo, W.T.; Lai, C.H.; Wu, C.W.; Fang, W.L.; Huang, K.H.; Lin, W.C. Urine miR-21-5p as a potential non-invasive biomarker for gastric cancer. *Oncol. Lett.* **2015**, in press.

19. Osaki, M.; Kosaka, N.; Okada, F.; Ochiya, T. Circulating microRNAs in drug safety assessment for hepatic and cardiovascular toxicity: The latest biomarker frontier? *Mol. Diagn. Ther.* **2014**, *18*, 121–126. [CrossRef] [PubMed]

20. Haldrup, C.; Kosaka, N.; Ochiya, T.; Borre, M.; Hoyer, S.; Orntoft, T.F.; Sorensen, K.D. Profiling of circulating microRNAs for prostate cancer biomarker discovery. *Drug Deliv. Transl. Res.* **2014**, *4*, 19–30. [CrossRef] [PubMed]

21. Gregory, R.I.; Chendrimada, T.P.; Cooch, N.; Shiekhattar, R. Human RISC couples microRNA biogenesis and posttranscriptional gene silencing. *Cell* **2005**, *123*, 631–640. [CrossRef] [PubMed]

22. Han, J.; Lee, Y.; Yeom, K.H.; Nam, J.W.; Heo, I.; Rhee, J.K.; Sohn, S.Y.; Cho, Y.; Zhang, B.T.; Kim, V.N. Molecular basis for the recognition of primary microRNAs by the Drosha-DGCR8 complex. *Cell* **2006**, *125*, 887–901. [CrossRef] [PubMed]

23. Lee, Y.; Ahn, C.; Han, J.; Choi, H.; Kim, J.; Yim, J.; Lee, J.; Provost, P.; Radmark, O.; Kim, S.; *et al.* The nuclear RNAse III Drosha initiates microRNA processing. *Nature* **2003**, *425*, 415–419. [CrossRef] [PubMed]

24. Khvorova, A.; Reynolds, A.; Jayasena, S.D. Functional siRNAs and miRNAs exhibit strand bias. *Cell* **2003**, *115*, 209–216. [CrossRef]

25. Li, S.C.; Liao, Y.L.; Ho, M.R.; Tsai, K.W.; Lai, C.H.; Lin, W.C. miRNA arm selection and isomiR distribution in gastric cancer. *BMC Genomics* **2012**, *13* (Suppl. 1). [CrossRef] [PubMed]

26. Zhou, H.; Arcila, M.L.; Li, Z.; Lee, E.J.; Henzler, C.; Liu, J.; Rana, T.M.; Kosik, K.S. Deep annotation of mouse iso-miR and iso-moR variation. *Nucleic Acids Res.* **2012**, *40*, 5864–5875. [CrossRef] [PubMed]

27. Kuo, W.T.; Ho, M.R.; Wu, C.W.; Fang, W.L.; Huang, K.H.; Lin, W.C. Interrogation of microRNAs involved in gastric cancer using 5p-arm and 3p-arm annotated microRNAs. *Anticancer Res.* **2015**, *35*, 1345–1352. [PubMed]

28. The Cancer Genome Atlas Data Portal. Available online: https://tcga-data.nci.nih.gov/tcga/tcgaHome2.jsp (accessed on 13 September 2015).

29. Griffiths-Jones, S.; Grocock, R.J.; van Dongen, S.; Bateman, A.; Enright, A.J. miRBase: MicroRNA sequences, targets and gene nomenclature. *Nucleic Acids Res.* **2006**, *34*, D140–D144. [CrossRef] [PubMed]

30. Griffiths-Jones, S.; Saini, H.K.; van Dongen, S.; Enright, A.J. miRBase: Tools for microRNA genomics. *Nucleic Acids Res.* **2008**, *36*, D154–D158. [CrossRef] [PubMed]

31. Gailhouste, L.; Ochiya, T. Cancer-related microRNAs and their role as tumor suppressors and oncogenes in hepatocellular carcinoma. *Histol. Histopathol.* **2013**, *28*, 437–451. [PubMed]

32. Neilsen, C.T.; Goodall, G.J.; Bracken, C.P. IsomiRs—The overlooked repertoire in the dynamic microRNAome. *Trends Genet.* **2012**, *28*, 544–549. [CrossRef] [PubMed]

33. Chan, S.H.; Wu, C.W.; Li, A.F.; Chi, C.W.; Lin, W.C. miR-21 microRNA expression in human gastric carcinomas and its clinical association. *Anticancer Res.* **2008**, *28*, 907–911. [PubMed]

34. Cancer Genome Atlas Research Network. Comprehensive molecular characterization of gastric adenocarcinoma. *Nature* **2014**, *513*, 202–209.

*J. Clin. Med.* **2015**, *4*, 1798–1814

35. Kang, S.M.; Choi, J.W.; Hong, S.H.; Lee, H.J. Up-regulation of microRNA* strands by their target transcripts. *Int. J. Mol. Sci.* **2013**, *14*, 13231–13240. [CrossRef] [PubMed]

36. Ro, S.; Park, C.; Young, D.; Sanders, K.M.; Yan, W. Tissue-dependent paired expression of miRNAs. *Nucleic Acids Res.* **2007**, *35*, 5944–5953. [CrossRef] [PubMed]

37. Schwarz, D.S.; Hutvagner, G.; Du, T.; Xu, Z.; Aronin, N.; Zamore, P.D. Asymmetry in the assembly of the RNAi enzyme complex. *Cell* **2003**, *115*, 199–208. [CrossRef]

38. Guo, L.; Zhang, H.; Zhao, Y.; Yang, S.; Chen, F. Selected isomiR expression profiles via arm switching? *Gene* **2014**, *533*, 149–155. [CrossRef] [PubMed]

39. Griffiths-Jones, S.; Hui, J.H.; Marco, A.; Ronshaugen, M. MicroRNA evolution by arm switching. *EMBO Rep.* **2011**, *12*, 172–177. [CrossRef] [PubMed]

40. Auyeung, V.C.; Ulitsky, I.; McGeary, S.E.; Bartel, D.P. Beyond secondary structure: Primary-sequence determinants license pri-miRNA hairpins for processing. *Cell* **2013**, *152*, 844–858. [CrossRef] [PubMed]

41. Larne, O.; Ostling, P.; Haflidadottir, B.S.; Hagman, Z.; Aakula, A.; Kohonen, P.; Kallioniemi, O.; Edsjo, A.; Bjartell, A.; Lilja, H.; *et al.* miR-183 in prostate cancer cells positively regulates synthesis and serum levels of prostate-specific antigen. *Eur. Urol.* **2015**, *68*, 581–588. [CrossRef] [PubMed]

42. Noh, J.H.; Chang, Y.G.; Kim, M.G.; Jung, K.H.; Kim, J.K.; Bae, H.J.; Eun, J.W.; Shen, Q.; Kim, S.J.; Kwon, S.H.; *et al.* miR-145 functions as a tumor suppressor by directly targeting histone deacetylase 2 in liver cancer. *Cancer Lett.* **2013**, *335*, 455–462. [CrossRef] [PubMed]

43. Tsai, K.W.; Hu, L.Y.; Wu, C.W.; Li, S.C.; Lai, C.H.; Kao, H.W.; Fang, W.L.; Lin, W.C. Epigenetic regulation of miR-196b expression in gastric cancer. *Genes Chromosomes Cancer* **2010**, *49*, 969–980. [CrossRef] [PubMed]

44. Wang, T.H.; Yeh, C.T.; Ho, J.Y.; Ng, K.F.; Chen, T.C. OncomiR miR-96 and miR-182 promote cell proliferation and invasion through targeting ephrinA5 in hepatocellular carcinoma. *Mol. Carcinog.* **2015**. [CrossRef] [PubMed]

45. Zhang, H.D.; Jiang, L.H.; Sun, D.W.; Li, J.; Tang, J.H. miR-139-5p: Promising biomarker for cancer. *Tumour. Biol.* **2015**, *36*, 1355–1365. [CrossRef] [PubMed]

46. Krishnan, K.; Steptoe, A.L.; Martin, H.C.; Pattabiraman, D.R.; Nones, K.; Waddell, N.; Mariasegaram, M.; Simpson, P.T.; Lakhani, S.R.; Vlassov, A.; *et al.* miR-139-5p is a regulator of metastatic pathways in breast cancer. *RNA* **2013**, *19*, 1767–1780. [CrossRef] [PubMed]

47. Uchino, K.; Takeshita, F.; Takahashi, R.U.; Kosaka, N.; Fujiwara, K.; Naruoka, H.; Sonoke, S.; Yano, J.; Sasaki, H.; Nozawa, S.; *et al.* Therapeutic effects of microRNA-582-5p and -3p on the inhibition of bladder cancer progression. *Mol. Ther.* **2013**, *21*, 610–619. [CrossRef] [PubMed]

48. Baraniskin, A.; Birkenkamp-Demtroder, K.; Maghnouj, A.; Zollner, H.; Munding, J.; Klein-Scory, S.; Reinacher-Schick, A.; Schwarte-Waldhoff, I.; Schmiegel, W.; Hahn, S.A. miR-30a-5p suppresses tumor growth in colon carcinoma by targeting DTL. *Carcinogenesis* **2012**, *33*, 732–739. [CrossRef] [PubMed]

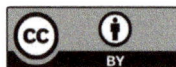

Journal of
*Clinical Medicine*

MDPI

*Article*

# Identification of Recurrence-Related microRNAs from Bone Marrow in Hepatocellular Carcinoma Patients

Keishi Sugimachi [1,2], Shotaro Sakimura [1], Akira Tomokuni [3], Ryutaro Uchi [1], Hidenari Hirata [1], Hisateru Komatsu [1], Yoshiaki Shinden [1], Tomohiro Iguchi [1], Hidetoshi Eguchi [1], Takaaki Masuda [1], Kazutoyo Morita [2], Ken Shirabe [4], Hidetoshi Eguchi [3], Yoshihiko Maehara [4], Masaki Mori [3] and Koshi Mimori [1,*]

[1] Department of Surgery, Kyushu University Beppu Hospital, 4546 Tsurumihara, Beppu 874-0838, Japan; sugimachi@beppu.kyushu-u.ac.jp (K.S.); z33sho2000@yahoo.co.jp (S.S.); ryuuchi@beppu.kyushu-u.ac.jp (R.U.); shusei_1300g7m7s@yahoo.co.jp (H.H.); komateru8312@gmail.com (H.K.); yshinden@beppu.kyushu-u.ac.jp (Y.S.); tomo@surg2.med.kyushu-u.ac.jp (T.I.); heguchi@beppu.kyushu-u.ac.jp (H.E.); takaakimas@yahoo.co.jp (T.M.)

[2] Department of Surgery, Fukuoka City Hospital, 13-1 Yoshizukahonmachi, Fukuoka 812-0046, Japan; kamorita@surg2.med.kyushu-u.ac.jp

[3] Department of Gastroenterological Surgery, Graduate School of Medicine, Osaka University, 2-2 Yamadaoka, Suita, Osaka 565-0871, Japan; akiratomokuni@gmail.com (A.T.); heguchi@gesurg.med.osaka-u.ac.jp (H.E.); mmori@gesurg.med.osaka-u.ac.jp (M.M.)

[4] Department of Surgery and Science Graduate School of Medical Sciences Kyushu University 3-1-1 Maidashi, Higashi-ku, Fukuoka 812-8582, Japan; kshirabe@surg2.med.kyushu-u.ac.jp (K.S.); maehara@surg2.med.kyushu-u.ac.jp (Y.M.)

\* Author to whom correspondence should be addressed; kmimori@beppu.kyushu-u.ac.jp; Tel.: +81-977-27-1650; Fax: +81-977-27-1651.

Academic Editors: Takahiro Ochiya and Ryou-u Takahashi
Received: 30 June 2015; Accepted: 5 August 2015; Published: 14 August 2015

**Abstract:** Hepatocellular carcinoma (HCC) is a poor-prognosis cancer due to its high rate of recurrence. microRNAs (miRNAs) are a class of small non-coding RNA molecules that affect crucial processes in cancer development. The objective of this study is to identify the role of miRNAs in patient bone marrow (BM) and explore the function of these molecules during HCC progression. We purified miRNAs from bone marrow cells of seven HCC patients, and divided them into three fractions by cell surface markers as follows: $CD14^+$ (macrophage), $CD14^-/CD45^+$ (lymphocyte), and $CD14^-/CD45^-/EpCAM^+$ (epithelial cell). We employed microarray-based profiling to analyze miRNA expression in the bone marrow of patients with HCC. Differentially expressed miRNAs were significantly different between fractions from whole bone marrow, macrophages, and lymphocytes, and depended on stages in tumor progression. Differences in expression of miRNAs associated with cell proliferation also varied significantly between HCC patients with recurrence, multiple tumors, and advanced clinical stages. These results suggest that miRNA profiles in separated fractions of BM cells are associated with HCC progression.

**Keywords:** bone marrow; microRNA; hepatocellular carcinoma; recurrence

## 1. Introduction

Hepatocellular carcinoma (HCC) is the fourth most common malignancy in Japan and the fifth worldwide. The mainstay of its treatment is hepatic resection with improved outcomes; however, HCC is still characterized by frequent recurrence [1,2]. microRNAs (miRNAs) are small (17–21 nt), non-coding RNAs that regulate gene expression at the post-transcriptional level through the RNA interference pathway. Currently, ~2000 miRNAs have been described in humans, and a single miRNA may regulate many mRNAs. Through this mechanism, miRNAs are essential components in the regulation of many cellular and developmental processes, including developmental timing, organ development, differentiation, proliferation, immune regulation, and cancer development and progression [3]. Depending upon their target gene(s) and level of expression, miRNAs may function as either oncogenes or tumor suppressors and assist in the promotion or suppression of cancer growth and progression [4,5].

We previously demonstrated that circulating miRNAs in serum extracellular vesicles (exosomes) could be novel biomarkers for predicting the recurrence and therapeutic targets of HCC [6,7]. Exosomes are small membrane vesicles (30–100 nm) derived from the luminal membranes of multivesicular bodies and are constitutively released by fusion with the cell membrane [8]. Exosomes transfer not only membrane components but also nucleic acids to other cells; therefore, cell-derived exosomes have recently been described as a new mode of cell-to-cell communication [9]. To date, 764 microRNAs (miRs) have been identified in exosomes derived from several different cell types and from multiple organisms [10]. In this light, exosomally transported miRNAs have found a place in cancer research as carriers of genetic information [11,12]. Functional exosomal miRs both from cancer cells and bone marrow (BM) mesenchymal stem cells have been reported [13,14], but in a previous study we could not show direct evidence that exosomal serum miRNA was secreted from either HCC cells or other host cells, such as BM-derived cells [6]. Here we briefly report the miRNA profile of BM cells to understand the role of miRNAs in the progression of HCC.

## 2. Materials and Methods

Seven patients who consecutively underwent hepatectomy for primary HCC were selected from records of the Department of Gastroenterological Surgery, Osaka University. The institutional review board approved this study and we obtained written informed consent from each patient. The median age of the seven patients was 60 years (range 37–72); the etiologies were hepatitis C infection in four cases, hepatitis B in two, and alcoholism in one. The number of tumors was single in five cases and multiple in two cases. After the median follow-up time of 22 months, three cases had recurrence of HCC while four cases had no recurrence. On the basis of the UICC classification (7th edition), three cases were classified as stage I, two cases as stage II, and two cases as stage IIIA.

Aspiration of BM was conducted under general anesthesia immediately before surgery, as previously described [15]. The BM aspirate was obtained from the sternum using a BM aspiration needle. A volume of 3 mL of BM was added to 4.0 mL of Isogen-LS (Nippon Gene, Toyama, Japan), which was shaken vigorously and stored at −80 °C until RNA extraction. BM cells were separated into three fractions using a three-step automagnetic-activated cell separation system (MACS) by MACS Cell Separators (Miltenyi Biotec, Bergisch Gladbach, Germany). CD45$^+$, CD14$^+$, and CD45$^-$/EpCAM$^+$ cell fractions were collected using CD45, CD14, and EpCAM (CD326) microbeads according to the manufacturer's instructions (Miltenyi Biotec).

RNA was extracted from each BM fraction separated by the Auto MACS system using the miRNeasy Mini Kit (Qiagen, Venlo, The Netherlands) according to the manufacturer's protocol. Extracted total RNA was labeled with Cy3 using the miRCURY LNA Array miR labeling kit (Exiqon, Vedbaek, Denmark). Labeled RNAs were hybridized onto 3D-Gene Human microRNA Oligo chips containing 837 anti-sense probes printed in duplicate spots (Toray, Kamakura, Japan). The annotation and oligonucleotide sequences of the probes conformed to the miRBase microRNA database (Faculty of Life Sciences, University of Manchester, Manchester, UK). After stringent washes, fluorescent signals were scanned with the 3D-Gene Scanner (Toray) and analyzed using GenePix Pro version 5.0 (Molecular Devices, Sunnyvale, CA, USA). The raw data from each spot were normalized by subtraction of the background signal mean intensity, determined by the 95% confidence intervals of the signal intensities of all blank spots. Valid measurements were considered those in which the signal intensity of both duplicate spots was greater than two standard deviations of the background signal intensity. MicroRNAs differentially expressed between groups were statistically identified using the Welch *t*-test. Data was uploaded in Gene Expression Omnibus datasets (GSE71762, National Center for Biotechnology Information, Bethesda, MD, USA).

## 3. Results and Discussion

### 3.1. Whole BM Fraction

miRNA profiles in the whole BM fraction are shown in Figure 1, depending on the recurrence factor, number of tumors, and clinical stage. Differentially expressed miRNAs were significantly different between fractions from whole bone marrow, macrophages, and lymphocytes (Table 1). Therefore, we further analyzed the miRNA profiles of macrophage and lymphocyte fractions. Our present data showed that miRNAs of selected fractions had to be independently analyzed with respect to the origin of the microRNAs present in the BM of HCC patients. miRNA processing may occur in the cancer cells themselves or in cells within the BM microenvironment, such as hematopoietic progenitor cells, endothelial cells, progenitor cells, and macrophages [16–18].

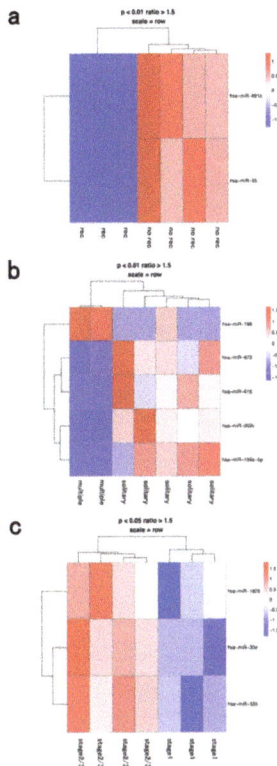

**Figure 1.** Hierarchical clustering analysis of microRNAs of whole bone marrow cells in seven patients with hepatocellular carcinoma. Heat map of the miRNA profile in bone marrow cells from hepatocellular carcinoma patients with (**a**) recurrence (*n* = 3) and no recurrence (*n* = 4); (**b**) solitary (*n* = 5) and multiple tumors (*n* = 2); (**c**) stage 1 (*n* = 3) and ≥stage 2 (*n* = 4). Cluster analysis showed two, five, and three miRNAs that were significantly differentially expressed between the two groups with a >1.50-fold change, respectively. Colors range from blue to red, corresponding to low to high expression, respectively. *p* values <0.01 or <0.05, unpaired *t* test. rec: recurrence.

**Table 1.** MicroRNAs in the bone marrow cells that were significantly correlated with clinical significance of HCC patients.

| BM Fraction | Clinical Significance | Upregulated microRNA | Downregulated microRNA |
|---|---|---|---|
| whole BM | recurrence | | hsa-mir-891b |
| | recurrence | | hsa-mir-95 |
| | multiple | hsa-mir-198 | hsa-mir-873 |
| | multiple | | hsa-mir-618 |
| | multiple | | hsa-mir-302c |
| | multiple | | hsa-mir-199a-5p |
| | stage 2≥ | hsa-mir-1825 | |
| | stage 2≥ | hsa-mir-30e | |
| | stage 2≥ | hsa-mir-335 | |
| lymphocyte | recurrence | hsa-mir-148a | hsa-mir-190 |
| | recurrence | hsa-mir-361-5p | hsa-mir-503 |
| | recurrence | hsa-mir-320d | hsa-mir-544 |
| | multiple | hsa-mir-654-5p | hsa-mir-517a |
| | multiple | | hsa-mir-497 |
| | multiple | | hsa-mir-454 |
| | multiple | | hsa-mir-22 |
| | stage 2≥ | hsa-mir-1537 | hsa-mir-345 |
| | stage 2≥ | hsa-mir-513b | hsa-mir-553 |
| | stage 2≥ | hsa-mir-15a | hsa-mir-653 |
| | stage 2≥ | hsa-mir-517a | hsa-mir-577 |
| | stage 2≥ | hsa-mir-28-5p | |
| macrophage | recurrence | hsa-mir-1207-3p | hsa-mir-1277 |
| | recurrence | hsa-mir-937 | hsa-mir-1279 |
| | recurrence | | hsa-mir-184 |
| | recurrence | | hsa-mir-563 |
| | recurrence | | hsa-mir-96 |
| | recurrence | | hsa-mir-302b |
| | multiple | hsa-mir-1 | hsa-mir-10b |
| | multiple | hsa-mir-889 | hsa-mir-204 |
| | multiple | hsa-mir-658 | hsa-mir-654-3p |
| | multiple | | hsa-mir-302a |
| | stage 2≥ | hsa-mir-555 | hsa-mir-942 |
| | stage 2≥ | hsa-mir-1293 | hsa-mir-1227 |
| | stage 2≥ | | hsa-mir-598 |
| | stage 2≥ | | hsa-mir-518d-3p |

BM: bone marrow.

### 3.2. Lymphocyte Fraction

Inflammation appears to be a crucial factor in hepatocarcinogenesis since HCC typically occurs in patients with chronic inflammatory liver diseases, such as viral hepatitis or non-alcoholic steatohepatitis [19,20]. One miR (hsa-miR-654-5p) was upregulated and four miRs (hsa-miR-517a, 497, 454, 22) were downregulated in the lymphocyte fraction of cases with multiple tumors compared to ones with a solitary tumor (Figure 2 and Table 1). miR-517a is located in the chromosome 19 miRNA cluster, and is considered to be a tumor-suppressive miRNA that is suppressed by epigenetic modifications [21]. miR-517a inhibited cell proliferation by blocking G2/M transition in HCC [21], and markedly induced bladder cancer cell apoptosis [22]. One of the target genes of miR-517a in HCC was reported to be Pyk2, which was associated with MAP kinase signaling pathways [23]. miR-497, clustered at 17p13.1, is also reported to be a tumor suppressor and shows significant growth-suppressive activity with induction of G1 arrest in HCC [24]. Potential target genes of miR-497 in cancers had been reported to be insulin-like growth factor 1 receptor, WEE1, HDGF, VEGF-A, Akt, and IKKβ [25–28].

*3.3. Macrophage Fraction*

Two miRNAs were upregulated (hsa-miR-1207-3p, 937) and six miRNAs (hsa-miR-1277, 1279, 184, 563, 96, 302b) were downregulated in the macrophage fractions from cases with post-operative recurrence compared to fractions from cases with no recurrence (Figure 3 and Table 1).

Previous studies have shown that miR-184 can act either as an oncogenic- or a tumor suppressive-miRNA in various human cancers, depending on cellular context [29,30]. Lin *et al.* reported that decreased miR-184 promotes cancer cell invasiveness by an increase in CDC25A and c-myc expression [31]. In HCC, miR-302b acts as a tumor suppressor by targeting AKT2, suppressing G1 regulators (Cyclin A, Cyclin D1, CDK2) and increasing p27Kip1 phosphorylation at Ser10 [32]. Recent studies have revealed that tumor-associated macrophages (TAMs) are an important component of the tumor microenvironment and can promote tumor progression [35,36]. TAMs were reported to be associated with metastasis, angiogenesis, epithelial-mesenchymal transition (EMT), and poor prognosis in HCC [35,37,38]. Macrophages have multiple biological roles, including antigen presentation, target cell cytotoxicity, removal of foreign bodies, tissue remodeling, regulation of inflammation, induction of immunity, thrombosis, and endocytosis. Aucher *et al.* recently reported that transfer of miRNAs from macrophages functionally inhibited proliferation of HCC cells [39]. Although the mechanisms by which TAMs promote tumor progression are poorly understood, our data implied that they might act through altered miRNA expression.

## 4. Conclusions

These results suggest that miRNA profiles in separated fractions of bone marrow cells are associated with metastasis, angiogenesis, epithelial-mesenchymal transition (EMT), and poor prognosis in HCC. In this study, the number of cases was small, therefore our data are preliminary and further analysis including validation studies with large cohorts and *in vitro* studies to search target genes and pathways of identified miRNAs are warranted. We revealed the miR profiling of BM cells associated with stage/recurrence of HCC in this study. It is possible that miR profiling of BM niche was affected by the progression of HCC or disseminated cancer cells. On the other hand, altered miR expression of BM cells might help the survival or proliferation of cancer cells in BM. At present, it is difficult to conclude that one specific mechanism is superior to others, and further studies are recommended. Our data could provide a database to seek new concepts in immunotherapy targeting miRNAs of BM cells to improve the outcome of patients with HCC in the near future.

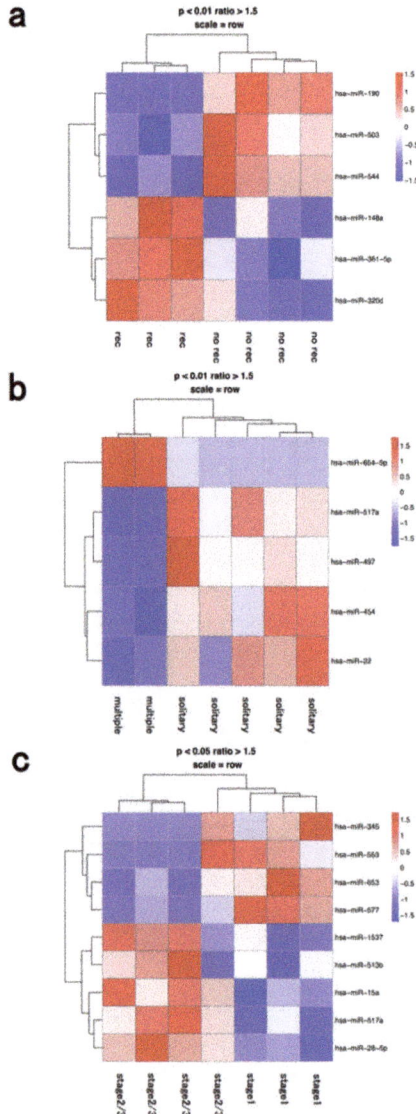

**Figure 2.** Hierarchical clustering analysis of microRNAs of lymphocyte fraction in seven patients with hepatocellular carcinoma. Heat map of the miRNA profile in macrophages from hepatocellular carcinoma patients with (**a**) recurrence (*n* = 3) and no recurrence (*n* = 4); (**b**) solitary (*n* = 5) and multiple tumors (*n* = 2); (**c**) stage 1 (*n* = 3) and ≥stage 2 (*n* = 4). Cluster analysis showed six, five, and nine miRNAs that were significantly differentially expressed between the two groups with a >1.50-fold change, respectively. Colors range from blue to red, corresponding to low to high expression, respectively. *p* values <0.01 or <0.05, unpaired *t* test. rec: recurrence.

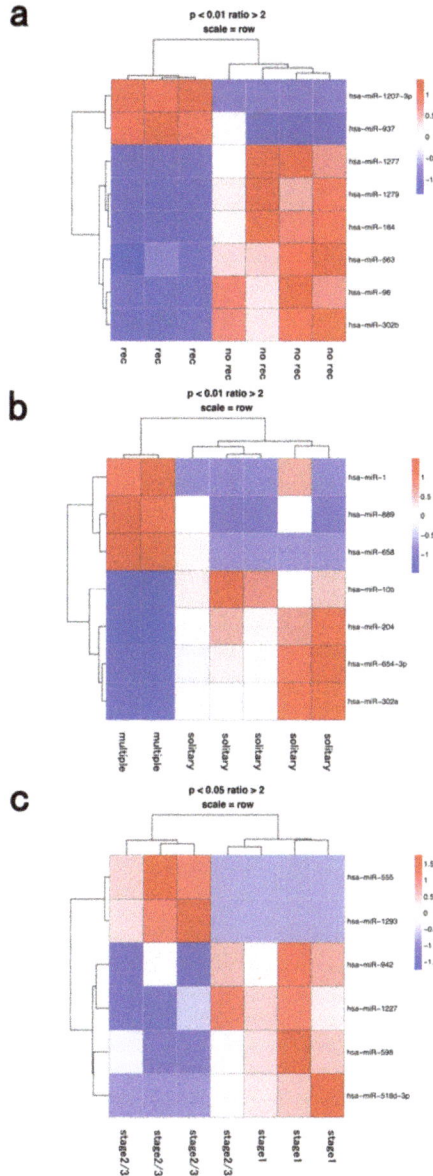

**Figure 3.** Hierarchical clustering analysis of microRNAs of macrophage fraction in seven patients with hepatocellular carcinoma. Heat map of the miRNA profile in lymphocytes from hepatocellular carcinoma patients with (**a**) recurrence (*n* = 3) and no recurrence (*n* = 4); (**b**) solitary (*n* = 5) and multiple tumors (*n* = 2); (**c**) stage 1 (*n* = 3) and ≥stage 2 (*n* = 4). Cluster analysis showed eight, seven, and six miRNAs that were significantly differentially expressed between the two groups with a >2-fold change, respectively. Colors range from blue to red, corresponding to low to high expression, respectively. *p* values <0.01 or <0.05, unpaired *t* test. rec: recurrence.

**Acknowledgments:** We thank Kazumi Oda, Michiko Kasagi, Satoko Kohno, and Tomoko Kawano for their technical assistance. This work was supported in part by the following grants and foundations: Japan Society for the Promotion of Science (JSPS) Grant-in-Aid for Scientific Research, grant number 24592005, and Grant-in Aid for Young Scientists S, grant number 21679006.

**Author Contributions:** Keishi Sugimachi, Shotaro Sakimura and Koshi Mimori contribute to conception and design of the study, the acquisition of data and writing the manuscript. Akira Tomokuni and Hidetoshi Eguchi (Osaka University) contribute to the collection of samples and the acquisition of data. Ryutaro Uchi, Hidenari Hirata, Hisateru Komatsu, Yoshiaki Shinden, Tomohiro Iguchi, Hidetoshi Eguchi (Kyushu University), Takaaki Masuda and Kazutoyo Morita contribute to the analysis of data. Ken Shirabe, Yoshihiko Maehara and Masaki Mori contribute to the interpretation of data.

**Conflicts of Interest:** Keishi Sugimachi and co-authors have no conflicts of interest.

## References

1. Okita, K. Clinical aspects of hepatocellular carcinoma in japan. *Intern. Med.* **2006**, *45*, 229–233. [CrossRef] [PubMed]
2. Llovet, J.M. Updated treatment approach to hepatocellular carcinoma. *J. Gastroenterol.* **2005**, *40*, 225–235. [CrossRef] [PubMed]
3. Croce, C.M. Causes and consequences of microRNA dysregulation in cancer. *Nat. Rev. Genet.* **2009**, *10*, 704–714. [CrossRef] [PubMed]
4. Morita, K.; Taketomi, A.; Shirabe, K.; Umeda, K.; Kayashima, H.; Ninomiya, M.; Uchiyama, H.; Soejima, Y.; Maehara, Y. Clinical significance and potential of hepatic microRNA-122 expression in hepatitis c. *Liver Int.* **2011**, *31*, 474–484. [CrossRef] [PubMed]
5. Calin, G.A.; Croce, C.M. MicroRNA signatures in human cancers. *Nat. Revi. Cancer* **2006**, *6*, 857–866. [CrossRef] [PubMed]
6. Sugimachi, K.; Matsumura, T.; Hirata, H.; Uchi, R.; Ueda, M.; Ueo, H.; Shinden, Y.; Iguchi, T.; Eguchi, H.; Shirabe, K.; *et al.* Identification of a bona fide microRNA biomarker in serum exosomes that predicts hepatocellular carcinoma recurrence after liver transplantation. *Br. J. Cancer* **2015**, *112*, 532–538. [CrossRef] [PubMed]
7. Matsumura, T.; Sugimachi, K.; Iinuma, H.; Takahashi, Y.; Kurashige, J.; Sawada, G.; Ueda, M.; Uchi, R.; Ueo, H.; Takano, Y.; *et al.* Exosomal microRNA in serum is a novel biomarker of recurrence in human colorectal cancer. *Br. J. Cancer* **2015**, *113*, 275–281. [CrossRef] [PubMed]
8. Simons, M.; Raposo, G. Exosomes—Vesicular carriers for intercellular communication. *Curr. Opin. Cell Biol.* **2009**, *21*, 575–581. [CrossRef] [PubMed]
9. Peinado, H.; Aleckovic, M.; Lavotshkin, S.; Matei, I.; Costa-Silva, B.; Moreno-Bueno, G.; Hergueta-Redondo, M.; Williams, C.; Garcia-Santos, G.; Ghajar, C.; *et al.* Melanoma exosomes educate bone marrow progenitor cells toward a pro-metastatic phenotype through met. *Nat. Med.* **2012**, *18*, 883–891. [CrossRef] [PubMed]
10. Mathivanan, S.; Fahner, C.J.; Reid, G.E.; Simpson, R.J. Exocarta 2012: Database of exosomal proteins, RNA and lipids. *Nucleic Acids Res.* **2012**, *40*, D1241–D1244. [CrossRef] [PubMed]
11. Valadi, H.; Ekstrom, K.; Bossios, A.; Sjostrand, M.; Lee, J.J.; Lotvall, J.O. Exosome-mediated transfer of mRNAs and microRNAs is a novel mechanism of genetic exchange between cells. *Nat. Cell Biol.* **2007**, *9*, 654–659. [CrossRef] [PubMed]
12. Hannafon, B.N.; Ding, W.Q. Intercellular communication by exosome-derived microRNAs in cancer. *Int. J. Mol. Sci.* **2013**, *14*, 14240–14269. [CrossRef] [PubMed]
13. Cereghetti, D.M.; Lee, P.P. Tumor-derived exosomes contain microRNAs with immunological function: Implications for a novel immunosuppression mechanism. *MicroRNA (Shariqah, United Arab Emirates)* **2014**, *2*, 194–204. [CrossRef]
14. Ono, M.; Kosaka, N.; Tominaga, N.; Yoshioka, Y.; Takeshita, F.; Takahashi, R.U.; Yoshida, M.; Tsuda, H.; Tamura, K.; Ochiya, T. Exosomes from bone marrow mesenchymal stem cells contain a microRNA that promotes dormancy in metastatic breast cancer cells. *Sci. Signal.* **2014**, *7*, ra63. [CrossRef] [PubMed]
15. Mimori, K.; Fukagawa, T.; Kosaka, Y.; Ishikawa, K.; Iwatsuki, M.; Yokobori, T.; Hirasaki, S.; Takatsuno, Y.; Sakashita, H.; Ishii, H.; *et al.* A large-scale study of mt1-mmp as a marker for isolated tumor cells in peripheral blood and bone marrow in gastric cancer cases. *Ann. Surg. Oncol.* **2008**, *15*, 2934–2942. [CrossRef] [PubMed]

16. Ota, D.; Mimori, K.; Yokobori, T.; Iwatsuki, M.; Kataoka, A.; Masuda, N.; Ishii, H.; Ohno, S.; Mori, M. Identification of recurrence-related microRNAs in the bone marrow of breast cancer patients. *Int. J. Oncol.* **2011**, *38*, 955–962. [PubMed]

17. Akiyoshi, S.; Fukagawa, T.; Ueo, H.; Ishibashi, M.; Takahashi, Y.; Fabbri, M.; Sasako, M.; Maehara, Y.; Mimori, K.; Mori, M. Clinical significance of mir-144-zfx axis in disseminated tumour cells in bone marrow in gastric cancer cases. *Br. J. Cancer* **2012**, *107*, 1345–1353. [CrossRef] [PubMed]

18. Takeyama, H.; Yamamoto, H.; Yamashita, S.; Wu, X.; Takahashi, H.; Nishimura, J.; Haraguchi, N.; Miyake, Y.; Suzuki, R.; Murata, K.; *et al.* Decreased mir-340 expression in bone marrow is associated with liver metastasis of colorectal cancer. *Mol. Cancer Ther.* **2014**, *13*, 976–985. [CrossRef] [PubMed]

19. Shirabe, K.; Mano, Y.; Muto, J.; Matono, R.; Motomura, T.; Toshima, T.; Takeishi, K.; Uchiyama, H.; Yoshizumi, T.; Taketomi, A.; *et al.* Role of tumor-associated macrophages in the progression of hepatocellular carcinoma. *Surg. Today* **2012**, *42*, 1–7. [CrossRef] [PubMed]

20. Mossanen, J.C.; Tacke, F. Role of lymphocytes in liver cancer. *Oncoimmunology* **2013**, *2*, e26468. [CrossRef] [PubMed]

21. Liu, R.F.; Xu, X.; Huang, J.; Fei, Q.L.; Chen, F.; Li, Y.D.; Han, Z.G. Down-regulation of mir-517a and mir-517c promotes proliferation of hepatocellular carcinoma cells via targeting pyk2. *Cancer Lett.* **2013**, *329*, 164–173. [CrossRef] [PubMed]

22. Yoshitomi, T.; Kawakami, K.; Enokida, H.; Chiyomaru, T.; Kagara, I.; Tatarano, S.; Yoshino, H.; Arimura, H.; Nishiyama, K.; Seki, N.; *et al.* Restoration of mir-517a expression induces cell apoptosis in bladder cancer cell lines. *Oncol. Rep.* **2011**, *25*, 1661–1668. [PubMed]

23. Sun, C.K.; Man, K.; Ng, K.T.; Ho, J.W.; Lim, Z.X.; Cheng, Q.; Lo, C.M.; Poon, R.T.; Fan, S.T. Proline-rich tyrosine kinase 2 (pyk2) promotes proliferation and invasiveness of hepatocellular carcinoma cells through c-src/erk activation. *Carcinogenesis* **2008**, *29*, 2096–2105. [CrossRef] [PubMed]

24. Furuta, M.; Kozaki, K.; Tanimoto, K.; Tanaka, S.; Arii, S.; Shimamura, T.; Niida, A.; Miyano, S.; Inazawa, J. The tumor-suppressive mir-497-195 cluster targets multiple cell-cycle regulators in hepatocellular carcinoma. *PLoS ONE* **2013**, *8*, e60155. [CrossRef] [PubMed]

25. Creevey, L.; Ryan, J.; Harvey, H.; Bray, I.M.; Meehan, M.; Khan, A.R.; Stallings, R.L. MicroRNA-497 increases apoptosis in mycn amplified neuroblastoma cells by targeting the key cell cycle regulator wee1. *Mol. Cancer* **2013**, *12*, 23. [CrossRef] [PubMed]

26. Guo, S.T.; Jiang, C.C.; Wang, G.P.; Li, Y.P.; Wang, C.Y.; Guo, X.Y.; Yang, R.H.; Feng, Y.; Wang, F.H.; Tseng, H.Y.; *et al.* MicroRNA-497 targets insulin-like growth factor 1 receptor and has a tumour suppressive role in human colorectal cancer. *Oncogene* **2013**, *32*, 1910–1920. [CrossRef] [PubMed]

27. Kong, X.J.; Duan, L.J.; Qian, X.Q.; Xu, D.; Liu, H.L.; Zhu, Y.J.; Qi, J. Tumor-suppressive microRNA-497 targets ikkbeta to regulate NF-kappab signaling pathway in human prostate cancer cells. *Am. J. Cancer Res.* **2015**, *5*, 1795–1804. [PubMed]

28. Shao, X.J.; Miao, M.H.; Xue, J.; Xue, J.; Ji, X.Q.; Zhu, H. The down-regulation of microRNA-497 contributes to cell growth and cisplatin resistance through pi3k/akt pathway in osteosarcoma. *Cell Physiol. Biochem.* **2015**, *36*, 2051–2062. [CrossRef] [PubMed]

29. Phua, Y.W.; Nguyen, A.; Roden, D.L.; Elsworth, B.; Deng, N.; Nikolic, I.; Yang, J.; McFarland, A.; Russell, R.; Kaplan, W.; *et al.* MicroRNA profiling of the pubertal mouse mammary gland identifies mir-184 as a candidate breast tumour suppressor gene. *Breast Cancer Res.* **2015**, *17*, 83. [CrossRef] [PubMed]

30. Wong, T.S.; Liu, X.B.; Wong, B.Y.; Ng, R.W.; Yuen, A.P.; Wei, W.I. Mature mir-184 as potential oncogenic microRNA of squamous cell carcinoma of tongue. *Clinical cancer research : an official journal of the American Association for Cancer Research* **2008**, *14*, 2588–2592. [CrossRef] [PubMed]

31. Lin, T.C.; Lin, P.L.; Cheng, Y.W.; Wu, T.C.; Chou, M.C.; Chen, C.Y.; Lee, H. MicroRNA-184 deregulated by the microRNA-21 promotes tumor malignancy and poor outcomes in non-small cell lung cancer via targeting cdc25a and c-myc. *Ann. Surg. Oncol.* **2015**. [CrossRef] [PubMed]

32. Wang, L.; Yao, J.; Zhang, X.; Guo, B.; Le, X.; Cubberly, M.; Li, Z.; Nan, K.; Song, T.; Huang, C. MiRNA-302b suppresses human hepatocellular carcinoma by targeting akt2. *Mol. Cancer Res.* **2014**, *12*, 190–202. [CrossRef] [PubMed]

33. Wang, L.; Zhu, M.J.; Ren, A.M.; Wu, H.F.; Han, W.M.; Tan, R.Y.; Tu, R.Q. A ten-microRNA signature identified from a genome-wide microRNA expression profiling in human epithelial ovarian cancer. *PLoS ONE* **2014**, *9*, e96472. [CrossRef] [PubMed]

34. Ujihira, T.; Ikeda, K.; Suzuki, T.; Yamaga, R.; Sato, W.; Horie-Inoue, K.; Shigekawa, T.; Osaki, A.; Saeki, T.; Okamoto, K.; *et al.* MicroRNA-574-3p, identified by microRNA library-based functional screening, modulates tamoxifen response in breast cancer. *Sci. Rep.* **2015**, *5*, 7641. [CrossRef] [PubMed]

35. Shirabe, K.; Motomura, T.; Muto, J.; Toshima, T.; Matono, R.; Mano, Y.; Takeishi, K.; Ijichi, H.; Harada, N.; Uchiyama, H.; *et al.* Tumor-infiltrating lymphocytes and hepatocellular carcinoma: Pathology and clinical management. *Int. J. Clin. Oncol.* **2010**, *15*, 552–558. [CrossRef] [PubMed]

36. De Visser, K.E.; Eichten, A.; Coussens, L.M. Paradoxical roles of the immune system during cancer development. *Nat. Rev. Cancer* **2006**, *6*, 24–37. [CrossRef] [PubMed]

37. Rolny, C.; Capparuccia, L.; Casazza, A.; Mazzone, M.; Vallario, A.; Cignetti, A.; Medico, E.; Carmeliet, P.; Comoglio, P.M.; Tamagnone, L. The tumor suppressor semaphorin 3b triggers a prometastatic program mediated by interleukin 8 and the tumor microenvironment. *J. Exp. Med.* **2008**, *205*, 1155–1171. [CrossRef] [PubMed]

38. Van Zijl, F.; Mair, M.; Csiszar, A.; Schneller, D.; Zulehner, G.; Huber, H.; Eferl, R.; Beug, H.; Dolznig, H.; Mikulits, W. Hepatic tumor-stroma crosstalk guides epithelial to mesenchymal transition at the tumor edge. *Oncogene* **2009**, *28*, 4022–4033. [CrossRef] [PubMed]

39. Aucher, A.; Rudnicka, D.; Davis, D.M. MicroRNAs transfer from human macrophages to hepato-carcinoma cells and inhibit proliferation. *J. Immunol. (Baltimore, Md.: 1950)* **2013**, *191*, 6250–6260. [CrossRef] [PubMed]

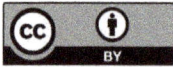

Journal of
*Clinical Medicine*

MDPI

*Article*

# A Circulating MicroRNA Signature as a Biomarker for Prostate Cancer in a High Risk Group

Brian D. Kelly [1,2,*], Nicola Miller [1], Karl J. Sweeney [1], Garrett C. Durkan [2], Eamon Rogers [2], Killian Walsh [2] and Michael J. Kerin [1]

[1] Department of Surgery, Clinical Science Institute, National University of Ireland, Galway, Ireland;
nicola.miller@nuigalway.ie (N.M.); karljsweeney@gmail.com (K.J.S.); michael.kerin@nuigalway.ie (M.J.K.)

[2] Department of Urology, Galway University Hospital, Galway, Ireland;
Garrett.Durkan@mailn.hse.ie (G.C.D.); emacruairi@me.com (E.R.); kilian.walsh@gmail.com (K.W.)

* Author to whom correspondence should be addressed; drbriankelly@hotmail.com;
Tel.: +353-85-7212337; Fax: +353-91-544130.

Academic Editors: Takahiro Ochiya and Ryou-u Takahashi
Received: 12 April 2015; Accepted: 18 June 2015; Published: 7 July 2015

**Abstract:** Introduction: Mi(cro)RNAs are small non-coding RNAs whose differential expression in tissue has been implicated in the development and progression of many malignancies, including prostate cancer. The discovery of miRNAs in the blood of patients with a variety of malignancies makes them an ideal, novel biomarker for prostate cancer diagnosis. The aim of this study was to identify a unique expression profile of circulating miRNAs in patients with prostate cancer attending a rapid access prostate assessment clinic. Methods: To conduct this study blood and tissue samples were collected from 102 patients (75 with biopsy confirmed cancer and 27 benign samples) following ethical approval and informed consent. These patients were attending a prostate assessment clinic. Samples were reverse-transcribed using stem-loop primers and expression levels of each of 12 candidate miRNAs were determined using real-time quantitative polymerase chain reaction. miRNA expression levels were then correlated with clinicopathological data and subsequently analysed using qBasePlus software and Minitab. Results: Circulating miRNAs were detected and quantified in all subjects. The analysis of miRNA mean expression levels revealed that four miRNAs were significantly dysregulated, including *let-7a* ($p = 0.005$) which has known tumour suppressor characteristics, along with *miR-141* ($p = 0.01$) which has oncogenic characteristics. In 20 patients undergoing a radical retropubic-prostatectomy, the expression levels of *miR-141* returned to normal at day 10 post-operatively. A panel of four miRNAs could be used in combination to detect prostate cancer with an area under the curve (AUC) of 0.783 and a PPV of 80%. Conclusion: These findings identify a unique expression profile of miRNA detectable in the blood of prostate cancer patients. This confirms their use as a novel, diagnostic biomarker for prostate cancer.

**Keywords:** prostate cancer; circulation; microRNA

## 1. Introduction

Prostate cancer is the most commonly diagnosed non-cutaneous malignancy in men and is the second leading cause of cancer death [1]. It is estimated that up to one in six men will be diagnosed with prostate cancer during their lifetime [2]. Clinicians use a combination of a digital rectal examination (DRE) and a prostate specific antigen (PSA) and a transrectal ultrasound guided prostate biopsy (TRUS) to detect prostate cancer. However, prostate cancer screening trials, such as The Prostate, Lung, Colorectal and Ovarian cancer screening trial (PLCO) and the European Randomised Study of Screening for Prostate cancer (ERSPC) trials, have highlighted that despite an increase in the diagnosis of prostate cancer using these tests, there is still no clear improvement in mortality [3,4]. In addition,

*J. Clin. Med.* **2015**, *4*, 1369–1379

PSA, a frequently used biomarker for the detection of prostate cancer, is limited by its lack of sensitivity and specificity for prostate cancer and therefore not considered an ideal biomarker. As a result, a search for a novel, minimally invasive, clinically relevant biomarkers for the detection of prostate cancer is required.

mi(cro)RNAs are small non-coding endogenous RNA molecules that vary in length from 18–25 nucleotides. There are numerous dysregulated miRNAs that are implicated in the pathogenesis of cancer and have been shown to regulate gene expression and function at the transcriptional and post-transcriptional level. They play a pivotal role in the expression of up to 60% of human genes [5]. miRNAs can be up or down-regulated, with up-regulation of oncogenic miRNAs and down-regulation of tumour suppressor miRNAs are demonstrated in a variety of malignancies. Dysregulation of miRNA has been associated with the pathogenesis of different cancers and approximately up to 50% of miRNA genes are located in cancer-related genomic regions [6]. Despite their small size miRNAs are extremely stable molecules and have been identified and quantified in RNA extracted from formalin fixed paraffin embedded tissue samples that have been stored for many years [7]. miRNAs are remarkably stable in the circulation and are protected from endogenous ribonuclease (RNase) activity and from variations in pH and temperature [8].

A number of studies have identified that there are numerous miRNAs that are dysregulated in prostate cancer tissue [9–12]. More recently, studies have identified that dysregulated miRNAs are also detectable in the circulation of patients with differing malignancies [13,14]. Specific to prostate cancer, Mitchell *et al.* identified that epithelial cancers release miRNAs into the circulation and that *miR-141* could identify those patients with metastatic prostate cancer from healthy controls [8]. As a result, miRNAs have the potential to be a novel, stable, non-invasive biomarker.

The primary aim of this study was to investigate if a miRNA signature was detectable that was unique to patients with prostate cancer in comparison with patients with benign prostatic histology attending a prostate assessment clinic. Secondary aims were to assess if there is a correlation between circulating levels of miRNAs and increasing risk stratification of prostate cancer as per the D'Amico risk stratification and also if the miRNA signature returned to normal after a radical prostatectomy [15].

## 2. Materials and Methods

### 2.1. Patients

Ethical approval was granted for the collection of blood samples and tissue samples by the Ethics committee at Galway University Hospital. Patients were recruited from the rapid access prostate assessment clinic (RAPAC) at Galway University Hospital tertiary referral cancer centre. Informed written consent was obtained from each patient prior to the collection of samples. Men were referred to the RAPAC if they had an elevated PSA, an abnormal DRE or a family history of prostate cancer. Histological diagnosis was made following a 12 core TRUS biopsy of the prostate.

### 2.2. Blood Collection and Storage

Whole blood samples were prospectively obtained from patients prior to TRUS biopsy and collected in 10 mL Ethylenediaminetetraacetic acid (EDTA) tubes. Samples were collected between September 2009 and March 2011 and stored at 4 °C until RNA extraction occurred. Whole blood was selected for analysis as this has previously been shown to have high yields of RNA and higher expression levels of miRNAs [16]. Relevant clinicopathological data was obtained from a prospectively maintained prostate cancer database.

### 2.3. Selected miRNA Targets

miRNAs are ideal molecules for a blood-based biomarkers for the detection of cancer, as they are dysregulated in carcinogenesis and are highly stable in both tissue and in blood samples. Various studies have documented the differential expression of miRNAs in the circulation of patients with cancer when compared with non-cancer patients and healthy controls, making miRNA an ideal non-invasive biomarker. Not all miRNAs that are dysregulated in prostate cancer tissue are released into the circulation. The exact mechanism by which miRNAs are released still remains unclear. miRNAs could be passively leaked or actively secreted into the circulation. Passive leakage can occur by tissue degradation associated with malignancy, through this mechanism miRNAs could be released into the circulation in an energy free mechanism.

A panel of 12 miRNAs were selected for miRNA expression profiling. They were selected on the basis of previously reported dysregulated expression levels in prostate tumour samples and in the circulation of prostate and other cancers and also based on information gleaned from previous studies within the Discipline of Surgery at NUI Galway [8,11,14,17–19]. The miRNAs investigated included *miR-16, -21, -34a, -141, -143, -145, -155, -125b, -221, -375, -425* and *let7a* (see Table 1).

**Table 1.** The 12 miRNAs selected for the expression profiling in the circulation.

| Dysregulated miRNA | Source | References |
|---|---|---|
| *let-7a* | Blood, Tissue | Heneghan *et al.* [14]; Volinia *et al.* [19]; Porkka *et al.* [11]; Tong *et al.* [31] |
| *miR-21* | Blood, Tissue | Zhang *et al.* [30]; Yaman Agaoglu *et al.* [26]; Volinia *et al.* [19]; Ozen *et al.* [32] |
| *miR-34a* | Tissue | Ambs *et al.* [18]; Ozen *et al.* [32] |
| *miR-125b* | Blood, Tissue | Mitchell *et al.* [8]; Porkka *et al.* [11]; Ozen *et al.* [32]; Tong *et al.* [31]; Schaefer *et al.* [33]; Spahn *et al.* [34] |
| *miR-141* | Blood, Tissue | Mitchell *et al.* [8]; Brase *et al.* [17]; Porkka *et al.* [11] |
| *miR-143* | Blood, Tissue | Mitchell *et al.* [8]; Porkka *et al.* [11]; Tong *et al.* [31] |
| *miR-145* | Blood, Tissue | Heneghan *et al.* [14]; Porkka *et al.* [11]; Ozen *et al.* [32], Ambs *et al.* [18]; Tong *et al.* [31]; Schaefer *et al.* [33] |
| *miR-155* | Blood | Heneghan *et al.* [14] |
| *miR-221* | Blood, Tissue | Yaman Agaoglu *et al.* [26]; Zheng *et al.* [35]; Porkka *et al.* [11]; Ambs *et al.* [18]; Ozen *et al.* [32]; Tong *et al.* [31]; Schaefer *et al.* [33]; Spahn *et al.* [34] |
| *miR-375* | Blood, Tissue | Brase *et al.* [17]; Schaefer *et al.* [33] |
| *miR-16* | Blood, Tissue | Lawrie *et al.* [21]; Heneghan *et al.* [14]; Huang *et al.* [22]; Liu *et al.* [20]; Wong *et al.* [24] |
| *miR-425* | Tissue | Chang *et al.* [25] |

*2.4. RNA Extraction*

Total RNA was extracted from 102 samples using TRI Reagent BD (Molecular Research Centre Inc., Cincinnati, OH, USA), from 1 mL of whole blood. The concentration of the RNA was ascertained using Nanodrop spectrophotometry (Nanodrop ND-1000 Technologies Inc., Wilmington, DE, USA). Extracted RNA was subsequently stored at −80 °C.

*2.5. Reverse Transcription and RQ-PCR*

100 ng of total RNA was reversed transcribed to cDNA using stem loop primers specific to each target miRNA of interest. RQ-PCR was performed using Taqman primers and probes (Applied Biosystems, Foster City, USA) on a 7900 HT Fast Real-Time PCR System (Applied Biosystems). RQ-PCR was performed on all samples in triplicate and interassay controls were used throughout. The threshold standard deviation for each of the replicates was taken at 0.3 for both samples and interassay controls.

PCR amplification efficiencies were calculated for each individual miRNA using the following equation: $E = (10^{-1/slope} - 1) \times 100$. The efficiency threshold was calculated at $+/-10\%$ across a 10-fold dilution series across five points. The relative miRNA expression levels ($\Delta\Delta Ct$) were calculated relative to endogenous controls, *miR-16* and *miR-425*. These were selected from a panel of miRNAs based on their stability and minimal variation across 66 benign and malignant blood samples (data not shown).

*2.6. Statistical Analysis*

QBasePlus was utilised to calculate the miRNA expression levels. Statistical analysis was performed using Minitab v16. The 2 sample t-test was used to compare the miRNA expression levels of cancer cases with benign cases. An analysis of variance (ANOVA) was used to analyse miRNA expression levels across factors of interest. A *p*-value of <0.05 was considered as significant with a Bonferroni correction. Binary logistic regression analysis was used to calculate an area under the curve (AUC) for combined miRNAs to determine their sensitivity and specificity.

## 3. Results

*3.1. Patient Demographics*

A total of 102 patients were selected at random and included in this study. Following TRUS biopsy 75 men were subsequently diagnosed with prostate cancer (median age 64 years, median PSA 7.4 μg/L) and 27 had a benign histological finding (median age 65 years, median PSA 7.45 μg/L). There was no significant difference between the PSA levels of the benign or cancer group, as most patients were referred with an elevated PSA level (see Table 2). Twenty eight patients had Gleason score 6, 34 had Gleason score 7, six had Gleason score 8 and seven patients had Gleason score 9 prostate cancer. In terms of risk stratification, there were 28 men with low-risk, 11 with intermediate-risk and 36 with high-risk prostate cancer (see Table 3). Within the benign group, men with a persistently elevated PSA underwent a second biopsy. We appreciate that there is a high cancer detection rate within this group and there is a high incidence of high grade disease which is a fair representation of the men referred to our service.

**Table 2.** Patient demographics.

|  | Benign | Cancer |
|---|---|---|
| Numbers (102) | 27 | 75 |
| Age |  |  |
| Median | 65 years | 64 years |
| Range | 48–80 years | 48–85 years |
| PSA (prostate specific antigen) |  |  |
| Median | 7.45 μg/L | 7.4 μg/L |
| Range | 1–77 μg/L | 1.42–52.24 μg/L |

**Table 3.** Histology, D'Amico risk stratification and dysregulated miRNAs.

| Histology | Numbers (102) | Risk Stratification | Numbers (75) |
|---|---|---|---|
| Benign | 27 | Low | 28 |
| 3 + 3 | 28 | Intermediate | 11 |
| 3 + 4 | 20 | | |
| 4 + 3 | 14 | High | 36 |
| 4 + 4 | 6 | | |
| 4 + 5 | 7 | | |

| miRNA | Up or Down Regulated | *p* Value | AUC (area under the curve) |
|---|---|---|---|
| *let-7a* | ↓ | 0.005 | 0.678 |
| *miR-141* | ↑ | 0.014 | 0.655 |
| *miR-145* | ↑ | 0.01 | 0.634 |
| *miR-155* | ↑ | 0.01 | 0.624 |
| *miR-375* | ↑ | 0.075 | 0.651 |

Of the 12 miRNAs quantified, there were four significant miRNAs ($p < 0.05$) (see Table 3). Three of these miRNAs were up-regulation of oncomirs (*miR-141, -145* and *-155*) and down-regulation of the tumour-suppressor *let7a* in patients with prostate cancer as compared with benign disease (see Figure 1). There was a trend towards significance for the oncomir *miR-375*, which was upregulated in patients with prostate cancer ($p = 0.07$).

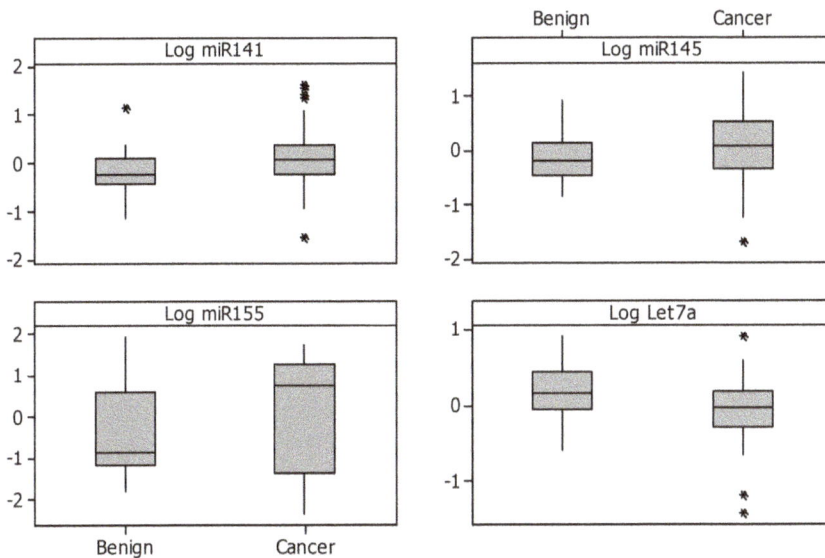

**Figure 1.** Boxplots of the four dysregulated miRNAs.

### 3.2. miRNAs as a Predictive Marker of Prostate Cancer

Of the 12 miRNAs investigated, four miRNAs were able to distinguish those with prostate cancer ($n = 75$) from those without ($n = 27$). To further investigate the diagnostic potential of these miRNAs, receiver operator curves (ROC) were generated for each and the AUCs were calculated as the measure of their accuracy. These include *let7a*, *miR-141, -145* and *-155*, with an AUC of 0.678, 0.655, 0.634 and 0.624 respectively (see Table 3). The oncomir *miR-141* had a sensitivity of 94% and a positive predictive value (PPV) of 73%. The tumour-suppressor *let7a* had a sensitivity of 93% and a positive predictive value (PPV) of 70%.

### 3.3. miRNAs in Combination

Using regression analysis, expression patterns were analysed in combination using the miRNAs as a diagnostic panel to improve upon the sensitivity. Using the four miRNAs mentioned above (*let-7a*, *miR-141*, *-145* and *miR-155*) the sensitivity improved to 97%, with a PPV of 80% and an AUC of 0.783.

### 3.4. Risk Stratification

The expression levels of *let7a* decreased from benign to low-risk and to intermediate-risk prostate cancer, as per the D'Amico risk stratification, with a similar mean expression levels for both intermediate-risk and high-risk prostate cancer were observed ($p = 0.04$). There was a significant upregulation of *miR-141* in relation to D'Amico risk stratification ($p = 0.023$). The expression levels of *miR-145* and *miR-155* increased as the risk increased, however, this only approached significance ($p = 0.1$ and $p = 0.115$, respectively).

### 3.5. Post-Operative miRNAs

Twenty men had pre-operative and post-operative blood taken to quantify miRNA levels. The four miRNAs mentioned above were also quantified post-operatively. The blood was collected the day prior to surgery and at mean post-operative day 10 (range day 7–22). The post-operative expression levels of *miR-141* reduced considerably to levels similar to those of the patients with benign histological findings. However, the other three miRNAs did not return to the benign levels.

## 4. Discussion

This study demonstrates that four miRNAs are significantly dysregulated in the circulation of patients with prostate cancer. Combining these miRNAs to identify a unique prostate cancer miRNA signature revealed a biomarker panel with an AUC of 0.783. A study investigating the expression profile of patients with gastric cancer using five circulating miRNAs in combination had a sensitivity of 80%, a specificity of 81% and an AUC of 0.879 [20].

To date there are a limited number of studies examining the expression profile of miRNAs in the circulation of patients with prostate cancer. Examining these papers reveals that there are a variety of different techniques used for RNA extraction and from different blood mediums such as whole blood, serum and plasma. Our institution has recently published on the variability of miRNA levels in whole blood, serum and plasma, and identified that whole blood contains a higher yield of miRNAs by RQ-PCR [16].

*Mir-16* and *miR-425* were found to be stably expressed in the circulation of all patients with little variability. As a result both were selected for use as endogenous controls. *miR-16* has been used as a normaliser in a many studies investigating levels of miRNAs in whole blood, serum, plasma and tissue [16,21–24]. To our knowledge, this is the first published evidence of *miR-425* being used as an endogenous control in the circulation, but has previously been described as a suitable endogenous control in tissue [25].

The oncomir *miR-141*, when quantified in circulation, Ha the ability to identify those men with prostate cancer with an AUC of 0.655. This highlights a potential clinical use of miRNAs in the identification of patients with malignancy in a group deemed to be clinically high risk due to an elevated PSA. Mitchell *et al.* have previously reported that *miR-141* could differentiate those with prostate cancer with an AUC of 0.9, although all 25 of the prostate cancer patients had metastatic disease [8]. Levels of *miR-141* has been shown to increase as the stage of disease progresses from organ confined disease, to locally advanced disease and on to metastatic prostate cancer [17,26]. However, similar to Mitchell *et al.* and using a RNA extraction technique from serum, Mahn *et al.* encountered difficulties in the detection of *miR-141* in the sera [27]. This further highlights the variability in results from different extraction methods, different blood products and the use of different endogenous controls. There is also evidence to support that RNAse activity is increased in the serum of prostate cancer patients however Mitchell *et al.* identified that circulating miRNAs are stable against RNAse activity [8,28].

In this study *let7a* was found to be significantly downregulated in prostate cancer patients. *Let7a* has the ability to act as both a oncogene and tumour suppressor and is dysregulated in a number of malignancies [14]. This is first reported downregulation of *let-7a* in the circulation of patients with prostate cancer, this also concurs with previous papers citing *let-7a* as downregulated in prostate cancer tumour tissue [11,19].

We have identified that mean expression levels of *miR-141* significantly reduce post-operatively. Previous studies have also highlighted that the expression levels of oncomirs return to normal after oncological surgery, this has been identified in patients undergoing radical prostatectomy, mastectomy and colonic resection [16,27,29]. Zhang *et al.* identified that *miR-21* was upregulated in patients with hormone refractory prostate cancer and *miR-21* levels were reduced in patients who responded to docetaxel chemotherapy as compared to those hormone refractory patients who were resistant to chemotherapy [30]. This highlights the potential use for miRNAs as biomarkers for treatment response and also as prognostic markers.

Using the four miRNAs (*miR-141, -145, -155* and *let7a*) in combination yielded a sensitive biomarker panel with an AUC of 0.783. Given a sensitivity of 97%, with few false negative results, illustrates that quantifying a panel of miRNAs in the circulation has the potential to reduce unnecessary TRUS biopsies from being performed, allows for risk stratification in active surveillance protocols and in the future may help with choices of therapeutic intervention for physicians, surgeons and patients. A limitation of this study is that men within the benign group with a high PSA may indeed have an undiagnosed prostate cancer.

## 5. Conclusions

This study has identified a panel of four miRNAs that have diagnostic potential superior to that of PSA and DRE for the detection of prostate cancer. Three miRNAs were observed to be upregulated and one miRNA downregulated in association with prostate cancer. The expression levels of two of these miRNAs were altered as stage of disease increased. miRNAs, due to their detection, dysregulation and stability in blood, hold immense promise as future, novel, non-invasive biomarkers for prostate cancer.

**Author Contributions:** Brian D. Kelly drafted manuscipt, statisitcal analyis and concept, design and performance. Nicola Miller editing manuscript and techical expimental supervision. Karl J. Sweeney concept of study. Garrett C. Durkan concept of study. Eamon Rogers concept of study. Killian Walsh concept of study and editing manuscript. Michael J. Kerin editing manuscript and concept of study.

**Conflicts of Interest:** The authors declare no conflict of interest.

## References

1. Jemal, A.; Siegel, R.; Ward, E.; Hao, Y.; Xu, J.; Murray, T.; Thun, M.J. Cancer statistics, 2008. *CA Cancer J. Clin.* **2008**, *58*, 71–96. [CrossRef] [PubMed]

2. van Leeuwen, P.J.; van Vugt, H.A.; Bangma, C.H. The implementation of screening for prostate cancer. *Prostate Cancer Prostatic Dis.* **2010**, *13*, 218–227. [CrossRef] [PubMed]

3. Andriole, G.L.; Crawford, E.D.; Grubb, R.L., 3rd; Buys, S.S.; Chia, D.; Church, T.R.; Fouad, M.N.; Gelmann, E.P.; Kvale, P.A.; Reding, D.J.; *et al.* Mortality results from a randomized prostate-cancer screening trial. *N. Engl. J. Med.* **2009**, *360*, 1310–1319. [CrossRef] [PubMed]

4. Schroder, F.H.; Hugosson, J.; Roobol, M.J.; Tammela, T.L.; Ciatto, S.; Nelen, V.; Kwiatkowski, M.; Lujan, M.; Lilja, H.; Zappa, M.; *et al.* Screening and prostate-cancer mortality in a randomized European study. *N. Engl. J. Med.* **2009**, *360*, 1320–1328. [CrossRef] [PubMed]

5. Friedman, R.C.; Farh, K.K.; Burge, C.B.; Bartel, D.P. Most mammalian mRNAs are conserved targets of microRNAs. *Genome Res.* **2009**, *19*, 92–105. [CrossRef] [PubMed]

6.  Vrba, L.; Jensen, T.J.; Garbe, J.C.; Heimark, R.L.; Cress, A.E.; Dickinson, S.; Stampfer, M.R.; Futscher, B.W. Role for DNA methylation in the regulation of miR-200c and miR-141 expression in normal and cancer cells. *PLoS ONE* **2010**, *5*, e8697. [CrossRef] [PubMed]

7.  Li, J.; Smyth, P.; Flavin, R.; Cahill, S.; Denning, K.; Aherne, S.; Guenther, S.M.; O'Leary, J.J.; Sheils, O. Comparison of miRNA expression patterns using total RNA extracted from matched samples of formalin-fixed paraffin-embedded (FFPE) cells and snap frozen cells. *BMC Biotechnol.* **2007**, *7*. [CrossRef] [PubMed]

8.  Mitchell, P.S.; Parkin, R.K.; Kroh, E.M.; Fritz, B.R.; Wyman, S.K.; Pogosova-Agadjanyan, E.L.; Peterson, A.; Noteboom, J.; O'Briant, K.C.; Allen, A.; *et al.* Circulating microRNAs as stable blood-based markers for cancer detection. *Proc. Natl. Acad. Sci. USA* **2008**, *105*, 10513–10518. [CrossRef] [PubMed]

9.  Lu, J.; Getz, G.; Miska, E.A.; Alvarez-Saavedra, E.; Lamb, J.; Peck, D.; Sweet-Cordero, A.; Ebert, B.L.; Mak, R.H.; Ferrando, A.A.; *et al.* MicroRNA expression profiles classify human cancers. *Nature* **2005**, *435*, 834–838. [CrossRef] [PubMed]

10. Mattie, M.D.; Benz, C.C.; Bowers, J.; Sensinger, K.; Wong, L.; Scott, G.K.; Fedele, V.; Ginzinger, D.; Getts, R.; Haqq, C. Optimized high-throughput microRNA expression profiling provides novel biomarker assessment of clinical prostate and breast cancer biopsies. *Mol. Cancer* **2006**, *5*. [CrossRef] [PubMed]

11. Porkka, K.P.; Pfeiffer, M.J.; Waltering, K.K.; Sensinger, K.; Wong, L.; Scott, G.K.; Fedele, V.; Ginzinger, D.; Getts, R.; Haqq, C. MicroRNA expression profiling in prostate cancer. *Cancer Res.* **2007**, *67*, 6130–6135. [CrossRef] [PubMed]

12. Prueitt, R.L.; Yi, M.; Hudson, R.S.; Wallace, T.A.; Howe, T.M.; Yfantis, H.G.; Lee, D.H.; Stephens, R.M.; Liu, C.G.; Calin, G.A.; *et al.* Expression of microRNAs and protein-coding genes associated with perineural invasion in prostate cancer. *Prostate* **2008**, *68*, 1152–1164. [CrossRef] [PubMed]

13. Lodes, M.J.; Caraballo, M.; Suciu, D.; Munro, S.; Kumar, A.; Anderson, B. Detection of cancer with serum miRNAs on an oligonucleotide microarray. *PLoS ONE* **2009**, *4*, e6229. [CrossRef] [PubMed]

14. Heneghan, H.M.; Miller, N.; Kelly, R.; Newell, J.; Kerin, M.J. Systemic miRNA-195 differentiates breast cancer from other malignancies and is a potential biomarker for detecting noninvasive and early stage disease. *Oncologist* **2010**, *15*, 673–682. [CrossRef] [PubMed]

15. D'Amico, A.V.; Whittington, R.; Malkowicz, S.B.; Schultz, D.; Blank, K.; Broderick, G.A.; Tomaszewski, J.E.; Renshaw, A.A.; Kaplan, I.; Beard, C.J.; *et al.* Biochemical outcome after radical prostatectomy, external beam radiation therapy, or interstitial radiation therapy for clinically localized prostate cancer. *JAMA* **1998**, *280*, 969–974. [CrossRef] [PubMed]

16. Heneghan, H.M.; Miller, N.; Lowery, A.J.; Sweeney, K.J.; Newell, J.; Kerin, M.J. Circulating microRNAs as novel minimally invasive biomarkers for breast cancer. *Ann. Surg.* **2010**, *251*, 499–505. [CrossRef] [PubMed]

17. Brase, J.C.; Johannes, M.; Schlomm, T.; Fälth, M.; Haese, A.; Steuber, T.; Beissbarth, T.; Kuner, R.; Sültmann, H. Circulating miRNAs are correlated with tumor progression in prostate cancer. *Int. J. Cancer* **2011**, *128*, 608–616. [CrossRef] [PubMed]

18. Ambs, S.; Prueitt, R.L.; Yi, M.; Hudson, R.S.; Howe, T.M.; Petrocca, F.; Wallace, T.A.; Liu, C.G.; Volinia, S.; Calin, G.A.; *et al.* Genomic profiling of microRNA and messenger RNA reveals deregulated microRNA expression in prostate cancer. *Cancer Res.* **2008**, *68*, 6162–6170. [CrossRef] [PubMed]

19. Volinia, S.; Calin, G.A.; Liu, C.G.; Ambs, S.; Cimmino, A.; Petrocca, F.; Visone, R.; Iorio, M.; Roldo, C.; Ferracin, M.; *et al.* A microRNA expression signature of human solid tumors defines cancer gene targets. *Proc. Natl. Acad. Sci. USA* **2006**, *103*, 2257–2261. [CrossRef] [PubMed]

20. Liu, R.; Zhang, C.; Hu, Z.; Li, G.; Wang, C.; Yang, C.; Huang, D.; Chen, X.; Zhang, H.; Zhuang, R.; *et al.* A five-microRNA signature identified from genome-wide serum microRNA expression profiling serves as a fingerprint for gastric cancer diagnosis. *Eur. J. Cancer* **2011**, *47*, 784–791. [CrossRef] [PubMed]

21. Lawrie, C.H.; Gal, S.; Dunlop, H.M.; Pushkaran, B.; Liggins, A.P.; Pulford, K.; Banham, A.H.; Pezzella, F.; Boultwood, J.; Wainscoat, J.S.; *et al.* Detection of elevated levels of tumour-associated microRNAs in serum of patients with diffuse large B-cell lymphoma. *Br. J. Haematol.* **2008**, *141*, 672–675. [CrossRef] [PubMed]

22. Huang, Z.; Huang, D.; Ni, S.; Peng, Z.; Sheng, W.; Du, X. Plasma microRNAs are promising novel biomarkers for early detection of colorectal cancer. *Int. J. Cancer* **2010**, *127*, 118–126. [CrossRef] [PubMed]

23. Liu, C.J.; Kao, S.Y.; Tu, H.F.; Tsai, M.M.; Chang, K.W.; Lin, S.C. Increase of microRNA miR-31 level in plasma could be a potential marker of oral cancer. *Oral Dis.* **2010**, *16*, 360–364. [CrossRef] [PubMed]

24. Wong, T.S.; Liu, X.B.; Wong, B.Y.; Ng, R.W.; Yuen, A.P.; Wei, W.I. Mature miR-184 as potential oncogenic microRNA of squamous cell carcinoma of tongue. *Clin. Cancer Res.* **2008**, *14*, 2588–2592. [CrossRef] [PubMed]

25. Chang, K.H.; Mestdagh, P.; Vandesompele, J.; Kerin, M.J.; Miller, N. MicroRNA expression profiling to identify and validate reference genes for relative quantification in colorectal cancer. *BMC Cancer* **2010**, *10*. [CrossRef] [PubMed]

26. Yaman Agaoglu, F.; Kovancilar, M.; Dizdar, Y.; Darendeliler, E.; Holdenrieder, S.; Dalay, N.; Gezer, U. Investigation of miR-21, miR-141, and miR-221 in blood circulation of patients with prostate cancer. *Tumour Biol.* **2011**, *32*, 583–588. [CrossRef] [PubMed]

27. Mahn, R.; Heukamp, L.C.; Rogenhofer, S.; von Ruecker, A.; Müller, S.C.; Ellinger, J. Circulating microRNAs (miRNA) in serum of patients with prostate cancer. *Urology* **2011**, *77*, 1265.e9–e16. [CrossRef] [PubMed]

28. Eskicorapci, S.Y.; Ozkara, H.A.; Onder, E.; Akdogan, B.; Erkan, I.; Ciliv, G.; Ozen, H. Serum ribonuclease activity in the diagnosis of prostate cancer in men with serum prostate-specific antigen levels between 2.5 and 20 ng/mL. *Clin. Biochem.* **2006**, *39*, 363–366. [CrossRef] [PubMed]

29. Ng, E.K.; Chong, W.W.; Jin, H.; Lam, E.K.; Shin, V.Y.; Yu, J.; Poon, T.C.; Ng, S.S.; Sung, J.J. Differential expression of microRNAs in plasma of patients with colorectal cancer: A potential marker for colorectal cancer screening. *Gut* **2009**, *58*, 1375–1381. [CrossRef] [PubMed]

30. Zhang, H.L.; Yang, L.F.; Zhu, Y.; Yao, X.D.; Zhang, S.L.; Dai, B.; Zhu, Y.P.; Shen, Y.J.; Shi, G.H.; Ye, D.W. Serum miRNA-21: Elevated levels in patients with metastatic hormone-refractory prostate cancer and potential predictive factor for the efficacy of docetaxel-based chemotherapy. *Prostate* **2011**, *71*, 326–331. [CrossRef] [PubMed]

31. Tong, A.W.; Fulgham, P.; Jay, C.; Chen, P.; Khalil, I.; Liu, S.; Senzer, N.; Eklund, A.C.; Han, J.; Nemunaitis, J. MicroRNA profile analysis of human prostate cancers. *Cancer Gene Ther.* **2009**, *16*, 206–216. [CrossRef] [PubMed]

32. Ozen, M.; Creighton, C.J.; Ozdemir, M.; Ittmann, M. Widespread deregulation of microRNA expression in human prostate cancer. *Oncogene* **2008**, *27*, 1788–1793. [CrossRef] [PubMed]

33. Schaefer, A.; Jung, M.; Mollenkopf, H.J.; Wagner, I.; Stephan, C.; Jentzmik, F.; Miller, K.; Lein, M.; Kristiansen, G.; Jung, K. Diagnostic and prognostic implications of microRNA profiling in prostate carcinoma. *Int. J. Cancer* **2010**, *126*, 1166–1176. [CrossRef] [PubMed]

34. Spahn, M.; Kneitz, S.; Scholz, C.J.; Stenger, N.; Rüdiger, T.; Ströbel, P.; Riedmiller, H.; Kneitz, B. Expression of microRNA-221 is progressively reduced in aggressive prostate cancer and metastasis and predicts clinical recurrence. *Int. J. Cancer* **2010**, *127*, 394–403. [PubMed]

35. Zheng, C.; Yinghao, S.; Li, J. miR-221 expression affects invasion potential of human prostate carcinoma cell lines by targeting DVL2. *Med. Oncol.* **2012**, *29*, 815–822. [CrossRef] [PubMed]

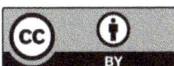

Journal of
*Clinical Medicine*

MDPI

*Review*

# The Role of microRNAs in the Diagnosis and Treatment of Pancreatic Adenocarcinoma

Maria Diab [1], Irfana Muqbil [2], Ramzi M. Mohammad [2], Asfar S. Azmi [2] and Philip A. Philip [2,*]

[1] Department of Internal Medicine, School of Medicine, Wayne State University, Detroit, MI 48201, USA; diab.maria@gmail.com
[2] Department of Oncology, Karmanos Cancer institute, Wayne State University, Detroit, MI 48201, USA; irfana.muqbil@wayne.edu (I.M.); mohammar@karmanos.org (R.M.M.); azmia@karmanos.org (A.S.A.)
* Correspondence: philipp@karmanos.org; Tel.: +1-313-575-8746

Academic Editors: Takahiro Ochiya and Ryou-u Takahashi
Received: 31 March 2016; Accepted: 13 June 2016; Published: 16 June 2016

**Abstract:** Pancreatic ductal adenocarcinoma (PDAC) remains a very challenging malignancy. Disease is diagnosed in an advanced stage in the vast majority of patients, and PDAC cells are often resistant to conventional cytotoxic drugs. Targeted therapies have made no progress in the management of this disease, unlike other cancers. microRNAs (miRs) are small non-coding RNAs that regulate the expression of multitude number of genes by targeting their 3′-UTR mRNA region. Aberrant expression of miRNAs has been linked to the development of various malignancies, including PDAC. In PDAC, a series of miRs have been defined as holding promise for early diagnostics, as indicators of therapy resistance, and even as markers for therapeutic response in patients. In this mini-review, we present an update on the various different miRs that have been defined in PDAC biology.

**Keywords:** pancreatic ductal adenocarcinoma; micro-RNA; biology; diagnosis; therapy; prognosis

## 1. Introduction

Pancreatic cancer is the fourth leading cause of cancer-related deaths in the United States, with 53,070 new cases expected in 2016, of which 41,780 are expected to die from disease [1]. Surgery remains the only potentially curative treatment. However, a majority of patients present with non-resectable disease; only 15%–20% are surgical candidates at the time of diagnosis [2]. Surgery has an overall morbidity and mortality of 24% and 5.3%, respectively [3]. Tumor size less than 3 cm, negative surgical resection margins, well-differentiated histology and absence of lymph node involvement are favorable prognostic indicators [4]. Following a pancreaticoduodenectomy (Whipple procedure), the five-year survival rate is 25%–30% for node-negative [5] and 10% for node-positive disease [6]. This can be explained, in part, by the tumor's high resistance to chemotherapy, as well as its propensity to recur and metastasize early, which may be related to the persistence of cancer stem cells (CSCs). Gemcitabine remains a commonly used drug in this disease [7]. Nab-paclitaxel has recently been shown to add to the benefit of gemcitabine in patients with favorable performance status [8]. The combination of fluorouracil, leucovorin, irinotecan, and oxalipatin (FOLFIRINOX) was also shown to be superior to gemcitabine, but, due to its side effect profile, it is reserved for patients with good performance [9]. More recently, monotherapy with S-1, an oral fluoropyrimidine derivative, demonstrated noninferiority to gemcitabine [10].

In light of the disappointing statistics in the prognosis of pancreatic ductal adenocarcinoma (PDAC), early detection of malignant and premalignant lesions is key. Unfortunately, no effective screening tool has been identified to date [11]. The tumors markers carcinoembryonic antigen (CEA) and carbohydrate antigen 19-9 (CA 19-9) are neither sensitive nor specific for screening but are used to follow known disease if they were initially elevated [12,13].

microRNAs (miRNA) are small (19–25 nucleotides) non-coding ribonucleic acids (RNAs) that interact with messenger RNA (mRNA) and serve as negative regulators of gene expression [14,15] by binding to imperfect complementary regions in the 3' untranslated region of the target messenger RNA (mRNAs), inhibiting their translation or leading to their degradation. They have been shown to influence cell differentiation, proliferation, and apoptosis [16]. They represent only 3% of the human genome, but regulate 20%–30% of the protein coding genes [17,18]. They were first described in *C. elegans* in 1993 [19], and have a tissue-specific expression that is modified in a number of different conditions, including malignancy. They have been profiled in many different malignancies including breast [20], lung [21], and colorectal cancer [22] and differential expression was detected with those malignancies, all of which have made miRNAs promising biomarkers. The aim of this review is to present the evidence on the utility of miRNA in the diagnosis, treatment, and prognosis of PDAC.

## 2. microRNA in PDAC Biology

An understanding of the processes that govern the development of PDAC is crucial as it sheds light on potential biomarkers of early diagnosis and rational systemic therapeutic approaches. Multiple mutations in the evolution of PDAC are influenced by miRNAs, which serve as tumor promoters or suppressors by silencing or promoting of downstream pathways [23].

Activating mutations in *KRAS* are present in more than 90% of PDAC [24]. miRNA-96, 126, and 217, all of which target *KRAS*, were found to be downregulated in PDAC compared to other noncancerous, as well as normal, pancreatic tissues [25–27]. Furthermore, re-expression of miR-96 and 217 suppressed *KRAS* activity and resulted in reduced tumor migration and invasion, suggesting their role as tumor suppressors [26,27]. Additionally, miR-217 overexpression phosphorylated AKT levels, suggesting that miR-217 also influences downstream signaling involving cell survival and proliferation [27]. In another study, Kent *et al.* showed that RAS-responsive element-binding protein (RREB1) repressed the expression of miR-143/145 by binding to the promoter of the cluster [28]. Interestingly, oncogenic *KRAS* G12D mutations induce expression of RREB1 in PDAC to check the expression of miR-143/145 cluster. As the miR-143/145 cluster expression targets RREB1 protein to inhibit a feed forward circuit of *KRAS* signals through RREB1, the *KRAS* (G12D) mediated overexpression of RREB1 simultaneously represses the miR143/145 cluster expression, resulting in promotion of *KRAS* mediated signaling. Loss of expression of let-7 family miRNAs was described for the first time by Torrisani *et al.* [29]. Expression of let-7 suppressed *KRAS* expression and mitogen-activated protein kinase activation (MAPK), and inhibited cell proliferation but failed to hinder tumor progression [29].

Inactivation of *p53* occurs in 50%–75% of PDAC, predominantly through missense mutations in the TP53 tumor suppressor gene [30]. Several studies showed that mutant p53 regulates the transcription of certain miRNAs, and, subsequently, influence the expression of their target genes either by degrading their messenger RNA or by inhibiting their translation [31,32]. miR-15a, a known transcriptional target of *p53*, was shown to be downregulated in PDAC [33]. The overexpression of miR-15a downregulated WNT3A and FGF7, resulting in reduced proliferation and survival of pancreatic cancer cells [33]. p53 has also been shown to induce the expression of miR-200 and repress that of Zeb1 and Zeb2, both of which are known activators of epithelial to mesenchymal transformation (EMT) [34]. In chemoresistant pancreatic cancer cell lines, miR-200 family was downregulated, suggesting a deregulated p53 signaling in those cell lines [34]. Furthermore, upregulation of Zeb1 was associated with downregulation of the miR-200 family expression [35]. The overexpression of miR-200 family led to the downregulation of Jag1, a target of Zeb1 and a ligand of the Notch pathway [35]. p53 not only regulates the expression of certain miRs but also is in turn modulated by specific miRs. miR-491-5p inhibited the expression of both TP53 and Bcl-XL genes, as well as mitogenic signaling pathways, such as STAT3 and PI-3K/Akt, resulting in decreased cell proliferation and induction of apoptosis [36]. Furthermore, Neault showed that miR-137 targets KMD4A messenger RNA during Ras-induced senescence, a tumor suppressor response, and activates both p53 and retinoblastoma tumor suppressor pathways [37]. miR-137 levels were found to be significantly reduced in PDAC; restoring its expression inhibited proliferation and promoted senescence of pancreatic cancer cells [37].

Aberrations in the expression of the *p16* genes have been described in PDAC [38]. Also known as cyclin dependent kinase inhibitor 2A, p16 functions as a tumor suppressor gene by regulating cell cycle and cellular senescence. Studies have shown the inhibitory role of miR-10b and -24 on the expression of p16 in malignancies other than pancreatic cancer [39,40]. Both miR-10 and -24 were overexpressed in pancreatic cancer [41,42].

The TGFβ/SMAD pathway has been implicated in EMT. Through binding with their receptors, transforming growth factor β (TGFβ) isoforms transduce the phosphorylation of SMAD2 and SMAD3, which in turn bind to SMAD4 and translocate to the nucleus, where they regulate the transcription of target genes [43]. Other SMADs include SMAD-1, SMAD-5, and SMAD-8, and are collectively referred to as R-SMAD. On the other hand, SMAD-6 and SMAD-7 are negative regulators of R-SMADs and referred to as I-SMADs, or inhibitory SMADs [44]. While TGFβ acts as a tumor suppressant in normal cells by inhibiting cell growth, in cancer cells, the TGFβ/SMAD axis is modified resulting in impaired mediation of growth arrest [45]. Overexpression of the messenger RNAs encoding for TGFβ was observed PDAC and was associated with poor prognosis [46]. There is evidence suggesting that various microRNAs are regulated by the TGFβ/SMAD pathway, while others serve as regulators of that same pathway. The 130a/301a/454 microRNA family regulates TGFβ signaling through suppressing SMAD-4 expression by directly binding to its 3'UTR sequence [47]. This cluster was found to be upregulated in PDAC [48]. In another study, miR-421 and -483-3p promoted PDAC progression through directly regulating the tumor suppressor DPC4/SMAD4 [49,50]. Furthermore, aberrant expression of miR-146a on dendritic cells from PDAC patients was observed, and repression of SMAD-4 resulted in impaired differentiation as well as inhibition of antigen presenting function of dendritic cells, suggesting a role of microRNAs in modulating the immune response in PDAC patients through regulating TGFβ/SMAD signaling [51]. Overexpression of miR-192 was associated with a reduction in the expression of SMAD-interacting protein 1 (SIP1) [52]. Through direct suppression of SMAD2 and SMAD3, miR-323-3p inhibited TGFβ signaling, resulting in decreased cell motility and metastasis [53].

### 3. microRNA in PDAC Diagnosis

Accumulating evidence is showing that miRNA profiles are cell-specific and tumor-specific [54,55]. miRNAs have been so far isolated from the pancreatic tissue, pancreatic juices, bile, stool, blood, plasma, and sera of patients with pancreatic cancer [56]. Circulating miRNAs, specifically, have several exceptionally appealing characteristics: they are abundant, they are strongly resistant to degradation or modification compared to protein or carbohydrate-based tumor markers, their isolation is non-invasive and their amplification is technically easy and inexpensive [57,58]. Several miRNA profiles were observed to discriminate pancreatic cancer from benign pancreatic pathology and healthy samples. Circulating miRNA-483-3p levels are overexpressed in PDAC compared to intrapapillary mucinous neoplasms and healthy controls, and plasma levels of miR-483-3p differentiated PDAC from intraductal papillary mucinous neoplasm (IPMN) with a sensitivity (Sn) of 43.8%, similar to that of CA19-9 (45%) [59]. Elevated serum miR-200a and -200b levels were associated with silencing of SIP1 and overexpression of E-cadherin in patients with pancreatic cancer and chronic pancreatitis compared to healthy controls [60]. Serum miR-200a and -200b distinguished patients with PDAC from healthy controls with a Sn and specificity (Sp) of 84.4% and 87.5% for miR-200a and 71.1% and 96.9% for miR-200b, respectively [60].

Compared to traditionally used markers, serum miR-1290 distinguished patients with low-stage pancreatic cancer from controls better than CA19-9 did, and it was also found to influence pancreatic cancer cell invasion capability [61]. miR-16 and -196a independently discriminated pancreatic cancer patients from those with chronic pancreatitis or healthy controls. When CA 19-9 was added to the analysis, the discrimination was more sensitive and specific compared to microRNA panel or CA19-9 alone, with a Sn of 92% and Sp 95.6% for the discrimination of pancreatic cancer from healthy controls, and 88.4% and 96.3% for discriminating pancreatic cancer from chronic pancreatitis [62].

Specific alterations in miRNA expression are also noted in metastatic disease. Singh *et al.* showed at least a two-fold downregulation of miRNA-205 compared to nonmetastatic disease [63]. On the other hand, miR-146a was upregulated. Diagnostic kits profiling differentially expressed miRNAs were investigated to distinguish benign, premalignant, and malignant pancreatic lesions [64]. Szafranska *et al.* developed the first miR diagnostic, miRInform Pancreas, which utilized miR-196a and -217 to differentiate chronic pancreatitis from PDAC; their diagnostic Sn and Sp were 95% [64]. Lee *et al.* identified a panel of four miRs (miR-21-5p, 485-3p, 708-5p, and 375) that distinguished PDAC from IPMN with a Sn and Sp or 95% and 85%, respectively [65].

Tables 1 and 2 list miRs that were shown to be upregulated and downregulated, respectively, in patients with pancreatic cancer, compared to benign pancreatic pathology and/or healthy samples.

**Table 1.** miRNAs upregulated in pancreatic ductal adenocarcinoma (PDAC) compared to benign pancreatic pathology and/or healthy pancreas.

| miRNA | Source | Reference |
|---|---|---|
| miR-10a, miR-10b, miR-146a, miR-204, miR-372 | PDAC tissue | [41] |
| miR-16, miR-21, miR-155, miR-181a, miR-181b, miR-196a, miR-210 | plasma | [62] |
| miR-155, miR-181a, miR-181b, miR–181b-1, miR-181c, miR-181d, miR-21, miR-221 | PDAC tissue | [66] |
| miR-196a, miR-196b, miR-203, miR-210, miR-222 | PDAC tissue | [67] |
| miR-196a, miR-155, miR-143, miR-145, miR-223, miR-31 | PDAC tissue | [68] |
| miR-196a, miR-221, miR-222, miR-15b, miR-95, miR-186, miR-190, miR-200b | PDAC tissue | [69] |
| miR-221, miR-181a, miR-181c, miR-155, miR-21, miR-100 | PDAC tissue | [70] |
| miR-132, miR-212 | PDAC tissue | [71] |
| miR-223, miR-143, miR-27a, miR-21, let-7i, miR-145, miR-142-5p, miR-142-3p, miR-10a, miR-150, miR-214, miR-107, miR-146b, miR-100, miR-23a, miR-199a-5p, miR-222, miR-155, miR-103, miR-221, miR34a, miR130a, miR-331-3p, miR-24, miR-505 | PDAC tissue | [72] |
| miR-107, miR-103, miR-23a, miR-1207-5p, miR-125a-5p, miR-140-5p, miR-221, miR-143, miR-146, let-7, let-7d, let-7e, miR-145, miR-199b-3p, miR-199a-3p, miR-138-1, miR-92b, miR-181, miR1246, miR-31, miR-155, miR-26a, miR-17, miR-23b, miR-24, miR-500, miR-331-3p, miR-939 | PDAC tissue | [73] |
| miR-196a, miR-200a, miR-21, miR-27a, miR-146a | PDAC tissue | [74] |
| miR-155, miR-203, miR-210, miR-222 | PDAC tissue | [75] |
| miR-21, miR-221, miR-100, miR-155, miR-181b, miR-196a | PDAC tissue | [76] |
| miR-21, miR-210, miR-221, miR-222, miR-155 | PDAC tissue | [77] |
| miR-21, miR-196a | PDAC tissue | [78] |
| miR-21, miR-155 | pancreatic juice | [79] |
| miR-205, miR-210, miR-492, miR-1247 | pancreatic juice | [80] |
| miR-26b, miR-34a, miR-122, miR-126, miR-145, miR-150, miR-223, miR-505, miR-636, miR-885-5p | whole blood | [81] |
| miR-483-3p, miR-21 | plasma | [59] |
| miR-21, 210, 155, 196a | plasma | [82] |
| miR-21 | plasma | [83] |
| miR-210 | plasma | [84] |
| miR-100a, miR-10 | plasma | [85] |
| miR-18a | plasma | [86] |
| miR-182 | plasma | [87] |
| miR-10b, miR-30c, miR-106b, miR-132, miR-155, miR-181a, miR-181b, miR-196a, miR-212 | plasma | [88] |
| miR-642b, miR-885-5p, miR-22 | plasma | [89] |
| miR-221 | plasma | [90] |
| miR-200a, 200b | serum | [60] |
| miR-24, miR-134, miR-146a, miR-378, miR-484, miR-628-3p, miR-1290, miR-1825 | serum | [61] |

**Table 1.** *Cont.*

| miRNA | Source | Reference |
|---|---|---|
| miR-6826-5p, mi-6757-5p, miR-miR-3131, miR-1343-3p, | serum | [91] |
| miR-20a, miR-21, miR-24, miR-25, miR-99a, miR-185, miR-191 | serum | [92] |
| miR-10b, miR-30c, miR-106b, miR-155, miR-181a, miR-196a, miR-212 | bile | [88] |
| miR-21, miR-155 | stool | [93] |

**Table 2.** miRNAs downregulated in PDAC compared to benign pancreatic pathology and/or healthy pancreas.

| miRNA | Source | Reference |
|---|---|---|
| miR-148a, miR-148b, miR-375 | PDAC tissue | [66] |
| miR-216, miR-217, miR-375 | PDAC tissue | [67] |
| miR-96, miR-130b, miR-148a, miR-217, miR-375 | PDAC tissue | [68] |
| miR-375 | PDAC tissue | [69] |
| miR-30d, miR-381, miR-29c, miR-30a, miR-874, miR-324-3p, miR-33b, miR-30c-1, miR-139-3p, miR-887, miR-141, miR-575, miR-28-3p, miR-665, miR-494, miR- 617, miR-564, miR-217, miR-130b, miR-148a, miR-708, miR-648, miR-148b, miR-345, miR216a | PDAC tissue | [72] |
| miR-1254, miR-559, miR-1274a, let-7f-1 | PDAC tissue | [73] |
| miR-217, miR-20a, miR-96 | PDAC tissue | [74] |
| miR-216, miR-217 | PDAC tissue | [75] |
| miR-31, miR-122, miR-145, miR-146a | PDAC tissue | [77] |
| miR-148a, miR-217 | PDAC tissue | [78] |
| let-7d, miR-146a | plasma | [83] |
| miR-375 | plasma | [90] |
| miR-6075, miR-4294, miR-6880-5p, miR-6799-5p, miR-125a-3p, miR-4530, miR-6836-3p, miR-4634, miR-7114-5p, miR-4476 | serum | [91] |
| miR-492, miR-663a | serum | [94] |
| miR-216 | stool | [93] |

## 4. microRNA in Therapy

### 4.1. Role of miRNAs in PDAC Therapy Resistance

The poor prognosis of pancreatic cancer is in part attributed to the high resistance rates to conventional chemotherapy. Accumulating evidence shows that most solid tumors are composed of two portions: the bulk and the cancer stem cell population. The latter survive the initial chemotherapy and utilize their self-renewal capabilities to regenerate a secondary population of tumor cells that is resistance to therapy. This inherent characteristic of CSCs might be controlled by specific miRNAs [63]. Jung *et al.* detected differentially expressed miRNAs in CSCs, including miR-99a, miR-100, miR-125b, miR-192, and miR-429 [95]. Certain alterations in miRNA expression are associated with chemoresistance. miRNA-200 family expression downregulation was observed in gemcitabine-resistant pancreatic cancer cells [96]. The mechanisms through which miRNAs induce chemoresistance have been elucidated in some studies. Hamada *et al.* showed that miR-365 induced chemoresistance through directly targeting the adaptor protein Src Homology 2 Domain Containing 1 (SHC1) and apoptosis-promoting protein BAX. It also upregulated S100P and Inhibitor of DNA binding 2, both of which are cancer-promoting molecules [97]. On the other hand, miRNA-34 regulated Notch signaling, leading to reduction in pancreatic CSC population [97]. Another study showed that miR-1246 expression induced chemoresistance through downregulating CCNG2 [98].

### 4.2. Potential of miRNAs as PDAC Therapeutics

As miRNAs regulate multiple gene expressions and signaling pathways, miRNA-based therapies are at an advantage over single-gene therapy, and, at least hypothetically, targeting miRNAs is expected to produce more effective anti-cancer activities. To that goal, multiple approaches have been utilized *in vitro* and *in vivo*, aiming for the downregulation of oncogenic miRNAs and/or the restoration of tumor suppressor ones. Approaches included introducing a miR antagonist or use of an miR mimic agent [55]. Transfecting pancreatic CSCs with a miR-200c mimic decreased colony formation, invasion and chemoresistance of pancreatic CSCs by regulating EMT [99]. Lu *et al.* reached similar results with transfection of miR-200a [100]. On the same note, transfecting gemcitabine-resistant pancreatic cells with miRNA-205 and miR-7 reduced the expression of TUBB3 and Pak-1, respectively, and reduced the CSC population [63]. Administering complexed micelles of gemcitabine and the tumor suppressor miRNA-205 achieved significant inhibition of tumor growth in a pancreatic tumor model; immuno-histochemical analysis showed decreased tumor cell proliferation and increased apoptosis [101]. Transfection efficiency was >90%. In another study, targeting miR-21 with lentiviral vectors inhibited cell proliferation [102]. Pancreatic stellate cells (PSCs) represent the precursor cells for cancer-associated fibroblasts in pancreatic tumor stroma [103]. Kuninty *et al.* showed that suppressing miR-199a and -214 in PSCs abolished the PSC-driven pro-tumor effects and resulted in decreased tumor cell growth [103].

Using treatment with the demethylating agent 5-Aza-2′-deoxycytidine (5-Aza-dC) and HDAC inhibitor vorinostat (SAHA), Nalls *et al.* restored the expression of miR-34, a transcriptional target of p53, which induced apoptosis and inhibited cell cycle progression and epithelial to mesenchymal transition [104]. Systemic intravenous delivery with miR-34a and miR-143/145 nanovectors inhibited the growth of MiaPsCa-2 subcutaneous xenografts in mouse models; this was displayed even in the orthotopic setting [105]. Treatment with a synthetic (fluorinated) curcumin analogue, CDF, led to the downregulation of miR-21, restoration of miR-200 and tumor suppressor PTEN, and the killing of the CSC population, resulting in suppressed tumor growth [106]. This was previously observed in the work of Ali *et al.*, as well as others [96,107–111]. Oral curcumin was well tolerated and showed some response in one phase II trial [112]. In another study, treatment with isoflavone or 3,3′-diindolylmethane (DIM) reversed the EMT, restored expression of the miRNA-200 family, and resensitized pancreatic cancer cells to gemcitabine [113].

Following miR expression patterns over the course of treatment provides a tool to monitor tumor burden, as well as the emergence of resistant strains of cancer cells, which would prompt modifying therapy [114]. In two studies, plasma levels of miR-18a and 221 dropped postoperatively in nine and eight patients, respectively [86,90]; furthermore, in one patient who had recurrence after surgery, miR-18a levels re-elevated with no similar change in the levels of CA19-9.

## 5. microRNAs as Prognostic Biomarkers

Evidence shows that certain miR profiles are associated with a more aggressive disease and worse survival. In a meta-analysis involving 1525 patients, overall and disease-free survivals were significantly shorter in patients with high tumoral miR-21 [115]. This was further shown in the work of Abue *et al.* [59]. Poor survival was also linked to high miR-155, 203, 222, and 10b, and low miR-34a levels [115]. Similarly, lower expression of miR-183 reduced survival compared to higher levels, and was significantly associated with tumor grade, metastasis, and TNM stage [116]. Overexpression of miR-1290 was also associated with worse outcomes [61].

## 6. Other Noncoding RNAs

Although miRNAs have gained a lot of praise as future biomarkers for PDAC, other less popular small noncoding RNAs (snRNAs), as well as long noncoding RNAs (lnRNAs), are also being studied as diagnostic and prognostic biomarkers. Circulating U2 snRNA identified PDAC from controls with high sensitivity and specificity [117]. Overexpression of lncRNAs HOTAIR, HULC, MALAT1, and PVT1 were observed in PDAC compared to non-cancerous controls, and was associated with more aggressive disease [118–121]. In another study, overexpression of lncRNA was associated with inhibition of cell proliferation [122].

## 7. Conclusions

Accumulating evidence supports the strong involvement of microRNAs in the pathogenesis of PDAC, highlighting their many different roles in the KRAS, p53, and TGFβ/SMAD pathways, among others. Whether it is their abundance, their resistance to degradation, the feasibility of isolating them noninvasively, or the ease of amplifying them, miRNAs represent appealing biomarkers that have so far been linked to the diagnosis, therapy, as well as the prognosis of PDAC. However, despite the many efforts that have occurred, a practical application to be used in the clinic is still lacking.

**Acknowledgments:** Work in the lab of A.S.A. is supported by NIH NCI 1R21CA188818-01A1. The authors acknowledge the support from Perri Foundation and SKY foundation.

**Author Contributions:** All authors are aware of the content of this manuscript. Maria Diab wrote significant portions of the text and all co-authors have read and edited the manuscript.

**Conflicts of Interest:** None of the authors have any conflicts of interest to disclose. This manuscript received no sources of funding.

## References

1. Siegel, R.L.; Miller, K.D.; Jemal, A. Cancer statistics, 2016. *CA: Cancer J. Clin.* **2016**, *66*, 7–30. [CrossRef] [PubMed]
2. Yeo, C.J.; Cameron, J.L. Prognostic factors in ductal pancreatic cancer. *Langenbeck's Arch. Surg. Deutsche Ges. Chir.* **1998**, *383*, 129–133. [CrossRef]
3. Benassai, G.; Mastrorilli, M.; Quarto, G.; Cappiello, A.; Giani, U.; Mosella, G. Survival after pancreaticoduodenectomy for ductal adenocarcinoma of the head of the pancreas. *Chir. Ital.* **2000**, *52*, 263–270. [PubMed]
4. Yeo, C.J.; Cameron, J.L.; Sohn, T.A.; Lillemoe, K.D.; Pitt, H.A.; Talamini, M.A.; Hruban, R.H.; Ord, S.E.; Sauter, P.K.; Coleman, J.; *et al.* Six hundred fifty consecutive pancreaticoduodenectomies in the 1990s: Pathology, complications, and outcomes. *Ann. Surg.* **1997**, *226*, 248–257, discussion 257–260. [CrossRef] [PubMed]
5. Trede, M.; Schwall, G.; Saeger, H.D. Survival after pancreatoduodenectomy. 118 consecutive resections without an operative mortality. *Ann. Surg.* **1990**, *211*, 447–458. [CrossRef] [PubMed]
6. Kang, M.J.; Jang, J.Y.; Chang, Y.R.; Kwon, W.; Jung, W.; Kim, S.W. Revisiting the concept of lymph node metastases of pancreatic head cancer: Number of metastatic lymph nodes and lymph node ratio according to n stage. *Ann. Surg. Oncol.* **2014**, *21*, 1545–1551. [CrossRef] [PubMed]
7. Heinemann, V.; Haas, M.; Boeck, S. Systemic treatment of advanced pancreatic cancer. *Cancer Treat. Rev.* **2012**, *38*, 843–853. [CrossRef] [PubMed]
8. Von Hoff, D.D.; Ervin, T.; Arena, F.P.; Chiorean, E.G.; Infante, J.; Moore, M.; Seay, T.; Tjulandin, S.A.; Ma, W.W.; Saleh, M.N.; *et al.* Increased survival in pancreatic cancer with nab-paclitaxel plus gemcitabine. *N. Engl. J. Med.* **2013**, *369*, 1691–1703. [CrossRef] [PubMed]
9. Conroy, T.; Desseigne, F.; Ychou, M.; Bouche, O.; Guimbaud, R.; Becouarn, Y.; Adenis, A.; Raoul, J.L.; Gourgou-Bourgade, S.; de la Fouchardiere, C.; *et al.* Folfirinox *versus* gemcitabine for metastatic pancreatic cancer. *N. Engl. J. Med.* **2011**, *364*, 1817–1825. [CrossRef] [PubMed]
10. Ueno, H.; Ioka, T.; Ikeda, M.; Ohkawa, S.; Yanagimoto, H.; Boku, N.; Fukutomi, A.; Sugimori, K.; Baba, H.; Yamao, K.; *et al.* Randomized phase iii study of gemcitabine plus s-1, s-1 alone, or gemcitabine alone in patients with locally advanced and metastatic pancreatic cancer in japan and taiwan: Gest study. *J. Clin. Oncol.* **2013**, *31*, 1640–1648. [CrossRef] [PubMed]
11. Ryan, D.P.; Hong, T.S.; Bardeesy, N. Pancreatic adenocarcinoma. *N. Engl. J. Med.* **2014**, *371*, 1039–1049. [CrossRef] [PubMed]
12. DiMagno, E.P.; Reber, H.A.; Tempero, M.A. Aga technical review on the epidemiology, diagnosis, and treatment of pancreatic ductal adenocarcinoma. American gastroenterological association. *Gastroenterology* **1999**, *117*, 1464–1484. [CrossRef]
13. Lamerz, R. Role of tumour markers, cytogenetics. *Ann. Oncol.* **1999**, *10* (Suppl. 4), 145–149. [CrossRef] [PubMed]

14. Galasso, M.; Sandhu, S.K.; Volinia, S. MicroRNA expression signatures in solid malignancies. *Cancer J. (Sudbury Mass.)* **2012**, *18*, 238–243. [CrossRef] [PubMed]

15. Zhang, B.; Pan, X.; Cobb, G.P.; Anderson, T.A. MicroRNAs as oncogenes and tumor suppressors. *Dev. Biol.* **2007**, *302*, 1–12. [CrossRef] [PubMed]

16. Iorio, M.V.; Croce, C.M. MicroRNAs in cancer: Small molecules with a huge impact. *J. Clin. Oncol.* **2009**, *27*, 5848–5856. [CrossRef] [PubMed]

17. Bentwich, I.; Avniel, A.; Karov, Y.; Aharonov, R.; Gilad, S.; Barad, O.; Barzilai, A.; Einat, P.; Einav, U.; Meiri, E.; *et al.* Identification of hundreds of conserved and nonconserved human microRNAs. *Nat. Genet.* **2005**, *37*, 766–770. [CrossRef] [PubMed]

18. Carthew, R.W. Gene regulation by microRNAs. *Curr. Opin. Genet. Dev.* **2006**, *16*, 203–208. [CrossRef] [PubMed]

19. Lee, R.C.; Feinbaum, R.L.; Ambros, V. The c. Elegans heterochronic gene lin-4 encodes small RNAs with antisense complementarity to lin-14. *Cell* **1993**, *75*, 843–854. [CrossRef]

20. Iorio, M.V.; Ferracin, M.; Liu, C.G.; Veronese, A.; Spizzo, R.; Sabbioni, S.; Magri, E.; Pedriali, M.; Fabbri, M.; Campiglio, M.; *et al.* MicroRNA gene expression deregulation in human breast cancer. *Cancer Res.* **2005**, *65*, 7065–7070. [CrossRef] [PubMed]

21. Johnson, S.M.; Grosshans, H.; Shingara, J.; Byrom, M.; Jarvis, R.; Cheng, A.; Labourier, E.; Reinert, K.L.; Brown, D.; Slack, F.J. Ras is regulated by the let-7 microRNA family. *Cell* **2005**, *120*, 635–647. [CrossRef] [PubMed]

22. Michael, M.Z.; SM, O.C.; van Holst Pellekaan, N.G.; Young, G.P.; James, R.J. Reduced accumulation of specific microRNAs in colorectal neoplasia. *Mol. Cancer Res. MCR* **2003**, *1*, 882–891. [PubMed]

23. Bhardwaj, A.; Arora, S.; Prajapati, V.K.; Singh, S.; Singh, A.P. Cancer "stemness"- regulating microRNAs: Role, mechanisms and therapeutic potential. *Curr. Drug Targets* **2013**, *14*, 1175–1184. [CrossRef] [PubMed]

24. Almoguera, C.; Shibata, D.; Forrester, K.; Martin, J.; Arnheim, N.; Perucho, M. Most human carcinomas of the exocrine pancreas contain mutant c-k-ras genes. *Cell* **1988**, *53*, 549–554. [CrossRef]

25. Jiao, L.R.; Frampton, A.E.; Jacob, J.; Pellegrino, L.; Krell, J.; Giamas, G.; Tsim, N.; Vlavianos, P.; Cohen, P.; Ahmad, R.; *et al.* MicroRNAs targeting oncogenes are down-regulated in pancreatic malignant transformation from benign tumors. *PLoS ONE* **2012**, *7*, e32068. [CrossRef] [PubMed]

26. Yu, S.; Lu, Z.; Liu, C.; Meng, Y.; Ma, Y.; Zhao, W.; Liu, J.; Yu, J.; Chen, J. MiRNA-96 suppresses kras and functions as a tumor suppressor gene in pancreatic cancer. *Cancer Res.* **2010**, *70*, 6015–6025. [CrossRef] [PubMed]

27. Zhao, W.G.; Yu, S.N.; Lu, Z.H.; Ma, Y.H.; Gu, Y.M.; Chen, J. The mir-217 microRNA functions as a potential tumor suppressor in pancreatic ductal adenocarcinoma by targeting kras. *Carcinogenesis* **2010**, *31*, 1726–1733. [CrossRef] [PubMed]

28. Kent, O.A.; Chivukula, R.R.; Mullendore, M.; Wentzel, E.A.; Feldmann, G.; Lee, K.H.; Liu, S.; Leach, S.D.; Maitra, A.; Mendell, J.T. Repression of the mir-143/145 cluster by oncogenic ras initiates a tumor-promoting feed-forward pathway. *Genes Dev.* **2010**, *24*, 2754–2759. [CrossRef] [PubMed]

29. Torrisani, J.; Bournet, B.; du Rieu, M.C.; Bouisson, M.; Souque, A.; Escourrou, J.; Buscail, L.; Cordelier, P. Let-7 microRNA transfer in pancreatic cancer-derived cells inhibits *in vitro* cell proliferation but fails to alter tumor progression. *Hum. Gene Ther.* **2009**, *20*, 831–844. [CrossRef] [PubMed]

30. Scarpa, A.; Capelli, P.; Mukai, K.; Zamboni, G.; Oda, T.; Iacono, C.; Hirohashi, S. Pancreatic adenocarcinomas frequently show p53 gene mutations. *Am. J. Pathol.* **1993**, *142*, 1534–1543. [PubMed]

31. Dong, P.; Karaayvaz, M.; Jia, N.; Kaneuchi, M.; Hamada, J.; Watari, H.; Sudo, S.; Ju, J.; Sakuragi, N. Mutant p53 gain-of-function induces epithelial-mesenchymal transition through modulation of the mir-130b-zeb1 axis. *Oncogene* **2013**, *32*, 3286–3295. [CrossRef] [PubMed]

32. Neilsen, P.M.; Noll, J.E.; Mattiske, S.; Bracken, C.P.; Gregory, P.A.; Schulz, R.B.; Lim, S.P.; Kumar, R.; Suetani, R.J.; Goodall, G.J.; *et al.* Mutant p53 drives invasion in breast tumors through up-regulation of mir-155. *Oncogene* **2013**, *32*, 2992–3000. [CrossRef] [PubMed]

33. Zhang, X.J.; Ye, H.; Zeng, C.W.; He, B.; Zhang, H.; Chen, Y.Q. Dysregulation of mir-15a and mir-214 in human pancreatic cancer. *J. Hematol. Oncol.* **2010**, *3*, 46. [CrossRef] [PubMed]

34. Soubani, O.; Ali, A.S.; Logna, F.; Ali, S.; Philip, P.A.; Sarkar, F.H. Re-expression of mir-200 by novel approaches regulates the expression of pten and mt1-mmp in pancreatic cancer. *Carcinogenesis* **2012**, *33*, 1563–1571. [CrossRef] [PubMed]

35. Brabletz, S.; Bajdak, K.; Meidhof, S.; Burk, U.; Niedermann, G.; Firat, E.; Wellner, U.; Dimmler, A.; Faller, G.; Schubert, J.; *et al.* The zeb1/mir-200 feedback loop controls notch signalling in cancer cells. *EMBO J.* **2011**, *30*, 770–782. [CrossRef] [PubMed]

36. Guo, R.; Wang, Y.; Shi, W.Y.; Liu, B.; Hou, S.Q.; Liu, L. MicroRNA mir-491–5p targeting both tp53 and bcl-xl induces cell apoptosis in sw1990 pancreatic cancer cells through mitochondria mediated pathway. *Molecules (Basel Switzerland)* **2012**, *17*, 14733–14747. [CrossRef] [PubMed]

37. Neault, M.; Mallette, F.A.; Richard, S. Mir-137 modulates a tumor suppressor network-inducing senescence in pancreatic cancer cells. *Cell Rep.* **2016**, *14*, 1966–1978. [CrossRef] [PubMed]

38. Okamoto, A.; Demetrick, D.J.; Spillare, E.A.; Hagiwara, K.; Hussain, S.P.; Bennett, W.P.; Forrester, K.; Gerwin, B.; Serrano, M.; Beach, D.H.; *et al.* Mutations and altered expression of p16ink4 in human cancer. *Proc. Natl. Acad. Sci. USA* **1994**, *91*, 11045–11049. [CrossRef] [PubMed]

39. Lal, A.; Kim, H.H.; Abdelmohsen, K.; Kuwano, Y.; Pullmann, R., Jr.; Srikantan, S.; Subrahmanyam, R.; Martindale, J.L.; Yang, X.; Ahmed, F.; *et al.* P16(ink4a) translation suppressed by mir-24. *PLoS ONE* **2008**, *3*, e1864. [CrossRef] [PubMed]

40. Venkataraman, S.; Alimova, I.; Fan, R.; Harris, P.; Foreman, N.; Vibhakar, R. MicroRNA 128a increases intracellular ros level by targeting bmi-1 and inhibits medulloblastoma cancer cell growth by promoting senescence. *PLoS ONE* **2010**, *5*, e10748. [CrossRef] [PubMed]

41. Nakata, K.; Ohuchida, K.; Mizumoto, K.; Kayashima, T.; Ikenaga, N.; Sakai, H.; Lin, C.; Fujita, H.; Otsuka, T.; Aishima, S.; *et al.* MicroRNA-10b is overexpressed in pancreatic cancer, promotes its invasiveness, and correlates with a poor prognosis. *Surgery* **2011**, *150*, 916–922. [CrossRef] [PubMed]

42. Zhang, L.; Jamaluddin, M.S.; Weakley, S.M.; Yao, Q.; Chen, C. Roles and mechanisms of microRNAs in pancreatic cancer. *World J. Surg.* **2011**, *35*, 1725–1731. [CrossRef] [PubMed]

43. Cano, C.E.; Motoo, Y.; Iovanna, J.L. Epithelial-to-mesenchymal transition in pancreatic adenocarcinoma. *Sci. World J.* **2010**, *10*, 1947–1957. [CrossRef] [PubMed]

44. Rachagani, S.; Macha, M.A.; Heimann, N.; Seshacharyulu, P.; Haridas, D.; Chugh, S.; Batra, S.K. Clinical implications of miRNAs in the pathogenesis, diagnosis and therapy of pancreatic cancer. *Adv. Drug Deliv. Rev.* **2015**, *81*, 16–33. [CrossRef] [PubMed]

45. Nicolas, F.J.; Hill, C.S. Attenuation of the tgf-beta-smad signaling pathway in pancreatic tumor cells confers resistance to tgf-beta-induced growth arrest. *Oncogene* **2003**, *22*, 3698–3711. [CrossRef] [PubMed]

46. Friess, H.; Yamanaka, Y.; Buchler, M.; Ebert, M.; Beger, H.G.; Gold, L.I.; Korc, M. Enhanced expression of transforming growth factor beta isoforms in pancreatic cancer correlates with decreased survival. *Gastroenterology* **1993**, *105*, 1846–1856. [CrossRef]

47. Liu, L.; Nie, J.; Chen, L.; Dong, G.; Du, X.; Wu, X.; Tang, Y.; Han, W. The oncogenic role of microRNA-130a/301a/454 in human colorectal cancer via targeting smad4 expression. *PLoS ONE* **2013**, *8*, e55532. [CrossRef] [PubMed]

48. Chen, Z.; Chen, L.Y.; Dai, H.Y.; Wang, P.; Gao, S.; Wang, K. Mir-301a promotes pancreatic cancer cell proliferation by directly inhibiting bim expression. *J. Cell. Biochem.* **2012**, *113*, 3229–3235. [CrossRef] [PubMed]

49. Hao, J.; Zhang, S.; Zhou, Y.; Hu, X.; Shao, C. MicroRNA 483–3p suppresses the expression of dpc4/smad4 in pancreatic cancer. *FEBS Lett.* **2011**, *585*, 207–213. [CrossRef] [PubMed]

50. Hao, J.; Zhang, S.; Zhou, Y.; Liu, C.; Hu, X.; Shao, C. MicroRNA 421 suppresses dpc4/smad4 in pancreatic cancer. *Biochem. Biophys. Res. Commun.* **2011**, *406*, 552–557. [CrossRef] [PubMed]

51. Du, J.; Wang, J.; Tan, G.; Cai, Z.; Zhang, L.; Tang, B.; Wang, Z. Aberrant elevated microRNA-146a in dendritic cells (dc) induced by human pancreatic cancer cell line bxpc-3-conditioned medium inhibits dc maturation and activation. *Med. Oncol. (Northwood Lond. Engl.)* **2012**, *29*, 2814–2823. [CrossRef] [PubMed]

52. Zhao, C.; Zhang, J.; Zhang, S.; Yu, D.; Chen, Y.; Liu, Q.; Shi, M.; Ni, C.; Zhu, M. Diagnostic and biological significance of microRNA-192 in pancreatic ductal adenocarcinoma. *Oncol. Rep.* **2013**, *30*, 276–284. [CrossRef] [PubMed]

53. Wang, C.; Liu, P.; Wu, H.; Cui, H.; Li, Y.; Liu, Y.; Liu, Z.; Gou, S. MicroRNA-323–3p inhibits cell invasion and metastasis in pancreatic ductal adenocarcinoma via direct suppression of SMAD2 and SMAD3. *Oncotarget* **2016**, *7*, 14912–14924. [PubMed]

54. Lu, J.; Getz, G.; Miska, E.A.; Alvarez-Saavedra, E.; Lamb, J.; Peck, D.; Sweet-Cordero, A.; Ebert, B.L.; Mak, R.H.; Ferrando, A.A.; *et al.* MicroRNA expression profiles classify human cancers. *Nature* **2005**, *435*, 834–838. [CrossRef] [PubMed]

55. Rosenfeld, N.; Aharonov, R.; Meiri, E.; Rosenwald, S.; Spector, Y.; Zepeniuk, M.; Benjamin, H.; Shabes, N.; Tabak, S.; Levy, A.; *et al.* MicroRNAs accurately identify cancer tissue origin. *Nat. Biotechnol.* **2008**, *26*, 462–469. [CrossRef] [PubMed]

56. Visani, M.; Acquaviva, G.; Fiorino, S.; Bacchi Reggiani, M.L.; Masetti, M.; Franceschi, E.; Fornelli, A.; Jovine, E.; Fabbri, C.; Brandes, A.A.; *et al.* Contribution of microRNA analysis to characterisation of pancreatic lesions: A review. *J. Clinical Pathol.* **2015**, *68*, 859–869. [CrossRef] [PubMed]

57. Kishikawa, T.; Otsuka, M.; Ohno, M.; Yoshikawa, T.; Takata, A.; Koike, K. Circulating RNAs as new biomarkers for detecting pancreatic cancer. *World J. Gastroenterol.* **2015**, *21*, 8527–8540. [CrossRef] [PubMed]

58. Schwarzenbach, H.; Nishida, N.; Calin, G.A.; Pantel, K. Clinical relevance of circulating cell-free microRNAs in cancer. *Nat. Rev. Clin. Oncol.* **2014**, *11*, 145–156. [CrossRef] [PubMed]

59. Abue, M.; Yokoyama, M.; Shibuya, R.; Tamai, K.; Yamaguchi, K.; Sato, I.; Tanaka, N.; Hamada, S.; Shimosegawa, T.; Sugamura, K.; *et al.* Circulating mir-483-3p and mir-21 is highly expressed in plasma of pancreatic cancer. *Int. J. Oncol.* **2015**, *46*, 539–547. [CrossRef] [PubMed]

60. Li, A.; Omura, N.; Hong, S.M.; Vincent, A.; Walter, K.; Griffith, M.; Borges, M.; Goggins, M. Pancreatic cancers epigenetically silence sip1 and hypomethylate and overexpress mir-200a/200b in association with elevated circulating mir-200a and mir-200b levels. *Cancer Res.* **2010**, *70*, 5226–5237. [CrossRef] [PubMed]

61. Li, A.; Yu, J.; Kim, H.; Wolfgang, C.L.; Canto, M.I.; Hruban, R.H.; Goggins, M. MicroRNA array analysis finds elevated serum mir-1290 accurately distinguishes patients with low-stage pancreatic cancer from healthy and disease controls. *Clin. Cancer Res.* **2013**, *19*, 3600–3610. [CrossRef] [PubMed]

62. Liu, J.; Gao, J.; Du, Y.; Li, Z.; Ren, Y.; Gu, J.; Wang, X.; Gong, Y.; Wang, W.; Kong, X. Combination of plasma microRNAs with serum ca19–9 for early detection of pancreatic cancer. *Int. J. Cancer* **2012**, *131*, 683–691. [CrossRef] [PubMed]

63. Singh, S.; Chitkara, D.; Kumar, V.; Behrman, S.W.; Mahato, R.I. MiRNA profiling in pancreatic cancer and restoration of chemosensitivity. *Cancer Lett.* **2013**, *334*, 211–220. [CrossRef] [PubMed]

64. Szafranska-Schwarzbach, A.E.; Adai, A.T.; Lee, L.S.; Conwell, D.L.; Andruss, B.F. Development of a miRNA-based diagnostic assay for pancreatic ductal adenocarcinoma. *Expert Rev. Mol. Diagn.* **2011**, *11*, 249–257. [PubMed]

65. Lee, L.S.; Szafranska-Schwarzbach, A.E.; Wylie, D.; Doyle, L.A.; Bellizzi, A.M.; Kadiyala, V.; Suleiman, S.; Banks, P.A.; Andruss, B.F.; Conwell, D.L. Investigating microRNA expression profiles in pancreatic cystic neoplasms. *Clin. Transl. Gastroenterol.* **2014**, *5*, e47. [CrossRef] [PubMed]

66. Bloomston, M.; Frankel, W.L.; Petrocca, F.; Volinia, S.; Alder, H.; Hagan, J.P.; Liu, C.G.; Bhatt, D.; Taccioli, C.; Croce, C.M. MicroRNA expression patterns to differentiate pancreatic adenocarcinoma from normal pancreas and chronic pancreatitis. *Jama* **2007**, *297*, 1901–1908. [CrossRef] [PubMed]

67. Szafranska, A.E.; Davison, T.S.; John, J.; Cannon, T.; Sipos, B.; Maghnouj, A.; Labourier, E.; Hahn, S.A. MicroRNA expression alterations are linked to tumorigenesis and non-neoplastic processes in pancreatic ductal adenocarcinoma. *Oncogene* **2007**, *26*, 4442–4452. [CrossRef] [PubMed]

68. Szafranska, A.E.; Doleshal, M.; Edmunds, H.S.; Gordon, S.; Luttges, J.; Munding, J.B.; Barth, R.J., Jr.; Gutmann, E.J.; Suriawinata, A.A.; Marc Pipas, J.; *et al.* Analysis of microRNAs in pancreatic fine-needle aspirates can classify benign and malignant tissues. *Clin. Chem.* **2008**, *54*, 1716–1724. [CrossRef] [PubMed]

69. Zhang, Y.; Li, M.; Wang, H.; Fisher, W.E.; Lin, P.H.; Yao, Q.; Chen, C. Profiling of 95 microRNAs in pancreatic cancer cell lines and surgical specimens by real-time pcr analysis. *World J. Surg.* **2009**, *33*, 698–709. [CrossRef] [PubMed]

70. Lee, E.J.; Gusev, Y.; Jiang, J.; Nuovo, G.J.; Lerner, M.R.; Frankel, W.L.; Morgan, D.L.; Postier, R.G.; Brackett, D.J.; Schmittgen, T.D. Expression profiling identifies microRNA signature in pancreatic cancer. *Int. J. Cancer* **2007**, *120*, 1046–1054. [CrossRef] [PubMed]

71. Park, J.K.; Henry, J.C.; Jiang, J.; Esau, C.; Gusev, Y.; Lerner, M.R.; Postier, R.G.; Brackett, D.J.; Schmittgen, T.D. Mir-132 and mir-212 are increased in pancreatic cancer and target the retinoblastoma tumor suppressor. *Biochem. Biophys. Res. Commun.* **2011**, *406*, 518–523. [CrossRef] [PubMed]

72. Jamieson, N.B.; Morran, D.C.; Morton, J.P.; Ali, A.; Dickson, E.J.; Carter, C.R.; Sansom, O.J.; Evans, T.R.; McKay, C.J.; Oien, K.A. MicroRNA molecular profiles associated with diagnosis, clinicopathologic criteria, and overall survival in patients with resectable pancreatic ductal adenocarcinoma. *Clin. Cancer Res.* **2012**, *18*, 534–545. [CrossRef] [PubMed]

73. Piepoli, A.; Tavano, F.; Copetti, M.; Mazza, T.; Palumbo, O.; Panza, A.; di Mola, F.F.; Pazienza, V.; Mazzoccoli, G.; Biscaglia, G.; *et al.* MiRNA expression profiles identify drivers in colorectal and pancreatic cancers. *PLoS ONE* **2012**, *7*, e33663. [CrossRef] [PubMed]

74. Hong, T.H.; Park, I.Y. MicroRNA expression profiling of diagnostic needle aspirates from surgical pancreatic cancer specimens. *Ann. Surg. Treat. Res.* **2014**, *87*, 290–297. [CrossRef] [PubMed]

75. Greither, T.; Grochola, L.F.; Udelnow, A.; Lautenschlager, C.; Wurl, P.; Taubert, H. Elevated expression of microRNAs 155, 203, 210 and 222 in pancreatic tumors is associated with poorer survival. *Int. J. Cancer* **2010**, *126*, 73–80. [CrossRef] [PubMed]

76. Panarelli, N.C.; Chen, Y.T.; Zhou, X.K.; Kitabayashi, N.; Yantiss, R.K. MicroRNA expression aids the preoperative diagnosis of pancreatic ductal adenocarcinoma. *Pancreas* **2012**, *41*, 685–690. [CrossRef] [PubMed]

77. Papaconstantinou, I.G.; Manta, A.; Gazouli, M.; Lyberopoulou, A.; Lykoudis, P.M.; Polymeneas, G.; Voros, D. Expression of microRNAs in patients with pancreatic cancer and its prognostic significance. *Pancreas* **2013**, *42*, 67–71. [CrossRef] [PubMed]

78. Xue, Y.; Abou Tayoun, A.N.; Abo, K.M.; Pipas, J.M.; Gordon, S.R.; Gardner, T.B.; Barth, R.J., Jr.; Suriawinata, A.A.; Tsongalis, G.J. MicroRNAs as diagnostic markers for pancreatic ductal adenocarcinoma and its precursor, pancreatic intraepithelial neoplasm. *Cancer Genet.* **2013**, *206*, 217–221. [CrossRef] [PubMed]

79. Sadakari, Y.; Ohtsuka, T.; Ohuchida, K.; Tsutsumi, K.; Takahata, S.; Nakamura, M.; Mizumoto, K.; Tanaka, M. MicroRNA expression analyses in preoperative pancreatic juice samples of pancreatic ductal adenocarcinoma. *JOP* **2010**, *11*, 587–592. [PubMed]

80. Wang, J.; Raimondo, M.; Guha, S.; Chen, J.; Diao, L.; Dong, X.; Wallace, M.B.; Killary, A.M.; Frazier, M.L.; Woodward, T.A.; *et al.* Circulating microRNAs in pancreatic juice as candidate biomarkers of pancreatic cancer. *J. Cancer* **2014**, *5*, 696–705. [CrossRef] [PubMed]

81. Schultz, N.A.; Dehlendorff, C.; Jensen, B.V.; Bjerregaard, J.K.; Nielsen, K.R.; Bojesen, S.E.; Calatayud, D.; Nielsen, S.E.; Yilmaz, M.; Hollander, N.H.; *et al.* MicroRNA biomarkers in whole blood for detection of pancreatic cancer. *Jama* **2014**, *311*, 392–404. [CrossRef] [PubMed]

82. Wang, J.; Chen, J.; Chang, P.; LeBlanc, A.; Li, D.; Abbruzzesse, J.L.; Frazier, M.L.; Killary, A.M.; Sen, S. MicroRNAs in plasma of pancreatic ductal adenocarcinoma patients as novel blood-based biomarkers of disease. *Cancer Prev. Res. (Philadelphia Pa.)* **2009**, *2*, 807–813. [CrossRef] [PubMed]

83. Ali, S.; Almhanna, K.; Chen, W.; Philip, P.A.; Sarkar, F.H. Differentially expressed miRNAs in the plasma may provide a molecular signature for aggressive pancreatic cancer. *Am. J. Transl. Res.* **2010**, *3*, 28–47. [PubMed]

84. Ho, A.S.; Huang, X.; Cao, H.; Christman-Skieller, C.; Bennewith, K.; Le, Q.T.; Koong, A.C. Circulating mir-210 as a novel hypoxia marker in pancreatic cancer. *Transl. Oncol.* **2010**, *3*, 109–113. [CrossRef] [PubMed]

85. LaConti, J.J.; Shivapurkar, N.; Preet, A.; Deslattes Mays, A.; Peran, I.; Kim, S.E.; Marshall, J.L.; Riegel, A.T.; Wellstein, A. Tissue and serum microRNAs in the kras(g12d) transgenic animal model and in patients with pancreatic cancer. *PLoS ONE* **2011**, *6*, e20687. [CrossRef] [PubMed]

86. Morimura, R.; Komatsu, S.; Ichikawa, D.; Takeshita, H.; Tsujiura, M.; Nagata, H.; Konishi, H.; Shiozaki, A.; Ikoma, H.; Okamoto, K.; *et al.* Novel diagnostic value of circulating mir-18a in plasma of patients with pancreatic cancer. *Br. J. Cancer* **2011**, *105*, 1733–1740. [CrossRef] [PubMed]

87. Chen, Q.; Yang, L.; Xiao, Y.; Zhu, J.; Li, Z. Circulating microRNA-182 in plasma and its potential diagnostic and prognostic value for pancreatic cancer. *Med. Oncol. (Northwood Lond. Engl.)* **2014**, *31*, 225. [CrossRef] [PubMed]

88. Cote, G.A.; Gore, A.J.; McElyea, S.D.; Heathers, L.E.; Xu, H.; Sherman, S.; Korc, M. A pilot study to develop a diagnostic test for pancreatic ductal adenocarcinoma based on differential expression of select miRNA in plasma and bile. *Am. J. Gastroenterol.* **2014**, *109*, 1942–1952. [CrossRef] [PubMed]

89. Ganepola, G.A.; Rutledge, J.R.; Suman, P.; Yiengpruksawan, A.; Chang, D.H. Novel blood-based microRNA biomarker panel for early diagnosis of pancreatic cancer. *World J. Gastrointest. Oncol.* **2014**, *6*, 22–33. [CrossRef] [PubMed]

90. Kawaguchi, T.; Komatsu, S.; Ichikawa, D.; Morimura, R.; Tsujiura, M.; Konishi, H.; Takeshita, H.; Nagata, H.; Arita, T.; Hirajima, S.; *et al.* Clinical impact of circulating mir-221 in plasma of patients with pancreatic cancer. *Br. J. Cancer* **2013**, *108*, 361–369. [CrossRef] [PubMed]

91. Kojima, M.; Sudo, H.; Kawauchi, J.; Takizawa, S.; Kondou, S.; Nobumasa, H.; Ochiai, A. MicroRNA markers for the diagnosis of pancreatic and biliary-tract cancers. *PLoS ONE* **2015**, *10*, e0118220. [CrossRef] [PubMed]

92. Liu, R.; Chen, X.; Du, Y.; Yao, W.; Shen, L.; Wang, C.; Hu, Z.; Zhuang, R.; Ning, G.; Zhang, C.; *et al.* Serum microRNA expression profile as a biomarker in the diagnosis and prognosis of pancreatic cancer. *Clin. Chem.* **2012**, *58*, 610–618. [CrossRef] [PubMed]

93. Yang, J.Y.; Sun, Y.W.; Liu, D.J.; Zhang, J.F.; Li, J.; Hua, R. MicroRNAs in stool samples as potential screening biomarkers for pancreatic ductal adenocarcinoma cancer. *Am. J. Cancer Res.* **2014**, *4*, 663–673. [PubMed]

94. Lin, M.S.; Chen, W.C.; Huang, J.X.; Gao, H.J.; Sheng, H.H. Aberrant expression of microRNAs in serum may identify individuals with pancreatic cancer. *Int. J. Clin. Exp. Med.* **2014**, *7*, 5226–5234. [PubMed]

95. Jung, D.E.; Wen, J.; Oh, T.; Song, S.Y. Differentially expressed microRNAs in pancreatic cancer stem cells. *Pancreas* **2011**, *40*, 1180–1187. [CrossRef] [PubMed]

96. Park, J.K.; Lee, E.J.; Esau, C.; Schmittgen, T.D. Antisense inhibition of microRNA-21 or -221 arrests cell cycle, induces apoptosis, and sensitizes the effects of gemcitabine in pancreatic adenocarcinoma. *Pancreas* **2009**, *38*, e190–e199. [CrossRef] [PubMed]

97. Ji, Q.; Hao, X.; Zhang, M.; Tang, W.; Yang, M.; Li, L.; Xiang, D.; Desano, J.T.; Bommer, G.T.; Fan, D.; *et al.* MicroRNA mir-34 inhibits human pancreatic cancer tumor-initiating cells. *PLoS ONE* **2009**, *4*, e6816. [CrossRef] [PubMed]

98. Hasegawa, S.; Eguchi, H.; Nagano, H.; Konno, M.; Tomimaru, Y.; Wada, H.; Hama, N.; Kawamoto, K.; Kobayashi, S.; Nishida, N.; *et al.* MicroRNA-1246 expression associated with ccng2-mediated chemoresistance and stemness in pancreatic cancer. *Br. J. Cancer* **2014**, *111*, 1572–1580. [CrossRef] [PubMed]

99. Ma, C.; Huang, T.; Ding, Y.C.; Yu, W.; Wang, Q.; Meng, B.; Luo, S.X. MicroRNA-200c overexpression inhibits chemoresistance, invasion and colony formation of human pancreatic cancer stem cells. *Int. J. Clin. Exp. Pathol.* **2015**, *8*, 6533–6539. [PubMed]

100. Lu, Y.; Lu, J.; Li, X.; Zhu, H.; Fan, X.; Zhu, S.; Wang, Y.; Guo, Q.; Wang, L.; Huang, Y.; *et al.* Mir-200a inhibits epithelial-mesenchymal transition of pancreatic cancer stem cell. *BMC Cancer* **2014**, *14*, 85. [CrossRef] [PubMed]

101. Mittal, A.; Chitkara, D.; Behrman, S.W.; Mahato, R.I. Efficacy of gemcitabine conjugated and miRNA-205 complexed micelles for treatment of advanced pancreatic cancer. *Biomaterials* **2014**, *35*, 7077–7087. [CrossRef] [PubMed]

102. Sicard, F.; Gayral, M.; Lulka, H.; Buscail, L.; Cordelier, P. Targeting mir-21 for the therapy of pancreatic cancer. *Mol. Ther.* **2013**, *21*, 986–994. [CrossRef] [PubMed]

103. Kuninty, P.R.; Bojmar, L.; Tjomsland, V.; Larsson, M.; Storm, G.; Ostman, A.; Sandstrom, P.; Prakash, J. MicroRNA-199a and -214 as potential therapeutic targets in pancreatic stellate cells in pancreatic tumor. *Oncotarget* **2016**, *7*, 1949–2553. [CrossRef] [PubMed]

104. Nalls, D.; Tang, S.N.; Rodova, M.; Srivastava, R.K.; Shankar, S. Targeting epigenetic regulation of mir-34a for treatment of pancreatic cancer by inhibition of pancreatic cancer stem cells. *PLoS ONE* **2011**, *6*, e24099. [CrossRef] [PubMed]

105. Pramanik, D.; Campbell, N.R.; Karikari, C.; Chivukula, R.; Kent, O.A.; Mendell, J.T.; Maitra, A. Restitution of tumor suppressor microRNAs using a systemic nanovector inhibits pancreatic cancer growth in mice. *Mol. Cancer Ther.* **2011**, *10*, 1470–1480. [CrossRef] [PubMed]

106. Bao, B.; Ali, S.; Kong, D.; Sarkar, S.H.; Wang, Z.; Banerjee, S.; Aboukameel, A.; Padhye, S.; Philip, P.A.; Sarkar, F.H. Anti-tumor activity of a novel compound-cdf is mediated by regulating mir-21, mir-200, and pten in pancreatic cancer. *PLoS ONE* **2011**, *6*, e17850. [CrossRef] [PubMed]

107. Ali, S.; Ahmad, A.; Banerjee, S.; Padhye, S.; Dominiak, K.; Schaffert, J.M.; Wang, Z.; Philip, P.A.; Sarkar, F.H. Gemcitabine sensitivity can be induced in pancreatic cancer cells through modulation of mir-200 and mir-21 expression by curcumin or its analogue cdf. *Cancer Res.* **2010**, *70*, 3606–3617. [CrossRef] [PubMed]

108. Giovannetti, E.; Funel, N.; Peters, G.J.; Del Chiaro, M.; Erozenci, L.A.; Vasile, E.; Leon, L.G.; Pollina, L.E.; Groen, A.; Falcone, A.; *et al.* MicroRNA-21 in pancreatic cancer: Correlation with clinical outcome and pharmacologic aspects underlying its role in the modulation of gemcitabine activity. *Cancer Res.* **2010**, *70*, 4528–4538. [CrossRef] [PubMed]

109. Hwang, J.H.; Voortman, J.; Giovannetti, E.; Steinberg, S.M.; Leon, L.G.; Kim, Y.T.; Funel, N.; Park, J.K.; Kim, M.A.; Kang, G.H.; *et al.* Identification of microRNA-21 as a biomarker for chemoresistance and clinical outcome following adjuvant therapy in resectable pancreatic cancer. *PLoS ONE* **2010**, *5*, e10630. [CrossRef] [PubMed]

110. Moriyama, T.; Ohuchida, K.; Mizumoto, K.; Yu, J.; Sato, N.; Nabae, T.; Takahata, S.; Toma, H.; Nagai, E.; Tanaka, M. MicroRNA-21 modulates biological functions of pancreatic cancer cells including their proliferation, invasion, and chemoresistance. *Mol. Cancer Ther.* **2009**, *8*, 1067–1074. [CrossRef] [PubMed]

111. Wang, P.; Zhuang, L.; Zhang, J.; Fan, J.; Luo, J.; Chen, H.; Wang, K.; Liu, L.; Chen, Z.; Meng, Z. The serum mir-21 level serves as a predictor for the chemosensitivity of advanced pancreatic cancer, and mir-21 expression confers chemoresistance by targeting fasl. *Mol. Oncol.* **2013**, *7*, 334–345. [CrossRef] [PubMed]

112. Dhillon, N.; Aggarwal, B.B.; Newman, R.A.; Wolff, R.A.; Kunnumakkara, A.B.; Abbruzzese, J.L.; Ng, C.S.; Badmaev, V.; Kurzrock, R. Phase ii trial of curcumin in patients with advanced pancreatic cancer. *Clin. Cancer Res.* **2008**, *14*, 4491–4499. [CrossRef] [PubMed]

113. Li, Y.; VandenBoom, T.G., 2nd; Kong, D.; Wang, Z.; Ali, S.; Philip, P.A.; Sarkar, F.H. Up-regulation of mir-200 and let-7 by natural agents leads to the reversal of epithelial-to-mesenchymal transition in gemcitabine-resistant pancreatic cancer cells. *Cancer Res.* **2009**, *69*, 6704–6712. [CrossRef] [PubMed]

114. Vietsch, E.E.; van Eijck, C.H.; Wellstein, A. Circulating DNA and micro-RNA in patients with pancreatic cancer. *Pancreat. Disord. Ther.* **2015**, *5*. [CrossRef]

115. Frampton, A.E.; Krell, J.; Jamieson, N.B.; Gall, T.M.; Giovannetti, E.; Funel, N.; Mato Prado, M.; Krell, D.; Habib, N.A.; Castellano, L.; *et al.* MicroRNAs with prognostic significance in pancreatic ductal adenocarcinoma: A meta-analysis. *Eur. J. Cancer* **2015**, *51*, 1389–1404. [CrossRef] [PubMed]

116. Zhou, L.; Zhang, W.G.; Wang, D.S.; Tao, K.S.; Song, W.J.; Dou, K.F. MicroRNA-183 is involved in cell proliferation, survival and poor prognosis in pancreatic ductal adenocarcinoma by regulating bmi-1. *Oncol. Rep.* **2014**, *32*, 1734–1740. [CrossRef] [PubMed]

117. Baraniskin, A.; Nopel-Dunnebacke, S.; Ahrens, M.; Jensen, S.G.; Zollner, H.; Maghnouj, A.; Wos, A.; Mayerle, J.; Munding, J.; Kost, D.; *et al.* Circulating u2 small nuclear RNA fragments as a novel diagnostic biomarker for pancreatic and colorectal adenocarcinoma. *Int. J. Cancer* **2013**, *132*, E48–E57. [CrossRef] [PubMed]

118. Huang, C.; Yu, W.; Wang, Q.; Cui, H.; Wang, Y.; Zhang, L.; Han, F.; Huang, T. Increased expression of the lncRNA pvt1 is associated with poor prognosis in pancreatic cancer patients. *Minerva Med.* **2015**, *106*, 143–149. [PubMed]

119. Kim, K.; Jutooru, I.; Chadalapaka, G.; Johnson, G.; Frank, J.; Burghardt, R.; Kim, S.; Safe, S. Hotair is a negative prognostic factor and exhibits pro-oncogenic activity in pancreatic cancer. *Oncogene* **2013**, *32*, 1616–1625. [CrossRef] [PubMed]

120. Pang, E.J.; Yang, R.; Fu, X.B.; Liu, Y.F. Overexpression of long non-coding RNA malat1 is correlated with clinical progression and unfavorable prognosis in pancreatic cancer. *Tumour Biol.* **2015**, *36*, 2403–2407. [CrossRef] [PubMed]

121. Peng, W.; Gao, W.; Feng, J. Long noncoding RNA hulc is a novel biomarker of poor prognosis in patients with pancreatic cancer. *Med. Oncol. (Northwood Lond. Engl.)* **2014**, *31*, 346. [CrossRef] [PubMed]

122. Lu, X.; Fang, Y.; Wang, Z.; Xie, J.; Zhan, Q.; Deng, X.; Chen, H.; Jin, J.; Peng, C.; Li, H.; *et al.* Downregulation of gas5 increases pancreatic cancer cell proliferation by regulating cdk6. *Cell Tissue Res.* **2013**, *354*, 891–896. [CrossRef] [PubMed]

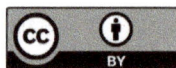

Journal of
*Clinical Medicine*

MDPI

*Review*

# Considering Exosomal miR-21 as a Biomarker for Cancer

Jian Shi

Department of Neurology, Department of Veterans Affairs Medical Center,
San Francisco and University of California, San Francisco, CA 94121, USA;
jian.shi@ucsf.edu; Tel.: +1-415-221-4810; Fax: +1-415-750-2273

Academic Editors: Takahiro Ochiya and Ryou-u Takahashi
Received: 29 November 2015; Accepted: 23 March 2016; Published: 29 March 2016

**Abstract:** Cancer is a fatal human disease. Early diagnosis of cancer is the most effective method to prevent cancer development and to achieve higher survival rates for patients. Many traditional diagnostic methods for cancer are still not sufficient for early, more convenient and accurate, and noninvasive diagnosis. Recently, the use of microRNAs (miRNAs), such as exosomal microRNA-21(miR-21), as potential biomarkers was widely reported. This initial systematic review analyzes the potential role of exosomal miR-21 as a general biomarker for cancers. A total of 10 studies involving 318 patients and 215 healthy controls have covered 10 types of cancers. The sensitivity and specificity of pooled studies were 75% (0.70–0.80) and 85% (0.81–0.91), with their 95% confidence intervals (CIs), while the area under the summary receiver operating characteristic curve (AUC) was 0.93. Additionally, we examined and evaluated almost all other issues about biomarkers, including cutoff points, internal controls and detection methods, from the literature. This initial meta-analysis indicates that exosomal miR-21 has a strong potential to be used as a universal biomarker to identify cancers, although as a general biomarker the case number for each cancer type is small. Based on the literature, a combination of miRNA panels and other cancer antigens, as well as a selection of appropriate internal controls, has the potential to serve as a more sensitive and accurate cancer diagnosis tool. Additional information on miR-21 would further support its use as a biomarker in cancer.

**Keywords:** miR-21; cancer; biomarker; meta-analysis; sensitivity; specificity; miRNAs

## 1. Introduction

Cancer is a major public health problem and is a leading cause of deaths worldwide. Since there is no effective treatment for advanced-stage cancer patients, the five-year survival rate may improve significantly with early diagnosis of cancer such as breast, cervical and prostate cancers. However, some cancer patients have a very poor five-year survival rate, as in the case of lung cancer where the disease is not detected until the late stages. The overall five-year survival rate of lung cancer is approximately 0%–14% [1], while the overall five-year survival rate of breast cancer at stages I and II is 100% (www.cancer.org). Therefore, it is essential to diagnose cancers in the early stages in order to improve the outcomes for patients. Over the past few decades, several biomarkers have been identified as circulating biomarkers in cancer diagnosis, including carcinoembryonic antigen (CEA) and carbohydrate antigen 19-9 (CA 19-9) [2,3]. Nevertheless, these are not capable of diagnosing most types of cancers with high accuracy, which is likely the major reason that limits their usage in cancer diagnosis.

MicroRNAs (miRNAs) are small non-coding RNA molecules of approximately 20–22 nucleotides, which post-transcriptionally regulate the production of proteins from their messenger RNAs. Their biological processes and regulatory pathways have been summarized very well in several reviews [4–6], and hence will not be discussed again in this review. These reviews have noted that miRNAs mediate growth, development, invasion, differentiation and progression of cancers as tumor-suppressing genes or oncogenes [7–9]. Additionally, miRNAs exist in several body fluids, including serum, cerebrospinal fluid, peritoneal lavage fluid, and urine, which makes them serve as robust and reproducible biomarkers for cancer diagnosis. For example, in the circulation system, miRNA levels have recently been used to identify various carcinomas [10,11]. In fact, miRNAs circulating in the serum are present in a variety of forms including within exosomes. Exosomes are 30–100 nm extracellular vesicles that are secreted from cells by exocytosis and are present in most circulating body fluids. Exosomes contain proteins, messenger RNAs and miRNAs [12]. Compared to other miRNA forms, exosomal miRNAs are more stable because they are protected from endogenous RNase degradation. Therefore, exosomal miRNAs may have significant potential as cancer-specific biomarkers.

Since the discovery of several regulatory regions of miR-21 in 2004 [13–15], miR-21 has been found to be over-expressed in many pathological conditions including most types of cancer analyzed so far [16]. As an oncomiR, miR-21 affects all major hallmarks of tumor-developing pathways, which include sustained proliferation through PTEN (phosphatase and tensin homolog) [17], Sprouty [18], PI3K (phosphoinositide 3-kinase) [19] and PDCD4 (tumor suppressor gene tropomyosin 4) [20,21]; impaired apoptosis through BTG2 (B-cell translocation gene 2) [22], FasL (pro-apoptotic FAS ligand) [23], FBXO11 (a member of the F-box subfamily 1) [24], and TIMP3 (inhibitor of metalloproteinases 3) [25]; and angiogenesis and invasion through PTEN [26], TIMP3 [27], and TPM1 (tropomyosin 1) [28], as well as some other pathways related to inflammation and genetic instability [29]. Importantly, a large number of studies have explored the function of miR-21 as a biomarker for cancer diagnosis. While several studies have published meta-analyses on this topic [10,11,16,30], an exosomal miR-21 meta-analysis has not been evaluated yet. In this systematic review, we perform the initial meta-analysis for exosomal miR-21 and discuss major issues related to the use of miR-21 as a potential biomarker for cancer.

## 2. Materials and Methods

### 2.1. Search Formula

For the literature search, we used two search formulas: (1) ("exosomal") AND ("miR-21" OR "miRNA-21") AND ("biomarker") AND ("cancer" OR "tumor"); (2) ("miR-21" OR "miRNA-21") AND ("biomarker") AND ("cancer"). We performed a literature search for relevant studies using the following databases: PubMed, CNKI, and Web of Science (updated to July 13 2015).

### 2.2. Inclusion Criteria and Data Extraction

We chose studies that met the following criteria: (1) investigated the diagnostic potential of exosomal miR-21 for human cancers; (2) used the gold standard to confirm the diagnosis of cancer patients; and (3) provided sufficient data to construct a diagnostic 2 × 2 table. This table contains true positives (TP), false positives (FP), false negatives (FN), and true negatives (TN). Conversely, studies were excluded if they (1) were obviously not related to our topic or focused on other miRNAs; (2) did not have enough data to construct the diagnostic 2 × 2 table; (3) were in the forms of letters, editorials, case reports, or reviews; and (4) used types of samples other than exosomes or extracellular vesicle (EV).

### 2.3. Statistics Analysis

The SAS software (SAS Institute Inc. Cary, NC, USA) and SigmaPlot (11.0) were performed to analyze the statistics. We calculated the pooled sensitivity (TP/(TP + FN)), specificity (TN/(TN + FP)) and 95% confidence intervals (CIs) using the bivariate regression model [31]. Based on the sensitivity and specificity of eligible studies, we constructed summary receiver operating characteristic (SROC) curves by using the Moses' fixed effects method [32]; meanwhile, the corresponding area under the SROC curve (AUC—area under the curve) was calculated.

## 3. Results

### 3.1. Literature Search Results and Summary of Studies

Only 10 of 346 records were selected [33–42] after the primary, secondary and tertiary searches following the strategy shown in the methods. Figure 1 shows the search process. Because the studies of exosomal miRNAs are in the initial stages, we used more general keywords in the second formula in order to obtain more studies. In the primary search, 346 records were gained, and 107 were excluded for duplicates and reviews after careful reading of all those titles and abstracts. In the secondary search, 201 records were excluded because they were neither related to the diagnostic study nor related to miR-21. Two records were excluded because of the unavailability of full articles. In the tertiary search, 26 records were excluded after reading 36 full articles because of the lack of data for the construction of 2 × 2 tables or the absence of exosomal miR-21 data. Finally, only 10 records were related to our topic, in which seven exosomes were from blood, two exosomes were from peritoneal lavage fluid (PLF) [42] or cervicovaginal lavage specimens (CLF) [40], and one extracellular vesicle (EV) was from the cerebrospinal fluid (CSF) [41].

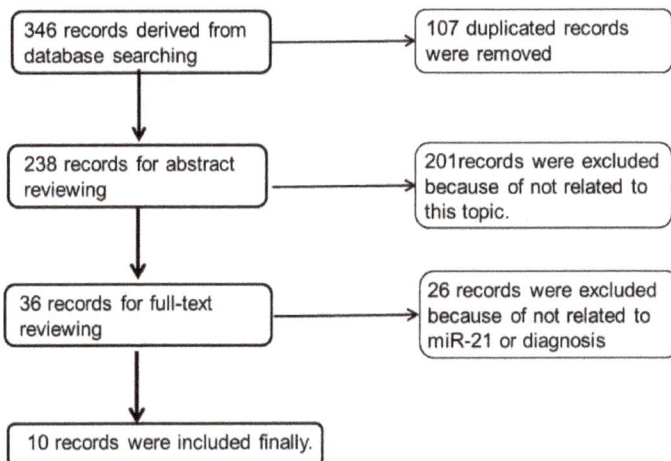

**Figure 1.** Flow diagram of the literature search process.

Table 1 summarized the characteristics of studies that we obtained from the search process. We used the data to perform initial meta-analysis for exosomal miR-21 as a biomarker for cancer. From 2008 to 2015, these studies covered 215 non-cancer controls and 318 cancer patients. Cancers included laryngeal squamous cell carcinoma (LSCC), hepatocellular cancer (HCC), esophageal squamous cell carcinoma (ESCC), colorectal cancer (CC), gastric cancer (GC), ovarian cancer (OC), breast cancer (BC), pancreatic adenocarcinoma (PC), cervical cancer, and glioblastoma. Among these studies, seven exosomal miR-21 samples were from serum, one EV miR-21 was from CSF, and two exosomal miR-21 samples were from cervicovaginal lavage specimens (CLF) and peritoneal lavage fluid (PLF). All information from these studies is listed in Table 1, including the numbers of patients and controls, the types of cancer and sample, and 2 × 2 tables.

**Table 1.** Characteristics of diagnostic clinical studies included in this analysis.

| Study ID | Patients | Controls | Cancer | Specimen | 2 × 2 Table | | | |
|---|---|---|---|---|---|---|---|---|
| | | | | | TP | FN | FP | TN |
| Wang 2014 [33] | 52 | 49 | LSCC | Serum exosome | 36 | 16 | 6 | 43 |
| Wang 2014 [34] | 13 | 30 | HCC (III-IV) | Serum exosome | 9 | 4 | 12 | 18 |
| Tanaka 2013 [37] | 44 | 41 | ESCC | Serum exosome | 28 | 16 | 6 | 35 |
| Taylor 2008 [38] | 30 | 10 | OC | Serum exosome | 30 | 0 | 0 | 10 |
| Tokuhisa 2015 [42] | 9 | 9 | GC | PLF exosome | 8 | 1 | 2 | 7 |
| Ogata-Kawata 2013 [35] | 88 | 11 | CC | Serum exosome | 54 | 34 | 2 | 9 |
| Que 2013 [36] | 22 | 27 | PC | Serum exosome | 21 | 1 | 5 | 22 |
| Liu 2014 [40] | 45 | 25 | Cervical cancer | CLF exosome | 40 | 5 | 0 | 25 |
| Melo 2014 [39] | 11 | 8 | BC | Serum exosome | 9 | 2 | 0 | 8 |
| Akers 2013 [41] | 13 | 14 | Glioblastoma | CSF-EV | 11 | 2 | 1 | 13 |

TP: true positives, FP: false positives, FN: false negatives, TN: true negatives.

### 3.2. The Sensitivity and Specificity of Pooled Studies

Sensitivity and specificity are the most important and widely used statistic indexes for a diagnostic test. It is widely accepted that the sensitivity of a test is its true positive response, and the specificity is its true negative response. As calculated by the bivariate meta-analysis, the overall sensitivity and specificity of these studies were 75% (0.70–0.80) and 85% (0.81–0.91) with 95% CIs. Figure 2A shows the forest plot of sensitivities of all included studies and the overall sensitivity. The red line represents overall sensitivity with hepatocellular cancer (HCC) [32], CC [34] and LSCC [33] studies on the left of the red line, indicating that their sensitivities were less than 75%, while other studies are on the right. In the HCC study, 13 patients in advanced tumor stages (III and IV) and 30 healthy volunteers as controls were included with high expression of miR-21 as the cutoff point [33]. In the ESCC study, there were two groups, which were difficult to combine. One group of 44 patients and 41 controls was included with 0.02-fold as the cutoff point [37]. The gastric cancer (GC) study had no healthy control, and thus, patients at stage T1-2 were used as controls for patients at stage T3–4 [42]. In the breast cancer (BC) study, after exosomes were harvested from the serum of healthy controls and breast cancer patients, they were left in cell-free culture conditions for 24 h or 72 h, followed by qPCR being performed for all samples at the two time points. The fold-change of exosome miR-21 at 72 h was quantified relative to the exosomal miRNA at 24 h [39]. We chose 1.5-fold as the cutoff points in this study.

Figure 2B shows the specificities of all included studies as well as the overall specificity. Notably, the specificity of the GC study [42] is on the left of the red line, which is the overall specificity position. The specificities of several other studies are also on the left of the red line, though close to it.

### 3.3. The SROC and AUC of Pooled Studies

In 1993, Moses *et al.* [32] developed the summary receiver operating characteristic (SROC) curve, which is used to summarize the results from several independent studies for the same biomarker or the same test. In fact, the ROC curve represents a diagnostic test's sensitivity *versus* its false positive rate (1-specificity). Although SROC and ROC curves are both plotted with sensitivity and 1-specificity, they are very different. The points of a ROC curve are usually obtained from a single study by changing the cutoff points continually, while the points of a SROC curve are from independent studies, and each point represents one study. After two decades of development, while there are more complex models for obtaining SROC curves to summarize independent studies, most curves are similar to the curve from Moses' model [43]. Therefore, to generate a SROC curve, Moses' model is still the most popular model. Following the process of Moses' model, in the first fitting process, two points were outliers. To keep HCC data, we chose HBsAg negative people (FP = 1, TN = 5) as controls from all healthy controls in this study [33]. In the second fitting process, only one data point was an outlier. Figure 3 shows the SROC curve of exosomal miR-21 fitted for this study, and those dots represent all pooled studies. The area under the curve (AUC) represents diagnostic accuracy. For the SROC of included studies, the AUC was 0.93, indicating a high level of diagnostic accuracy and the possibility of using exosomal miR-21 as an overall diagnostic biomarker for cancer.

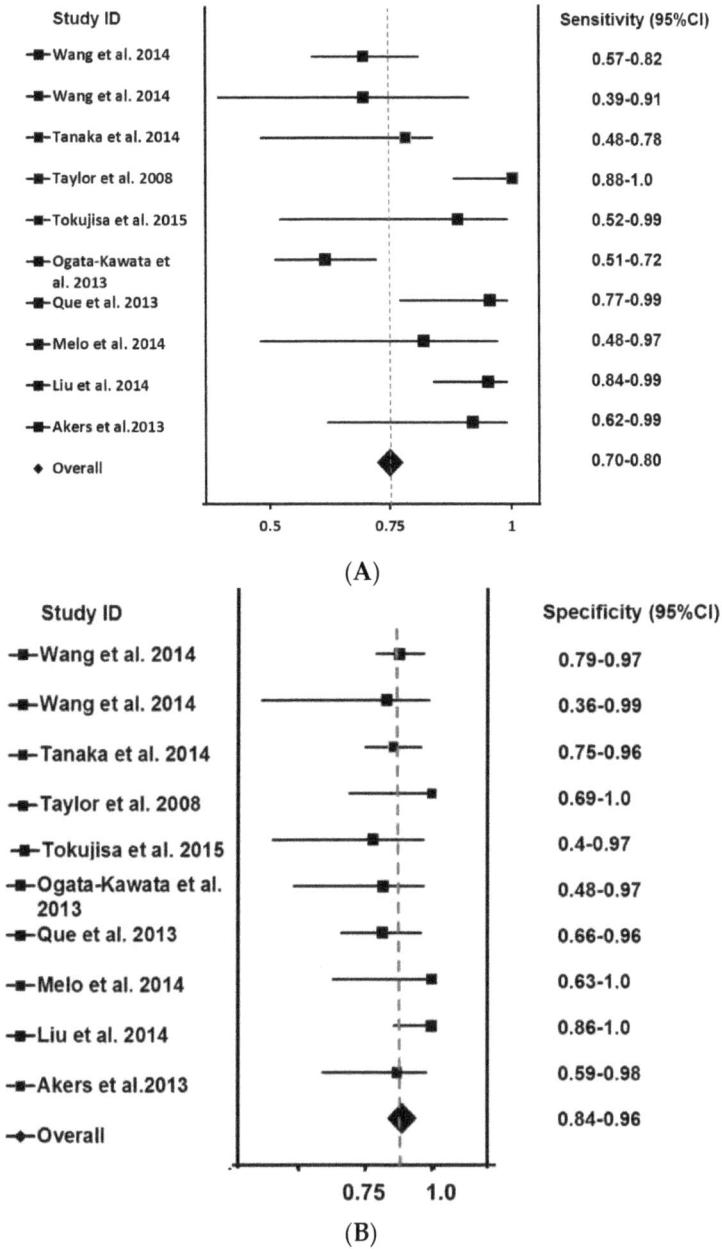

**Figure 2.** The forest plots of sensitivity (**A**) and specificity (**B**) of each included studies. In each picture, the left side shows the ID of studies, and the right side shows their 95% CIs.

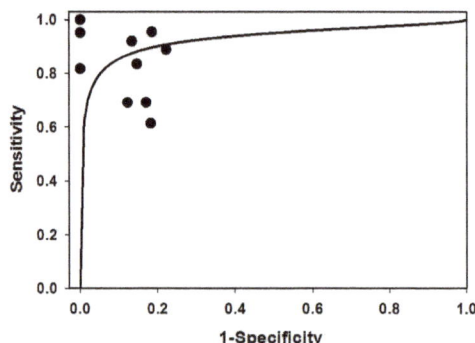

**Figure 3.** The SROC curve for different cancers with pooled studies of sensitivity and specificity. Exosomal miR-21 yielded an area under the SROC curve (AUC) of 0.93 with an overall sensitivity of 75% (0.70–0.80) and specificity of 85% (0.81–0.91) with their 95% CIs.

### 3.4. The Cutoff Values and Endogenous Controls

To consider exosomal miR-2 as a biomarker, we have to evaluate its cutoff value and endogenous control for cancer diagnosis. Although these studies used different methods for the isolation of exosomes, performing qPCR as well as internal controls, we could obtain pertinent information that would allow us to understand the characteristics of exosomal miR-21 as a biomarker for cancers in the future. In Table 2, we compare the cutoff values and internal controls from all studies, especially those five studies that used serum exosomal miR-21 and measured miR-21 by real-time PCR. The cutoff values were calculated using either the $-\Delta\Delta CT$ equation or the $2^{-\Delta\Delta CT}$ equation. The methods of exosome isolation and qPCR performance are also shown in Table 2.

**Table 2.** The cutoff value and internal control of exosomal miR-21.

| Cancer | Cutoff Point | | Internal Control | qPCR | Exosome Isolation |
|---|---|---|---|---|---|
| | Fold | $2^{-\Delta\Delta CT}$ | | | |
| HCC [33] | 5 | 0.03 ** | U6 | SYBR Green | Reagent (Life Tech.) |
| PC [36] | 4.05 | 0.06 ** | U6 | TaqMan | Ultracentrifugation |
| ESCC [37] | 5.66 * | 0.02 | miR-16 | TaqMan | ExoQuick (SBI) |
| LSCC [34] | 4.55 * | 0.043 | U6 | SYBR Green | ExoQuick (SBI) |
| CC [35] | 6.56 * | 0.0108 | miR-451 | TaqMan | Ultracentrifugation |
| GC [42] | 3.5 * | 0.088 | miR-16 | TagMan | Ultracentrifugation |
| OC [38] | 11 intensity | None | microarry | None | MACS |
| Cervical C. [40] cancer [40] | 3.0-fold | None | None | TaqMan | Ultracentrifugation |
| Glioblastoma [41] | 0.25/EV | None | None | absolute | Ultracentrifugation |

MACS: magnetic activated cell sorting; * The cutoff values were calculated using $\Delta\Delta CT$ (patients-controls);
** The cutoff values were calculated using the $2^{-\Delta\Delta CT}$ equation and then normalized to given internal control.

Usually, the $2^{-\Delta\Delta CT}$ formula is calculated for the quantification of miRNA expressions, where CT is the cycle threshold and $\Delta\Delta CT = ((CTmiRNA)tumor - (CTcontrol)tumor) - ((CTmiRNA)normal - (CTcontrol)normal)$. The values of $\Delta\Delta CT$ directly indicate fold changes, while $2^{-\Delta\Delta CT}$ indicates the changes in miRNA expression. In Table 2, the cutoff values without stars are original data from the listed studies, while the other cutoff points are those calculated by authors for easy comparison.

According to the upper five data points of Table 2, the cutoff point of exosomal miR-21 as a general biomarker may be close to 4.0 to 5.5 folds, between which the variation is very narrow, at least in serum-derived exosomal miR-21. The data could be compared because the studies used relative RT-PCR with all exosomes derived from blood. In the GC study, the 3.5-fold cutoff value is close to the range of 4.0 to 5.5 folds because relative RT-PCR methods were used, although the exosomes were derived from PLF and not from blood. In fact, differences in reagents for qPCR, internal controls and methods of exosome isolation would also influence the results of qPCR and the cutoff values. Therefore, it may be possible to obtain a universal cutoff point for the miR-21 in order to detect cancers after using standard reagent, internal controls, and methods and resources for the isolation of exosomes. Indeed, it is essential to obtain a universal cutoff point in order to establish a universal biomarker.

However, the cutoff values cannot be compared to each other upon using different experimental methods in the lower four rows of Table 2. For example, the ovarian cancer (OC) study used microarray analysis, whereas the BC study used values of miR-21 at 72 h *vs.* 24 h as the cutoff points. Their cutoff points had different meanings, so they could not be compared to each other. Likely, the absolute RT-PCR was performed in a glioblastoma study, while a relative RT-PCR without any internal control was used in the cervical cancer study. Although these two studies did not have internal controls, the cutoff values could not be compared because of the same reason. The cutoff value was a copy number per exosome in the glioblastoma study, whereas the cutoff value was relative folds in the cervical cancer study.

## 4. Discussion

### 4.1. The Exosomal miR-21 as a Universal Biomarker for Diagnostic Cancers

This initial meta-analysis, including 10 types of cancer, suggests that exosomal miR-21 may be a universal fluid biomarker for cancers. Compared to CA19-9 and CEA, which have widely been used as tumor biomarkers for detecting many types of cancer, exosomal miR-21 seems to be more accurate for the diagnosis of cancers. For example, the sensitivities of CEA, CA 19-9 and miR-21 for detecting colorectal cancer were 30.7%, 15.9% and 61.4%, respectively [35]. Additionally, the accuracy of exosomal miR-21 (AUC = 93) for diagnosis was likely to be better than that of circulating miR-21 in various carcinomas (AUC = 87) [10], lung cancer (AUC = 81) [1], non-small cell lung cancers (AUC = 0.775) [44], and all cancers (AUC = 88) [30]. However, we need to note that all of these meta-analyses were based on larger case numbers compared to our study. Therefore, higher patient numbers are needed for exosomal miR-21 to be compared and to confirm whether or not exosomal miR-21 is better than circulating miR-21. Importantly, several studies indicated that miR-21 may be an important regulatory molecule in carcinogenesis, and suggested that miR-21 may become a universal serum biomarker for carcinomas [36]. Conversely, there is still a lack of effective biomarkers for the early diagnosis of brain tumors even though there are many new advances in the understanding of the molecular pathogenesis of brain tumors. A miR-21 meta-analysis of brain tumors may explore the prognostic role of miR-21 expression in patients with brain tumors, in which miR-21 may be expressed in the tumor tissue or blood of patients. It has been suggested that high expression of miR-21 is associated with poor prognosis in patients with brain tumors [45]. Nevertheless, the expression levels of CSF-derived EV miR-21 from glioblastoma patients were 10-fold higher than those derived from non-tumor patients; the detected sensitivity, specificity, and accuracy were 87%, 93% and 91% (AUC = 0.91), respectively. In contrast, no significant differences in EV miR-21 levels could be detected between patients with or without glioblastoma when EVs were isolated from sera [41].

However, as an overall early biomarker, miR-21 is not appropriate for use in diagnosis of some cancers. For example, we can see in the HCC study that exosomal miR-21 could not detect HCC in stage I and II and it represented sensitivity not only in HCC patients but also in HBsAg-positive healthy controls [33]. Similarly, given that exosomal miR-21 expression increased in HPV-positive controls as well as in cervical cancer patients [40], HPV-positive patients could not be used as controls. Therefore, because the function of exosomal miR-21 in a number of diseases other than cancer is unclear, its usage is limited to being a general biomarker for cancers. In breast cancer, exosomal miR-21 was also more sensitive to the later stages of cancer [46]. Thus, some studies can use miR-21 as a progressive indicator.

### 4.2. The Combination of miRNA Panels and Cancer Antigens

Some combinations of miRNAs and cancer antigens may enhance the sensitivity and specificity of these biomarker panels for cancer diagnosis. In this regard, a combination of miR-21, miR-210 and miR-486-5p might be used to diagnose lung tumors because the miRNA panel distinguished lung tumors from benign pulmonary nodules, with the AUC of 0.86, sensitivity of 75% and specificity of 85% [47]. Additionally, another panel of plasma miRNAs, including miR-122, miR-192, miR-21, miR-223, miR-26a, miR-27a, and miR-801, provided high diagnostic accuracy (AUC = 0.89) to identify hepatocellular carcinoma (HCC) [48]. Moreover, a combination of miR-10b and miR-373 indicated that patients with lymph node–positive breast cancer, compared to those with node-negative breast cancer, had an enhanced diagnostic sensitivity and specificity up to 72% and 94%, which was better than miR-10b or miR-373 individual diagnosis [49]. In fact, this might be very helpful for surgeons to choose a breast-conserving surgery for patients with lymph node–negative breast cancer, which could greatly improve the quality of life in the post-surgery patients. Further, the aberrant serum levels of miRNAs in the panel, namely miR-21 (high), miR-126 (low), miR-155 (high), miR-199a (low) and miR-335 (low), could identify breast cancer with hormone-negative receptor status [46], in which the three common hormone receptors are not present in cancer tissues, so they are also called triple negative breast cancer. Mostly, triple negative breast cancer is more aggressive and difficult to treat, but in earlier stages, the cancer can respond to chemotherapy even better compared to other forms of breast cancers (www.nationalbreastcancer.org). Thus, this complex miRNA panel may have potential for diagnosing triple negative breast cancer in the earlier stages, and therefore, it may have potential to increase the five-year survival rate.

Furthermore, from the above example, we observed that if CEA and miR-21 were combined, the sensitivity would be 72.7%, which is better than 30.7% (CEA) or 61.4% (miR-21) individually [35]. In a pancreatic cancer study, the combination of miR-16, miR-196a and CA19-9 was even more effective in diagnosing the disease, with AUC, sensitivity, and specificity up to 0.98, 92% and 96%, respectively [50]. This study also showed that the AUC of miR-21 was 0.83, but the combination of miR-21 with CA19-9 did not significantly improve the AUC. Therefore, to achieve an effective diagnosis, not only do we need to use the combination of some miRNA panels and/or cancer antigens, but we also need to compare and choose the right combination of miRNAs and cancer antigens.

### 4.3. Choosing the Right Internal Controls

The endogenous control is very important for the normalization, reliability and reproducibility of diagnostic results because it helps to normalize differences among sample qualities and variations in detecting processes, including RNA extraction, reverse transcription procedures and reverse transcription quantitative PCR (RT-qPCR). In the pooled studies, internal controls included miR-16, U6 and miR-451, of which U6 and miR-16 seemed more popular. Recently, Xiang *et al.* compared the expressions of U6, miR-16 and miR-24 in serum following several freeze-thaw cycles, knowing that U6 expression gradually decreased after several cycles of freezing and thawing. In contrast, the expression of miR-16 and miR-24 remained relatively stable. This suggests that U6 is not an ideal internal control if freeze-thawing is required [51]. Additionally, U6 varied significantly from −1.03 to 8.12-fold in different tumors [52], and the expression levels of U6 showed a high degree of variability between the carcinoma tissues of the liver and the adjacent normal tissues [53]. Therefore, when selecting U6 as an internal control for evaluating profiles of miRNAs in freeze-thaw procedures as well as in carcinoma patients, we need to pay more attention.

Conversely, miR-16 is frequently used as a control because it is highly expressive and relatively invariant across large numbers of samples and tissues [54]; however, elevated levels of miR-16 were found in serum correlating with bone metastasis in breast cancer patients [55]. Additionally, in a pancreatic cancer study we discussed above, the combination of miR-16 and miR-24 was even used to diagnose this cancer [47]. Therefore, further investigation is required for selecting an internal normalization procedure in this scenario.

Recently, there have been several better choices for internal controls. Like miRNA panels, a panel of miR-16 and miR-425 was suggested as an internal control panel because of its more stable expressions in different cancers and controls that may lead to more accurate detection of altered target miRNA expression [56]. Conversely, for pancreatic ductal adenocarcinoma diagnostics, the internal control U91 was better than U6 or miR-16, but the most stable panel of internal controls was a combination of U6 and U91, compared to U6, miR-16 or U91 separately [52]. In addition, as internal controls of plasma miRNA research, the panel of U6 and miR-520d-5p was the best candidate after being compared with Let-7a, Let-7d, Let-7g, miR-16, U6, RNU48, miR-191, miR-223, miR-484, and miR-520d-5p. Accordingly, this control panel represented the consistency and high Ct in all studied samples and a very narrow and reproducible SD [57].

*4.4. Comparison of Exosomal miR-21 Expression in Other Diseases*

Understanding exosomal miR-21 expression in other diseases (non-cancer) would improve its use as a biomarker to distinguish cancers from other diseases. For example, the miR-21 expressed in HBsAg-positive people and live cirrhosis patients had very high true positive (TP) values, 45.8% and 52.2%, respectively, using the same cutoff points of HCC. Thus, we should treat the positive data very carefully when using miR-21 to detect HCC (69.2% TP) [33] in these people and patients. Additionally, we could not use these people and patients as negative controls when studying cancer diagnosis. Additionally, as discussed above, exosomal miR-21 expressed in HPV-positive people had 52% TP using the cutoff value of cervical cancer [40]; in fact, almost all CC cases are caused by HPV, so we should know that some people have a high expression of miR-21 and HPV positivity without cancer. In this situation, detecting high-risk HPV expression may be a useful method to distinguish some cervical cancer patients and people with a high risk of cervical cancer from regular HPV-positive people. Moreover, patents with vocal cord polyps or cholecystolithiasis were used as negative controls for the miR-21 detection of LSCC [34] or ESCC [37], knowing that exosomal miR-21 expression was lower in those patients. Further, a recent study showed that exosomal miR-21 was highly upregulated in the CSF of Japanese Encephalitis Virus (JEV) patients, in which the detected difference was approximately five folds between JEV-positive patients and JEV-negative controls using the RT-PCR method and miR-93, miR-24 and miR-103 as internal controls [58]. As shown above, exosomal miR-21 was highly upregulated (10-fold) in glioblastoma [45], but the cutoff values could not be compared here because their meanings were different. Even so, the upregulation of miR-21 in JEV patients may allow doctors to pay more attention to the false positive results generated by exosomal miR-21 when detecting glioblastoma in the virus-infected areas. Therefore, knowing more about miR-21 expression in other diseases may provide more supportive data for miR-21 use.

## 5. Conclusions and Prospect

Based on the accuracy of this initial meta-analysis and very close cutoff values from different experimental conditions, methods and internal controls, exosomal miR-21 has a very strong potential to be a good general biomarker for cancer diagnosis. The results of exosomal miR-21 seemed to be better than those of circulating miR-21 according to several comparisons we discussed above, but we know the case number was too small to give a very strong conclusion. Although the sample size was small in this study, determining and understanding the characteristics of different candidates as biomarkers for cancers are important topics in the development of the best diagnostic methods for early stages of cancers in order to increase the survival rates of the patients.

Prospectively, combining the right miRNA panels or cancer antigens may give better diagnostic results or prognostic predictions in most circumstances. To make a better diagnosis, we should also pay more attention to choosing correct, stable and consistent internal controls or internal control panels. For a general biomarker, other issues, including qPCR reagents and exosome-isolating methods, also need to be standardized. In addition, an in-depth study of various diseases for miR-21 would allow better application for cancer diagnosis.

**Acknowledgments:** Thanks to Tina Lam for her reading and revising one version of the manuscript.

**Conflicts of Interest:** The author declares no conflict of interest.

## References

1. Wu, R.; Jiang, Y.; Wu, Q.; Li, Q.; Cheng, D.; Xu, L.; Zhang, C.; Zhang, M.; Ye, L. Diagnostic value of microRNA-21 in the diagnosis of lung cancer: Evidence from a meta-analysis involving 11 studies. *Tumour Biol.* **2014**, *35*, 8829–8836. [CrossRef] [PubMed]

2. Duffy, M.J. Role of tumor markers in patients with solid cancers: A critical review. *Eur. J. Intern. Med.* **2007**, *18*, 175–184. [CrossRef] [PubMed]

3. O'Byrne, K.J.; Gatzemeier, U.; Bondarenko, I.; Barrios, C.; Eschbach, C.; Martens, U.M.; Hotko, Y.; Kortsik, C.; Paz-Ares, L.; Pereira, J.R.; *et al.* Molecular biomarkers in non-small-cell lung cancer: A retrospective analysis of data from the phase 3 flex study. *Lancet Oncol.* **2011**, *12*, 795–805.

4. Ambros, V. The functions of animal microRNAs. *Nature* **2004**, *431*, 350–355. [CrossRef] [PubMed]

5. Bartel, D.P. MicroRNAs: Genomics, biogenesis, mechanism, and function. *Cell* **2004**, *116*, 281–297. [CrossRef]

6. Shi, J. Regulatory networks between neurotrophins and miRNAs in brain diseases and cancers. *Actapharmacol. Sin.* **2015**, *36*, 149–157. [CrossRef] [PubMed]

7. Schwarzenbach, H.; Nishida, N.; Calin, G.A.; Pantel, K. Clinical relevance of circulating cell-free microRNAs in cancer. *Nat. Rev. Clin. Oncol.* **2014**, *11*, 145–156. [CrossRef] [PubMed]

8. Yoshino, H.; Seki, N.; Itesako, T.; Chiyomaru, T.; Nakagawa, M.; Enokida, H. Aberrant expression of microRNAs in bladder cancer. *Nat. Rev. Urol.* **2013**, *10*, 396–404. [CrossRef] [PubMed]

9. Takahashi, R.U.; Miyazaki, H.; Ochiya, T. The roles of microRNAs in breast cancer. *Cancers* **2015**, *7*, 598–616. [CrossRef] [PubMed]

10. Wu, K.; Li, L.; Li, S. Circulating microRNA-21 as a biomarker for the detection of various carcinomas: An updated meta-analysis based on 36 studies. *Tumour Biol.* **2015**, *36*, 1973–1981. [CrossRef] [PubMed]

11. Zeng, Z.; Wang, J.; Zhao, L.; Hu, P.; Zhang, H.; Tang, X.; He, D.; Tang, S.; Zeng, Z. Potential role of microRNA-21 in the diagnosis of gastric cancer: A meta-analysis. *PLoS ONE* **2013**, *8*, e73278. [CrossRef] [PubMed]

12. Colombo, M.; Raposo, G.; Thery, C. Biogenesis, secretion, and intercellular interactions of exosomes and other extracellular vesicles. *Annu. Rev. Cell Dev. Biol.* **2014**, *30*, 255–289. [CrossRef] [PubMed]

13. Cai, X.; Hagedorn, C.H.; Cullen, B.R. Human microRNAs are processed from capped, polyadenylated transcripts that can also function as miRNAs. *RNA* **2004**, *10*, 1957–1966. [CrossRef] [PubMed]

14. Loffler, D.; Brocke-Heidrich, K.; Pfeifer, G.; Stocsits, C.; Hackermuller, J.; Kretzschmar, A.K.; Burger, R.; Gramatzki, M.; Blumert, C.; Bauer, K.; *et al.* Interleukin-6 dependent survival of multiple myeloma cells involves the Stat3-mediated induction of microRNA-21 through a highly conserved enhancer. *Blood* **2007**, *110*, 1330–1333. [CrossRef] [PubMed]

15. Fujita, S.; Ito, T.; Mizutani, T.; Minoguchi, S.; Yamamichi, N.; Sakurai, K.; Iba, H. miR-21 gene expression triggered by AP-1 is sustained through a double-negative feedback mechanism. *J. Mol. Biol.* **2008**, *378*, 492–504. [CrossRef] [PubMed]

16. Shen, L.; Wan, Z.; Ma, Y.; Wu, L.; Liu, F.; Zang, H.; Xin, S. The clinical utility of microRNA-21 as novel biomarker for diagnosing human cancers. *Tumour Biol.* **2015**, *36*, 1993–2005. [CrossRef] [PubMed]

17. Meng, F.; Henson, R.; Wehbe-Janek, H.; Ghoshal, K.; Jacob, S.T.; Patel, T. microRNA-21 regulates expression of the pten tumor suppressor gene in human hepatocellular cancer. *Gastroenterology* **2007**, *133*, 647–658. [CrossRef] [PubMed]

18. Sayed, D.; Rane, S.; Lypowy, J.; He, M.; Chen, I.Y.; Vashistha, H.; Yan, L.; Malhotra, A.; Vatner, D.; Abdellatif, M. microRNA-21 targets sprouty2 and promotes cellular outgrowths. *Mol. Biol. Cell* **2008**, *19*, 3272–3282. [CrossRef] [PubMed]

19. Xiong, B.; Cheng, Y.; Ma, L.; Zhang, C. miR-21 regulates biological behavior through the PTEN/PI-3 k/Akt signaling pathway in human colorectal cancer cells. *Int. J. Oncol.* **2013**, *42*, 219–228. [CrossRef] [PubMed]

20. Asangani, I.A.; Rasheed, S.A.; Nikolova, D.A.; Leupold, J.H.; Colburn, N.H.; Post, S.; Allgayer, H. MicroRNA-21 (miR-21) post-transcriptionally downregulates tumor suppressor Pdcd4 and stimulates invasion, intravasation and metastasis in colorectal cancer. *Oncogene* **2008**, *27*, 2128–2136. [CrossRef] [PubMed]

21. Peacock, O.; Lee, A.C.; Cameron, F.; Tarbox, R.; Vafadar-Isfahani, N.; Tufarelli, C.; Lund, J.N. Inflammation and miR-21 pathways functionally interact to downregulate PDCD4 in colorectal cancer. *PLoS ONE* **2014**, *9*, e110267. [CrossRef] [PubMed]

22. Yang, C.H.; Yue, J.; Pfeffer, S.R.; Handorf, C.R.; Pfeffer, L.M. MicroRNA miR-21 regulates the metastatic behavior of B16 melanoma cells. *J. Biol. Chem.* **2011**, *286*, 39172–39178. [CrossRef] [PubMed]

23. Wang, K.; Li, P.F. Foxo3a regulates apoptosis by negatively targeting miR-21. *J. Biol. Chem.* **2010**, *285*, 16958–16966. [CrossRef] [PubMed]

24. Yang, C.H.; Pfeffer, S.R.; Sims, M.; Yue, J.; Wang, Y.; Linga, V.G.; Paulus, E.; Davidoff, A.M.; Pfeffer, L.M. The oncogenic microRNA-21 inhibits the tumor suppressive activity of FBXO11 to promote tumorigenesis. *J. Biol. Chem.* **2015**, *290*, 6037–6046. [CrossRef] [PubMed]

25. Martin del Campo, S.E.; Latchana, N.; Levine, K.M.; Grignol, V.P.; Fairchild, E.T.; Jaime-Ramirez, A.C.; Dao, T.V.; Karpa, V.I.; Carson, M.; Ganju, A.; *et al.* miR-21 enhances melanoma invasiveness *via* inhibition of tissue inhibitor of metalloproteinases 3 expression: In vivo effects of miR-21 inhibitor. *PLoS ONE* **2015**, *10*, e0115919.

26. Liu, L.Z.; Li, C.; Chen, Q.; Jing, Y.; Carpenter, R.; Jiang, Y.; Kung, H.F.; Lai, L.; Jiang, B.H. miR-21 induced angiogenesis through AKT and ERK activation and HIF-1α expression. *PLoS ONE* **2011**, *6*, e19139. [CrossRef] [PubMed]

27. Qi, J.H.; Ebrahem, Q.; Moore, N.; Murphy, G.; Claesson-Welsh, L.; Bond, M.; Baker, A.; Anand-Apte, B. A novel function for tissue inhibitor of metalloproteinases-3 (TIMP3): Inhibition of angiogenesis by blockage of VEGF binding to VEGF receptor-2. *Nat. Med.* **2003**, *9*, 407–415. [CrossRef] [PubMed]

28. Zhu, S.; Si, M.L.; Wu, H.; Mo, Y.Y. MicroRNA-21 targets the tumor suppressor gene tropomyosin 1 (TMP1). *J. Biol. Chem.* **2007**, *282*, 14328–14336. [CrossRef] [PubMed]

29. Melnik, B.C. Mir-21: An environmental driver of malignant melanoma? *J. Transl. Med.* **2015**, *13*, 202. [CrossRef] [PubMed]

30. Shen, J.; Todd, N.W.; Zhang, H.; Yu, L.; Lingxiao, X.; Mei, Y.; Guarnera, M.; Liao, J.; Chou, A.; Lu, C.L.; *et al.* Plasma microRNAs as potential biomarkers for non-small-cell lung cancer. *Labo. Investig.* **2011**, *91*, 579–587. [CrossRef] [PubMed]

31. Deville, W.L.; Buntinx, F.; Bouter, L.M.; Montori, V.M.; de Vet, H.C.; van der Windt, D.A.; Bezemer, P.D. Conducting systematic reviews of diagnostic studies: Didactic guidelines. *BMC Med. Res. Methodol.* **2002**, *2*, 9. [CrossRef] [PubMed]

32. Moses, L.E.; Shapiro, D.; Littenberg, B. Combining independent studies of a diagnostic test into a summary roc curve: Data-analytic approaches and some additional considerations. *Stat. Med.* **1993**, *12*, 1293–1316. [CrossRef] [PubMed]

33. Wang, H.; Hou, L.; Li, A.; Duan, Y.; Gao, H.; Song, X. Expression of serum exosomal microRNA-21 inhuman hepatocellular carcinoma. *BioMed Res. Int.* **2014**, *2014*, 864894. [CrossRef] [PubMed]

34. Wang, J.; Zhou, Y.; Lu, J.; Sun, Y.; Xiao, H.; Liu, M.; Tian, L. Combined detection of serum exosomal miR-21 and hotair as diagnostic and prognostic biomarkers for laryngeal squamous cell carcinoma. *Med. Oncol.* **2014**, *31*, 148. [CrossRef] [PubMed]

35. Ogata-Kawata, H.; Izumiya, M.; Kurioka, D.; Honma, Y.; Yamada, Y.; Furuta, K.; Gunji, T.; Ohta, H.; Okamoto, H.; Sonoda, H.; *et al.* Circulating exosomal microRNAs as biomarkers of colon cancer. *PLoS ONE* **2014**, *9*, e92921. [CrossRef] [PubMed]

36. Que, R.; Ding, G.; Chen, J.; Cao, L. Analysis of serum exosomal microRNAs and clinicopathologic features of patients with pancreatic adenocarcinoma. *World J. Surg. Oncol.* **2013**, *11*, 219. [CrossRef] [PubMed]

37. Tanaka, Y.; Kamohara, H.; Kinoshita, K.; Kurashige, J.; Ishimoto, T.; Iwatsuki, M.; Watanabe, M.; Baba, H. Clinical impact of serum exosomal microRNA-21 as a clinical biomarker in human esophageal squamous cell carcinoma. *Cancer* **2013**, *119*, 1159–1167. [CrossRef] [PubMed]

38. Taylor, D.D.; Gercel-Taylor, C. MicroRNA signatures of tumor-derived exosomes as diagnostic biomarkers of ovarian cancer. *Gynecol. Oncol.* **2008**, *110*, 13–21. [CrossRef] [PubMed]

39. Melo, S.A.; Sugimoto, H.; O'Connell, J.T.; Kato, N.; Villanueva, A.; Vidal, A.; Qiu, L.; Vitkin, E.; Perelman, L.T.; Melo, C.A.; *et al.* Cancer exosomes perform cell-independent microRNA biogenesis and promote tumorigenesis. *Cancer Cell* **2014**, *26*, 707–721. [CrossRef] [PubMed]

40. Liu, J.; Sun, H.; Wang, X.; Yu, Q.; Li, S.; Yu, X.; Gong, W. Increased exosomal microRNA-21 and microRNA-146a levels in the cervicovaginal lavage specimens of patients with cervical cancer. *Int. J. Mol. Sci.* **2014**, *15*, 758–773. [CrossRef] [PubMed]

41.    Akers, J.C.; Ramakrishnan, V.; Kim, R.; Skog, J.; Nakano, I.; Pingle, S.; Kalinina, J.; Hua, W.; Kesari, S.; Mao, Y.; *et al.* MiR-21 in the extracellular vesicles (EVs) of cerebrospinal fluid (CSF): A platform for glioblastoma biomarker development. *PLoS ONE* **2013**, *8*, e78115.

42.    Tokuhisa, M.; Ichikawa, Y.; Kosaka, N.; Ochiya, T.; Yashiro, M.; Hirakawa, K.; Kosaka, T.; Makino, H.; Akiyama, H.; Kunisaki, C.; *et al.* Exosomal miRNAs from peritoneum lavage fluid as potential prognostic biomarkers of peritoneal metastasis in gastric cancer. *PLoS ONE* **2015**, *10*, e0130472. [CrossRef] [PubMed]

43.    Dahabreh, I.J.; Trikalinos, T.A.; Lau, J.; Schmid, C. *An empirical Assessment of Bivariate Methods for Meta-Analysis of Test Accuracy*; Agency for Healthcare Research and Quality: Rockville, MD, USA, 2012.

44.    Wei, J.; Gao, W.; Zhu, C.; Liu, Y.; Mei, Z.; Cheng, T.; Shu, Y. Identification of plasma microRNA-21 as a biomarker for early detection and chemosensitivity of non-small lung cancer. *Chin. J. Caner* **2011**, *30*, 407–414. [CrossRef]

45.    He, X.Y.; Liao, Y.D.; Guo, X.Q.; Wang, R.; Xiao, Z.Y.; Wang, Y.G. Prognostic role of microRNA-21 expression in brain tumors: A meta-analysis. *Mol. Neurobiol.* **2016**, *53*, 1856–1861. [CrossRef] [PubMed]

46.    Wang, F.; Zheng, Z.; Guo, J.; Ding, X. Correlation and quantitation of microRNA aberrant expression in tissues and sera from patients with breast tumor. *Gynecol. Oncol.* **2010**, *119*, 586–593. [CrossRef] [PubMed]

47.    Shen, J.; Liu, Z.; Todd, N.W.; Zhang, H.; Liao, J.; Yu, L.; Guarnera, M.A.; Li, R.; Cai, L.; Zhan, M.; *et al.* Diagnosis of lung cancer in individuals with solitary pulmonary nodules by plasma microRNA biomarkers. *BMC Cancer* **2011**, *11*, 374. [CrossRef] [PubMed]

48.    Zhou, J.; Yu, L.; Gao, X.; Hu, J.; Wang, J.; Dai, Z.; Wang, J.F.; Zhang, Z.; Lu, S.; Huang, X.; *et al.* Plasma microRNA panel to diagnose hepatitis b virus-related hepatocellular carcinoma. *J. Clin. Oncol.* **2011**, *29*, 4781–4788. [CrossRef] [PubMed]

49.    Chen, W.; Cai, F.; Zhang, B.; Barekati, Z.; Zhong, X.Y. The level of circulating miRNA-10b and miRNA-373 in detecting lymph node metastasis of breast cancer: Potential biomarkers. *Tumour Biol.* **2013**, *34*, 455–462. [CrossRef] [PubMed]

50.    Liu, J.; Gao, J.; Du, Y.; Li, Z.; Ren, Y.; Gu, J.; Wang, X.; Gong, Y.; Wang, W.; Kong, X. Combination of plasma microRNAs with serum CA19-9 for early detection of pancreatic cancer. *Int. J. Cancer* **2012**, *131*, 683–691. [CrossRef] [PubMed]

51.    Xiang, M.; Zeng, Y.; Yang, R.; Xu, H.; Chen, Z.; Zhong, J.; Xie, H.; Xu, Y.; Zeng, X. U6 is not a suitable endogenous control for the quantification of circulating microRNAs. *Biochem. Biophys. Res. Commun.* **2014**, *454*, 210–214. [CrossRef] [PubMed]

52.    Popov, A.; Szabo, A.; Mandys, V. Small nucleolar RNA U91 is a new internal control for accurate microRNAs quantification in pancreatic cancer. *BMC Cancer* **2015**, *15*, 774. [CrossRef] [PubMed]

53.    Lou, G.; Ma, N.; Xu, Y.; Jiang, L.; Yang, J.; Wang, C.; Jiao, Y.; Gao, X. Differential distribution of U6 (RNU6–1) expression in human carcinoma tissues demonstrates the requirement for caution in the internal control gene selection for microRNA quantification. *Int. J. Mol. Med.* **2015**, *36*, 1400–1408. [CrossRef] [PubMed]

54.    Kroh, E.M.; Parkin, R.K.; Mitchell, P.S.; Tewari, M. Analysis of circulating microRNA biomarkers in plasma and serum using quantitative reverse transcription-PCR (qRT-PCR). *Methods* **2010**, *50*, 298–301. [CrossRef] [PubMed]

55.    Ell, B.; Mercatali, L.; Ibrahim, T.; Campbell, N.; Schwarzenbach, H.; Pantel, K.; Amadori, D.; Kang, Y. Tumor-induced osteoclast miRNA changes as regulators and biomarkers of osteolytic bone metastasis. *Cancer Cell* **2013**, *24*, 542–556. [CrossRef] [PubMed]

56.    McDermott, A.M.; Kerin, M.J.; Miller, N. Identification and validation of miRNAs as endogenous controls for RQ-PCR in blood specimens for breast cancer studies. *PLoS ONE* **2013**, *8*, e83718.

57.    Rice, J.; Roberts, H.; Rai, S.N.; Galandiuk, S. Housekeeping genes for studies of plasma microRNA: A need for more precise standardization. *Surgery* **2015**, *158*, 1345–1351. [CrossRef] [PubMed]

58.    Goswami, S.; Banerjee, A.; Kumari, B.; Bandopadhyay, B.; Bhattacharya, N.; Basu, N.; Vrati, S.; Banerjee, A. Differential expression and significance of circulating microRNAs in cerebrospinal fluid of acute encephalitis patients infected with Japanese Encephalitis Virus. *Mol. Neurobiol.* **2016**. [CrossRef] [PubMed]

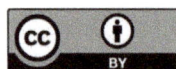

Journal of
*Clinical Medicine*

MDPI

*Review*

# MicroRNA In Lung Cancer: Novel Biomarkers and Potential Tools for Treatment

**Kentaro Inamura and Yuichi Ishikawa ***

Division of Pathology, The Cancer Institute, Japanese Foundation for Cancer Research, 3-8-31 Ariake, Koto-ku, Tokyo 135-8550, Japan; kentaro.inamura@jfcr.or.jp
* Correspondence: ishikawa@jfcr.or.jp; Tel.: +81-3-3570-0448; Fax: +81-3-3570-0558

Academic Editors: Takahiro Ochiya and Ryou-u Takahashi
Received: 4 December 2015; Accepted: 1 March 2016; Published: 9 March 2016

**Abstract:** Lung cancer is the leading cause of cancer death in men and women worldwide. The lack of specific and sensitive tools for early diagnosis as well as still-inadequate targeted therapies contribute to poor outcomes. MicroRNAs are small non-coding RNAs, which regulate gene expression post-transcriptionally by translational repression or degradation of target mRNAs. A growing body of evidence suggests various roles of microRNAs including development and progression of lung cancer. In lung cancer, several studies have showed that certain microRNA profiles classified lung cancer subtypes, and that specific microRNA expression signatures distinguished between better-prognosis and worse-prognosis lung cancers. Furthermore, microRNAs circulate in body fluids, and therefore may serve as promising biomarkers for early diagnosis of lung cancer as well as for predicting prognosis of patients. In the present review, we briefly summarize microRNAs in the development and progression of lung cancer, focusing on possible applications of microRNAs as novel biomarkers and tools for treatment.

**Keywords:** adenocarcinoma; carcinoma; driver mutation; histology; miRNA; molecular pathology; morphology; plasma; mutation; oncology; serum; sputum

## 1. Introduction

Lung cancer is the leading cause of cancer death in men and women worldwide, accounting for more than 1.5 million deaths per year [1]. Lung carcinoma is generally classified as either small-cell lung carcinoma (SCLC) (about 20% of all lung carcinomas) or non-small cell lung carcinoma (NSCLC) (about 80%). Within these groups, further distinctions are made, with NSCLC sub-divided into adenocarcinoma (about 50% of all lung carcinomas), squamous cell carcinoma (SqCC), and large cell carcinoma.

Although new molecular targeted therapies to some types of lung cancer have shown promising results, no potential targeted therapy can be applied to a large number of lung cancer patients. Despite improvements in early diagnosis of lung cancer, most lung cancers are diagnosed at an advanced stage. Therefore, the identification of novel diagnostic biomarkers or treatment strategies is critical and essential for the control of lung cancer.

MicroRNAs, which are small non-coding RNAs that range in size from 19 to 25 nucleotides, play important regulatory roles in animals and plants by targeting mRNAs for translational repression or degradation. MicroRNAs comprise one of the most abundant classes of gene regulatory molecules in multicellular organisms and likely influence the output of many protein-coding genes [2]. A growing body of evidence is emerging to suggest a wide range of fundamental cellular processes such as cell differentiation, proliferation, growth, mobility, and apoptosis, as well as carcinogenesis or cancer progression [3,4]. The expression patterns of microRNAs are likely to correlate with characteristic clinicopathological parameters in cancer subtypes [5], suggesting that microRNAs are potential biomarkers for different cancer subtypes, classified by origin, histology, aggressiveness, or chemosensitivity [6,7].

Public database, miRBase (http://www.mirbase.org/) (last access: 9 February 2016) provides various aspects of microRNA information, and the annotated human microRNAs of 1881 have been registered in miRBase 21. In general, the list of microRNAs involved in lung cancer is not limited to several microRNAs, but much wider, as well as the potential diagnostic microRNAs in tissues.

Of importance, an abundance of undegradated microRNAs exists not only in tissues but also in body fluids, including blood, plasma, serum, and sputum [8]. This nature of easy availability makes microRNAs promising biomarkers for non-invasive liquid biopsy in cancer practice. Biomarkers analyzed by liquid biopsy [9,10] include circulating tumor cells and exosomes (containing DNA, mRNA, microRNA, *etc.*) [11,12] as well as circulating cell-free DNA [13], mRNA [14], and microRNA [15]. Although, non-invasive liquid biopsy is promising, it has not been employed for multiclass cancer diagnostics due to non-specificity of these blood-based biosources to pinpoint the nature of the primary cancer [9,13,14].

In addition, microRNAs are far less degradated in formalin-fixed paraffin-embedded (FFPE) samples than mRNAs. Therefore, accurate measurements of microRNAs can be performed from FFPE samples, which are usually collected and preserved in hospitals. An availability of archived FFPE samples for the accurate measurement of microRNAs is a great advantage to conduct microRNA research or apply microRNA profiles for clinical practice.

Due to the characteristic nature of microRNAs, microRNAs have a potential to be used for the development of diagnostics, prognostics, and targeted therapeutics. In terms of treatment, microRNA expression profiles can predict chemotherapeutic response and serve as important biomarkers for the stratification of patients for personalized therapeutic strategies. Furthermore, microRNAs have the potential to serve as molecular targeted agents. Although the initial results from human-based studies revealed the promise of microRNA targeted therapies, several obstacles need to be overcome prior to the therapeutic application of microRNAs to the clinic [16].

In this review, we summarize recent works of microRNAs in lung cancer, focusing on microRNAs as novel biomarkers and potential tools for treatment.

## 2. MicroRNA Biogenesis

Biogenesis of microRNA (Figure 1) begins with the transcription of primary-microRNA by RNA polymerase II. Then, DROSHA/DGCR8 enzyme complex crops the primary-microRNA into precursor-microRNA, followed by exportin-5-mediated transport from the nucleus to the cytoplasm. Subsequently, DICER1 cleaves the precursor-microRNA to form the microRNA duplex. One strand of the microRNA duplex is selected to function as a mature microRNA and loaded into the RNA-induced silencing complex (RISC), whereas the partner microRNA* strand is preferentially degradated. The mature microRNA leads to translational repression or degradation of target mRNAs.

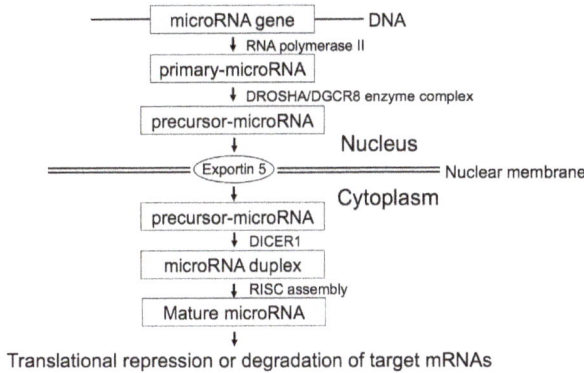

Figure 1. MicroRNA biogenesis. MicroRNAs are initially transcribed by RNA polymerase II as primary-microRNAs with hairpin structures. DROSHA/DGCR8 enzyme complex then cleaves primary-microRNAs into precursor-microRNAs, which are transported to cytoplasm by Exportin 5, and cleaved by DICER to form microRNA duplexes. One strand is selected to function as a mature microRNA and loaded into the RNA-induced silencing complex (RISC), whereas the partner microRNA* is preferentially degraded. The mature microRNA with RISC binds to 3′UTR of target mRNA resulting in translational repression or degradation.

## 3. MicroRNAs as Tumor Suppressor Genes and Oncogenes

MicroRNAs play important regulatory roles in carcinogenesis not only as tumor suppressor genes but also as oncogenes. Several microRNAs are dysregulated in lung cancer. Table 1 shows principal microRNAs involved in the development or progression of lung cancer, their gene targets, and associated biological processes.

Table 1. Principal microRNAs involved in the development or progression of lung cancer.

| microRNAs | Gene Targets | Biological Processes |
|---|---|---|
| Tumor suppressor microRNAs with down-regulation in lung cancer | | |
| *let-7 family* | *RAS, HMGA2, CDK6, MYC, DICER1* | (i) Cell proliferation (*RAS, MYC, HMGA2*) (ii) Cell cycle regulation (*CDK6*) (iii) microRNA maturation (*DICER1*) |
| *miR-34 family* | *MET, BCL2, PDGFRA, PDGFRB* | TRAIL-induced cell death and cell proliferation |
| *miR-200 family* | *ZEB1, ZEB2*, E-cadherin (*CDH1*), vimentin (*VIM*) | Promotion of EMT and metastasis |
| Oncogenic microRNAs with up-regulation in lung cancer | | |
| miR-21 | *PTEN, PDCD4, TPM1* | Apoptosis, cell proliferation, and migration |
| miR-17-92 cluster | *E2F1, PTEN, HIF1A* | Cell proliferation and carcinogenesis |
| miR-221/222 | *PTEN, TIMP3* | Apoptosis and cell migration |

TRAIL: TNF-related apoptosis-inducing ligand; EMT: epithelial-mesenchymal transition.

### 3.1. Tumor Suppressor microRNAs

3.1.1. *Let-7* Family

The *let-7* family was the first identified microRNA in humans [17]. In lung cancer, *let-7* has been shown to inhibit the expression of oncogenes involved in cellular proliferation, such as *RAS*, *MYC*, and *HMGA2* [18,19]. *Let-7* also inhibits the expression of *CDK6*, and the reduced expression of *let-7*, therefore, leads to the promotion of cell cycle progression [19]. Of interest, *let-7* directly down-regulates *DICER1* expression, suggesting that *let-7* may regulate the global production of microRNAs [20].

### 3.1.2. *miR-34* Family

The *miR-34* family (*miR-34a*, *miR-34b*, and *miR-34c*) is directly induced by TP53 in response to DNA damage, controlling cell cycle arrest and apoptosis in cancer [21]. The *miR-34* family is down-regulated in lung cancer, leading to the up-regulation of *miR-34* target genes, such as *MET*, *BCL2*, *PDGFR-α* (*PDGFRA*), and *PDGFR-β* (*PDGFRB*) [22–24]. The up-regulation of *MET* and *BCL2* by reduced *miR-34* expression leads to cell proliferation. *MiR-34* dependent PDGFR-α/β downregulation inhibits tumorigenesis and enhances TRAIL (TNF-related apoptosis-inducing ligand)-induced apoptosis in lung cancer [24].

### 3.1.3. *miR-200* Family

The *miR-200* family (*miR-200a*, *miR-200b*, *miR-200c*, and *miR-429*) plays an important role in the promotion of epithelial-mesenchymal transition (EMT). Through the regulation of ZEB (zinc finger E-box-binding homeobox) transcription factors (*ZEB1* and *ZEB2*), E-cadherin (*CDH1*), vimentin (*VIM*), the down-regulated *miR-200* family promotes EMT in the progression of lung cancer [25,26].

### 3.2. Oncogenic microRNAs

### 3.2.1. *miR-21*

*miR-21* is one of the most representative oncogenic microRNAs, being overexpressed in various types of solid tumors as well as leukemia. *miR-21* drives tumorigenesis through inhibition of negative regulators of RAS/MEK/ERK pathway and suppression of apoptosis. Overexpressed *miR-21* downregulates the expressions of *PTEN* [27], *PDCD4* [28–30], and *TPM1* [30], promoting cell proliferation and migration, and inhibiting apoptosis.

### 3.2.2. *miR-17-92* Cluster

The *miR-17-92* polycistronic cluster comprises seven different microRNAs (*miR-17-3p*, *miR-17-5p*, *miR-18a*, *miR-19a*, *miR-20a*, *miR-19b-1*, and *miR-92a*) and resides in intron 3 of the *C13orf25* gene at 13q31.3 [31]. The *miR-17-92* cluster was reported to be overexpressed in lung cancer, in particular SCLC [31]. Overexpression of *miR-17-92* cluster down-regulates *E2F1*, *HIF1A*, and *PTEN*, promoting cell proliferation and cancer progression [32,33].

### 3.2.3. *miR-221/222*

*miR-221* and *miR-222* are involved in the development and progression of lung cancer by targeting *PTEN* and *TIMP3* tumor suppressor genes [34,35]. Overexpressed *miR-221/222* inhibits apoptosis and promotes cell migration by down-regulating PTEN and TIMP3.

## 4. Diagnostic microRNAs

### 4.1. Diagnostic microRNAs in Tissues

Early detection of lung cancer is prerequisite to reduce lung cancer mortality, because lung cancers are often diagnosed at advanced stages, where clinical treatments are less (or least) effective. MicroRNA expression signatures of lung cancer have been reported by numerous studies, however the reported microRNA profiles were not so consistent. Vosa *et al.* performed a comprehensive meta-analysis of 20 published microRNA expression studies in lung cancer, including a total of 598 tumor and 528 normal lung tissues [36]. Using a recently published robust rank aggregation method, they identified a statistically significant microRNA meta-signature of seven up-regulated (*miR-21*, *miR-210*, *miR-182*, *miR-31*, *miR-200b*, *miR-205*, and *miR-183*) and eight down-regulated (*miR-126-3p*, *miR-30a*, *miR-30d*, *miR-486-5p*, *miR-451a*, *miR-126-5p*, *miR-143*, and *miR-145*) microRNAs.

*4.2. Diagnostic microRNAs in Body Fluids*

Importantly, microRNAs are present not only in tissues but also in body fluids, such as blood, plasma, serum, or sputum. By examining body fluids, we may be able to distinguish lung cancer patients from healthy individuals. Jiang's group conducted several studies to assess the usefulness of microRNAs in body fluids for the lung cancer screening [37–40]. Using sputum specimens, they examined the expression of *miR-21*, which is an overexpressed microRNA in lung cancer [37]. The expression of *miR-21* in sputum was higher in NSCLC patients, and the detection of *miR-21* expression produced 70% sensitivity and 100% specificity in the distinction between 23 NSCLC patients and 17 cancer-free individuals. In another study, using an independent set, they demonstrated that the expression profile of four sputum microRNAs (*miR-21*, *miR-486*, *miR-375*, and *miR-200b*) demonstrated 81% sensitivity and 92% specificity in the distinction between 64 NSCLC patients and 58 healthy individuals [40]. They also assessed the usefulness for plasma microRNAs as potential biomarkers for NSCLC [39]. They showed that the expression profile of four plasma microRNAs (*miR-21*, *miR-126*, *miR-210*, and *miR-486-5p*) yielded 86% sensitivity and 97% specificity in distinguishing 58 NSCLC patients from 29 healthy individuals. Furthermore, this panel of microRNAs produced 73% sensitivity and 97% specificity in identifying stage I NSCLC patients, suggesting the usefulness of plasma microRNAs as potential biomarkers to identify even early stage NSCLC patients [39]. In another study, they showed that the expression profile of three plasma microRNAs (*miR-21*, *miR-210*, and *miR-486-5p*) produced 75% sensitivity and 85% specificity in the distinction between 32 patients with malignant solitary pulmonary nodules (SPNs) and 33 individuals with benign SPNs. SPNs have been increasingly diagnosed with the advancement and widespread use of computed tomography (CT) scan. The combination of microRNA testing and CT scan may serve as a minimally invasive method of diagnosing individuals with SPNs. All of these four studies by Jiang's group [37–40] included *miR-21* as a biomarker to distinguish lung cancer patients from healthy individuals. Because *miR-21* is overexpressed in various types of cancer, further studies are warranted to examine *miR-21* expression for the distinction between lung cancer patients and patients of the other cancers.

## 5. MicroRNAs as Biomarkers for Histological Classification

Recent advances in the treatment of NSCLC with new drugs require an appropriate histological subtyping at diagnosis to avoid hazardous side effects. For instance, bevacizumab (brand name: Avastin), a monoclonal antibody which blocks angiogenesis by inhibiting vascular endothelial growth factor A (VEGFA), cannot be used for SqCC patients due to serious hemorrhagic complications. Similarly, pemetrexed (brand name: Alimta), a chemotherapy drug belonging to a class of chemotherapeutic drugs known as folate antimetabolites, cannot be used for SqCC patients due to adverse responses. Several studies have been conducted to distinguish between SqCC and non-SqCC NSCLC, utilizing microRNAs profiles [41–43]. Lebanony *et al.* found that higher expression of *miR-205* was specific to SqCC in a test set. In an independent validation set, *miR-205* expression in FFPE samples yielded 96% sensitivity and 90% specificity in the distinction between SqCCs and non-SqCC NSCLCs [41]. As a replication study, Bishop *et al.* showed that the measurement of *miR-205* expression in small biopsies/aspirates can distinguish between SqCCs and non-SqCC NSCLCs [42]. Recently, Hamamoto *et al.* have reported that the expression profile of three microRNAs (*miR-205*, *miR-196b*, and *miR-375*) distinguished between SqCCs and adenocarcinomas with 85% sensitivity and 83% specificity in a validation set [43].

SCLC, one of the neuroendocrine tumors, shows increased expression of *ASCL1*, which is a master gene of neuroendocrine differentiation. Nishikawa *et al.* demonstrated that *miR-357* expression was induced by ASCL1 in lung neuroendocrine carcinoma [44]. They showed that the increased expression of *miR-375* was prerequisite for the neuroendocrine differentiation by ASCL1, and suggested that *miR-375* might reduce the YAP1-related proliferative arrest by inhibiting YAP1.

## 6. Prognostic microRNAs

### 6.1. Investigation for Prognostic microRNAs

As is the case with mRNA, microRNA profiles have been investigated as potential prognostic biomarkers. In 2004, Takamizawa *et al.* focused on microRNA *let-7* [45], and reported that *let-7* expression is lower in lung cancer than in normal lung tissue, and that the lower expression of *let-7* in lung cancer was associated with poor prognosis. In addition, overexpression of *let-7* in A549 lung adenocarcinoma cell line inhibited cell growth. This study [45] is important with respect to the first report of reduced expression of *let-7* and the potential clinical and biological effects of such a microRNA alteration in lung cancer. We examined *let-7* expressions in adenocarcinoma *in situ* (AIS, the new name for BAC (bronchioloalveolar carcinoma) [46]) as well as in invasive adenocarcinoma to investigate the association of *let-7* expression with the progression of lung adenocarcinoma [47]. Of note, even in AIS, the expression of *let-7* was reduced in comparison to matched normal lung tissue, suggesting that *let-7* expression was reduced in the early stage of lung carcinogenesis. AIS is categorized into two subtypes, non-mucinous and mucinous AIS. Interestingly, the expression of *let-7* was lower in mucinous AIS than non-mucinous AIS. The differential expression of *let-7* between two morphological subtypes of AIS suggests an association between microRNA expression and morphology (even in the same category of AIS). According to this observation, complexity of microRNA expressions depending on morphology as well as cancer progression or driver mutations can be presumed.

In 2006, the first microRNA profiling in lung cancer was reported by Yanaihara *et al.* [48]. Using 104 NSCLCs (65 adenocarcinomas and 39 SqCCs) and matched normal lung tissues, they conducted profiling analyses of microRNA expression by microarray. They identified the higher expression of *miR-155* and the lower expression of *let-7a-2* as biomarkers of poor prognosis for NSCLC patients, and confirmed the validity using an independent set by real-time RT-PCR. Subsequently, in 2008, Yu *et al.* [49] identified a five-microRNA signature (*let-7a, miR-221*, miR-137, *miR-372*, and *miR-182**) that classified a training set of 56 NSCLC cases into good-prognosis and poor-prognosis group. Then, they confirmed that the five-microRNA signature divided 62 NSCLC testing cases into two groups with good and poor prognosis. Furthermore, they validated the five-microRNAs signature as a prognostic classifier using an independent cohort set of 62 NSCLCs. This five-microRNA signature worked as a prognostic classifier for NSCLCs even with the same stage or SqCCs as well as adenocarcinomas.

### 6.2. Integrated Prognostic Classifier for Stage I Lung Cancer

*MiR-21* is one of the overexpressed microRNAs in various types of cancer, and targets of *miR-21* include tumor suppressor genes, such as *PTEN* [27,50] and *PDCD4* [28–30]. Harris' group has identified an integrated prognostic classifier for stage I lung adenocarcinoma based on microRNA, mRNA, and DNA methylation biomarkers, using frozen specimens [51]. This integrated prognostic classifier consisted of *miR-21*, four protein-coding genes (*XPO1, BRCA1, HIF1A*, and *DLC1*), and *HOXA9* promoter methylation. *miR-21*, four protein-coding genes, or *HOXA9* promoter methylation could independently classified stage I adenocarcinomas into two groups with a different survival (hazard ratio (HR) = 2.3, $p = 0.01$; HR = 2.8, $p = 0.002$; HR = 2.4, $p = 0.005$, respectively). When combined, the integrated biomarker worked as a much more accurate prognostic classifier for stage I adenocarcinoma (HR = 10.2, $p = 3 \times 10^{-5}$).

Importantly, abundant undegradaded microRNAs circulate in body fluids, such as blood, plasma, serum, and sputum [8]. There have been several studies to predict survival in NSCLC patients, by using microRNA profiles in body fluids. In 2010, Hu *et al.* reported that a four-serum-microRNA signature (*miR-486, miR-30d, miR-1*, and *miR-499*) was associated with overall survival in NSCLC, utilizing 120 cases for the training set and 123 cases for the testing set [52]. Subsequently, Wang *et al.*

conducted pathway-based serum microRNA profiling and examined the prognostic association in advanced stage NSCLC patients [53]. They focused on microRNAs involved in TGF-β pathway, which plays crucial roles in control of cell proliferation, differentiation, apoptosis, and invasion. They identified 17 microRNAs which were significantly associated with two-year patient survival. Of these 17 microRNAs, *miR-16* exhibited the most statistically significant association; high expression of *miR-16* was associated with better survival (HR = 0.4, 95% confidence interval (CI), 0.3–0.5). They created 17-microRNA risk score to identify patients at the highest risk of death. NSCLC patients with a high-risk score had a 2.5-fold increased risk of death compared with those with a low-risk score (95% CI, 1.8–3.4; $p = 1.1 \times 10^{-7}$).

### 6.3. Let-7, DICER1, and Survival of Lung Cancer

DICER1 has an important role in microRNA biogenesis, converting precursor-microRNAs into mature microRNAs (Figure 1). Inversely, microRNA *let-7* directly down-regulates *DICER1* expression [20]. According to the study by Karube *et al.* [54], the reduced expression of *DICER1* was associated with poor prognosis in NSCLC, suggesting the involvement of reduced *DICER1* expression in the progression of lung cancer.

### 7. MicroRNA Associated with Driver Mutations and Therapeutic microRNAs

Somatic mutations in tyrosine kinases have recently emerged as driver mutations in carcinogenesis of lung cancer, especially in that of lung adenocarcinoma. Adenocarcinomas with activating mutations of *EGFR* are responsive to EGFR tyrosine kinase inhibitors (TKIs). However, T790M *EGFR* mutation and *MET* amplification lead to the resistance of EGFR TKIs [55]. Other mutually exclusive genetic alterations, which have been reported to work as driver mutations in lung adenocarcinoma, include translocations of *ALK, ROS1, RET, NTKR1, NRG2, ERBB4,* and *BRAF*, and mutations of *KRAS, BRAF, ERBB2, NRAS, HRAS, MAP2K1, NF1,* and *RIT1* [56–61]. Adenocarcinomas with specific driver mutations sometimes have characteristic clinicopathological features [62–67]. For example, *ALK*-translocation lung adenocarcinomas are characterized by young-onset, never/light smokers, and acinar morphology with mucin/signet-ring cell morphology [64–67].

There are several studies examining the association between microRNAs expression and driver mutations (especially *EGFR* and *KRAS* mutation). *miR-21* has been suggested to be an EGFR-regulated anti-apoptotic factor in never-smokers' lung adenocarcinoma [68]. Recently, Li *et al.* have reported an association of *miR-21* overexpression with acquired resistance of EGFR-TKI in NSCLCs [69]. Dacic *et al.* [70] examined the microRNA expressions in lung adenocarcinomas with different driver mutations, focusing on *EGFR* and *KRAS* mutation, using two *EGFR*-mutant, two *KRAS*-mutant, and two *EGFR*-wild-type/*KRAS*-wild-type adenocarcinomas and confirmed differentially expressed microRNAs in a validation set of 18 adenocarcinomas. They showed that *miR-155, miR-25,* and *miR-495* were up-regulated only in the *EGFR*-wild-type/*KRAS*-wild-type, *EGFR*-mutant, and *KRAS*-mutant lung adenocarcinomas, respectively. In 2014, Bjaanaes *et al.* also examined microRNA profiles according to mutation status of *EGFR* and *KRAS*, using 154 lung adenocarcinomas by microarray [71]. The identified profiles were confirmed by real-time RT-PCR, using 103 lung cancer cases. They identified 17 microRNAs that were differentially expressed between *EGFR*-mutant and *EGFR*-wild-type adenocarcinomas, and three microRNAs differentially expressed between *KRAS*-mutant and *KRAS*-wild-type adenocarcinomas. There was no overlap between Dacic's and Bjaanaes' study, possibly due to the small sample size of Dacic's study, differences in methodologies, or by chance. Further researches with a large sample size are required to elucidate the specific microRNA profiles according to the mutation status of *EGFR* or *KRAS*.

Weiss *et al.* [72] reported that *miR-128b* could directly regulate *EGFR*. The loss of heterozygosity (LOH) of *miR-128b* occurred frequently in NSCLC and correlated significantly with clinical response and survival after EGFR-TKI. Another study showed that *microRNA-146a* targeted *EGFR*, suppressed its downstream signaling and regulation of cell growth, and enhanced the cytotoxic effect of EGFR-TKI in five NSCLC cell lines [73].

To understand the role of microRNAs in TKI-resistant NSCLCs, Garofalo *et al.* examined microRNA changes that were mediated by tyrosine kinase receptors [74]. They demonstrated that this resistance could be overcome by anti-*miR-221/222* and anti-*miR-30c*, which recovered the expression of the pro-apoptotic protein BCL2L11 (BIM) and increased the gefitinib sensitivity of NSCLC both *in vitro* and *in vivo*.

Other aspects regarding the role of microRNAs in relation to EGFR-TKI deserve comment. Recently, plasma microRNA profiles (*miR-21*, *miR-27a*, and *miR-218*) have been identified for primary resistance to EGFR-TKIs in advanced NSCLCs with *EGFR* activating mutation [75]. Pak *et al.* have found unique microRNAs (*miR-34c*, *miR-183*, and *miR-210*) in lung adenocarcinoma groups according to major TKI sensitive *EGFR* mutation status [76]. A recent study by Wang *et al.* suggests that the modulation of specific microRNAs (*miR-374a* and *miR-548b*) may provide a therapeutic target to treat or reverse gefitinib resistance in NSCLC with high expression of the Axl kinase [77]. The review by Ricciuti *et al.* [78] is worth reading because it summarized the existing relationship between microRNAs and resistance to EGFR-TKIs, and also focusing on the possible clinical applications of microRNAs in reverting and overcoming such resistance.

For now, limited evidence can be available for the microRNA profiles of lung cancer with specific driver mutations. Further studies should be conducted to elucidate driver-mutation-specific microRNA profiles. MicroRNA signature may be used as a diagnostic biomarker of lung cancer with a specific driver mutation, and also the combination of TKI and microRNA-based treatment is promising.

## 8. Prospects from Basic to Clinical Application of microRNAs

Actually, despite enormous efforts, several obstacles remain to be solved for the transition of microRNAs from basic to clinical application as novel biomarkers or potential tools for treatment. These obstacles include the standardization of microRNA detection, improved understanding of how microRNAs interact with other components of the genome, and the development of non-toxic targeted delivery of microRNAs to the lung or metastatic lesions as well as the selection of the proper vehicle for delivery [79]. Therefore, we have a bunch of obstacles to clear away, however we are now trying to solve these issues strenuously [79].

## 9. Conclusions

In this review, we introduced recent works of microRNAs involved in the development and progression of lung cancer, with a particular interest in microRNAs as novel biomarkers and potential tools for treatment. Of importance, microRNAs are far less degraded in FFPE samples than mRNAs, and therefore, an easy availability of FFPE samples in hospitals enables us to measure accurate microRNA expressions. In addition, microRNAs are also present in body fluids, making microRNAs promising diagnostic biomarkers. Therefore, there exists a great potential in microRNA analyses for cancer research. Further studies are demanded in order to use microRNA profiles as diagnostic markers and conduct microRNA-based therapies in clinical practice.

**Acknowledgments:** This study was funded, in part, by Grants-in-Aid for scientific Research from the Ministry of Education, Culture, Sports, Science, and Technology, Japan, grants from the Japan Society for the Promotion of Science, the Ministry of Health, Labour, and Welfare, and the Smoking Research Foundation.

**Author Contributions:** Kentaro Inamura and Yuichi Ishikawa conceived the review, wrote the text, and created the tables and figures.

**Conflicts of Interest:** The authors declare no conflict of interest.

## References

1. Torre, L.A.; Bray, F.; Siegel, R.L.; Ferlay, J.; Lortet-Tieulent, J.; Jemal, A. Global cancer statistics, 2012. *CA Cancer J. Clin.* **2015**, *65*, 87–108. [CrossRef] [PubMed]
2. Bartel, D.P. MicroRNAs: Genomics, biogenesis, mechanism, and function. *Cell* **2004**, *116*, 281–297. [CrossRef]
3. Winter, J.; Jung, S.; Keller, S.; Gregory, R.I.; Diederichs, S. Many roads to maturity: MicroRNA biogenesis pathways and their regulation. *Nat. Cell Biol.* **2009**, *11*, 228–234. [CrossRef] [PubMed]
4. Joshi, P.; Middleton, J.; Jeon, Y.J.; Garofalo, M. MicroRNAs in lung cancer. *World J. Methodol.* **2014**, *4*, 59–72. [CrossRef] [PubMed]
5. Lu, J.; Getz, G.; Miska, E.A.; Alvarez-Saavedra, E.; Lamb, J.; Peck, D.; Sweet-Cordero, A.; Ebert, B.L.; Mak, R.H.; Ferrando, A.A.; *et al.* MicroRNA expression profiles classify human cancers. *Nature* **2005**, *435*, 834–838. [CrossRef] [PubMed]
6. Kishikawa, T.; Otsuka, M.; Ohno, M.; Yoshikawa, T.; Takata, A.; Koike, K. Circulating RNAs as new biomarkers for detecting pancreatic cancer. *World J. Gastroenterol.* **2015**, *21*, 8527–8540. [CrossRef] [PubMed]
7. Hollis, M.; Nair, K.; Vyas, A.; Chaturvedi, L.S.; Gambhir, S.; Vyas, D. MicroRNAs potential utility in colon cancer: Early detection, prognosis, and chemosensitivity. *World J. Gastroenterol.* **2015**, *21*, 8284–8292. [CrossRef] [PubMed]
8. Gilad, S.; Meiri, E.; Yogev, Y.; Benjamin, S.; Lebanony, D.; Yerushalmi, N.; Benjamin, H.; Kushnir, M.; Cholakh, H.; Melamed, N.; *et al.* Serum microRNAs are promising novel biomarkers. *PLoS ONE* **2008**, *3*, e3148. [CrossRef] [PubMed]
9. Alix-Panabieres, C.; Pantel, K. Challenges in circulating tumour cell research. *Nat. Rev. Cancer* **2014**, *14*, 623–631. [CrossRef] [PubMed]
10. Hyun, K.A.; Kim, J.; Gwak, H.; Jung, H.I. Isolation and enrichment of circulating biomarkers for cancer screening, detection, and diagnostics. *Analyst* **2016**, *141*, 382–392. [CrossRef] [PubMed]
11. Peterson, M.F.; Otoc, N.; Sethi, J.K.; Gupta, A.; Antes, T.J. Integrated systems for exosome investigation. *Methods* **2015**, *87*, 31–45. [CrossRef] [PubMed]
12. Hoshino, A.; Costa-Silva, B.; Shen, T.L.; Rodrigues, G.; Hashimoto, A.; Tesic Mark, M.; Molina, H.; Kohsaka, S.; Di Giannatale, A.; Ceder, S.; *et al.* Tumour exosome integrins determine organotropic metastasis. *Nature* **2015**, *527*, 329–335. [CrossRef] [PubMed]
13. Bettegowda, C.; Sausen, M.; Leary, R.J.; Kinde, I.; Wang, Y.; Agrawal, N.; Bartlett, B.R.; Wang, H.; Luber, B.; Alani, R.M.; *et al.* Detection of circulating tumor DNA in early- and late-stage human malignancies. *Sci. Transl. Med.* **2014**, *6*, 224ra24. [CrossRef] [PubMed]
14. Best, M.G.; Sol, N.; Kooi, I.; Tannous, J.; Westerman, B.A.; Rustenburg, F.; Schellen, P.; Verschueren, H.; Post, E.; Koster, J.; *et al.* RNA-Seq of Tumor-Educated Platelets Enables Blood-Based Pan-Cancer, Multiclass, and Molecular Pathway Cancer Diagnostics. *Cancer Cell* **2015**, *28*, 666–676. [CrossRef] [PubMed]
15. Kosaka, N.; Iguchi, H.; Ochiya, T. Circulating microRNA in body fluid: A new potential biomarker for cancer diagnosis and prognosis. *Cancer Sci.* **2010**, *101*, 2087–2092. [CrossRef] [PubMed]
16. Barger, J.F.; Nana-Sinkam, S.P. MicroRNA as tools and therapeutics in lung cancer. *Respir. Med.* **2015**, *109*, 803–812. [CrossRef] [PubMed]
17. Pasquinelli, A.E.; Reinhart, B.J.; Slack, F.; Martindale, M.Q.; Kuroda, M.I.; Maller, B.; Hayward, D.C.; Ball, E.E.; Degnan, B.; Muller, P.; *et al.* Conservation of the sequence and temporal expression of let-7 heterochronic regulatory RNA. *Nature* **2000**, *408*, 86–89. [PubMed]
18. Johnson, S.M.; Grosshans, H.; Shingara, J.; Byrom, M.; Jarvis, R.; Cheng, A.; Labourier, E.; Reinert, K.L.; Brown, D.; Slack, F.J. RAS is regulated by the let-7 microRNA family. *Cell* **2005**, *120*, 635–647. [CrossRef] [PubMed]
19. Johnson, C.D.; Esquela-Kerscher, A.; Stefani, G.; Byrom, M.; Kelnar, K.; Ovcharenko, D.; Wilson, M.; Wang, X.; Shelton, J.; Shingara, J.; *et al.* The let-7 microRNA represses cell proliferation pathways in human cells. *Cancer Res.* **2007**, *67*, 7713–7722. [CrossRef] [PubMed]
20. Tokumaru, S.; Suzuki, M.; Yamada, H.; Nagino, M.; Takahashi, T. let-7 regulates Dicer expression and constitutes a negative feedback loop. *Carcinogenesis* **2008**, *29*, 2073–2077. [CrossRef] [PubMed]
21. He, L.; He, X.; Lim, L.P.; de Stanchina, E.; Xuan, Z.; Liang, Y.; Xue, W.; Zender, L.; Magnus, J.; Ridzon, D.; *et al.* A microRNA component of the p53 tumour suppressor network. *Nature* **2007**, *447*, 1130–1134. [CrossRef] [PubMed]

22. Bommer, G.T.; Gerin, I.; Feng, Y.; Kaczorowski, A.J.; Kuick, R.; Love, R.E.; Zhai, Y.; Giordano, T.J.; Qin, Z.S.; Moore, B.B.; *et al.* p53-mediated activation of miRNA34 candidate tumor-suppressor genes. *Curr. Biol.* **2007**, *17*, 1298–1307. [CrossRef] [PubMed]

23. Kasinski, A.L.; Slack, F.J. MiRNA-34 prevents cancer initiation and progression in a therapeutically resistant K-ras and p53-induced mouse model of lung adenocarcinoma. *Cancer Res.* **2012**, *72*, 5576–5587. [CrossRef] [PubMed]

24. Garofalo, M.; Jeon, Y.J.; Nuovo, G.J.; Middleton, J.; Secchiero, P.; Joshi, P.; Alder, H.; Nazaryan, N.; di Leva, G.; Romano, G.; *et al.* miR-34a/c-Dependent PDGFR-alpha/beta Downregulation Inhibits Tumorigenesis and Enhances TRAIL-Induced Apoptosis in Lung Cancer. *PLoS ONE* **2013**, *8*, e67581. [CrossRef] [PubMed]

25. Ceppi, P.; Mudduluru, G.; Kumarswamy, R.; Rapa, I.; Scagliotti, G.V.; Papotti, M.; Allgayer, H. Loss of miR-200c expression induces an aggressive, invasive, and chemoresistant phenotype in non-small cell lung cancer. *Mol. Cancer Res.* **2010**, *8*, 1207–1216. [CrossRef] [PubMed]

26. Takeyama, Y.; Sato, M.; Horio, M.; Hase, T.; Yoshida, K.; Yokoyama, T.; Nakashima, H.; Hashimoto, N.; Sekido, Y.; Gazdar, A.F.; *et al.* Knockdown of ZEB1, a master epithelial-to-mesenchymal transition (EMT) gene, suppresses anchorage-independent cell growth of lung cancer cells. *Cancer Lett.* **2010**, *296*, 216–224. [CrossRef] [PubMed]

27. Zhang, J.G.; Wang, J.J.; Zhao, F.; Liu, Q.; Jiang, K.; Yang, G.H. MicroRNA-21 (miR-21) represses tumor suppressor PTEN and promotes growth and invasion in non-small cell lung cancer (NSCLC). *Clin. Chim. Acta* **2010**, *411*, 846–852. [CrossRef] [PubMed]

28. Bhatti, I.; Lee, A.; James, V.; Hall, R.I.; Lund, J.N.; Tufarelli, C.; Lobo, D.N.; Larvin, M. Knockdown of microRNA-21 inhibits proliferation and increases cell death by targeting programmed cell death 4 (PDCD4) in pancreatic ductal adenocarcinoma. *J. Gastrointest. Surg.* **2011**, *15*, 199–208. [CrossRef] [PubMed]

29. Asangani, I.A.; Rasheed, S.A.; Nikolova, D.A.; Leupold, J.H.; Colburn, N.H.; Post, S.; Allgayer, H. MicroRNA-21 (miR-21) post-transcriptionally downregulates tumor suppressor Pdcd4 and stimulates invasion, intravasation and metastasis in colorectal cancer. *Oncogene* **2008**, *27*, 2128–2136. [CrossRef] [PubMed]

30. Zhu, S.; Wu, H.; Wu, F.; Nie, D.; Sheng, S.; Mo, Y.Y. MicroRNA-21 targets tumor suppressor genes in invasion and metastasis. *Cell Res.* **2008**, *18*, 350–359. [CrossRef] [PubMed]

31. Hayashita, Y.; Osada, H.; Tatematsu, Y.; Yamada, H.; Yanagisawa, K.; Tomida, S.; Yatabe, Y.; Kawahara, K.; Sekido, Y.; Takahashi, T. A polycistronic microRNA cluster, miR-17-92, is overexpressed in human lung cancers and enhances cell proliferation. *Cancer Res.* **2005**, *65*, 9628–9632. [CrossRef] [PubMed]

32. Matsubara, H.; Takeuchi, T.; Nishikawa, E.; Yanagisawa, K.; Hayashita, Y.; Ebi, H.; Yamada, H.; Suzuki, M.; Nagino, M.; Nimura, Y.; *et al.* Apoptosis induction by antisense oligonucleotides against miR-17–5p and miR-20a in lung cancers overexpressing miR-17-92. *Oncogene* **2007**, *26*, 6099–6105. [CrossRef] [PubMed]

33. Osada, H.; Takahashi, T. let-7 and miR-17-92: Small-sized major players in lung cancer development. *Cancer Sci.* **2011**, *102*, 9–17. [CrossRef] [PubMed]

34. Garofalo, M.; Quintavalle, C.; di Leva, G.; Zanca, C.; Romano, G.; Taccioli, C.; Liu, C.G.; Croce, C.M.; Condorelli, G. MicroRNA signatures of TRAIL resistance in human non-small cell lung cancer. *Oncogene* **2008**, *27*, 3845–3855. [CrossRef] [PubMed]

35. Garofalo, M.; di Leva, G.; Romano, G.; Nuovo, G.; Suh, S.S.; Ngankeu, A.; Taccioli, C.; Pichiorri, F.; Alder, H.; Secchiero, P.; *et al.* miR-221&222 regulate TRAIL resistance and enhance tumorigenicity through PTEN and TIMP3 downregulation. *Cancer Cell* **2009**, *16*, 498–509. [PubMed]

36. Vosa, U.; Vooder, T.; Kolde, R.; Vilo, J.; Metspalu, A.; Annilo, T. Meta-analysis of microRNA expression in lung cancer. *Int. J. Cancer* **2013**, *132*, 2884–2893. [CrossRef] [PubMed]

37. Xie, Y.; Todd, N.W.; Liu, Z.; Zhan, M.; Fang, H.; Peng, H.; Alattar, M.; Deepak, J.; Stass, S.A.; Jiang, F. Altered miRNA expression in sputum for diagnosis of non-small cell lung cancer. *Lung Cancer* **2010**, *67*, 170–176. [CrossRef] [PubMed]

38. Shen, J.; Todd, N.W.; Zhang, H.; Yu, L.; Lingxiao, X.; Mei, Y.; Guarnera, M.; Liao, J.; Chou, A.; Lu, C.L.; *et al.* Plasma microRNAs as potential biomarkers for non-small-cell lung cancer. *Lab. Investig.* **2011**, *91*, 579–587. [CrossRef] [PubMed]

39. Shen, J.; Liu, Z.; Todd, N.W.; Zhang, H.; Liao, J.; Yu, L.; Guarnera, M.A.; Li, R.; Cai, L.; Zhan, M.; *et al.* Diagnosis of lung cancer in individuals with solitary pulmonary nodules by plasma microRNA biomarkers. *BMC Cancer* **2011**, *11*, 374. [CrossRef] [PubMed]

40. Yu, L.; Todd, N.W.; Xing, L.; Xie, Y.; Zhang, H.; Liu, Z.; Fang, H.; Zhang, J.; Katz, R.L.; Jiang, F. Early detection of lung adenocarcinoma in sputum by a panel of microRNA markers. *Int. J. Cancer* **2010**, *127*, 2870–2878. [CrossRef] [PubMed]

41. Lebanony, D.; Benjamin, H.; Gilad, S.; Ezagouri, M.; Dov, A.; Ashkenazi, K.; Gefen, N.; Izraeli, S.; Rechavi, G.; Pass, H.; *et al.* Diagnostic assay based on hsa-miR-205 expression distinguishes squamous from nonsquamous non-small-cell lung carcinoma. *J. Clin. Oncol.* **2009**, *27*, 2030–2037. [CrossRef] [PubMed]

42. Bishop, J.A.; Benjamin, H.; Cholakh, H.; Chajut, A.; Clark, D.P.; Westra, W.H. Accurate classification of non-small cell lung carcinoma using a novel microRNA-based approach. *Clin. Cancer Res.* **2010**, *16*, 610–619. [CrossRef] [PubMed]

43. Hamamoto, J.; Soejima, K.; Yoda, S.; Naoki, K.; Nakayama, S.; Satomi, R.; Terai, H.; Ikemura, S.; Sato, T.; Yasuda, H.; *et al.* Identification of microRNAs differentially expressed between lung squamous cell carcinoma and lung adenocarcinoma. *Mol. Med. Rep.* **2013**, *8*, 456–462. [PubMed]

44. Nishikawa, E.; Osada, H.; Okazaki, Y.; Arima, C.; Tomida, S.; Tatematsu, Y.; Taguchi, A.; Shimada, Y.; Yanagisawa, K.; Yatabe, Y.; *et al.* miR-375 is activated by ASH1 and inhibits YAP1 in a lineage-dependent manner in lung cancer. *Cancer Res.* **2011**, *71*, 6165–6173. [CrossRef] [PubMed]

45. Takamizawa, J.; Konishi, H.; Yanagisawa, K.; Tomida, S.; Osada, H.; Endoh, H.; Harano, T.; Yatabe, Y.; Nagino, M.; Nimura, Y.; *et al.* Reduced expression of the let-7 microRNAs in human lung cancers in association with shortened postoperative survival. *Cancer Res.* **2004**, *64*, 3753–3756. [CrossRef] [PubMed]

46. Travis, W.D.; Brambilla, E.; Burke, A.P.; Marx, A.; Nicholson, A.G. *WHO Classification of Tumours of the Lung, Pleura, Thymus and Heart*, 4th ed.; IARC: Lyon, France, 2015.

47. Inamura, K.; Togashi, Y.; Nomura, K.; Ninomiya, H.; Hiramatsu, M.; Satoh, Y.; Okumura, S.; Nakagawa, K.; Ishikawa, Y. let-7 microRNA expression is reduced in bronchioloalveolar carcinoma, a non-invasive carcinoma, and is not correlated with prognosis. *Lung Cancer* **2007**, *58*, 392–396. [CrossRef] [PubMed]

48. Yanaihara, N.; Caplen, N.; Bowman, E.; Seike, M.; Kumamoto, K.; Yi, M.; Stephens, R.M.; Okamoto, A.; Yokota, J.; Tanaka, T.; *et al.* Unique microRNA molecular profiles in lung cancer diagnosis and prognosis. *Cancer Cell* **2006**, *9*, 189–198. [CrossRef] [PubMed]

49. Yu, S.L.; Chen, H.Y.; Chang, G.C.; Chen, C.Y.; Chen, H.W.; Singh, S.; Cheng, C.L.; Yu, C.J.; Lee, Y.C.; Chen, H.S.; *et al.* MicroRNA signature predicts survival and relapse in lung cancer. *Cancer Cell* **2008**, *13*, 48–57. [CrossRef] [PubMed]

50. Inamura, K.; Togashi, Y.; Nomura, K.; Ninomiya, H.; Hiramatsu, M.; Okui, M.; Satoh, Y.; Okumura, S.; Nakagawa, K.; Tsuchiya, E.; *et al.* Up-regulation of PTEN at the transcriptional level is an adverse prognostic factor in female lung adenocarcinomas. *Lung Cancer* **2007**, *57*, 201–206. [CrossRef] [PubMed]

51. Robles, A.I.; Arai, E.; Mathe, E.A.; Okayama, H.; Schetter, A.J.; Brown, D.; Petersen, D.; Bowman, E.D.; Noro, R.; Welsh, J.A.; *et al.* An Integrated Prognostic Classifier for Stage I Lung Adenocarcinoma Based on mRNA, microRNA, and DNA Methylation Biomarkers. *J. Thorac. Oncol.* **2015**, *10*, 1037–1048. [CrossRef] [PubMed]

52. Hu, Z.; Chen, X.; Zhao, Y.; Tian, T.; Jin, G.; Shu, Y.; Chen, Y.; Xu, L.; Zen, K.; Zhang, C.; *et al.* Serum microRNA signatures identified in a genome-wide serum microRNA expression profiling predict survival of non-small-cell lung cancer. *J. Clin. Oncol.* **2010**, *28*, 1721–1726. [CrossRef] [PubMed]

53. Wang, Y.; Gu, J.; Roth, J.A.; Hildebrandt, M.A.; Lippman, S.M.; Ye, Y.; Minna, J.D.; Wu, X. Pathway-based serum microRNA profiling and survival in patients with advanced stage non-small cell lung cancer. *Cancer Res.* **2013**, *73*, 4801–4809. [CrossRef] [PubMed]

54. Karube, Y.; Tanaka, H.; Osada, H.; Tomida, S.; Tatematsu, Y.; Yanagisawa, K.; Yatabe, Y.; Takamizawa, J.; Miyoshi, S.; Mitsudomi, T.; *et al.* Reduced expression of Dicer associated with poor prognosis in lung cancer patients. *Cancer Sci.* **2005**, *96*, 111–115. [CrossRef] [PubMed]

55. Bean, J.; Brennan, C.; Shih, J.Y.; Riely, G.; Viale, A.; Wang, L.; Chitale, D.; Motoi, N.; Szoke, J.; Broderick, S.; *et al.* MET amplification occurs with or without T790M mutations in EGFR mutant lung tumors with acquired resistance to gefitinib or erlotinib. *Proc. Natl. Acad. Sci. USA* **2007**, *104*, 20932–20937. [CrossRef] [PubMed]

56. The Cancer Genome Atlas Research Network. Comprehensive molecular profiling of lung adenocarcinoma. *Nature* **2014**, *511*, 543–550.

57. Takeuchi, K.; Soda, M.; Togashi, Y.; Suzuki, R.; Sakata, S.; Hatano, S.; Asaka, R.; Hamanaka, W.; Ninomiya, H.; Uehara, H.; *et al.* RET, ROS1 and ALK fusions in lung cancer. *Nat. Med.* **2012**, *18*, 378–381. [CrossRef] [PubMed]

58. Kohno, T.; Ichikawa, H.; Totoki, Y.; Yasuda, K.; Hiramoto, M.; Nammo, T.; Sakamoto, H.; Tsuta, K.; Furuta, K.; Shimada, Y.; *et al.* KIF5B-RET fusions in lung adenocarcinoma. *Nat. Med.* **2012**, *18*, 375–377. [CrossRef] [PubMed]

59. Vaishnavi, A.; Capelletti, M.; Le, A.T.; Kako, S.; Butaney, M.; Ercan, D.; Mahale, S.; Davies, K.D.; Aisner, D.L.; Pilling, A.B.; *et al.* Oncogenic and drug-sensitive NTRK1 rearrangements in lung cancer. *Nat. Med.* **2013**, *19*, 1469–1472. [CrossRef] [PubMed]

60. Fernandez-Cuesta, L.; Plenker, D.; Osada, H.; Sun, R.; Menon, R.; Leenders, F.; Ortiz-Cuaran, S.; Peifer, M.; Bos, M.; Dassler, J.; *et al.* CD74-NRG1 fusions in lung adenocarcinoma. *Cancer Discov.* **2014**, *4*, 415–422. [CrossRef] [PubMed]

61. Nakaoku, T.; Tsuta, K.; Ichikawa, H.; Shiraishi, K.; Sakamoto, H.; Enari, M.; Furuta, K.; Shimada, Y.; Ogiwara, H.; Watanabe, S.; *et al.* Druggable oncogene fusions in invasive mucinous lung adenocarcinoma. *Clin. Cancer Res.* **2014**, *20*, 3087–3093. [CrossRef] [PubMed]

62. Ninomiya, H.; Hiramatsu, M.; Inamura, K.; Nomura, K.; Okui, M.; Miyoshi, T.; Okumura, S.; Satoh, Y.; Nakagawa, K.; Nishio, M.; *et al.* Correlation between morphology and EGFR mutations in lung adenocarcinomas significance of the micropapillary pattern and the hobnail cell type. *Lung Cancer* **2009**, *63*, 235–240. [CrossRef] [PubMed]

63. Inamura, K.; Ninomiya, H.; Ishikawa, Y.; Matsubara, O. Is the epidermal growth factor receptor status in lung cancers reflected in clinicopathologic features? *Arch. Pathol. Lab. Med.* **2010**, *134*, 66–72. [PubMed]

64. Inamura, K.; Takeuchi, K.; Togashi, Y.; Nomura, K.; Ninomiya, H.; Okui, M.; Satoh, Y.; Okumura, S.; Nakagawa, K.; Soda, M.; *et al.* EML4-ALK fusion is linked to histological characteristics in a subset of lung cancers. *J. Thorac. Oncol.* **2008**, *3*, 13–17. [CrossRef] [PubMed]

65. Inamura, K.; Takeuchi, K.; Togashi, Y.; Hatano, S.; Ninomiya, H.; Motoi, N.; Mun, M.Y.; Sakao, Y.; Okumura, S.; Nakagawa, K.; *et al.* EML4-ALK lung cancers are characterized by rare other mutations, a TTF-1 cell lineage, an acinar histology, and young onset. *Mod. Pathol.* **2009**, *22*, 508–515. [CrossRef] [PubMed]

66. Shaw, A.T.; Yeap, B.Y.; Mino-Kenudson, M.; Digumarthy, S.R.; Costa, D.B.; Heist, R.S.; Solomon, B.; Stubbs, H.; Admane, S.; McDermott, U.; *et al.* Clinical features and outcome of patients with non-small-cell lung cancer who harbor EML4-ALK. *J. Clin. Oncol.* **2009**, *27*, 4247–4253. [CrossRef] [PubMed]

67. Pan, Y.; Zhang, Y.; Li, Y.; Hu, H.; Wang, L.; Li, H.; Wang, R.; Ye, T.; Luo, X.; Zhang, Y.; *et al.* ALK, ROS1 and RET fusions in 1139 lung adenocarcinomas: A comprehensive study of common and fusion pattern-specific clinicopathologic, histologic and cytologic features. *Lung Cancer* **2014**, *84*, 121–126. [CrossRef] [PubMed]

68. Seike, M.; Goto, A.; Okano, T.; Bowman, E.D.; Schetter, A.J.; Horikawa, I.; Mathe, E.A.; Jen, J.; Yang, P.; Sugimura, H.; *et al.* miR-21 is an EGFR-regulated anti-apoptotic factor in lung cancer in never-smokers. *Proc. Natl. Acad. Sci. USA* **2009**, *106*, 12085–12090. [CrossRef] [PubMed]

69. Li, B.; Ren, S.; Li, X.; Wang, Y.; Garfield, D.; Zhou, S.; Chen, X.; Su, C.; Chen, M.; Kuang, P.; *et al.* miR-21 overexpression is associated with acquired resistance of EGFR-TKI in non-small cell lung cancer. *Lung Cancer* **2014**, *83*, 146–153. [CrossRef] [PubMed]

70. Dacic, S.; Kelly, L.; Shuai, Y.; Nikiforova, M.N. miRNA expression profiling of lung adenocarcinomas: Correlation with mutational status. *Mod. Pathol.* **2010**, *23*, 1577–1582. [CrossRef] [PubMed]

71. Bjaanaes, M.M.; Halvorsen, A.R.; Solberg, S.; Jorgensen, L.; Dragani, T.A.; Galvan, A.; Colombo, F.; Anderlini, M.; Pastorino, U.; Kure, E.; *et al.* Unique microRNA-profiles in EGFR-mutated lung adenocarcinomas. *Int. J. Cancer* **2014**, *135*, 1812–1821. [CrossRef] [PubMed]

72. Weiss, G.J.; Bemis, L.T.; Nakajima, E.; Sugita, M.; Birks, D.K.; Robinson, W.A.; Varella-Garcia, M.; Bunn, P.A., Jr.; Haney, J.; Helfrich, B.A.; *et al.* EGFR regulation by microRNA in lung cancer: Correlation with clinical response and survival to gefitinib and EGFR expression in cell lines. *Ann. Oncol.* **2008**, *19*, 1053–1059. [CrossRef] [PubMed]

73. Chen, G.; Umelo, I.A.; Lv, S.; Teugels, E.; Fostier, K.; Kronenberger, P.; Dewaele, A.; Sadones, J.; Geers, C.; de Greve, J. miR-146a inhibits cell growth, cell migration and induces apoptosis in non-small cell lung cancer cells. *PLoS ONE* **2013**, *8*, e60317. [CrossRef] [PubMed]

74. Garofalo, M.; Romano, G.; Di Leva, G.; Nuovo, G.; Jeon, Y.J.; Ngankeu, A.; Sun, J.; Lovat, F.; Alder, H.; Condorelli, G.; *et al.* EGFR and MET receptor tyrosine kinase-altered microRNA expression induces tumorigenesis and gefitinib resistance in lung cancers. *Nat. Med.* **2011**, *18*, 74–82. [CrossRef] [PubMed]

75. Wang, S.; Su, X.; Bai, H.; Zhao, J.; Duan, J.; An, T.; Zhuo, M.; Wang, Z.; Wu, M.; Li, Z.; *et al.* Identification of plasma microRNA profiles for primary resistance to EGFR-TKIs in advanced non-small cell lung cancer (NSCLC) patients with EGFR activating mutation. *J. Hematol. Oncol.* **2015**, *8*, 127. [CrossRef] [PubMed]

76. Pak, M.G.; Lee, C.H.; Lee, W.J.; Shin, D.H.; Roh, M.S. Unique microRNAs in lung adenocarcinoma groups according to major TKI sensitive EGFR mutation status. *Diagn. Pathol.* **2015**, *10*, 99. [CrossRef] [PubMed]

77. Wang, Y.; Xia, H.; Zhuang, Z.; Miao, L.; Chen, X.; Cai, H. Axl-altered microRNAs regulate tumorigenicity and gefitinib resistance in lung cancer. *Cell Death Dis.* **2014**, *5*, e1227. [CrossRef] [PubMed]

78. Ricciuti, B.; Mecca, C.; Cenci, M.; Leonardi, G.C.; Perrone, L.; Mencaroni, C.; Crino, L.; Grignani, F.; Baglivo, S.; Chiari, R.; *et al.* miRNAs and resistance to EGFR-TKIs in EGFR-mutant non-small cell lung cancer: Beyond "traditional mechanisms" of resistance. *Ecancermedicalscience* **2015**, *9*, 569. [CrossRef] [PubMed]

79. Brown, D.; Rahman, M.; Nana-Sinkam, S.P. MicroRNAs in respiratory disease. A clinician's overview. *Ann. Am. Thorac. Soc.* **2014**, *11*, 1277–1285. [CrossRef] [PubMed]

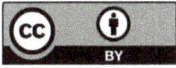

Journal of
*Clinical Medicine*

MDPI

Review

# Decoding the Secret of Cancer by Means of Extracellular Vesicles

Nobuyoshi Kosaka [1,2,3]

[1]  Division of Molecular and Cellular Medicine, National Cancer Center Research Institute, 5-1-1, Tsukiji, Chuo-ku, Tokyo 104-0045, Japan; nkosaka@ncc.go.jp; Tel.: +81-3-3542-2511 (ext. 4809)
[2]  Department of Zoology, University of Oxford, Tinbergen Building, South Parks Road, Oxford OX1 3PS, UK
[3]  JSPS Postdoctoral Fellow for Research Abroad, 5-3-1, Kojimachi, Chiyoda-ku, Tokyo 102-0083, Japan

Academic Editors: Takahiro Ochiya and Ryou-u Takahashi
Received: 2 August 2015; Accepted: 26 January 2016; Published: 4 February 2016

**Abstract:** One of the recent outstanding developments in cancer biology is the emergence of extracellular vesicles (EVs). EVs, which are small membrane vesicles that contain proteins, mRNAs, long non-coding RNAs, and microRNAs (miRNAs), are secreted by a variety of cells and have been revealed to play an important role in intercellular communications. These molecules function in the recipient cells; this has brought new insight into cell-cell communication. Recent reports have shown that EVs contribute to cancer cell development, including tumor initiation, angiogenesis, immune surveillance, drug resistance, invasion, metastasis, maintenance of cancer stem cells, and EMT phenotype. In this review, I will summarize recent studies on EV-mediated miRNA transfer in cancer biology. Furthermore, I will also highlight the possibility of novel diagnostics and therapy using miRNAs in EVs against cancer.

**Keywords:** extracellular vesicles; exosomes; microRNA; microenvironment cell; metastasis; dormancy; cancer initiation; recurrence; brain metastasis; biomarker

## 1. Introduction

Dr. Jan Lotvall's group was the first to discover microRNA (miRNA) transfer [1]. In their 2007 paper, the authors showed the transfer of variable RNA, such as mRNA, long non-coding RNA (lncRNA), and microRNA (miRNA), between cells through extracellular vesicles (EVs). EVs are small membranous vesicles that are secreted from numerous types of cells and function in intercellular communication by transporting intracellular contents, such as protein and RNA [2]. EVs, including exosomes, microvesicles, and other types of membrane vesicles found in various body fluids such as blood, urine, and saliva, are differentiated by their mechanisms of biogenesis and secretion [3]. miRNA, which is the small RNA molecule inhibiting the gene function by interacting with the 3′UTR of those genes [4,5], had been thought to function only inside the cells that expressed those miRNAs. After this, three papers, including ours, first showed the function of transferred miRNAs in the recipient cells, such as immune cells [6], cancer cells [7], or endothelial cells [8]. These papers opened up a novel research field in which miRNAs may serve as novel humoral factors in cell–cell communication. Indeed, the current focus in this field is on the roles of exosomal miRNA between cancer cells and microenvironmental cells in cancer development [9].

In this review, I will summarize current knowledge regarding the contribution of miRNAs in EVs during cancer development, such as initiation, invasion, metastasis, and recurrence. Furthermore, I will discuss therapeutic approaches using EVs and miRNAs, which are originally from cancer cells and/or microenvironmental cells, in EVs for diagnosis and treatment of cancer (Figure 1).

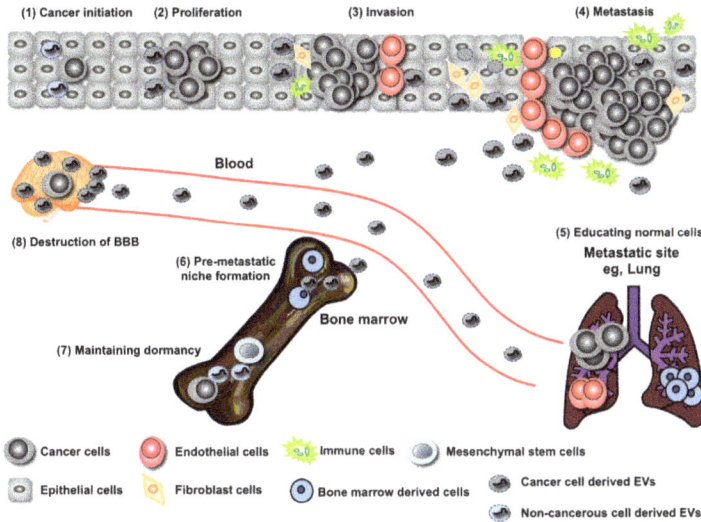

**Figure 1.** EVs from cancer cells manipulate the cells in their microenvironment. EVs are involved in every step of cancer development. In cancer's initiation stage, normal cells prevent the outgrowth of cancer cells by secreting tumor suppressive miRNAs through EVs (1); however, the cancer cells can avoid this inhibitory machinery, finally resulting in a tumor expansion (2). Cancer cells exhibit horizontal transfer of genes that promote proliferation by EVs from cancer cells harboring those genes to cancer cells that do not harbor those genes (2); Many reports have shown that cancer cell-derived EVs promote cancer malignancy (3,4). In addition, cancer cell-derived EVs activate fibroblasts, leading to extracellular matrix degradation and the induction of cancer-promoting cytokines (3,4). When the tumor microenvironment is hypoxic, cancer cells secrete angiogenesis-inducing EVs that help to overcome oxygen and nutrition deficiency by activating endothelial cells to form the vascular system (3,4). These will contribute to further cancer development, such as metastasis (4); EVs derived from cancer cells infiltrate bone marrow cells, leading to the formation of a pre-metastatic niche that is prepared by bone marrow cells (5); In addition, EVs from cancer cells directly affect the metastatic site to induce angiogenesis (6). Transfer of miRNAs by EVs from the bone marrow mesenchymal stem cells regulate breast cancer cell dormancy in a metastatic niche (7). Furthermore, mechanism of brain metastasis mediated by EVs triggers the destruction of BBB (8).

## 2. EV miRNA's Contribution to Both the Promotion and Suppression of Cancer Initiation

Numerous studies have shown a broad variety of mechanisms for tumor initiation, including gene amplification/deletion/mutation, cellular stress, metabolic alteration, and epigenetic changes [10]. In addition to those cell-autonomous mechanisms, non-cell-autonomous mechanisms also contribute to cancer initiation. Recent research has shown that the EVs from noncancerous neighboring epithelial cells have the capacity to suppress the expansion of cancer initiation [11]. It has been shown that one tumor-suppressive miRNA, miR-143, whose expression in normal prostate cell lines is higher than that in prostate cancer cell lines [12], transfers growth-inhibitory signals to cancerous cells *in vitro* and *in vivo* in EVs released from noncancerous cells. During cancer initiation, it has been shown that there are some fights between newly emerged cancerous cells and the surrounding epithelial cells [13,14]. Taken together with these results and publications, I hypothesized that growth inhibitory miRNAs are actively released from noncancerous cells to suppress the growth of abnormal cells with a partial oncogenic ability, thereby restoring them to a healthy state [11]. Because abundantly existing healthy cells continuously provide nascent overproliferative cells with tumor-suppressive miRNAs for a long period, it can be assumed that a local concentration of secretory miRNAs can become high enough to restrain tumor initiation. Indeed, employing the copy number analysis of miRNA in EVs, it has been proposed that the large numbers of EVs produced per cell allows for the loading of low miRNA numbers per EVs to achieve functional relevance [15]. In many cases, the expression of tumor-suppressive miRNAs is downregulated in cancer cells [16]; therefore, this continuous provision of tumor-suppressive miRNA through the EVs could be a homeostatic mechanism that tumor cells need to overcome. Although further studies are essential to clarify this hypothesis, understanding the preventing mechanisms of cancer initiation by surrounding cells might be important to realize the prevention of cancer.

Furthermore, this biological process has been confirmed between other combinations of cells, such as multiple myeloma and bone marrow mesenchymal stromal cells (BM-MSCs) [17]. In this case, EVs isolated from BM-MSCs of patients with multiple myeloma induced multiple myeloma tumor growth *in vivo* and promoted dissemination of tumor cells to the BM in an *in vivo* translational model of multiple myeloma. Moreover, the levels of miR-15a were significantly higher in EVs from normal BM-MSC-derived EVs than those in EVs from multiple myeloma BM-MSCs, suggesting the tumor-suppressive role of MSC-derived miR-15a from EVs against multiple myeloma. It has been known that miR-15a acts as a tumor-suppressive miRNA and that multiple myeloma growth can also be suppressed by miR-15a [18,19]. As in the relationship between prostate epithelial cells and prostate cancer cells shown above [11], BM-MSCs seem to guard against cancer cells by providing tumor-suppressive miR-15a against multiple myeloma; however, for some reason, the expression of miR-15a is downregulated in BM-MSCs, and the EVs from those BM-MSCs are no longer able to suppress the expansion of multiple myeloma. One of the main reasons for downregulation of tumor-suppressive miRNAs, such as miR-143 and miR-15a, is deletion from the genome [18]; however, this deletion has been reported in cancer cells. Thus, other downregulation mechanisms of tumor-suppressive miRNA should exist in those normal cells. As shown above, the secretion of miR-143 or miR-15a in EVs from noncancerous cells is important for suppressing cancer initiation; revealing the regulatory mechanisms of miRNAs in noncancerous cells might also lead to answers regarding the mechanisms of cancer initiation.

Although a variety of noncancerous cells surround cancer cells, because of the low secretion level of EVs from noncancerous cells, a single species of miRNA in EVs is insufficient for suppressing the expansion of cancer cells. However, considering that EVs carry a variety of molecules, not only the many tumor-suppressive miRNAs but also another protein with anti-cancer activity that does exist in EVs might contribute greatly to the suppression of cancer cell expansion by surrounding noncancerous cells. In EVs, for instance, PTEN, one of the most commonly lost tumor suppressors in human cancer, can transfer into other cells and reduce phosphorylation of the serine and threonine kinase Akt, resulting in the reduction of cellular proliferation in recipient cells [20]. The role of EV miRNAs in cancer initiation has not yet been clarified; however, considering the current incidence of cancer, how to prevent cancer is a question that must be answered.

## 3. Regulation of Cancer Progression by miRNAs in EVs

EVs from cancer cells affect other cancer cells in the heterogeneous population of a tumor, resulting in the transfer of metastatic capability. Most cancer cells release a variety of EV types, and the transfer of EVs dictates the behavior of the recipient cell for their benefit. Much of this research involved *in vitro* studies; however, the behavior of EVs *in vivo* needs to be addressed. Recently, significant work was published regarding the EV exchange between tumor cells by combining high-resolution intravital imaging with a Cre-LoxP system to trace the behavior of EVs *in vivo* [21]. Less malignant breast cancer cells located within the same and within distant tumors take up EVs secreted by highly metastatic breast cancer cell lines. These EVs carry mRNAs involved in migration and metastasis, resulting in the promotion of migratory behavior and metastatic capacity. For instance, the miR-200 family, which regulates the mesenchymal-to-epithelial transition, was secreted in EVs from metastatic breast cancer cell lines; this miR-200 transfer to the non-metastatic cancer cells altered gene expression and promoted mesenchymal-to-epithelial transition [22]. Drug resistance in neuroblastoma (NBL) is another example of the role of miRNA in EVs [23]. Co-culture experiments were performed that showed the transfer of miR-21 from NBL cells to human monocytes and miR-155 from human monocytes to NBL cells by EVs. miR-21 in EVs secreted from NBL cells bind to TLR8 in human monocytes, resulting the activation of NF-κB pathway activation in monocytes. On the other hands, miR-155 levels in human monocytes were progressively increased by the NBL-derived EVs and this led to the accumulation of miR-155 in EVs from human monocytes. This miR-155 suppresses the expression of TERF1, which is an inhibitor of telomerase, resulting in the promotion of chemoresistance in NBL [24]. These data indicate a unique role of miR-21 and miR-155 in the crosstalk between NBL cells and human monocytes in their resistance to chemotherapy. In addition to NBL, it has been shown that miRNAs in EVs contribute to the growth of HCC (hepatocellular carcinoma) [25]. In this report, the miRNAs that were highly expressed in EVs from HCC can modulate TAK1 expression, resulting in the enhancement of transformed cell growth in recipient cells.

It is already clear that microenvironmental cells contribute greatly to cancer development, which enhances the cancer cell's capacity to metastasize to other organs [10]. The microenvironment contains many factors and cell types, such as immune cells, fibroblasts, and endothelial cells, which influence cancer progression. The secretion of humoral factors from microenvironmental cells to cancer cells is essential for metastasis during cancer development.

Endothelial cells contribute to vascular generation and provide cancer cells with oxygen and nutrition, which are difficult to obtain in a tumor [26]. In this case, cytokines, such as VEGF or bFGF, are the molecules responsible for communication between cancer cells and endothelial cells. Recently, it has been shown that EVs from cancer cells contain various molecules that promote angiogenic cytokines, such as VEGF, bFGF, and TGF-beta. In addition to these angiogenic cytokines, there are multiple secretory miRNAs in EVs that have been reported to promote angiogenesis. For instance, miR-9 in EVs from cancer cells educed SOCS5 levels, leading to the activated JAK-STAT pathway, resulting in the promotion of endothelial cell migration and tumor angiogenesis [27]. In addition, miR-210, which was known to act as angiogenic miRNA, transfers from cancer cells to the endothelial cells through the EVs and promotes angiogenesis under the regulation of nSMase2 [28], which has known to regulate EV production [7,29]. In endothelial cells, the expression of Ephrin A, the target gene of miR-210 [30], was downregulated after the transfer of EVs from cancer cells. In addition, *in vivo* studies showed the effect of miRNA transfers from cancer cells. Indeed, manipulating the expression of nSMase2 can affect EV production, and this manipulation affects the metastatic ability as well. Indeed, miR-210 has been known to regulate angiogenesis in endothelial cells [30] and iron homeostasis in cancer cells [31] and was upregulated by a hypoxic condition [30].

## 4. Long-Distance Regulation of Metastasis by miRNAs in EVs

EVs affect not only cells close to cancer cells but also cells in distant tissues. For instance, highly metastatic melanoma-derived EVs increased the metastasis of primary tumors by educating the bone marrow [32]. In addition, miR-122 in EVs from cancer cells downregulated the glycolytic enzyme pyruvate kinase in non-tumor cells located in the pre-metastatic niche, resulting in the suppression of glucose uptake by non-tumor cells in the pre-metastatic niche and increased nutrient availability to cancer cells in the pre-metastatic niche [33].

EVs seem to tightly associate with brain metastasis, an important cause of mortality in cancer patients. Brain metastasis is associated with a particularly poor prognosis for cancer patients; however, the detailed molecular mechanisms have not yet been clarified. One of the key features of brain metastasis is the destruction of the blood–brain barrier (BBB) and the migration of cancer cells through the BBB [34,35], which consists of the endothelium and surrounding cells including pericytes and astrocytes [36,37] and limits the passive diffusion of molecules. Tumor cells recognize and bind to components of the vascular membrane, thereby initiating extravasation, invasion of cancer cells through the BBB, and the beginning of new growth at secondary organ sites [38,39]. Variable potential molecules promote or disturb BBB destruction. The contribution of EVs in brain metastasis was also reported. EVs from brain metastatic cancer cells contained miR-181c, and it transferred to brain endothelial cells, resulting in the destruction of tight junction proteins of BBB, such as Claudin-5, Occludin, and ZO-1 [40]. The primary cytoskeletal protein, actin, has been known to bind all ZO proteins, claudin, and occludin. Phosphorylation of cofilin through 3-phosphoinositide-dependent protein kinase-1 (PDPK1), which is the target gene of miR-181c, is thought to inactivate cofilin in a spatial manner, in which local activation occurs in the cell membrane [40]. In addition, tight junction proteins are also the direct targets of miRNA in EVs. Indeed, miR-105 in EVs from breast cancer cells suppressed ZO-1 expression in endothelial cells, resulting in the loss of cell–cell adhesion and leading to the promotion of metastasis [41].

These reports suggest that miRNAs in EVs from brain metastatic cancer cells targeted tight junction proteins and regulators of actin proteins simultaneously, resulting in the efficient destruction of the BBB for metastasis.

## 5. Recurrence Rebooted by EVs

Recent successful early detection and effective systemic adjuvant therapy has caused a decrease in mortality from breast cancer. However, breast cancer often recurs, typically within five years but even up to 10 to 20 years after surgery [42]. In addition, breast cancer recurrence is often more aggressive and untreatable. The usual explanation is that breast cancer cells survive for a long time somewhere in the body in a state of cancer dormancy. Dormant cancer cells cease dividing but survive in a quiescent state while waiting for appropriate environmental conditions to resume proliferation. It has been shown that breast cancer cells can be detected in the bone marrow (BM) in early stages of breast cancer [43]. It is thought that micrometastases form in the bone marrow and then recirculate to invade other, distant organs [44], thus understanding the molecular mechanisms for keeping cancer cells dormant by interacting with their microenvironmental cells is essential for diagnosing and preventing the recurrence of cancer. However, little is understood about this molecular mechanism. Recently, it was revealed that BM-MSCs play an important role in inducing dormancy in breast cancer cells in bone marrow through the transfer of a cell cycle inhibitory miRNA by EVs [45]. In this situation, miR-23b in EVs from BM-MSCs promoted dormancy through the downregulation of MARCKS, which is a target gene of miR-23b in breast cancer cells. Therefore, transfer of miR-23b by EVs and its suppression of MARCKS, one of the mechanisms for cancer recurrence, result in the suppression of the cell cycle and the transition to dormancy in breast cancer cells.

It is tempting to postulate the possibility of answering the following questions: (1) What is the physiological effect of miR-23b in EVs? (2) What is the molecular mechanism for avoiding dormancy of breast cancer cells? Answering these questions will lead to predicting the existence of breast cancer cells in bone marrow, or allow us to make drugs that target breast cancer cells in the bone marrow.

## 6. EVs as a New Diagnostic Tool

It has been shown that EVs reflect the physiological state of their cells of origin [46], and almost all types of cells, including cancer cells, secrete EVs that contain specific proteins and miRNAs into their microenvironment and circulation [3,47]. Because of this, EVs can be found in various body fluids, such as blood, urine, and saliva [2,48]. Taking these facts into account, EVs provide a rich source of potential biomarkers.

As shown above, the first indication regarding circulating RNA as a biomarker was the discovery of mRNA and miRNA in EVs [1]. After this, it was shown that miR-21 in EVs enriched in the serum of glioblastoma patients was expressed at higher levels in the serum of patients compared with normal controls [49]. This report became an impetus for research into biomarkers that use exosomal miRNAs in various types of cancer, and a specific miRNA profile has been published [3,50]. Moreover, miRNAs can be readily detected in small sample volumes using specific and sensitive quantitative real-time PCR (qRT-PCR) [51]. Many studies have evaluated the feasibility of circulating miRNAs for detecting cancer for diagnosis and for prognostic/predictive markers [49,52–61]. For instance, the amount of circulating miR-210 is significantly higher in serum from circulating tumor cell (CTC)-positive metastatic breast cancer patients compared with that in plasma from CTC-negative metastatic breast cancer patients and controls [62]. In addition, circulating miR-210 levels were significantly higher in individuals with residual disease than in those who achieved a pathologically complete response to trastuzumab [63], suggesting that circulating miR-210 can be used to predict and perhaps monitor responses to therapies involving the use of trastuzumab. As shown above, EVs isolated from metastatic breast cancer cells promote metastasis via the induction of angiogenesis in the tumor [28]. These EVs contain multiple miRNAs that promote angiogenesis by regulating the gene expressed in endothelial cells, and it has been shown that miR-210 was included in this type of miRNAs [30]. Furthermore, as shown above, circulating miR-181c [40] and miR-105 [41] can be found in the serum from brain metastatic cancer patients. These data give hope for the treatment of brain metastasis, as the detection of circulating miRNA, such as miR-181c or miR-105, leads to the finding of brain metastasis.

This kind of approach against sera from patients with cancers, such as prostate cancer, colorectal cancer, and pancreatic cancer, has been widely investigated recently. Although there are still some issues to be resolved in using miRNA in EVs from serum, such as isolation methods, inner control, and detection methods, miRNA in EVs from serum/plasma will be a great help in the diagnosis of cancer or the monitoring of cancer during treatment. Combined with other cancer biomarkers that have already been used, this might be the earliest method for clinical usage of miRNAs in EVs as a cancer biomarker.

## 7. EVs Are Novel Therapeutic Target in Cancer

The great contribution of EVs and miRNAs during cancer development has been shown, and their utilization for diagnosing or monitoring cancer is now a promising method for preemptive or personalized medicine. In addition to the diagnostic usage of EVs, targeting EVs for cancer treatment is becoming realistic as well (Figure 2).

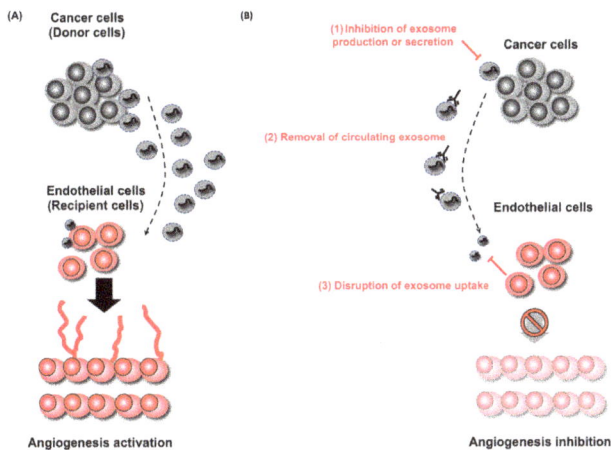

**Figure 2.** Therapeutic strategies against cancer-derived EVs. EVs are secreted from cancer cells and delivered to recipient cells, modulating the phenotype of the recipient cells. For instance, EVs from cancer cells are delivered to endothelial cells, which enhance angiogenesis (**A**). In this case, there are three therapeutic applications (**B**): (1) inhibition of EVs production from cancer cells; (2) elimination of circulating EVs from cancer cells; and disruption of EVs uptake by recipient cells (3). These therapeutic applications will prevent the delivery of EVs from cancer cells to endothelial cells, leading to the suppression of development of cancer cells.

Targeting molecules secreted through EVs from metastatic niches may prevent or delay cancer recurrence. In this situation, targeting the molecules related to EV secretion and/or production will be good candidates for EV-targeting treatment, such as nSMase2 [22,28,64,65], RAB27A, RAB27B [32,66,67], and RAB22A [68]. The suppression of these molecules leads to the inhibition of EV production, which results in the disruption of cancer development; however, it is essential to understand the contribution of these molecules in the secretion of EVs from not only cancer cells but also normal cells. Otherwise, disturbing the secretion of EVs from normal cells might influence the homeostatic function of EVs as shown above.

Another method for targeting EVs for cancer treatment involves capturing the circulating EVs from cancer cells. As shown above, cancer cells secrete some EVs from outside of the original tumor position. Thus, the complete elimination of circulating EVs will be a great benefit to cancer patients. For instance, EVs with human epidermal growth factor receptor type 2 (HER2) isolated from HER2 over-express breast cancer cells; this interferes with the activity of the therapeutic antibody Herceptin in the breast cancer patient. From this point of view, a device that could eliminate target EVs from the entire circulatory system would be a great benefit in cancer treatment. Indeed, this type of device has already been proposed and developed [69]. This technology immobilizes exosome-binding lectins and antibodies in the outer-capillary space of plasma filtration membranes that integrate into existing kidney dialysis systems.

Another possible therapeutic approach against EVs is to disturb EV absorption in recipient cells. Based on current reports, there are some tropisms for receiving EVs. For example, EVs from brain metastatic breast cancer cells tend to incorporate into endothelial cells but not into astrocytes or pericytes [40]. Only a few reports deal with the recipient mechanisms for EVs; however, understanding this process will give us another way to disturb the progression of cancer.

As shown above, tumor-suppressive miRNAs can attenuate the growth of cancer cell proliferation. Indeed, miR-143-tansduced EVs can suppress the proliferation of cancer cells *in vivo* [9]. Thus, it is tempting to postulate that this tumor-suppressive miRNA and EV combination might be useful for cancer treatment. In addition, EVs can efficiently deliver another tumor-suppressive miRNA, let-7, to epidermal growth factor receptor (EGFR)-expressing breast cancer cells [70]. Targeting has been achieved by engineering the donor cells to express the transmembrane domain of platelet-derived growth factor receptor fused to the GE11 peptide. These reports suggest that EVs can be a vehicle for tumor-suppressive miRNAs to attack cancer cells in patients.

## 8. Conclusions

Unlike the first discovery of exosomes in the 1980s [71], which thought of exosomes as the garbage of the cells, current research indicates that EVs including exosomes might be central mediators of cell–cell communication. Much research has been done in the past several years; however, we need to continue so that we can understand EV function and character in more detail. Then, we will be able to use EVs freely in clinical situations.

**Acknowledgments:** I thank members of the Molecular and Cellular Medicine laboratory, National Cancer Center Research Institute, especially Yusuke Yoshioka for critically reading the manuscript. Nobuyoshi Kosaka is supported by the Japan Society for the Promotion of Science.

**Conflicts of Interest:** The author declares no conflict of interest.

## References

1. Valadi, H.; Ekstrom, K.; Bossios, A.; Sjostrand, M.; Lee, J.J.; Lotvall, J.O. Exosome-mediated transfer of mRNAs and microRNAs is a novel mechanism of genetic exchange between cells. *Nat. Cell Biol.* **2007**, *9*, 654–659. [PubMed]
2. Raposo, G.; Stoorvogel, W. Extracellular vesicles: Exosomes, microvesicles, and friends. *J. Cell Biol.* **2013**, *200*, 373–383. [PubMed]

3. Kosaka, N.; Iguchi, H.; Ochiya, T. Circulating microRNA in body fluid: A new potential biomarker for cancer diagnosis and prognosis. *Cancer Sci.* **2010**, *101*, 2087–2092. [PubMed]
4. Suzuki, H.I.; Katsura, A.; Matsuyama, H.; Miyazono, K. MicroRNA regulons in tumor microenvironment. *Oncogene* **2014**, *34*, 3085–3094. [PubMed]
5. Mendell, J.T.; Olson, E.N. MicroRNAs in Stress Signaling and Human Disease. *Cell* **2012**, *148*, 1172–1187. [PubMed]
6. Pegtel, D.M.; Cosmopoulos, K.; Thorley-Lawson, D.A.; van Eijndhoven, M.A.J.; Hopmans, E.S.; Lindenberg, J.L.; de Gruijl, T.D.; Würdinger, T.; Middeldorp, J.M. Functional delivery of viral miRNAs via exosomes. *Proc. Natl. Acad. Sci. USA* **2010**, *107*, 6328–6333. [PubMed]
7. Kosaka, N.; Iguchi, H.; Yoshioka, Y.; Takeshita, F.; Matsuki, Y.; Ochiya, T. Secretory mechanisms and intercellular transfer of microRNAs in living cells. *J. Biol. Chem.* **2010**, *285*, 17442–17452. [PubMed]
8. Zhang, Y.; Liu, D.; Chen, X.; Li, J.; Li, L.; Bian, Z.; Sun, F.; Lu, J.; Yin, Y.; Cai, X.; *et al.* Secreted monocytic miR-150 enhances targeted endothelial cell migration. *Mol. Cell.* **2010**, *39*, 133–144. [CrossRef] [PubMed]
9. Kosaka, N.; Yoshioka, Y.; Tominaga, N.; Hagiwara, K.; Katsuda, T.; Ochiya, T. Dark side of the exosome: The role of the exosome in cancer metastasis and targeting the exosome as a strategy for cancer therapy. *Future Oncol. (Lond. Engl.)* **2014**, *10*, 671–681. [CrossRef] [PubMed]
10. Hanahan, D.; Weinberg, R.A. Hallmarks of Cancer: The Next Generation. *Cell* **2011**, *144*, 646–674. [PubMed]
11. Kosaka, N.; Iguchi, H.; Yoshioka, Y.; Hagiwara, K.; Takeshita, F.; Ochiya, T. Competitive Interactions of Cancer Cells and Normal Cells via Secretory MicroRNAs. *J. Biol. Chem.* **2012**, *287*, 1397–1405. [PubMed]
12. Clapé, C.; Fritz, V.; Henriquet, C.; Apparailly, F.; Fernandez, P.L.; Iborra, F.; Avancès, C.; Villalba, M.; Culline, S.; Fajas, L. miR-143 interferes with ERK5 signaling, and abrogates prostate cancer progression in mice. *PLoS ONE* **2009**, *4*, e7542.
13. Wagstaff, L.; Kolahgar, G.; Piddini, E. Competitive cell interactions in cancer: A cellular tug of war. *Trends Cell Biol.* **2012**, *23*, 160–167. [PubMed]
14. Moreno, E. Is cell competition relevant to cancer? *Nat. Rev. Cancer* **2008**, *8*, 141–147. [PubMed]
15. Alexander, M.; Hu, R.; Runtsch, M.C.; Kagele, D.A.; Mosbruger, T.L.; Tolmachova, T.; Seabra, M.C.; Round, J.L.; Ward, D.M.; O'Connell, R.M. Exosome-delivered microRNAs modulate the inflammatory response to endotoxin. *Nat. Commun.* **2015**, *6*. [CrossRef]
16. Calin, G.A.; Croce, C.M. MicroRNA signatures in human cancers. *Nat. Rev. Cancer* **2006**, *11*, 857–866. [CrossRef] [PubMed]
17. Roccaro, A.M.; Sacco, A.; Maiso, P.; Azab, A.K.; Tai, Y.; Reagan, M.; Azab, F.; Flores, L.M.; Campigotto, F.; Weller, E.; *et al.* BM mesenchymal stromal cell—Derived exosomes facilitate multiple myeloma progression. *J. Clin. Investig.* **2013**, *123*, 1542–1555. [PubMed]
18. Pekarsky, Y.; Croce, C.M. Role of miR-15/16 in CLL. *Cell Death Differ.* **2014**, *22*, 6–11. [CrossRef] [PubMed]
19. Corthals, S.L.; Jongen-Lavrencic, M.; de Knegt, Y.; Peeters, J.K.; Beverloo, H.B.; Lokhorst, H.M.; Sonneveld, P. Micro-RNA-15a and micro-RNA-16 expression and chromosome 13 deletions in multiple myeloma. *Leuk. Res.* **2010**, *34*, 677–681. [PubMed]
20. Putz, U.; Howitt, J.; Doan, A.; Goh, C.-P.; Low, L.-H.; Silke, J.; Tan, S.-S. The Tumor Suppressor PTEN Is Exported in Exosomes and Has Phosphatase Activity in Recipient Cells. *Sci. Signal.* **2012**, *5*. [CrossRef] [PubMed]
21. Zomer, A.; Maynard, C.; Verweij, F.J.; Kamermans, A.; Schäfer, R.; Beerling, E.; Schiffelers, R.M.; de Wit, E.; Berenguer, J.; Ellenbroek, S.I.J.; *et al.* In Vivo Imaging Reveals Extracellular Vesicle-Mediated Phenocopying of Metastatic Behavior. *Cell* **2015**, *161*, 1046–1057. [PubMed]
22. Le, M.T.N.; Hamar, P.; Guo, C.; Basar, E.; Perdigão-henriques, R.; Balaj, L.; Lieberman, J. miR-200-containing extracellular vesicles promote breast cancer cell metastasis. *J. Clin. Investig.* **2014**, *124*, 5109–5128. [CrossRef] [PubMed]
23. Challagundla, K.B.; Wise, P.M.; Neviani, P.; Chava, H.; Murtadha, M.; Xu, T.; Kennedy, R.; Ivan, C.; Zhang, X.; Vannini, I.; *et al.* Exosome-Mediated Transfer of microRNAs Within the Tumor Microenvironment and Neuroblastoma Resistance to Chemotherapy. *JNCI J. Natl. Cancer Inst.* **2015**, *107*. [CrossRef] [PubMed]
24. Dinami, R.; Ercolani, C.; Petti, E.; Piazza, S.; Ciani, Y.; Sestito, R.; Sacconi, A.; Biagioni, F.; le Sage, C.; Agami, R.; *et al.* miR-155 drives telomere fragility in human breast cancer by targeting TRF1. *Cancer Res.* **2014**, *74*, 4145–4156. [PubMed]

25. Kogure, T.; Lin, W.-L.; Yan, I.K.; Braconi, C.; Patel, T. Inter-cellular nanovesicle mediated microRNA transfer: A mechanism of environmental modulation of hepatocellular cancer cell growth. *Hepatology (Baltim. MD)* **2011**, *54*, 1237–1248.

26. Weis, S.M.; Cheresh, D.A. Tumor angiogenesis: Molecular pathways and therapeutic targets. *Nat. Med.* **2011**, *17*, 1359–1370. [PubMed]

27. Zhuang, G.; Wu, X.; Jiang, Z.; Kasman, I.; Yao, J.; Guan, Y.; Oeh, J.; Modrusan, Z.; Bais, C.; Sampath, D.; *et al.* Tumour-secreted miR-9 promotes endothelial cell migration and angiogenesis by activating the JAK-STAT pathway. *EMBO J.* **2012**, *31*, 3513–3523. [PubMed]

28. Kosaka, N.; Iguchi, H.; Hagiwara, K.; Yoshioka, Y.; Takeshita, F.; Ochiya, T. Neutral sphingomyelinase 2 (nSMase2)-dependent exosomal transfer of angiogenic micrornas regulate cancer cell metastasis. *J. Biol. Chem.* **2013**, *288*, 10849–10859. [PubMed]

29. Trajkovic, K.; Hsu, C.; Chiantia, S.; Rajendran, L.; Wenzel, D.; Wieland, F.; Schwille, P.; Brügger, B.; Simons, M. Ceramide triggers budding of exosome vesicles into multivesicular endosomes. *Science (N. Y. NY)* **2008**, *319*, 1244–1247. [CrossRef] [PubMed]

30. Fasanaro, P.; D'Alessandra, Y.; di Stefano, V.; Melchionna, R.; Romani, S.; Pompilio, G.; Capogrossi, M.C.; Martelli, F. MicroRNA-210 modulates endothelial cell response to hypoxia and inhibits the receptor tyrosine kinase ligand ephrin-A3. *J. Biol. Chem.* **2008**, *283*, 15878–15883. [PubMed]

31. Yoshioka, Y.; Kosaka, N.; Ochiya, T.; Kato, T. Micromanaging iron homeostasis: Hypoxia-inducible micro-RNA-210 suppresses iron homeostasis-related proteins. *J. Biol. Chem.* **2012**, *287*, 34110–34119. [PubMed]

32. Peinado, H.; Alečković, M.; Lavotshkin, S.; Matei, I.; Costa-Silva, B.; Moreno-Bueno, G.; Hergueta-Redondo, M.; Williams, C.; García-Santos, G.; Ghajar, C.M.; *et al.* Melanoma exosomes educate bone marrow progenitor cells toward a pro-metastatic phenotype through MET. *Nat. Med.* **2012**, *18*, 883–891. [PubMed]

33. Fong, M.Y.; Zhou, W.; Liu, L.; Alontaga, A.Y.; Chandra, M.; Ashby, J.; Chow, A.; O'Connor, S.T.F.; Li, S.; Chin, A.R.; *et al.* Breast-cancer-secreted miR-122 reprograms glucose metabolism in premetastatic niche to promote metastasis. *Nat. Cell Biol.* **2015**, *17*, 183–194. [PubMed]

34. Arshad, F.; Wang, L.; Sy, C.; Avraham, S.; Avraham, H.K. Blood-brain barrier integrity and breast cancer metastasis to the brain. *Pathol. Res. Int.* **2010**, *2011*, 920509. [CrossRef] [PubMed]

35. Bos, P.D.; Nguyen, D.X.; Massagué, J. Modeling metastasis in the mouse. *Curr. Opin. Pharmacol.* **2010**, *10*, 571–577. [PubMed]

36. Ballabh, P.; Braun, A.; Nedergaard, M. The blood-brain barrier: An overview: Structure, regulation, and clinical implications. *Neurobiol. Dis.* **2004**, *16*, 1–13. [CrossRef] [PubMed]

37. Winkler, E.A.; Bell, R.D.; Zlokovic, B.V. Central nervous system pericytes in health and disease. *Nat. Neurosci.* **2011**, *14*, 1398–1405. [PubMed]

38. Nicolson, G.L. Organ specificity of tumor metastasis: Role of preferential adhesion, invasion and growth of malignant cells at specific secondary sites. *Cancer Metastasis Rev.* **1988**, *7*, 143–188. [PubMed]

39. Orr, F.W.; Wang, H.H.; Lafrenie, R.M.; Scherbarth, S.; Nance, D.M. Interactions between cancer cells and the endothelium in metastasis. *J. Pathol.* **2000**, *190*, 310–329. [CrossRef]

40. Tominaga, N.; Kosaka, N.; Ono, M.; Katsuda, T.; Yoshioka, Y.; Tamura, K.; Lötvall, J.; Nakagama, H.; Ochiya, T. Brain metastatic cancer cells release microRNA-181c-containing extracellular vesicles capable of destructing blood-brain barrier. *Nat. Commun.* **2015**, *6*. [CrossRef]

41. Zhou, W.; Fong, M.Y.; Min, Y.; Somlo, G.; Liu, L.; Palomares, M.R.; Yu, Y.; Chow, A.; O'Connor, S.T.F.; Chin, A.R.; *et al.* Cancer-Secreted miR-105 destroys vascular endothelial barriers to promote metastasis. *Cancer Cell* **2014**, *25*, 501–515. [PubMed]

42. Kurtz, J.M.; Spitalier, J.M.; Amalric, R. Late breast recurrence after lumpectomy and irradiation. *Int. J. Radiat. Oncol. Biol. Phys.* **1983**, *9*, 1191–1194. [PubMed]

43. Braun, S.; Vogl, F.D.; Naume, B.; Janni, W.; Osborne, M.P.; Coombes, R.C.; Schlimok, G.; Diel, I.J.; Gerber, B.; Gebauer, G.; *et al.* A pooled analysis of bone marrow micrometastasis in breast cancer. *N. Engl. J. Med.* **2005**, *353*, 793–802. [PubMed]

44. Pantel, K.; Alix-Panabières, C.; Riethdorf, S. Cancer micrometastases. *Nat. Rev. Clin. Oncol.* **2009**, *6*, 339–351. [PubMed]

45. Ono, M.; Kosaka, N.; Tominaga, N.; Yoshioka, Y.; Takeshita, F.; Takahashi, R.-U.; Yoshida, M.; Tsuda, H.; Tamura, K.; Ochiya, T. Exosomes from bone marrow mesenchymal stem cells contain a microRNA that promotes dormancy in metastatic breast cancer cells. *Sci. Signal.* **2014**, *7*. [CrossRef]

46. Yáñez-Mó, M.; Siljander, P.R.-M.; Andreu, Z.; Zavec, A.B.; Borràs, F.E.; Buzas, E.I.; Buzas, K.; Casal, E.; Cappello, F.; Carvalho, J.; *et al.* Biological properties of extracellular vesicles and their physiological functions. *J. Extracell. Vesicles* **2015**, *4*. [CrossRef] [PubMed]

47. Katsuda, T.; Kosaka, N.; Ochiya, T. The roles of extracellular vesicles in cancer biology: Toward the development of novel cancer biomarkers. *Proteomics* **2014**, *14*, 412–425. [CrossRef] [PubMed]

48. Thery, C. Exosomes: Secreted vesicles and intercellular communications. *F1000 Biol. Rep.* **2011**, *3*. [CrossRef] [PubMed]

49. Skog, J.; Wurdinger, T.; Rijn, S.V.; Meijer, D.H.; Gainche, L.; Sena-esteves, M.; Curry, W.T., Jr.; Carter, B.S.; Krichevsky, A.M.; Breakefield, X.O. Glioblastoma microvesicles transport RNA and proteins that promote tumour growth and provide diagnostic biomarkers. *Nat. Cell Biol.* **2008**, *10*, 1470–1476. [PubMed]

50. Wittmann, J.; Jäck, H.-M. Serum microRNAs as powerful cancer biomarkers. *Biochim. Biophys. Acta* **2010**, *1806*, 200–207. [CrossRef] [PubMed]

51. Chen, C.; Ridzon, D.A.; Broomer, A.J.; Zhou, Z.; Lee, D.H.; Nguyen, J.T.; Barbisin, M.; Xu, N.L.; Mahuvakar, V.R.; Andersen, M.R.; *et al.* Real-time quantification of microRNAs by stem-loop RT-PCR. *Nucleic Acids Res.* **2005**, *33*, e179. [PubMed]

52. Que, R.; Ding, G.; Chen, J.; Cao, L. Analysis of serum exosomal microRNAs and clinicopathologic features of patients with pancreatic adenocarcinoma. *World J. Surg. Oncol.* **2013**, *11*. [CrossRef]

53. Bryant, R.J.; Pawlowski, T.; Catto, J.W.F.; Marsden, G.; Vessella, R.L.; Rhees, B.; Kuslich, C.; Visakorpi, T.; Hamdy, F.C. Changes in circulating microRNA levels associated with prostate cancer. *Br. J. Cancer* **2012**, *106*, 768–774. [PubMed]

54. Liu, J.; Sun, H.; Wang, X.; Yu, Q.; Li, S.; Yu, X.; Gong, W. Increased exosomal microRNA-21 and microRNA-146a levels in the cervicovaginal lavage specimens of patients with cervical cancer. *Int. J. Mol. Sci.* **2014**, *15*, 758–773. [CrossRef] [PubMed]

55. Wang, H.; Hou, L.; Li, A.; Duan, Y.; Gao, H.; Song, X. Expression of serum exosomal microRNA-21 in human hepatocellular carcinoma. *BioMed Res. Int.* **2014**, *2014*. [CrossRef]

56. Wang, J.; Zhou, Y.; Lu, J.; Sun, Y.; Xiao, H.; Liu, M.; Tian, L. Combined detection of serum exosomal miR-21 and HOTAIR as diagnostic and prognostic biomarkers for laryngeal squamous cell carcinoma. *Med. Oncol. (Northwood Lond. Engl.)* **2014**, *31*. [CrossRef]

57. Matsumura, T.; Sugimachi, K.; Iinuma, H.; Takahashi, Y.; Kurashige, J.; Sawada, G.; Ueda, M.; Uchi, R.; Ueo, H.; Takano, Y.; *et al.* Exosomal microRNA in serum is a novel biomarker of recurrence in human colorectal cancer. *Br. J. Cancer* **2015**, *113*, 275–281. [PubMed]

58. Chiam, K.; Wang, T.; Watson, D.I.; Mayne, G.C.; Irvine, T.S.; Bright, T.; Smith, L.; White, I.A.; Bowen, J.M.; Keefe, D.; *et al.* Circulating Serum Exosomal miRNAs as Potential Biomarkers for Esophageal Adenocarcinoma. *J. Gastrointest. Surg.* **2015**, *19*, 1208–1215. [PubMed]

59. Madhavan, B.; Yue, S.; Galli, U.; Rana, S.; Gross, W.; Muller, M.; Giese, N.A.; Kalthoff, H.; Becker, T.; Buchler, M.W.; *et al.* Combined evaluation of a panel of protein and miRNA serum-exosome biomarkers for pancreatic cancer diagnosis increases sensitivity and specificity. *Int. J. Cancer.* **2015**, *136*, 2616–2627. [PubMed]

60. Huang, X.; Yuan, T.; Liang, M.; Du, M.; Xia, S.; Dittmar, R.; Wang, D.; See, W.; Costello, B.A.; Quevedo, F.; *et al.* Exosomal miR-1290 and miR-375 as prognostic markers in castration-resistant prostate cancer. *Eur. Urol.* **2015**, *67*, 33–41. [CrossRef] [PubMed]

61. Manterola, L.; Guruceaga, E.; Gallego Perez-Larraya, J.; Gonzalez-Huarriz, M.; Jauregui, P.; Tejada, S.; Diez-Valle, R.; Segura, V.; Sampron, N.; Barrena, C.; *et al.* A small noncoding RNA signature found in exosomes of GBM patient serum as a diagnostic tool. *Neuro-Oncol.* **2014**, *16*, 520–527. [CrossRef] [PubMed]

62. Madhavan, D.; Zucknick, M.; Wallwiener, M.; Cuk, K.; Modugno, C.; Scharpff, M.; Schott, S.; Heil, J.; Turchinovich, A.; Yang, R.; *et al.* Circulating miRNAs as surrogate markers for circulating tumor cells and prognostic markers in metastatic breast cancer. *Clin. Cancer Res.* **2012**, *18*, 5972–5982. [CrossRef] [PubMed]

63. Jung, E.J.; Santarpia, L.; Kim, J.; Esteva, F.J.; Moretti, E.; Buzdar, A.U.; di Leo, A.; le, X.F.; Bast, R.C.; Park, S.T.; *et al.* Plasma microRNA 210 levels correlate with sensitivity to trastuzumab and tumor presence in breast cancer patients. *Cancer* **2012**, *118*, 2603–2614. [PubMed]

64.  Singh, R.; Pochampally, R.; Watabe, K.; Lu, Z.; Mo, Y.-Y. Exosome-mediated transfer of miR-10b promotes cell invasion in breast cancer. *Mol. Cancer* **2014**, *13*. [CrossRef] [PubMed]
65.  Hu, Y.; Yan, C.; Mu, L.; Huang, K.; Li, X.; Tao, D.; Wu, Y.; Qin, J. Fibroblast-Derived Exosomes Contribute to Chemoresistance through Priming Cancer Stem Cells in Colorectal Cancer. *PLoS ONE* **2015**, *10*, e0125625.
66.  Ostrowski, M.; Carmo, N.B.; Krumeich, S.; Fanget, I.; Raposo, G.; Savina, A.; Moita, C.F.; Schauer, K.; Hume, A.N.; Freitas, R.P.; *et al.* Rab27a and Rab27b control different steps of the exosome secretion pathway. *Nat. Cell Biol.* **2010**, *12*, 19–30. [PubMed]
67.  Ostenfeld, M.S.; Jeppesen, D.K.; Laurberg, J.R.; Boysen, A.T.; Bramsen, J.B.; Primdal-Bengtson, B.; Hendrix, A.; Lamy, P.; Dagnaes-Hansen, F.; Rasmussen, M.H.; *et al.* Cellular disposal of miR23b by RAB27-dependent exosome release is linked to acquisition of metastatic properties. *Cancer Res.* **2014**, *74*, 5758–5771. [PubMed]
68.  Wang, T.; Gilkes, D.M.; Takano, N.; Xiang, L.; Luo, W.; Bishop, C.J.; Chaturvedi, P.; Green, J.J.; Semenza, G.L. Hypoxia-inducible factors and RAB22A mediate formation of microvesicles that stimulate breast cancer invasion and metastasis. *Proc. Natl. Acad. Sci. USA* **2014**, *111*, E3234–E3242. [CrossRef] [PubMed]
69.  Marleau, A.M.; Chen, C.S.; Joyce, J.A.; Tullis, R.H. Exosome removal as a therapeutic adjuvant in cancer. *J. Transl. Med.* **2012**, *10*. [CrossRef]
70.  Ohno, S.; Takanashi, M.; Sudo, K.; Ueda, S.; Ishikawa, A.; Matsuyama, N.; Fujita, K.; Mizutani, T.; Ohgi, T.; Ochiya, T.; *et al.* Systemically Injected Exosomes Targeted to EGFR Deliver Antitumor MicroRNA to Breast Cancer Cells. *Mol. Ther.* **2013**, *21*, 185–191. [PubMed]
71.  Johnstone, R.M. Revisiting the road to the discovery of exosomes. *Blood Cells Mol. Dis.* **2005**, *34*, 214–219. [CrossRef]

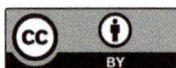

Journal of
*Clinical Medicine*

MDPI

*Review*

# MicroRNA Regulation of Human Breast Cancer Stem Cells

**Yohei Shimono [1,3,\*], Junko Mukohyama [1], Shun-ichi Nakamura [1,2] and Hironobu Minami [3]**

[1]  Division of Molecular and Cellular Biology, Kobe University Graduate School of Medicine, Kobe 650-0017, Japan; junkom@med.kobe-u.ac.jp (J.M.); snakamur@kobe-u.ac.jp (S.N.)
[2]  Division of Biochemistry, Kobe University Graduate School of Medicine, Kobe 650-0017, Japan
[3]  Division of Medical Oncology/Hematology, Kobe University Graduate School of Medicine, Kobe 650-0017, Japan; hminami@med.kobe-u.ac.jp
\*  Correspondence: yshimono@med.kobe-u.ac.jp; Tel.: +81-78-382-5820; Fax: +81-78-382-5821

Academic Editors: Takahiro Ochiya and Ryou-u Takahashi
Received: 22 October 2015; Accepted: 21 December 2015; Published: 25 December 2015

**Abstract:** MicroRNAs (miRNAs) are involved in virtually all biological processes, including stem cell maintenance, differentiation, and development. The dysregulation of miRNAs is associated with many human diseases including cancer. We have identified a set of miRNAs differentially expressed between human breast cancer stem cells (CSCs) and non-tumorigenic cancer cells. In addition, these miRNAs are similarly upregulated or downregulated in normal mammary stem/progenitor cells. In this review, we mainly describe the miRNAs that are dysregulated in human breast CSCs directly isolated from clinical specimens. The miRNAs and their clusters, such as the miR-200 clusters, miR-183 cluster, miR-221-222 cluster, let-7, miR-142 and miR-214, target the genes and pathways important for stem cell maintenance, such as the self-renewal gene BMI1, apoptosis, Wnt signaling, Notch signaling, and epithelial-to-mesenchymal transition. In addition, the current evidence shows that metastatic breast CSCs acquire a phenotype that is different from the CSCs in a primary site. Thus, clarifying the miRNA regulation of the metastatic breast CSCs will further advance our understanding of the roles of human breast CSCs in tumor progression.

**Keywords:** cancer stem cells; microRNA; Bmi1; Wnt signaling; epithelial-to-mesenchymal transition (EMT); metastasis

## 1. Breast Cancer Stem Cells

The heterogeneity of tumor cells and the presence of cancer cells with stem cell properties have long been appreciated. For example, the histological resemblance of the tissue of teratocarcinoma to that of the developing fetus was suggested by Virchow in the mid-1800s. The hypothesis that cancers arise from "embryonic rests", cells leftover from embryogenesis, was proposed in 1875 [1,2]. The genetic studies in leukemia patients demonstrated that a primitive leukemia cell can give rise to fully mature non-replicating progeny, showing that not all cancer cells have the ability to form tumors [3–5]. Existence of cancer stem cells (CSCs) was prospectively presented first in leukemia in 1997 [6]. However, evidence for the existence of CSCs in solid tumors has been more difficult to obtain because cells within solid tumors are less accessible, and functional assays suitable for detecting and quantifying normal stem cells from many organs have not been developed. The breast CSCs are the first CSCs prospectively identified from human solid tumors [7]. In 2003, the cells that can cause breast cancer in immunodeficient NOD/SCID mice through serial transplantations were identified. These cells are $CD44^+CD24^{-/low}$ cancer cells and they establish tumors in recipient animals when as few as one hundred cells are transplanted, whereas tens of thousands of cancer cells with a different marker set fail to form tumors. Then the CSCs are prospectively isolated in various cancers including glioblastoma, colon cancers, and prostate cancers [8].

The CSC hypothesis proposes that tumors are complex systems that recapitulate the complexity of organs or tissues during tumor initiation, maintenance and progression. The CSCs are proposed to have the ability to self-renew and generate differentiated progeny in the same way as normal stem cells in the tissue do. As the cells within a solid tumor are heterogeneous, the cells with CSC properties are still composed of heterogeneous cells. To date, many terms have been used instead of using CSCs, such as tumor-initiating cells and stem-like cells, because of the controversy on the CSC hypothesis or when analyzing the cells whose stem cell abilities are not fully confirmed.

The term CSCs led to some confusion. CSCs do not necessarily arise from normal stem cells by mutations of genes that make the stem cells cancerous [9]. CSCs capable of forming a tumor at one point in time might change during the progression of the disease [9,10]. Genetic and epigenetic factors, such as the acquisition of gene mutations and/or induction of epithelial-to-mesenchymal transition (EMT), affect the generation of CSCs during tumor progression. For example, during the progression to blast crisis in chronic myelogenous leukemia, additional events, including the activation of β-catenin, occur in the granulocyte–macrophage progenitor population, allowing the progenitor cells, not hematopoietic stem cells (HSCs), to become leukemic stem cells [11]. In contrast, in chronic lymphocytic leukemia, the HSCs are involved in leukemogenesis by acquiring the propensity to generate clonal B cells [12]. Thus, the CSCs within an individual tumor may constitute a moving target and the cells that drive growth at one point in time may not be identical to those during tumor progression.

Several experimental methods to characterize CSCs are proposed, including sphere culture, side-population, ALDH1 activity (ALDFLUOR), and limiting dilution assays. Among them, the limiting dilution xenotransplantation assay is considered to be a gold standard to characterize and identify CSCs within a tumor. Because the CSC populations identified by each method contain heterogeneous cancer cells with variable self-renewal and tumorigenic abilities, there will be a little overlap between the CSCs isolated by different purification methods [13]. In addition, it is reported that the gene expression profile changes when the cancer cells in the primary cancer specimens are cultured *in vitro* and/or passaged by xenotransplantation [14]. Breast cancer tissue contains heterogeneous cancer cell populations and clonal selection is observed during the passages by xenotransplantation [15]. Considering that the growth and maintenance of breast CSCs depend on their microenvironment, it is reasonable to speculate that the presence or absence of niche cells, their species differences, and difference of CSC culture methods affect properties and gene expression profiles of breast CSCs. In this review, we mainly focus on the miRNAs specifically expressed in the human breast CSCs directly isolated from the surgical specimens of human breast cancer patients. These miRNAs will help to delineate the molecular regulation of human breast CSCs in breast cancer patients.

## 2. Shared Properties between Breast CSCs and Normal Mammary Stem/Progenitor Cells

Human tissues maintain their architecture over time through a tightly regulated process of renovation. Under physiological conditions, this process is sustained by a minority of tissue stem cells. The mammary gland develops from a thickening in the ventral skin during embryogenesis that grows into a rudimentary ductal tree by birth [16–18]. Then, ductal morphogenesis of the mammary gland occurs largely in the early pubertal period. Pregnancy enhances elongation and side branching of ducts and induces alveologenesis with lactational differentiation. In the murine mammary tissue, *in vitro* and *in vivo* clonality and implantation studies showed that even a single cell within the mammary repopulating unit (MRU) population is able to regenerate whole epithelial tissues of the mammary gland, showing that MRU cells are responsible for the development and maintenance of mammary tissues [19,20].

The mammary epithelium is composed of the inner luminal cell and outer myoepithelium cell layers. The lineage tracing experiments in the mouse identified the luminal and myoepithelial stem/progenitor cells in each layer of the mammary epithelium [21,22]. Thus, it is possible that distinct stem/progenitor cells are responsible for the initial development, homeostasis, and remodeling of the mammary epithelium. In the human mammary epithelium, putative mammary epithelial progenitors have been identified using clonogenicity assays and transplantation assays [23].

Breast CSCs and normal mammary stem cells share a part of the genetic and epigenetic properties that are associated with the regulation of tissue stem cells. We identified that the profile of a set of the 37 miRNAs is shared between human breast CSCs and the stem/progenitor cells of human or murine normal mammary tissues [24]. The findings that transcriptional regulation by SLUG and SOX9 works in both human breast CSCs and normal mammary stem/progenitor cells further show the part of genetic programs shared between these cells [25].

Origin of breast CSCs will differ depending on the tumor subtypes [26]. Comprehensive gene expression profiling revealed the five major molecular subtypes of breast cancer: basal-like, luminal A, luminal B, HER2+/ER−, and normal breast-like. It is generally considered that the luminal compartment or its reprogrammed equivalent will provide breast CSCs. On the other hand, breast CSCs with the gene expression profile similar to basal stem cells exist across the different molecular subtypes of breast cancer [13], suggesting that human breast CSCs use the genetic program for the maintenance of basal stem cells irrespective of tumor subtypes. Understanding the similarity and difference of stem cell properties between human breast CSCs and normal mammary stem/progenitor cells will clarify the roles of CSCs in human breast cancer development and progression.

## 3. miRNAs Specific for Breast CSCs

miRNAs are non-coding RNAs with less than 25 nucleotides and base pairs to their target mRNAs to suppress their translation and/or accelerate degradation. Most miRNAs are evolutionarily conserved and have been implicated in a wide variety of cellular processes in both invertebrates and vertebrates [27]. miRNAs are located within intergenic regions, or introns of pre-mRNAs or non-coding RNAs [28,29]. Intergenic miRNAs are located in the regions that are distant from previously annotated genes and constitute an independent transcription unit with a promoter of their own. A minority of miRNAs are derived from the introns of pre-mRNAs or encoded within non-coding RNA genes, suggesting that these miRNAs are dependent on the promoter region of the associated gene and their RNA splicing mechanisms.

miRNAs typically function by base pairing with the 3′ untranslated regions (3′-UTRs) of their target mRNAs through the seed sequences of the miRNAs. The base pairing between a miRNA and its target mRNAs can result in translational inhibition, mRNA destabilization and/or degradation. In this way, miRNAs function as a switch and a fine-tuner of the gene regulatory network [30]. It is also shown that miRNAs can interact with other non-coding RNAs. Competing endogenous RNAs (ceRNAs) are the non-coding RNAs that have multiple binding sites for miRNAs. The interactions of miRNAs with ceRNAs play important roles in the regulation of gene expression, including oncogenes and tumor suppressor genes [31].

miRNAs are especially attractive candidates for regulating stem cell self-renewal and cell fate decisions, as their ability to simultaneously regulate many targets provides a means for coordinated control of concerned gene action [32]. The first two miRNAs to be identified, the *lin-4* and *let-7* in nematode *C. elegans*, control cell divisions in the hypodermal blast lineage and serve as a developmental switch during normal temporal regulation of post-embryonic developmental events [33–35]. *lin-4*, the first miRNA identified, mediates translational repression of its target mRNA lin-14, which facilitates the switching of lava of *C. elegans* from stage L1 to L2 and then to L3 [34]. In the absence of either gene, this stem cell lineage fails to differentiate and continues its proliferative cycle. *let-7* is involved in the regulation of the timing of the developmental switch from larval to adult cell fates during *C. elegans* development [35]. Embryonic stem (ES) cell-specific miRNAs, such as miR-302 family, miR-371 cluster, and miR-290 cluster miRNAs, regulate the maintenance and differentiation of ES cells [36–39].

Cancer cells within a tumor are heterogeneous and miRNAs are differentially expressed between CSCs and other non-tumorigenic cancer cells. Because CSCs are in the minority of cell population in human breast cancers (usually less than 10%), analyses of bulk tumor are unable to identify the miRNAs involved in the regulation of breast CSCs. We isolated breast CSCs directly from the surgically resected specimens of human breast cancer patients and identified a set of miRNAs that are differentially expressed between CSCs and the remaining non-tumorigenic cancer cells [24]. Among them, eight miRNAs are selectively downregulated in the human breast CSC population of 11 human breast cancers. These eight miRNAs are located on the three miRNA clusters and two of the three clusters are the miR-200 clusters, suggesting that the suppression of miR-200 family miRNAs is critically important in the maintenance of stem cell functions.

In addition, other miRNAs, including let-7, miR-1 and miR-27, are among the miRNAs that are differentially expressed between breast CSCs and non-tumorigenic cancer cells ([24,40–43], for review [8,44,45]). Let-7 family miRNAs are undetectable in ES cells and upregulated upon differentiation [46]. Microprocessor-mediated cleavage and maturation of pri-let-7 miRNAs are blocked by lin-28, a conserved RNA-binding protein and an oncogene [47]. In human breast CSCs, let-7 targets H-RAS and HMGA2 and suppresses self-renewal and differentiation [40]. miR-1 targets the Wnt signaling and suppresses proliferation and migration of breast CSCs [41]. The expression of miR-27 is upregulated by VEGF in breast CSCs and promotes angiogenesis and metastasis [43]. Furthermore, miR-27 targets ectonucleotide pyrophosphatase/phosphodiesterase family member 1 (ENPP1) and regulates the tumorigenicity and drug resistance of breast cancer cells [42]. Downregulation of miR-200 family miRNAs and let-7 family miRNAs is observed in the CSCs of other cancers, such as colon cancer and Wilms tumor, and is associated with cancer progression [48,49]. These evidences suggest that breast CSC-specific miRNAs play important roles in the regulation of self-renewal ability, tumorigenicity, and metastasis.

### 3.1. miR-200 Clusters

Some miRNA genes are clustered in the genome and transcribed as a multi-cistronic primary transcript [50]. Usually, there are between two to three miRNA genes in a cluster. However, larger clusters are also identified, such as the human miR-17-92 and miR-106a-363 clusters, and both of them are composed of six members, which are also conserved in other mammals. It is predicted that a total of 15%–35% of known and predicted miRNA genes in nine selected species constitute clusters under the inter-miRNA distances ranging from 1 kb to 50 kb [51]. miRNAs within a cluster are often, but not always, paralogous with high sequence homology, indicating that they may be the result of genomic duplications.

The polycistronic miR-17-92 cluster is the first microRNA cluster shown to play a role in tumorigenesis [52]. It has two other paralogs in the human genome, the miR-106b-25 cluster and the miR-106a-363 cluster. miR-17-92 and miR-106b-25 are expressed abundantly in a wide spectrum of tissues, but miR-106a-363 is expressed at lower levels. The bicistronic miR-143-145 cluster functions as a tumor suppressor and regulates vascular smooth-muscle cells and mesenchymal cells in the intestine [53,54].

The miR-200 cluster is an extensively studied tumor-suppressive miRNA cluster in the genome (Figure 1). The miR-200 family miRNAs have been highly conserved in deuterostome from Echinodermata and Chordata to all Vertebrata classes, including fish, amphibians, reptiles, birds and mammals [55]. The miR-200 family in mammals is composed of five miRNAs: miR-200a, miR-200b, miR-200c, miR-141, and miR-429. Among them, miR-200a, miR-200b and miR-429 are found in all deuterostomes including Echinodermata, Chordata and Vertebrata, but miR-200c and miR-141 are only detected in cephalochordates, teleosts and mammals or in tunicates, teleosts and mammals, respectively. Invertebrate species such as the fruit fly *D. melanogaster* possess only one orthologue of this family, miR-8 [55,56].

The mammalian miR-200 family clusters are expressed as two separate polycistronic pri-miRNA transcripts: miR-200b-200a-429 and miR-200c-141 clusters (Figure 1). The tricistronic miR-200b-200a-429 cluster is located on mouse chromosome 4 and human chromosome 1p36, whose length of transcript is 6464 bp [57]. The bicistronic miR-200c-141 cluster is located on mouse chromosome 6 and human chromosome 12p13, whose length of transcript is 1211 bp [57]. The miR-200 family members can also be divided into two subgroups based upon their seed sequences that differ by only 1 nt between the subgroups: miR-200b, -200c, and -429 (AA<u>U</u>ACUG) and miR-200a and -141 (AA<u>C</u>ACUG). Furthermore, miR-200 family members belonging to either seed sequence subgroup do not show a clear phylogenetic relationship, suggesting that the 1 nt difference between the two subgroups arose independently in different lineages [56].

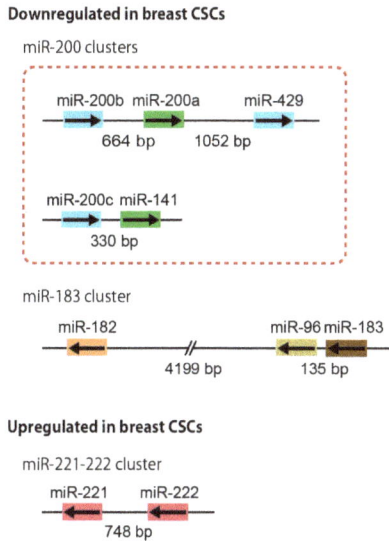

**Figure 1.** A schematic representation of the miRNA clusters dysregulated in human breast CSCs. The miRNAs sharing the same seed sequence (nucleotides from two to seven) are marked by the same color. The mammalian miR-200 clusters are expressed as two separate polycistronic pri-miRNA transcripts. The miRNAs coded in the miR-200b-200a-429, miR-200c-141 and miR-183-96-182 clusters are downregulated, and those in the miR-221-222 cluster are upregulated in the human breast CSCs. The arrows indicate the direction of the pri-miRNA transcription.

The expression of the miR-200 family members can be regulated through interactions with transcriptional factors, modifications of their promoter regions, and Polycomb-group-gene-mediated repression. The promoter regions of the miR-200 family are bound by multiple transcription factors, including zinc finger E-box binding homeobox 1 (ZEB1) and 2 (ZEB2, also known as SIP1), specificity protein 1 (Sp1), Smad3, Wnt inhibitory factor 1 (WIF1) and p53. ZEB1 and ZEB2 can inhibit the transcription of the entire miR-200 family [58]. Sp1 activates the transcription of the miR-200b-200a-429 [59]. p53, Smad3, and WIF1 activate the transcription of miR-200c-141 [60–63]. The modifications to the promoter regions of each of the miR-200 clusters cause the loss of the expression of the miR-200 family miRNAs in cancer. The miR-200c-141 cluster is silenced by promoter hypermethylation, whereas the miR-200b-200a-429 cluster is silenced primarily through Polycomb-group–mediated histone modifications [64]. miR-22 targets the methylcytosine dioxygenase TET (ten-eleven translocation) family members, inhibits the demethylation of the miR-200 promoter, and suppresses the expression of miR-200 [65].

The mammalian miR-200 family gained particular prominence because it is involved in the regulation of EMT, EGF signaling, regulation of stem cell characters, and somatic cell reprogramming into induced pluripotent stem cells [24,56,66–72]. EGF signaling induces EMT, and EGF is also targeted by miR-96 which is downregulated in breast CSCs [73]. A large number of studies demonstrate the strong suppressive effects of miR-200 on cell transformation, cancer cell proliferation, migration, invasion, tumor growth and metastasis [61]. The roles of miR-200 family miRNAs in breast CSCs are described in more detail later in Section 4.

*3.2. miR-183 Cluster*

The miR-183 cluster, which is comprised of miRNA-183, -96 and -182, is a miRNA family with sequence homology (Figure 1). The tricistronic miR-183 cluster is located on mouse chromosome 6 and human chromosome 7, whose length of transcript is 19121 bp [57]. Despite the strong similarity in the sequences of these miRNAs, minute differences in their seed sequences result in both overlapping and distinct targets, which are often within the same pathway. These miRNAs have tightly synchronized expression during development and are required for maturation of sensory organs [74]. The miR-183 cluster is highly and widely conserved in protostomes and deuterostomes [74,75]. Although the chromosomal order of miR-183, -96, -182 is conserved in deuterostomes, their location and the intergenic spacing between the miRNA genes vary between species.

The miR-183 cluster miRNAs are frequently upregulated in a variety of non-sensory diseases, including cancer. However, the miR-183 cluster miRNAs are downregulated in the human breast CSCs, suggesting that suppression of the miR-183 cluster is required for the maintenance of CSC properties. The fact that common targets of miR-183 cluster miRNAs include SNAI2, SMAD4, β-catenin and Bmi1 suggests that the downregulation of miR-183 cluster in breast CSCs is associated with activation of EMT, self-renewal and Wnt signaling [67,74,76]. The transcription of the miR-183 cluster is upregulated by transcription factors, such as β-catenin/TCF/LEF and TGF-β, and is downregulated by GATA-3, ZEB1 and DNA methylation [76–79]. There are several CpG islands before the miR-183 transcription start site (3.5, 8 and 10 kb) that are epigenetically regulated by DNA methylation. In addition, secondary transcription start sites are identified, suggesting that the independent regulation for each miRNA exists in the miR-183 cluster.

*3.3. miR-221-222 Cluster*

The miR-222-221 cluster, which is composed of miR-221 and miR-222, is located in tandem on human chromosome Xp11 and is transcribed as a single RNA precursor with RNA polymerase II [80]. The expression of the miR-221-222 cluster is upregulated by angiotensin II, HMGB1, NF-kB, HOXB7/pBX2, and microphthalmia-associated transcription factor (MITF), and is downregulated by promyelocytic leukemia zinc finger (PLZF) and a repressive complex formed by estrogen receptor α (ERα) and two nuclear receptor corepressors, NCOR1 and NCOR2 [80–83]. The miR-222-221 cluster is highly conserved in Vertebrata classes, including mouse, rat and human [84].

miR-221 and miR-222 have the same seed sequence, and they mostly function as oncogenes in human epithelial tumors [84,85]. They also function as tumor suppressors in some tumors, such as erythroleukemia [86]. miR-221 and miR-222 regulate cell cycle progression, apoptosis, cell migration and stemness by targeting cell cycle inhibitors CDKN1B (p27$^{Kip1}$) and CDKN1C(p57$^{Kip2}$), PUMA, FOXO3, PTEN, Bim, c-Kit, TIMP3, ER-α and DNA methyltransferase DNMT3b [82,84,87].

The miR-222-221 cluster miRNAs are upregulated in the human breast CSCs and normal mammary stem/progenitor cells (Figure 1) [24]. Upregulation of miR-221 and/or miR-222 is observed in CSCs isolated from pancreas and glioblastoma cancer cells [88,89]. miR-221 is involved in the promotion of an aggressive basal-like phenotype in breast cancer, functions downstream of the RAS pathway and triggers EMT [90,91].

*3.4. miR-142*

miR-142 is broadly expressed in various hematopoietic lineages, and plays important functions in hematopoiesis, immune responses, and T cell differentiation [92–95]. miR-142 is located at a genomic locus associated with t(8;17) translocation in B-cell leukemia and is mutated in diffuse large B-cell lymphoma [96]. In contrast, miR-142 is expressed at low levels in many other cell types. Consistent with these findings, miR-142-null mice and miR-142 gene trap mice show the impairment of hematopoietic lineage formation [97,98]. The transcription start site of miR-142 is located 1205 base pairs upstream of the precursor sequence within a highly conserved CpG island and the transcription of the pri-miR-142 is epigenetically repressed by DNA methylation [99]. In addition, a second CpG island overlapped with the precursor.

miR-142 is very highly expressed in a human breast CSC population, but is undetectable in a normal mammary stem cell population [24,100]. We and others show that miR-142 targets APC and activates the canonical Wnt signaling pathway and further activates the transcription of miR-150 which is also upregulated in human breast CSCs. The regulation of the Wnt signaling pathway by miR-142 and other miRNAs is described in more detail later in Section 4.3.

### 3.5. miR-214

miR-214, together with miR-199a-2, is located inside the sequence of the long non-coding Dynamin 3 opposite strand (Dnm3os) transcript on mouse and human chromosome 1. miR-214 is upregulated or downregulated in human tumors [101]. miR-214 is one of the miRNAs highly upregulated in human breast CSCs. And the miR-214 locus is frequently amplified in breast cancers [102]. miR-214 is upregulated in luminal A, normal-like and triple-negative subtypes, but it is not upregulated in other subtypes [101,103,104]. Ubiquitous miR-214-specific knockout mice are viable and fertile, but following ischemia-reperfusion injury, show impaired cardiac function and progression to heart failure [105]. In contrast, mice lacking Dnm3os, which encodes miR-214 and miR-199a-2, display severe skeletal defects and die within the first month of birth [106]. Further studies are required to clarify the roles of miR-214, miR-199a-2, and long non-coding Dnm3os in development.

miR-214 regulates cell differentiation, stemness, apoptosis, and invasion by targeting Ezh2, p53, transcription factor TFAP2, PTEN, BIM, and β-catenin [107–110]. In ovarian cancer, miR-214 increases CSCs by upregulating the Nanog expression [107]. miR-214 induces cell survival by targeting PTEN and BIM [108]. miR-214 induces cell invasion by targeting p53 [109]. In contrast, miR-214 suppresses stem-like traits in human hepatocellular carcinoma cells by directly targeting Ezh2 and β-catenin [110], suggesting that the roles of miR-214 will be different depending on the tumor types. Thus, miR-214 seems to have important roles in the regulation of proliferation, differentiation, stemness, apoptosis, invasion and metastasis [101].

## 4. Signaling Pathways and Genes Targeted by miRNAs Specific to the Breast CSCs

Multiple miRNAs and miRNA clusters specifically dysregulated in human breast CSCs coordinately target the signaling pathways and genes that have important roles in the maintenance and regulation of breast CSCs and normal mammary stem/progenitor cells. These signaling pathways and genes include a self-renewal factor Bmi-1, the apoptosis signaling pathway, the canonical Wnt signaling pathway, the Notch signaling pathway, and EMT.

### 4.1. Self-Renewal Factor Bmi1

Many tissues are maintained throughout the lifespan of an organism by a small number of adult stem cells. These cells are unique in that they have both the ability to give rise to new stem cells via self-renewal and the ability to differentiate into the mature cells of a tissue. To maintain tissue homeostasis, stem cells have developed strict regulatory mechanisms to self-renew, differentiate, and prevent premature senescence and apoptosis.

Bmi1 is a component of Polycomb repressive complex 1 (PRC1). Analyses of Bmi1 knockout mice showed that Bmi1 is involved in the stem cell maintenance in multiple tissues and organs, including hematopoiesis, skeletal patterning, neurological functions, and development of the cerebellum [111]. Bmi1 is also essential for the self-renewal of multiple tissues and organs including mammary tissues [112]. To support self-renewal of somatic stem cells, PRC1 suppresses the expression of the Ink4a locus that encodes the $p16^{Ink4a}$ and the $p19^{Arf}$ genes and other genomic loci through specific biochemical histone modifications, the addition of trimethyl groups to the H3-K27 amino acid residue and of ubiquitin protein to H2A-K119 (Figure 2). The deubiquitinating enzyme USP16 removes the ubiquitin protein from H2A-K119, and upregulates the transcription of the Ink4a locus [113]. In this way, USP16 antagonizes the self-renewal and senescence pathways in multiple tissues.

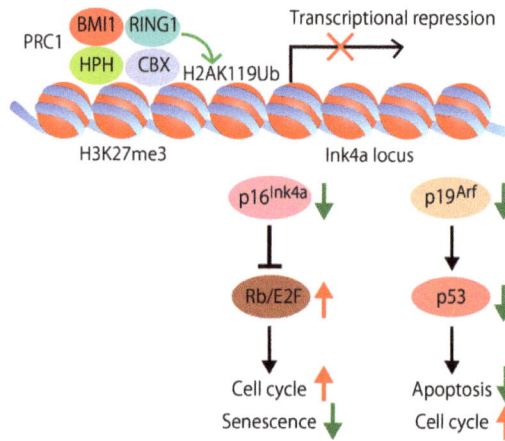

**Figure 2.** Regulation of cell cycle, apoptosis, and senescence by self-renewal factor Bmi1. Bmi1, a component of PRC1, is involved in the stem cell maintenance in multiple tissues and organs. PRC1 suppresses the Ink4a locus that encodes the *p16^Ink4a* and the *p19^Arf* genes through the specific biochemical histone modifications, such as the trimethylation of the H3-K27 (H3K27me3) and the ubiquitination of H2A-K119 (H2AK119Ub). The chromodomain of CBX binds to H3K27me3 and RING1 deposits monoubiquitin on H2AK119. In the absence of p16^Ink4a, the cyclin D/Cdk4/6 complex can phosphorylate RB, allowing the E2F-dependent transcription which leads to cell cycle progression. In the absence of p19^Arf, MDM2-mediated p53 degradation causes low p53 levels, thus preventing cell cycle arrest and apoptosis. In addition, the gradual accumulation of p16^Ink4a expression during physiological aging implicates that p16^Ink4a is involved in the regulation of senescence.

Bmi1 was initially identified as an oncogene cooperating with c-myc in a murine model of lymphoma ([114,115], for review [116]). Bmi1 suppresses the *p16^Ink4a* and the *p19^Arf* genes coded in the Ink4a locus and regulates senescence, cell cycle, and apoptosis (Figure 2) [116,117]. In the absence of Bmi1, p16^Ink4a is upregulated and prevents binding of Cdk4/6 to cyclin D. The inhibition of the kinase activity of Cdk4/6 results in hypophosphorylation of pRB, leading to cell cycle arrest and senescence [117]. The gradual accumulation of p16^Ink4a expression during physiological aging and several aging-associated diseases directly implicates that p16^Ink4a is involved in the aging process [118]. p19^Arf is another target suppressed by Bmi1 (Figure 2). p19^Arf sequesters mouse double minute 2 (MDM2) and inhibits p53 degradation. In the absence of Bmi1, p19^Arf and p53 are upregulated, resulting in p53-mediated cell cycle arrest and apoptosis [119,120]. Point mutations and deletion of *p16^Ink4a* and *p19^Arf* are frequently found in many types of human cancers, which implicate them as key regulators of immortalization and/or senescence checkpoints. The observation that Bmi1 is essential for the self-renewal of multiple adult tissues and organs in part via repression of the genes involved in senescence, apoptosis, and cell cycle progression suggests that stem cells have evolved specific mechanisms to repress senescence and to prolong their capacity to proliferate [116].

The expression of Bmi1 is regulated by miRNAs, such as miR-128, miR-200b/c, miR-141, miR-15, miR-16, miR-203, miR-183, miR-194, and miR-218 [24,67,121–125]. Among them, miR-200b, miR-200c, miR-141, and miR-183 are specifically downregulated in the human breast CSCs and normal mammary stem/progenitor cells [24], suggesting that miRNAs are important regulators of self-renewal abilities in breast CSCs and normal mammary stem/progenitor cells (Figure 3). miR-200c strongly suppresses the ability of human breast CSCs to form tumor when engrafted into the mammary fat pad region of immunodeficient mice [24]. miR-200c also suppresses the ability of normal mammary stem cells to form mammary ducts when engrafted into the mammary fat pad of the syngeneic mice. These findings suggest that the three miRNA clusters, namely two miR-200 clusters and one miR-183 cluster, coordinately upregulate the expression of Bmi1 to enhance the stem cell self-renewal abilities in both breast CSCs and normal mammary stem/progenitor cells.

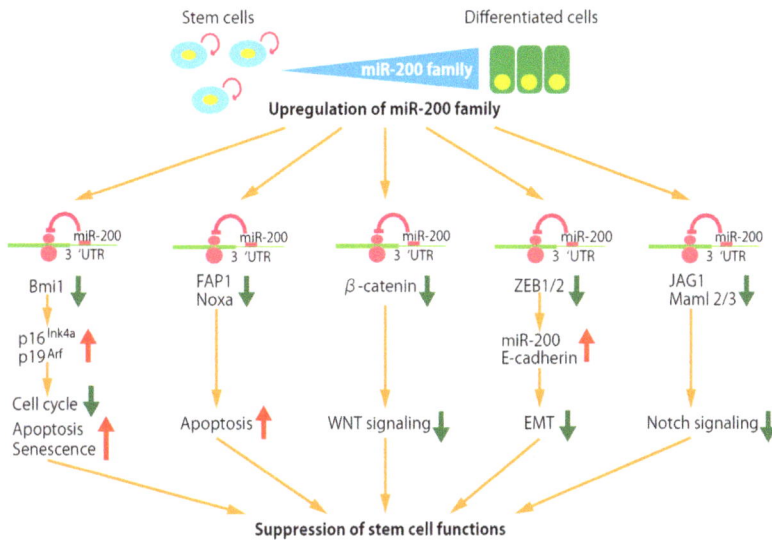

**Figure 3.** Targeting of the genes and pathways for stem cell maintenance by miR-200 family miRNAs. Expression of the miR-200 family miRNAs is downregulated in the breast CSCs and normal mammary stem/progenitor cells, and is upregulated in the more differentiated counterparts. The miR-200 family miRNAs are involved in the regulation stem cell functions by targeting the genes and pathways important for stem cell maintenance, such as self-renewal factor Bmi-1, the apoptosis signaling pathway, the canonical Wnt signaling pathway, EMT and the Notch signaling pathway.

### 4.2. Apoptosis Signaling Pathway

miR-200b, miR-200c and miR-141 target Bmi1 which suppresses p53-mediated cell cycle arrest and apoptosis by repressing p19$^{\mathrm{Arf}}$(Figures 2 and 3). In addition, miR-200c functions as an enhancer of apoptosis by targeting molecules such as FAP-1, a known inhibitor of CD95-mediated apoptosis, and Noxa, a member of the Bcl-2 family (Figure 3) [126,127]. The miR-200b, -200c and -429 subgroup miRNAs, but not the miR-200a and -141 subgroup miRNAs, target PLCγ1, reduce cell viability and induce apoptosis [71].

The miR-221-222 miRNA cluster is upregulated in the human breast CSCs and normal mammary stem/progenitor cells. miR-221 and miR-222 induce cell cycle progression and suppression of apoptosis by targeting cell cycle inhibitors p27 and p57, and Bcl-2 homology 3 (BH3)-only Bcl-2 family member PUMA [128–130]. These findings suggest that dysregulation of the three miRNA clusters, namely the downregulation of the miR-200 clusters and the upregulation of the miR-221-222 cluster, is involved in the suppression of apoptosis in both breast CSCs and normal mammary stem/progenitor cells.

### 4.3. Wnt Signaling

The fact that some cancer cells share the extended self-renewal ability with normal stem cells and that the canonical Wnt signaling pathway is implicated in both stem cell self-renewal and cancer suggest that the normal physiological regulator of stem cell functions might be "hijacked" in cancer [131]. In 1982, Nusse and Varmus identified the mouse proto-oncogene Wnt1 (Int1) in Wnt signaling [132]. Wnt regulates cell proliferation, differentiation, adhesion, migration and stem cell self-renewal through β-catenin-dependent (canonical) and β-catenin-independent (non-canonical) Wnt signaling pathways [133]. In human colon cancers, mutations in the *Adenomatous polyposis coli* (*APC*) gene are the most common known acquired genetic change for the aberrant activation of the canonical Wnt signaling pathway during tumor development and progression [134–136]. APC is a component of the destruction complex that destabilizes β-catenin and suppresses the activity of the canonical Wnt signaling pathway. In a model for the stepwise progression of colon tumorigenesis, *APC* gene mutations play an important role in the initiation step, followed by successive mutations in other genes, including *K-Ras* and *p53* [137].

The expression of APC is not limited to the intestine, but is widely observed in many other tissues, including lung, liver, kidney, and mammary tissue. However, the role of the suppression of APC and the activation of the canonical Wnt signaling in the tumor initiation process of the tissues other than the colon largely remain unknown, because *APC* mutations are less frequent in tumors originating from these tissues. For example, recent data from The Cancer Genome Atlas (TCGA) reveals a ~2% incidence of *APC* mutations in human breast cancer (the TCGA Research Network: http://cancergenome.nih.gov/).

miRNAs target Wnt signaling components and dysregulate the activity of the canonical Wnt signaling. For example, miRNAs, such as miR-135, miR-27, mir-155, miR-129, miR-106b, let-7, miR-125, miR-663, and miR-142, target APC and activate canonical Wnt signaling [100,138–146]. miR-29 targets the negative regulators of Wnt signaling, such as Dikkopf-1 (Dkk1), Kremen2, and secreted frizzled related protein 2 (sFRP2) and activates the Wnt signaling pathway [147]. Furthermore, the Wnt signaling pathway is activated by the miRNAs that target other inhibitors of the Wnt signaling pathway [148].

The profile of a set of the 37 miRNAs is mostly shared between human breast CSCs and the stem/progenitor cells of human or murine normal mammary tissues, but miR-142 is exceptional; miR-142 is very highly expressed in the human breast CSC population, but is undetectable in a normal mammary stem cell population [24,100]. We and others show that miR-142 targets APC and activates the canonical Wnt signaling pathway (Figure 4) [97,100,141,146,148]. Knockdown of miR-142 upregulates the APC expression, reduces the clonogenicity of human breast CSCs *in vitro*, and suppresses the tumor growth initiated by the human breast CSCs *in vivo* [100]. Furthermore, aberrantly proliferating dysplastic mammary tissues are formed when the mammary stem cells overexpressing miR-142 are transplanted into the mammary fat pad of the syngeneic mouse.

These findings propose a novel mechanism for the activation of the Wnt signaling in breast cancers in which the gene mutations involved in the activation of the Wnt signaling pathway are less frequent; the Wnt signaling pathway is epigenetically transactivated by miR-142 in human breast CSCs. Analyses of bulk tumor will be unable to identify the important roles of miR-142 in breast cancer because CSCs are a minority population in human breast cancers (usually less than 10%). Thus, focusing on the CSCs that are a minority population in breast cancer tissue will have a potential to uncover molecular mechanisms that are important for cancer development and progression.

miR-150 is a miRNA specifically expressed in mature lymphocytes and its premature expression blocks B-cell development [149]. We identified that miR-150 is expressed in the mammary epithelium and its expression is higher in breast CSCs and normal mammary stem/progenitor cells [24,100]. The promoter region of miR-150 precursor is targeted by T-cell factor (TCF)/β-catenin and the transcription of miR-150 is activated by miR-142 which activates the canonical Wnt signaling pathway (Figure 4) [100]. Mammary cells overexpressing miR-150 form a hyperplastic mammary tree with extremely increased branching and thick mammary ducts. However, unlike miR-142, miR150 does not induce the dysplastic change of the mammary tissue. A simple model to explain the upregulation of miR-142 and miR-150 in human breast CSCs is that suppression of the APC protein expression by miR-142 increases the activity of the canonical Wnt signaling pathway and thereby enhances miR-150 expression.

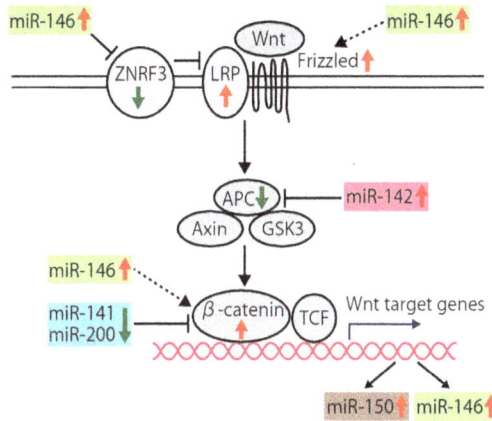

**Figure 4.** Activation of the canonical Wnt signaling pathway by the breast CSC-specific miRNAs. The canonical Wnt signaling pathway is implicated in both stem cell self-renewal and cancer. The multiple miRNAs dysregulated in the breast CSCs, such as miR-142, miR-146, miR-200, and miR-141, cooperatively activate the Wnt signaling pathway by targeting or upregulating the expression of its components. The activation of the Wnt signaling pathway induces the transcription of the Wnt target genes, including miR-146 and miR-150. miR-150 enhances the proliferation of mammary epithelial cells. Upregulation of miR-146 further enhances the activity of the Wnt signaling pathway in a positive feedback manner.

miR-200 family miRNAs that are downregulated in human breast CSCs and normal mammary stem/progenitor cells function as the suppressors of the Wnt signaling pathways (Figures 3 and 4). miR-200a and miR-141 suppress the Wnt signaling pathway by targeting β-catenin [150,151]. miR-8, a *Drosophila* homologue of miR-200, targets TCF transcription factor and suppresses the Wnt signaling activities [152].

miR-146 is a miRNA upregulated in human breast CSCs and functions as the enhancer of the Wnt signaling pathways (Figure 4) [24]. miR-146 targets Zinc RING finger 3 (ZNRF3), an E3 ubiquitin ligase and an antagonist of Wnt signaling in papillary thyroid carcinoma cells (Figure 4) [153]. ZNRF3 removes Wnt receptors from the stem cell surface [154]. In addition, cell membrane levels of FZD6 and LRP6 are increased by miR-146, which further activate the Wnt/β-catenin signaling [153]. Furthermore, miR-146a maintains the Wnt signaling activity by stabilizing β-catenin and induces symmetrical cell division of CSCs (Figure 4) [155]. Because the expression of miR-146a is induced by Snail and β-catenin, the Snail-miR-146a-β-catenin loop plays an important role in the maintenance of the activity of the Wnt signaling pathway. These findings suggest that the multiple miRNAs specific to the breast CSCs coordinately upregulate the Wnt signaling pathway in both breast CSCs and normal mammary stem/progenitor cells.

*4.4. EMT*

EMT is a process by which a normally polar, epithelial cell undergoes a change to a mesenchymal-like cell. By undergoing EMT, a cell is able to take on the characteristics of a mesenchymal cell and becomes more motile and invasive. In human breast cancer cells, the canonical Wnt signaling induces the expression of intracellular protein Axin2 to stabilize EMT-transcription factor Snail and induces EMT [156]. EMT is linked to the progression of cancer and increases stemness of breast CSCs and mammary stem/progenitor cells [157].

The miR-200 family is highly expressed within epithelial cells and miR-200c and miR-141 have both been strongly linked to epithelial integrity [158,159]. The miR-200 family miRNAs downregulate ZEB1 and ZEB2 expression, and effectively upregulate the cellular E-cadherin level to maintain a cell in a more epithelial-like state (Figure 3). ZEB1 suppresses the expression of all miR-200 family members (miR-141, miR-200a,b,c and miR-429), which in turn inhibits the translation of ZEB1 mRNA, resulting in the double-negative ZEB/miR-200 feedback loop [160]. Thus, ZEB1 and ZEB2 keep a cell in a mesenchymal phenotype by repressing the transcription of both E-cadherin and the miR-200 family miRNAs.

miR-22 targets the ten-eleven-translocation (TET) family of methylcytosine dioxygenases and demethylates the promoter region of the miR-200 precursor [161]. Interestingly, the cooperation between miR-22 and the miR-200 family results in EMT, an elevated pool of stem cells and increased tumorigenesis. Therefore, the interplay between the miR-200 family, miR-22, and ZEB1/ZEB2 plays an important role in the stemness regulation and EMT.

Slug, Snail, and Twist are the transcriptional factors that trigger EMT which is connected to the stem cell phenotype. Although these transcription factors induce EMT, they have distinct roles, especially during development. For example, Slug directly transactivates ZEB1, but Snail works indirectly in this transactivation [162]. Among these transcription factors, Slug cooperates the transcription factor Sox9 in breast cancer cells and normal mammary stem/progenitor cells [25]. Inhibition of either Slug or Sox9 blocks the activities of normal mammary stem/progenitor cells and that of breast cancer cells, suggesting that breast cancer cells and normal stem/progenitor cells are controlled by similar key regulators. Analyses of the genetically engineered knock-in reporter mouse lines confirmed that Slug regulates mammary stem cells [163]. In contrast, Snail serves as the regulator of CSCs of MMTV-PyMT mouse mammary tumor, whose formation appears to be driven primarily from luminal mammary epithelial cells. As discussed in Section 2, breast CSCs with a gene expression profile similar to basal stem cells exist across the different molecular subtypes of breast cancer [13], suggesting that human breast CSCs use the genetic program for the maintenance of basal stem cells irrespective of tumor subtypes. Therefore, understanding the roles of Snail and Slug in mammary basal stem cell-derived tumors is required to further clarify the roles of Snail and Slug in human breast CSCs.

We found that miR-199a, a miRNA upregulated in human breast CSCs, targets Snail and suppresses its expression [164]. And miR-182 targets Slug and induces mesenchymal-to-epithelial transition (MET) features in prostate cells [165]. Because miR-199a is highly upregulated and miR-182 is downregulated in human breast CSCs and mammary stem/progenitor cells, it is possible that miRNAs function as epigenetic regulators of the EMT transcription factors Snail and Slug to regulate the stem cell abilities of breast CSCs and normal mammary stem/progenitor cells.

### 4.5. Notch Signaling Pathway

The Notch signaling pathway is associated with the regulation of cell fate at several distinct developmental stages of the mammary gland and has been implicated in cancer initiation and progression [166–168]. In addition to its central role in development, the Notch signaling pathway is deregulated in a number of cancers. Nevertheless, mutations in Notch pathway components are rare in solid tumors.

The activation of the Notch signaling pathway occurs when Notch receptors bind to one of the membrane-bound Notch ligands, such as Jagged1 (JAG1), Jagged2 (JAG2), Delta-like 1 (DLL1), Delta-like 3 (DLL3), and Delta-like 4 (DLL4). Ligand binding causes a conformational change in the Notch receptor and leads to a sequence of proteolytic cleavage events in the receptor. A $\gamma$-secretase releases the intracellular domain of Notch (NICD), allowing it to translocate to the nucleus to activate the expression of target genes, including the Hairy/enhancer of split (Hes) family genes, the cell cycle regulator p21 and cyclin D1 [169].

miR-200 family miRNAs suppress the Notch signaling by targeting Notch pathway components, such as JAG1 and the mastermind-like Notch coactivators, Maml2 and Maml3 (Figure 3) [170]. miR-146a, a miRNA upregulated in human breast CSCs, also activates the Notch signaling pathway by targeting Numb, a suppressor of the Notch signaling pathway [171,172]. These findings suggest that the downregulation of miR-200 members and upregulation of miR-146 are involved in the activation of the Notch signaling pathway in the breast CSCs and normal mammary stem/progenitor cells.

## 5. Metastatic CSC Specific miRNAs

Systemic dissemination and metastasis are responsible for most cancer-related deaths. The breast cancer metastases appear years or even decades after the surgical removal of the primary tumor [173]. Current evidence shows that metastases are initiated by metastasis-initiating cells with stem cell abilities. The CSC marker CD44$^+$ breast cancer cells in the lung metastases are highly enriched for tumor-initiating abilities [174]. Similarly, CD133$^+$/CXCR4$^+$ cells, a subfraction of the putative pancreatic CSCs present at the invasive front of cell line-induced pancreatic tumors, are enriched for metastatic capabilities [175]. Along the same lines, CD26, in combination with the CSC marker CD133, has been proposed as a marker for the colorectal metastatic CSC population in primary tumor xenografts [176]. Furthermore, the early stage metastatic cells in the human breast cancer patient-derived xenograft (PDX) mice are characterized by the expression of the stem cell genes, together with EMT, prosurvival and dormant associated genes [177].

The breast tumor growth and metastasis are analyzed in the PDX models of human breast cancer. These tumor grafts illustrate the diversity of human breast cancer and maintain essential features of the original tumors, including metastasis to specific sites. Tumor engraftment into mice is a prognostic indicator of disease outcome for women with newly diagnosed breast cancer [178]. The tumor cells in the lung metastases of the PDX models exhibit the epithelial and differentiated statuses that are different from the cells in the primary site [179]. We found that metastatic cancer cells in the lung of the PDX mice are in the dormant state which is characterized by the reduced expression of cell surface CXCR4 expression [180,181]. Spontaneous metastases observed in these breast cancer PDX models potentially recapitulate the process of metastasis of cancer cells in human breast cancer patients.

Several miRNAs that are associated with metastatic CSCs are identified. miR-33b inhibits the stemness, migration and invasion of metastatic breast cancer cells is by targeting HMGA2, SALL4 and Twist1 [182]. miR-199a suppresses the expression of FOXP2 and promotes breast cancer CSC propagation, tumor initiation, and metastasis [183]. miR-20a downregulates MICA and MICB, two ligands for the stimulatory NK cell receptor NKG2D, in breast CSCs and enhances the metastatic abilities by promoting the resistance of breast CSC to NK cell cytotoxicity [184]. miR-7 inhibits the metastasis of breast CSCs by targeting SETDB1 and reducing the expression of c-myc, twist, and mir-9, the downstream target genes of the STAT3 pathway [185]. It is also shown that lncRNA linc-ROR enhanced breast cancer cell migration, invasion and stem cell properties [186]. linc-ROR is associated with miRNA ribonucleoprotein complexes (miRNPs) and functions as a ceRNA to mi-205, thereby preventing the degradation of mir-205 target genes, including EMT inducer ZEB2.

miRNAs are selectively incorporated in exosomes, membrane vesicles of an average 30–100 nm diameter. Exosomes are formed within the multivesicular bodies (MVBs), also known as late endosomes, and are released upon the fusion of MVBs with the plasma membrane [187]. The mechanism of exosome-mediated cell-to-cell communication is important in the regulation of cell growth and dissemination of cancer cells, since cancer cells constitutively secrete exosomes and can target both locally adjacent cells and cells located at distant organs [188]. For example, miR-181c in exosomes targets PDPK1 which regulates actin-dynamics by regulating the phosphorylation of cofilin, and promotes the destruction of the blood-brain barrier through the abnormal localization of actin [189]. Furthermore, the metastatic mouse mammary tumor 4T1 cells, but not the poorly metastatic mammary tumor 4TO7 cells, can secrete miR-200 family miRNAs into exosomes [190]. The poorly metastatic 4TO7 cells can take up miR-200 from the exosomes of 4T1 cells and become metastatic in a miR-200-dependent manner. This study provided novel evidence showing that metastatic capability can be transferred from metastatic to non-metastatic cancer cells through exosomes. In addition, this finding suggests that circulating miRNAs are not only just cancer biomarkers, but they are also functional, being capable of promoting metastasis *in vivo*.

Human metastatic CSCs will initiate metastatic colonization by adapting to a distant tissue microenvironment. [10]. For example, metastatic breast cancer cells express many osteoblast-related genes (osteomimicry) that promote its metastasis to the bone [191]. miRNAs play an important role in regulating osteoblast differentiation and also function as regulators of bone metastases [192,193]. miR-218 is significantly upregulated during osteoblast differentiation and targets the inhibitors of Wnt signaling [194]. Thus, miR-218 found in metastatic breast cancer cells is a potent activator of Wnt signaling and promotes the osteomimicry to facilitate bone metastasis of breast cancer cells. In addition, miR-200 family miRNAs are involved in colonization and metastases to distant organs [195]. Because the expression of miR-200 family is downregulated in breast CSCs, analyses of the metastatic CSCs will be required to further characterize the roles of miR-200 family miRNAs in colonization and metastases to distant organs. Uncovering the gene and miRNA expression in the metastatic CSCs is required to characterize the metastatic CSCs and find ways to target them.

## 6. Future Perspectives

miRNAs work as a part of the epigenetic program that regulates the stem cell abilities of both breast CSCs and normal mammary stem/progenitor cells. The miRNAs specifically expressed in breast CSCs target the genes and the signaling pathways important for the regulation of stem cell properties of CSCs. In addition, it will become clearer that miRNA regulation is involved in the initiation, dormancy, and establishment of metastases driven by the metastatic CSCs.

Several small RNA-based drugs are under clinical trials. Fomivirsen was the first RNA-based drug approved by the US Food and Drug Administration (FDA) in 1998 [196]. It is a synthetic, modified, 21-long antisense oligonucleotide used as an antiviral for the treatment of cytomegalovirus retinitis. MRX34 (Mirna therapeutics, Inc., Austin, TX, USA) is a liposomal miR-34 mimicis designed to deliver a mimic of the naturally occurring tumor suppressor miR-34 [197]. The most advanced miRNA trial involves the use of anti-miR-122 (miravirsen) for hepatitis C therapy, which shows a reduction in viral RNA with no evidence of resistance [198]. However, miRNA therapeutics are still in their infancy.

The CSC-targeting therapy has the potential to improve the prognosis of breast cancer patients by attaching the CSCs in the primary sites and suppressing recurrence driven by the metastatic CSCs. Considering that the miRNAs are important regulators of CSCs, miRNA therapeutics will be one of the therapeutic interventions for the CSC-targeting therapies that suppress tumor progression and metastasis.

**Acknowledgments:** We apologize to investigators whose work we were not able to discuss in this focused review. We thank present and previous colleagues and collaborators, for their great contributions and excellent achievements. This work is supported by Grants-in-Aid from the Japan Society for the Promotion of Science, and Japan Foundation for Applied Enzymology.

**Conflicts of Interest:** The authors declare no conflict of interest.

## References

1. Sell, S. Stem cell origin of cancer and differentiation therapy. *Crit. Rev. Oncol. Hematol.* **2004**, *51*, 1–28. [CrossRef] [PubMed]
2. Cohnheim, J. Congenitales, quergestreiftes muskelsarkom der nieren. *Arch. Pathol. Anatom. Physiol. Klin. Med.* **1875**, *65*, 64–69. [CrossRef]
3. Fialkow, P.J. Clonal origin of human tumors. *Biochim. Biophys. Acta* **1976**, *458*, 283–321. [CrossRef]
4. Fialkow, P.J. Human tumors studied with genetic markers. *Birth Defects Orig. Artic. Ser.* **1976**, *12*, 123–132. [PubMed]
5. Fialkow, P.J. Stem cell origin of human myeloid blood cell neoplasms. *Verh. Dtsch. Ges. Pathol.* **1990**, *74*, 43–47. [PubMed]
6. Bonnet, D.; Dick, J.E. Human acute myeloid leukemia is organized as a hierarchy that originates from a primitive hematopoietic cell. *Nat. Med.* **1997**, *3*, 730–737. [CrossRef] [PubMed]

7.  Al-Hajj, M.; Wicha, M.S.; Benito-Hernandez, A.; Morrison, S.J.; Clarke, M.F. Prospective identification of tumorigenic breast cancer cells. *Proc. Natl. Acad. Sci. USA* **2003**, *100*, 3983–3988. [CrossRef] [PubMed]
8.  Takahashi, R.U.; Miyazaki, H.; Ochiya, T. The role of microRNAs in the regulation of cancer stem cells. *Front. Genet.* **2014**, *4*, 295. [CrossRef] [PubMed]
9.  Clarke, M.F.; Dick, J.E.; Dirks, P.B.; Eaves, C.J.; Jamieson, C.H.; Jones, D.L.; Visvader, J.; Weissman, I.L.; Wahl, G.M. Cancer stem cells—perspectives on current status and future directions: AACR Workshop on cancer stem cells. *Cancer Res.* **2006**, *66*, 9339–9344. [CrossRef] [PubMed]
10. Baccelli, I.; Trumpp, A. The evolving concept of cancer and metastasis stem cells. *J. Cell Biol.* **2012**, *198*, 281–293. [CrossRef] [PubMed]
11. Jamieson, C.H.; Ailles, L.E.; Dylla, S.J.; Muijtjens, M.; Jones, C.; Zehnder, J.L.; Gotlib, J.; Li, K.; Manz, M.G.; Keating, A.; *et al.* Granulocyte-macrophage progenitors as candidate leukemic stem cells in blast-crisis CML. *N. Engl. J. Med.* **2004**, *351*, 657–667. [CrossRef] [PubMed]
12. Kikushige, Y.; Ishikawa, F.; Miyamoto, T.; Shima, T.; Urata, S.; Yoshimoto, G.; Mori, Y.; Iino, T.; Yamauchi, T.; Eto, T.; *et al.* Self-renewing hematopoietic stem cell is the primary target in pathogenesis of human chronic lymphocytic leukemia. *Cancer Cell* **2011**, *20*, 246–259. [CrossRef] [PubMed]
13. Liu, S.; Cong, Y.; Wang, D.; Sun, Y.; Deng, L.; Liu, Y.; Martin-Trevino, R.; Shang, L.; McDermott, S.P.; Landis, M.D.; *et al.* Breast cancer stem cells transition between epithelial and mesenchymal states reflective of their normal counterparts. *Stem Cell Rep.* **2014**, *2*, 78–91. [CrossRef] [PubMed]
14. Daniel, V.C.; Marchionni, L.; Hierman, J.S.; Rhodes, J.T.; Devereux, W.L.; Rudin, C.M.; Yung, R.; Parmigiani, G.; Dorsch, M.; Peacock, C.D.; *et al.* A primary xenograft model of small-cell lung cancer reveals irreversible changes in gene expression imposed by culture *in vitro. Cancer Res.* **2009**, *69*, 3364–3373. [CrossRef] [PubMed]
15. Eirew, P.; Steif, A.; Khattra, J.; Ha, G.; Yap, D.; Farahani, H.; Gelmon, K.; Chia, S.; Mar, C.; Wan, A.; *et al.* Dynamics of genomic clones in breast cancer patient xenografts at single-cell resolution. *Nature* **2015**, *518*, 422–426. [CrossRef] [PubMed]
16. Cowin, P.; Wysolmerski, J. Molecular mechanisms guiding embryonic mammary gland development. *Cold Spring Harb. Perspect. Biol.* **2010**, *2*, a003251. [CrossRef] [PubMed]
17. Lechner, R.B.; Gurll, N.J.; Reynolds, D.G. Effects of naloxone on regional blood flow distribution in canine hemorrhagic shock. *Proc. Soc. Exp. Biol. Med.* **1985**, *178*, 227–233. [CrossRef] [PubMed]
18. Watson, C.J.; Khaled, W.T. Mammary development in the embryo and adult: A journey of morphogenesis and commitment. *Development* **2008**, *135*, 995–1003. [CrossRef] [PubMed]
19. Shackleton, M.; Vaillant, F.; Simpson, K.J.; Stingl, J.; Smyth, G.K.; Asselin-Labat, M.L.; Wu, L.; Lindeman, G.J.; Visvader, J.E. Generation of a functional mammary gland from a single stem cell. *Nature* **2006**, *439*, 84–88. [CrossRef] [PubMed]
20. Stingl, J.; Eirew, P.; Ricketson, I.; Shackleton, M.; Vaillant, F.; Choi, D.; Li, H.I.; Eaves, C.J. Purification and unique properties of mammary epithelial stem cells. *Nature* **2006**, *439*, 993–997. [CrossRef] [PubMed]
21. Rios, A.C.; Fu, N.Y.; Lindeman, G.J.; Visvader, J.E. *In situ* identification of bipotent stem cells in the mammary gland. *Nature* **2014**, *506*, 322–327. [CrossRef] [PubMed]
22. Van Keymeulen, A.; Rocha, A.S.; Ousset, M.; Beck, B.; Bouvencourt, G.; Rock, J.; Sharma, N.; Dekoninck, S.; Blanpain, C. Distinct stem cells contribute to mammary gland development and maintenance. *Nature* **2011**, *479*, 189–193. [CrossRef] [PubMed]
23. Eirew, P.; Stingl, J.; Raouf, A.; Turashvili, G.; Aparicio, S.; Emerman, J.T.; Eaves, C.J. A method for quantifying normal human mammary epithelial stem cells with *in vivo* regenerative ability. *Nat. Med.* **2008**, *14*, 1384–1389. [CrossRef] [PubMed]
24. Shimono, Y.; Zabala, M.; Cho, R.W.; Lobo, N.; Dalerba, P.; Qian, D.; Diehn, M.; Liu, H.; Panula, S.P.; Chiao, E.; *et al.* Downregulation of miRNA-200c links breast cancer stem cells with normal stem cells. *Cell* **2009**, *138*, 592–603. [CrossRef] [PubMed]
25. Guo, W.; Keckesova, Z.; Donaher, J.L.; Shibue, T.; Tischler, V.; Reinhardt, F.; Itzkovitz, S.; Noske, A.; Zurrer-Hardi, U.; Bell, G.; *et al.* Slug and Sox9 cooperatively determine the mammary stem cell state. *Cell* **2012**, *148*, 1015–1028. [CrossRef] [PubMed]
26. Polyak, K. Breast cancer: Origins and evolution. *J. Clin. Invest.* **2007**, *117*, 3155–3163. [CrossRef] [PubMed]
27. Alvarez-Garcia, I.; Miska, E.A. MicroRNA functions in animal development and human disease. *Development* **2005**, *132*, 4653–4662. [CrossRef] [PubMed]

28. Saini, H.K.; Griffiths-Jones, S.; Enright, A.J. Genomic analysis of human microRNA transcripts. *Proc. Natl. Acad. Sci. USA* **2007**, *104*, 17719–17724. [CrossRef] [PubMed]
29. Rodriguez, A.; Griffiths-Jones, S.; Ashurst, J.L.; Bradley, A. Identification of mammalian microRNA host genes and transcription units. *Genome Res.* **2004**, *14*, 1902–1910. [CrossRef] [PubMed]
30. Bartel, D.P. MicroRNAs: Target recognition and regulatory functions. *Cell* **2009**, *136*, 215–233. [CrossRef] [PubMed]
31. Xia, T.; Liao, Q.; Jiang, X.; Shao, Y.; Xiao, B.; Xi, Y.; Guo, J. Long noncoding RNA associated-competing endogenous RNAs in gastric cancer. *Sci. Rep.* **2014**, *4*, 6088. [CrossRef] [PubMed]
32. Cheng, L.C.; Tavazoie, M.; Doetsch, F. Stem cells: From epigenetics to microRNAs. *Neuron* **2005**, *46*, 363–367. [CrossRef] [PubMed]
33. Chalfie, M.; Horvitz, H.R.; Sulston, J.E. Mutations that lead to reiterations in the cell lineages of *C. elegans*. *Cell* **1981**, *24*, 59–69. [CrossRef]
34. Ambros, V.; Horvitz, H.R. Heterochronic mutants of the nematode *Caenorhabditis elegans*. *Science* **1984**, *226*, 409–416. [CrossRef] [PubMed]
35. Reinhart, B.J.; Slack, F.J.; Basson, M.; Pasquinelli, A.E.; Bettinger, J.C.; Rougvie, A.E.; Horvitz, H.R.; Ruvkun, G. The 21-nucleotide *let-7* RNA regulates developmental timing in *Caenorhabditis elegans*. *Nature* **2000**, *403*, 901–906. [PubMed]
36. Suh, M.R.; Lee, Y.; Kim, J.Y.; Kim, S.K.; Moon, S.H.; Lee, J.Y.; Cha, K.Y.; Chung, H.M.; Yoon, H.S.; Moon, S.Y.; *et al.* Human embryonic stem cells express a unique set of microRNAs. *Dev. Biol.* **2004**, *270*, 488–498. [CrossRef] [PubMed]
37. Houbaviy, H.B.; Murray, M.F.; Sharp, P.A. Embryonic stem cell-specific microRNAs. *Dev. Cell* **2003**, *5*, 351–358. [CrossRef]
38. Sinkkonen, L.; Hugenschmidt, T.; Berninger, P.; Gaidatzis, D.; Mohn, F.; Artus-Revel, C.G.; Zavolan, M.; Svoboda, P.; Filipowicz, W. MicroRNAs control *de novo* DNA methylation through regulation of transcriptional repressors in mouse embryonic stem cells. *Nat. Struct. Mol. Biol.* **2008**, *15*, 259–267. [CrossRef] [PubMed]
39. Stadler, B.; Ivanovska, I.; Mehta, K.; Song, S.; Nelson, A.; Tan, Y.; Mathieu, J.; Darby, C.; Blau, C.A.; Ware, C.; *et al.* Characterization of microRNAs involved in embryonic stem cell states. *Stem Cells Dev.* **2010**, *19*, 935–950. [CrossRef] [PubMed]
40. Yu, F.; Yao, H.; Zhu, P.; Zhang, X.; Pan, Q.; Gong, C.; Huang, Y.; Hu, X.; Su, F.; Lieberman, J.; *et al.* Let-7 regulates self renewal and tumorigenicity of breast cancer cells. *Cell* **2007**, *131*, 1109–1123. [CrossRef] [PubMed]
41. Liu, T.; Hu, K.; Zhao, Z.; Chen, G.; Ou, X.; Zhang, H.; Zhang, X.; Wei, X.; Wang, D.; Cui, M.; *et al.* MicroRNA-1 down-regulates proliferation and migration of breast cancer stem cells by inhibiting the Wnt/β-catenin pathway. *Oncotarget* **2015**, *6*, 41638–41649. [PubMed]
42. Takahashi, R.U.; Miyazaki, H.; Takeshita, F.; Yamamoto, Y.; Minoura, K.; Ono, M.; Kodaira, M.; Tamura, K.; Mori, M.; Ochiya, T. Loss of microRNA-27b contributes to breast cancer stem cell generation by activating ENPP1. *Nat. Commun.* **2015**, *6*, 7318. [CrossRef] [PubMed]
43. Tang, W.; Yu, F.; Yao, H.; Cui, X.; Jiao, Y.; Lin, L.; Chen, J.; Yin, D.; Song, E.; Liu, Q. miR-27a regulates endothelial differentiation of breast cancer stem like cells. *Oncogene* **2014**, *33*, 2629–2638. [CrossRef] [PubMed]
44. Liu, C.; Tang, D.G. MicroRNA regulation of cancer stem cells. *Cancer Res.* **2011**, *71*, 5950–5954. [CrossRef] [PubMed]
45. Schwarzenbacher, D.; Balic, M.; Pichler, M. The role of microRNAs in breast cancer stem cells. *Int. J. Mol. Sci.* **2013**, *14*, 14712–14723. [CrossRef] [PubMed]
46. Thomson, J.M.; Newman, M.; Parker, J.S.; Morin-Kensicki, E.M.; Wright, T.; Hammond, S.M. Extensive post-transcriptional regulation of microRNAs and its implications for cancer. *Genes Dev.* **2006**, *20*, 2202–2207. [CrossRef] [PubMed]
47. Viswanathan, S.R.; Daley, G.Q.; Gregory, R.I. Selective blockade of microRNA processing by Lin28. *Science* **2008**, *320*, 97–100. [CrossRef] [PubMed]
48. Pode-Shakked, N.; Shukrun, R.; Mark-Danieli, M.; Tsvetkov, P.; Bahar, S.; Pri-Chen, S.; Goldstein, R.S.; Rom-Gross, E.; Mor, Y.; Fridman, E.; *et al.* The isolation and characterization of renal cancer initiating cells from human Wilms' tumour xenografts unveils new therapeutic targets. *EMBO Mol. Med.* **2013**, *5*, 18–37. [CrossRef] [PubMed]

49. Peter, M.E. Let-7 and miR-200 microRNAs: Guardians against pluripotency and cancer progression. *Cell Cycle* **2009**, *8*, 843–852. [CrossRef] [PubMed]

50. Altuvia, Y.; Landgraf, P.; Lithwick, G.; Elefant, N.; Pfeffer, S.; Aravin, A.; Brownstein, M.J.; Tuschl, T.; Margalit, H. Clustering and conservation patterns of human microRNAs. *Nucleic Acids Res.* **2005**, *33*, 2697–2706. [CrossRef] [PubMed]

51. Chan, W.C.; Ho, M.R.; Li, S.C.; Tsai, K.W.; Lai, C.H.; Hsu, C.N.; Lin, W.C. MetaMirClust: Discovery of miRNA cluster patterns using a data-mining approach. *Genomics* **2012**, *100*, 141–148. [CrossRef] [PubMed]

52. Mogilyansky, E.; Rigoutsos, I. The miR-17/92 cluster: A comprehensive update on its genomics, genetics, functions and increasingly important and numerous roles in health and disease. *Cell Death Differ.* **2013**, *20*, 1603–1614. [CrossRef] [PubMed]

53. Xin, M.; Small, E.M.; Sutherland, L.B.; Qi, X.; McAnally, J.; Plato, C.F.; Richardson, J.A.; Bassel-Duby, R.; Olson, E.N. MicroRNAs miR-143 and miR-145 modulate cytoskeletal dynamics and responsiveness of smooth muscle cells to injury. *Genes Dev.* **2009**, *23*, 2166–2178. [CrossRef] [PubMed]

54. Chivukula, R.R.; Shi, G.; Acharya, A.; Mills, E.W.; Zeitels, L.R.; Anandam, J.L.; Abdelnaby, A.A.; Balch, G.C.; Mansour, J.C.; Yopp, A.C.; *et al.* An essential mesenchymal function for miR-143/145 in intestinal epithelial regeneration. *Cell* **2014**, *157*, 1104–1116. [CrossRef] [PubMed]

55. Wheeler, B.M.; Heimberg, A.M.; Moy, V.N.; Sperling, E.A.; Holstein, T.W.; Heber, S.; Peterson, K.J. The deep evolution of metazoan microRNAs. *Evol. Dev.* **2009**, *11*, 50–68. [CrossRef] [PubMed]

56. Trumbach, D.; Prakash, N. The conserved miR-8/miR-200 microRNA family and their role in invertebrate and vertebrate neurogenesis. *Cell Tissue Res.* **2015**, *359*, 161–177. [CrossRef] [PubMed]

57. Saini, H.K.; Enright, A.J.; Griffiths-Jones, S. Annotation of mammalian primary microRNAs. *BMC Genomics* **2008**, *9*, 564. [CrossRef] [PubMed]

58. Burk, U.; Schubert, J.; Wellner, U.; Schmalhofer, O.; Vincan, E.; Spaderna, S.; Brabletz, T. A reciprocal repression between ZEB1 and members of the miR-200 family promotes EMT and invasion in cancer cells. *EMBO Rep.* **2008**, *9*, 582–589. [CrossRef] [PubMed]

59. Kolesnikoff, N.; Attema, J.L.; Roslan, S.; Bert, A.G.; Schwarz, Q.P.; Gregory, P.A.; Goodall, G.J. Specificity protein 1 (Sp1) maintains basal epithelial expression of the miR-200 family: Implications for epithelial-mesenchymal transition. *J. Biol. Chem.* **2014**, *289*, 11194–11205. [CrossRef] [PubMed]

60. Ahn, S.M.; Cha, J.Y.; Kim, J.; Kim, D.; Trang, H.T.; Kim, Y.M.; Cho, Y.H.; Park, D.; Hong, S. Smad3 regulates E-cadherin via miRNA-200 pathway. *Oncogene* **2012**, *31*, 3051–3059. [CrossRef] [PubMed]

61. Humphries, B.; Yang, C. The microRNA-200 family: Small molecules with novel roles in cancer development, progression and therapy. *Oncotarget* **2015**, *6*, 6472–6498. [CrossRef] [PubMed]

62. Ramachandran, I.; Ganapathy, V.; Gillies, E.; Fonseca, I.; Sureban, S.M.; Houchen, C.W.; Reis, A.; Queimado, L. Wnt inhibitory factor 1 suppresses cancer stemness and induces cellular senescence. *Cell Death Dis.* **2014**, *5*, e1246. [CrossRef] [PubMed]

63. Kim, T.; Veronese, A.; Pichiorri, F.; Lee, T.J.; Jeon, Y.J.; Volinia, S.; Pineau, P.; Marchio, A.; Palatini, J.; Suh, S.S.; *et al.* p53 Regulates epithelial-mesenchymal transition through microRNAs targeting ZEB1 and ZEB2. *J. Exp. Med.* **2011**, *208*, 875–883. [CrossRef] [PubMed]

64. Lim, Y.Y.; Wright, J.A.; Attema, J.L.; Gregory, P.A.; Bert, A.G.; Smith, E.; Thomas, D.; Lopez, A.F.; Drew, P.A.; Khew-Goodall, Y.; *et al.* Epigenetic modulation of the miR-200 family is associated with transition to a breast cancer stem-cell-like state. *J. Cell Sci.* **2013**, *126*, 2256–2266. [CrossRef] [PubMed]

65. Song, S.J.; Poliseno, L.; Song, M.S.; Ala, U.; Webster, K.; Ng, C.; Beringer, G.; Brikbak, N.J.; Yuan, X.; Cantley, L.C.; *et al.* MicroRNA-antagonism regulates breast cancer stemness and metastasis via TET-family-dependent chromatin remodeling. *Cell* **2013**, *154*, 311–324. [CrossRef] [PubMed]

66. Lin, C.H.; Jackson, A.L.; Guo, J.; Linsley, P.S.; Eisenman, R.N. Myc-regulated microRNAs attenuate embryonic stem cell differentiation. *EMBO J.* **2009**, *28*, 3157–3170. [CrossRef] [PubMed]

67. Wellner, U.; Schubert, J.; Burk, U.C.; Schmalhofer, O.; Zhu, F.; Sonntag, A.; Waldvogel, B.; Vannier, C.; Darling, D.; zur Hausen, A.; *et al.* The EMT-activator ZEB1 promotes tumorigenicity by repressing stemness-inhibiting microRNAs. *Nat. Cell Biol.* **2009**, *11*, 1487–1495. [CrossRef] [PubMed]

68. Gill, J.G.; Langer, E.M.; Lindsley, R.C.; Cai, M.; Murphy, T.L.; Kyba, M.; Murphy, K.M. Snail and the microRNA-200 family act in opposition to regulate epithelial-to-mesenchymal transition and germ layer fate restriction in differentiating ESCs. *Stem Cells* **2011**, *29*, 764–776. [CrossRef] [PubMed]

69. Chen, J.; Wang, G.; Lu, C.; Guo, X.; Hong, W.; Kang, J.; Wang, J. Synergetic cooperation of microRNAs with transcription factors in iPS cell generation. *PLoS ONE* **2012**, *7*, e40849. [CrossRef] [PubMed]

70. Wang, G.; Guo, X.; Hong, W.; Liu, Q.; Wei, T.; Lu, C.; Gao, L.; Ye, D.; Zhou, Y.; Chen, J.; *et al.* Critical regulation of miR-200/ZEB2 pathway in Oct4/Sox2-induced mesenchymal-to-epithelial transition and induced pluripotent stem cell generation. *Proc. Natl. Acad. Sci. USA* **2013**, *110*, 2858–2863. [CrossRef] [PubMed]

71. Uhlmann, S.; Zhang, J.D.; Schwager, A.; Mannsperger, H.; Riazalhosseini, Y.; Burmester, S.; Ward, A.; Korf, U.; Wiemann, S.; Sahin, O. miR-200bc/429 cluster targets PLCγ1 and differentially regulates proliferation and EGF-driven invasion than miR-200a/141 in breast cancer. *Oncogene* **2010**, *29*, 4297–4306. [CrossRef] [PubMed]

72. Zhang, B.; Zhang, Z.; Xia, S.; Xing, C.; Ci, X.; Li, X.; Zhao, R.; Tian, S.; Ma, G.; Zhu, Z.; *et al.* KLF5 activates microRNA 200 transcription to maintain epithelial characteristics and prevent induced epithelial-mesenchymal transition in epithelial cells. *Mol. Cell. Biol.* **2013**, *33*, 4919–4935. [CrossRef] [PubMed]

73. Yang, M.; Pan, Y.; Zhou, Y. miR-96 promotes osteogenic differentiation by suppressing HBEGF-EGFR signaling in osteoblastic cells. *FEBS Lett.* **2014**, *588*, 4761–4768. [CrossRef] [PubMed]

74. Dambal, S.; Shah, M.; Mihelich, B.; Nonn, L. The microRNA-183 cluster: The family that plays together stays together. *Nucleic Acids Res.* **2015**, *43*, 7173–7188. [CrossRef] [PubMed]

75. Pierce, M.L.; Weston, M.D.; Fritzsch, B.; Gabel, H.W.; Ruvkun, G.; Soukup, G.A. MicroRNA-183 family conservation and ciliated neurosensory organ expression. *Evol. Dev.* **2008**, *10*, 106–113. [CrossRef] [PubMed]

76. Leung, W.K.; He, M.; Chan, A.W.; Law, P.T.; Wong, N. Wnt/β-Catenin activates miR-183/96/182 expression in hepatocellular carcinoma that promotes cell invasion. *Cancer Lett.* **2015**, *362*, 97–105. [CrossRef] [PubMed]

77. Chen, C.; Xiang, H.; Peng, Y.L.; Peng, J.; Jiang, S.W. Mature miR-183, negatively regulated by transcription factor GATA3, promotes 3T3-L1 adipogenesis through inhibition of the canonical Wnt/β-catenin signaling pathway by targeting LRP6. *Cell. Signal.* **2014**, *26*, 1155–1165. [CrossRef] [PubMed]

78. Donatelli, S.S.; Zhou, J.M.; Gilvary, D.L.; Eksioglu, E.A.; Chen, X.; Cress, W.D.; Haura, E.B.; Schabath, M.B.; Coppola, D.; Wei, S.; *et al.* TGF-β-inducible microRNA-183 silences tumor-associated natural killer cells. *Proc. Natl. Acad Sci. USA* **2014**, *111*, 4203–4208. [CrossRef] [PubMed]

79. Li, X.L.; Hara, T.; Choi, Y.; Subramanian, M.; Francis, P.; Bilke, S.; Walker, R.L.; Pineda, M.; Zhu, Y.; Yang, Y.; *et al.* A p21-ZEB1 complex inhibits epithelial-mesenchymal transition through the microRNA 183-96-182 cluster. *Mol. Cell Biol.* **2014**, *34*, 533–550. [CrossRef] [PubMed]

80. Chistiakov, D.A.; Sobenin, I.A.; Orekhov, A.N.; Bobryshev, Y.V. Human miR-221/222 in physiological and atherosclerotic vascular remodeling. *Biomed. Res. Int.* **2015**, *2015*, 354517. [CrossRef] [PubMed]

81. Di Leva, G.; Gasparini, P.; Piovan, C.; Ngankeu, A.; Garofalo, M.; Taccioli, C.; Iorio, M.V.; Li, M.; Volinia, S.; Alder, H.; *et al.* MicroRNA cluster 221-222 and estrogen receptor α interactions in breast cancer. *J. Natl. Cancer Inst.* **2010**, *102*, 706–721. [CrossRef] [PubMed]

82. Zhao, J.J.; Lin, J.; Yang, H.; Kong, W.; He, L.; Ma, X.; Coppola, D.; Cheng, J.Q. MicroRNA-221/222 negatively regulates estrogen receptor α and is associated with tamoxifen resistance in breast cancer. *J. Biol. Chem.* **2008**, *283*, 31079–31086. [CrossRef] [PubMed]

83. Pallante, P.; Battista, S.; Pierantoni, G.M.; Fusco, A. Deregulation of microRNA expression in thyroid neoplasias. *Nat. Rev. Endocrinol.* **2014**, *10*, 88–101. [CrossRef] [PubMed]

84. Garofalo, M.; Quintavalle, C.; Romano, G.; Croce, C.M.; Condorelli, G. miR221/222 in cancer: Their role in tumor progression and response to therapy. *Curr. Mol. Med.* **2012**, *12*, 27–33. [CrossRef] [PubMed]

85. Volinia, S.; Calin, G.A.; Liu, C.G.; Ambs, S.; Cimmino, A.; Petrocca, F.; Visone, R.; Iorio, M.; Roldo, C.; Ferracin, M.; *et al.* A microRNA expression signature of human solid tumors defines cancer gene targets. *Proc. Natl. Acad. Sci. USA* **2006**, *103*, 2257–2261. [CrossRef] [PubMed]

86. Felli, N.; Fontana, L.; Pelosi, E.; Botta, R.; Bonci, D.; Facchiano, F.; Liuzzi, F.; Lulli, V.; Morsilli, O.; Santoro, S.; *et al.* MicroRNAs 221 and 222 inhibit normal erythropoiesis and erythroleukemic cell growth via kit receptor down-modulation. *Proc. Natl. Acad. Sci. USA* **2005**, *102*, 18081–18086. [CrossRef] [PubMed]

87. Roscigno, G.; Quintavalle, C.; Donnarumma, E.; Puoti, I.; Diaz-Lagares, A.; Iaboni, M.; Fiore, D.; Russo, V.; Todaro, M.; Romano, G.; *et al.* miR-221 promotes stemness of breast cancer cells by targeting DNMT3b. *Oncotarget* **2015**. [CrossRef]

88. Zhao, Y.; Zhao, L.; Ischenko, I.; Bao, Q.; Schwarz, B.; Niess, H.; Wang, Y.; Renner, A.; Mysliwietz, J.; Jauch, K.W.; *et al.* Antisense inhibition of microRNA-21 and microRNA-221 in tumor-initiating stem-like cells modulates tumorigenesis, metastasis, and chemotherapy resistance in pancreatic cancer. *Target. Oncol.* **2015**, *10*, 535–548. [CrossRef] [PubMed]

89. Aldaz, B.; Sagardoy, A.; Nogueira, L.; Guruceaga, E.; Grande, L.; Huse, J.T.; Aznar, M.A.; Diez-Valle, R.; Tejada-Solis, S.; Alonso, M.M.; *et al.* Involvement of miRNAs in the differentiation of human glioblastoma multiforme stem-like cells. *PLoS ONE* **2013**, *8*, e77098. [CrossRef] [PubMed]

90. Shah, M.Y.; Calin, G.A. MicroRNAs miR-221 and miR-222: A new level of regulation in aggressive breast cancer. *Genome Med.* **2011**, *3*, 56. [CrossRef] [PubMed]

91. Stinson, S.; Lackner, M.R.; Adai, A.T.; Yu, N.; Kim, H.J.; O'Brien, C.; Spoerke, J.; Jhunjhunwala, S.; Boyd, Z.; Januario, T.; *et al.* TRPS1 targeting by miR-221/222 promotes the epithelial-to-mesenchymal transition in breast cancer. *Sci. Signal.* **2011**, *4*, ra41. [CrossRef] [PubMed]

92. Chen, C.Z.; Lodish, H.F. MicroRNAs as regulators of mammalian hematopoiesis. *Semin. Immunol.* **2005**, *17*, 155–165. [CrossRef] [PubMed]

93. Ramkissoon, S.H.; Mainwaring, L.A.; Ogasawara, Y.; Keyvanfar, K.; McCoy, J.P., Jr.; Sloand, E.M.; Kajigaya, S.; Young, N.S. Hematopoietic-specific microRNA expression in human cells. *Leuk. Res.* **2006**, *30*, 643–647. [CrossRef] [PubMed]

94. Visone, R.; Rassenti, L.Z.; Veronese, A.; Taccioli, C.; Costinean, S.; Aguda, B.D.; Volinia, S.; Ferracin, M.; Palatini, J.; Balatti, V.; *et al.* Karyotype-specific microRNA signature in chronic lymphocytic leukemia. *Blood* **2009**, *114*, 3872–3879. [CrossRef] [PubMed]

95. Wu, H.; Neilson, J.R.; Kumar, P.; Manocha, M.; Shankar, P.; Sharp, P.A.; Manjunath, N. miRNA profiling of naive, effector and memory CD8 T cells. *PLoS ONE* **2007**, *2*, e1020. [CrossRef] [PubMed]

96. Kwanhian, W.; Lenze, D.; Alles, J.; Motsch, N.; Barth, S.; Doll, C.; Imig, J.; Hummel, M.; Tinguely, M.; Trivedi, P.; *et al.* MicroRNA-142 is mutated in about 20% of diffuse large B-cell lymphoma. *Cancer Med.* **2012**, *1*, 141–155. [CrossRef] [PubMed]

97. Shrestha, A.; Carraro, G.; El Agha, E.; Mukhametshina, R.; Chao, C.M.; Rizvanov, A.; Barreto, G.; Bellusci, S. Generation and validation of miR-142 knock out mice. *PLoS ONE* **2015**, *10*, e0136913. [CrossRef] [PubMed]

98. Chapnik, E.; Rivkin, N.; Mildner, A.; Beck, G.; Pasvolsky, R.; Metzl-Raz, E.; Birger, Y.; Amir, G.; Tirosh, I.; Porat, Z.; *et al.* miR-142 orchestrates a network of actin cytoskeleton regulators during megakaryopoiesis. *eLife* **2014**, *3*, e01964. [CrossRef] [PubMed]

99. Skarn, M.; Baroy, T.; Stratford, E.W.; Myklebost, O. Epigenetic regulation and functional characterization of microRNA-142 in mesenchymal cells. *PLoS ONE* **2013**, *8*, e79231. [CrossRef] [PubMed]

100. Isobe, T.; Hisamori, S.; Hogan, D.J.; Zabala, M.; Hendrickson, D.G.; Dalerba, P.; Cai, S.; Scheeren, F.; Kuo, A.H.; Sikandar, S.S.; *et al.* miR-142 regulates the tumorigenicity of human breast cancer stem cells through the canonical WNT signaling pathway. *eLife* **2014**, *3*. [CrossRef] [PubMed]

101. Penna, E.; Orso, F.; Taverna, D. miR-214 as a key hub that controls cancer networks: Small player, multiple functions. *J. Invest. Dermatol.* **2015**, *135*, 960–969. [CrossRef] [PubMed]

102. Zhang, L.; Huang, J.; Yang, N.; Greshock, J.; Megraw, M.S.; Giannakakis, A.; Liang, S.; Naylor, T.L.; Barchetti, A.; Ward, M.R.; *et al.* MicroRNAs exhibit high frequency genomic alterations in human cancer. *Proc. Natl. Acad. Sci. USA* **2006**, *103*, 9136–9141. [CrossRef] [PubMed]

103. Blenkiron, C.; Goldstein, L.D.; Thorne, N.P.; Spiteri, I.; Chin, S.F.; Dunning, M.J.; Barbosa-Morais, N.L.; Teschendorff, A.E.; Green, A.R.; Ellis, I.O.; *et al.* MicroRNA expression profiling of human breast cancer identifies new markers of tumor subtype. *Genome Biol.* **2007**, *8*, R214. [CrossRef] [PubMed]

104. Sempere, L.F.; Christensen, M.; Silahtaroglu, A.; Bak, M.; Heath, C.V.; Schwartz, G.; Wells, W.; Kauppinen, S.; Cole, C.N. Altered MicroRNA expression confined to specific epithelial cell subpopulations in breast cancer. *Cancer Res.* **2007**, *67*, 11612–11620. [CrossRef] [PubMed]

105. Aurora, A.B.; Mahmoud, A.I.; Luo, X.; Johnson, B.A.; van Rooij, E.; Matsuzaki, S.; Humphries, K.M.; Hill, J.A.; Bassel-Duby, R.; Sadek, H.A.; *et al.* MicroRNA-214 protects the mouse heart from ischemic injury by controlling $Ca^{2+}$ overload and cell death. *J. Clin. Invest.* **2012**, *122*, 1222–1232. [CrossRef] [PubMed]

106. Watanabe, T.; Sato, T.; Amano, T.; Kawamura, Y.; Kawamura, N.; Kawaguchi, H.; Yamashita, N.; Kurihara, H.; Nakaoka, T. Dnm3os, a non-coding RNA, is required for normal growth and skeletal development in mice. *Dev. Dyn.* **2008**, *237*, 3738–3748. [CrossRef] [PubMed]

107. Xu, C.X.; Xu, M.; Tan, L.; Yang, H.; Permuth-Wey, J.; Kruk, P.A.; Wenham, R.M.; Nicosia, S.V.; Lancaster, J.M.; Sellers, T.A.; *et al.* MicroRNA miR-214 regulates ovarian cancer cell stemness by targeting p53/Nanog. *J. Biol. Chem.* **2012**, *287*, 34970–34978. [CrossRef] [PubMed]

108. Zhang, Z.C.; Li, Y.Y.; Wang, H.Y.; Fu, S.; Wang, X.P.; Zeng, M.S.; Zeng, Y.X.; Shao, J.Y. Knockdown of miR-214 promotes apoptosis and inhibits cell proliferation in nasopharyngeal carcinoma. *PLoS ONE* **2014**, *9*, e86149. [CrossRef] [PubMed]

109. Wang, F.; Lv, P.; Liu, X.; Zhu, M.; Qiu, X. MicroRNA-214 enhances the invasion ability of breast cancer cells by targeting p53. *Int. J. Mol. Med.* **2015**, *35*, 1395–1402. [CrossRef] [PubMed]

110. Xia, H.; Ooi, L.L.; Hui, K.M. miR-214 targets β-catenin pathway to suppress invasion, stem-like traits and recurrence of human hepatocellular carcinoma. *PLoS ONE* **2012**, *7*, e44206. [CrossRef] [PubMed]

111. Van der Lugt, N.M.; Domen, J.; Linders, K.; van Roon, M.; Robanus-Maandag, E.; te Riele, H.; van der Valk, M.; Deschamps, J.; Sofroniew, M.; van Lohuizen, M.; *et al.* Posterior transformation, neurological abnormalities, and severe hematopoietic defects in mice with a targeted deletion of the *bmi-1* proto-oncogene. *Genes Dev.* **1994**, *8*, 757–769. [CrossRef] [PubMed]

112. Pietersen, A.M.; Evers, B.; Prasad, A.A.; Tanger, E.; Cornelissen-Steijger, P.; Jonkers, J.; van Lohuizen, M. Bmi1 regulates stem cells and proliferation and differentiation of committed cells in mammary epithelium. *Curr. Biol.* **2008**, *18*, 1094–1099. [CrossRef] [PubMed]

113. Adorno, M.; Sikandar, S.; Mitra, S.S.; Kuo, A.; Nicolis di Robilant, B.; Haro-Acosta, V.; Ouadah, Y.; Quarta, M.; Rodriguez, J.; Qian, D.; *et al.* Usp16 contributes to somatic stem-cell defects in Down's syndrome. *Nature* **2013**, *501*, 380–384. [CrossRef] [PubMed]

114. Haupt, Y.; Bath, M.L.; Harris, A.W.; Adams, J.M. Bmi-1 transgene induces lymphomas and collaborates with myc in tumorigenesis. *Oncogene* **1993**, *8*, 3161–3164. [PubMed]

115. Jacobs, J.J.; Kieboom, K.; Marino, S.; DePinho, R.A.; van Lohuizen, M. The oncogene and Polycomb-group gene *bmi-1* regulates cell proliferation and senescence through the *ink4a* locus. *Nature* **1999**, *397*, 164–168. [PubMed]

116. Park, I.K.; Morrison, S.J.; Clarke, M.F. Bmi1, stem cells, and senescence regulation. *J. Clin. Invest.* **2004**, *113*, 175–179. [CrossRef] [PubMed]

117. Sharpless, N.E.; DePinho, R.A. The *INK4A/ARF* locus and its two gene products. *Curr. Opin. Genet. Dev.* **1999**, *9*, 22–30. [CrossRef]

118. Zindy, F.; Quelle, D.E.; Roussel, M.F.; Sherr, C.J. Expression of the $p16^{INK4a}$ tumor suppressor *versus* other INK4 family members during mouse development and aging. *Oncogene* **1997**, *15*, 203–211. [CrossRef] [PubMed]

119. Honda, R.; Yasuda, H. Association of $p19^{ARF}$ with Mdm2 inhibits ubiquitin ligase activity of Mdm2 for tumor suppressor p53. *EMBO J.* **1999**, *18*, 22–27. [CrossRef] [PubMed]

120. Weber, J.D.; Taylor, L.J.; Roussel, M.F.; Sherr, C.J.; Bar-Sagi, D. Nucleolar Arf sequesters Mdm2 and activates p53. *Nat. Cell Biol.* **1999**, *1*, 20–26. [PubMed]

121. He, X.; Dong, Y.; Wu, C.W.; Zhao, Z.; Ng, S.S.; Chan, F.K.; Sung, J.J.; Yu, J. MicroRNA-218 inhibits cell cycle progression and promotes apoptosis in colon cancer by downregulating BMI1 polycomb ring finger oncogene. *Mol. Med.* **2012**, *18*, 1491–1498.

122. Dimri, M.; Carroll, J.D.; Cho, J.H.; Dimri, G.P. MicroRNA-141 regulates BMI1 expression and induces senescence in human diploid fibroblasts. *Cell Cycle* **2013**, *12*, 3537–3546. [CrossRef] [PubMed]

123. Dong, P.; Kaneuchi, M.; Watari, H.; Hamada, J.; Sudo, S.; Ju, J.; Sakuragi, N. MicroRNA-194 inhibits epithelial to mesenchymal transition of endometrial cancer cells by targeting oncogene BMI-1. *Mol. Cancer* **2011**, *10*, 99. [CrossRef] [PubMed]

124. Bhattacharya, R.; Nicoloso, M.; Arvizo, R.; Wang, E.; Cortez, A.; Rossi, S.; Calin, G.A.; Mukherjee, P. miR-15a and miR-16 control Bmi-1 expression in ovarian cancer. *Cancer Res.* **2009**, *69*, 9090–9095. [CrossRef] [PubMed]

125. Godlewski, J.; Nowicki, M.O.; Bronisz, A.; Williams, S.; Otsuki, A.; Nuovo, G.; Raychaudhury, A.; Newton, H.B.; Chiocca, E.A.; Lawler, S. Targeting of the Bmi-1 oncogene/stem cell renewal factor by microRNA-128 inhibits glioma proliferation and self-renewal. *Cancer Res.* **2008**, *68*, 9125–9130. [CrossRef] [PubMed]

126. Schickel, R.; Park, S.M.; Murmann, A.E.; Peter, M.E. miR-200c regulates induction of apoptosis through CD95 by targeting FAP-1. *Mol. Cell* **2010**, *38*, 908–915. [CrossRef] [PubMed]

127. Lerner, M.; Haneklaus, M.; Harada, M.; Grander, D. miR-200c regulates Noxa expression and sensitivity to proteasomal inhibitors. *PLoS ONE* **2012**, *7*, e36490. [CrossRef] [PubMed]

128. Medina, R.; Zaidi, S.K.; Liu, C.G.; Stein, J.L.; van Wijnen, A.J.; Croce, C.M.; Stein, G.S. MicroRNAs 221 and 222 bypass quiescence and compromise cell survival. *Cancer Res.* **2008**, *68*, 2773–2780. [CrossRef] [PubMed]

129. Le Sage, C.; Nagel, R.; Egan, D.A.; Schrier, M.; Mesman, E.; Mangiola, A.; Anile, C.; Maira, G.; Mercatelli, N.; Ciafre, S.A.; *et al.* Regulation of the p27$^{Kip1}$ tumor suppressor by miR-221 and miR-222 promotes cancer cell proliferation. *EMBO J.* **2007**, *26*, 3699–3708. [CrossRef] [PubMed]

130. Zhang, C.Z.; Zhang, J.X.; Zhang, A.L.; Shi, Z.D.; Han, L.; Jia, Z.F.; Yang, W.D.; Wang, G.X.; Jiang, T.; You, Y.P.; *et al.* miR-221 and miR-222 target PUMA to induce cell survival in glioblastoma. *Mol. Cancer* **2010**, *9*, 229. [CrossRef] [PubMed]

131. Reya, T.; Clevers, H. Wnt signalling in stem cells and cancer. *Nature* **2005**, *434*, 843–850. [CrossRef] [PubMed]

132. Nusse, R.; Fuerer, C.; Ching, W.; Harnish, K.; Logan, C.; Zeng, A.; Ten Berge, D.; Kalani, Y. Wnt signaling and stem cell control. *Cold Spring Harb. Symp. Quant. Biol.* **2008**, *73*, 59–66. [CrossRef] [PubMed]

133. Anastas, J.N.; Moon, R.T. WNT signalling pathways as therapeutic targets in cancer. *Nat. Rev. Cancer* **2013**, *13*, 11–26. [CrossRef] [PubMed]

134. Cottrell, S.; Bicknell, D.; Kaklamanis, L.; Bodmer, W.F. Molecular analysis of APC mutations in familial adenomatous polyposis and sporadic colon carcinomas. *Lancet* **1992**, *340*, 626–630. [CrossRef]

135. Kinzler, K.W.; Nilbert, M.C.; Su, L.K.; Vogelstein, B.; Bryan, T.M.; Levy, D.B.; Smith, K.J.; Preisinger, A.C.; Hedge, P.; McKechnie, D.; *et al.* Identification of FAP locus genes from chromosome 5q21. *Science* **1991**, *253*, 661–665. [CrossRef] [PubMed]

136. Nishisho, I.; Nakamura, Y.; Miyoshi, Y.; Miki, Y.; Ando, H.; Horii, A.; Koyama, K.; Utsunomiya, J.; Baba, S.; Hedge, P. Mutations of chromosome 5q21 genes in FAP and colorectal cancer patients. *Science* **1991**, *253*, 665–669. [CrossRef] [PubMed]

137. Fearon, E.R.; Vogelstein, B. A genetic model for colorectal tumorigenesis. *Cell* **1990**, *61*, 759–767. [CrossRef]

138. Nagel, R.; le Sage, C.; Diosdado, B.; van der Waal, M.; Oude Vrielink, J.A.; Bolijn, A.; Meijer, G.A.; Agami, R. Regulation of the adenomatous polyposis coli gene by the miR-135 family in colorectal cancer. *Cancer Res.* **2008**, *68*, 5795–5802. [CrossRef] [PubMed]

139. Wang, T.; Xu, Z. miR-27 promotes osteoblast differentiation by modulating Wnt signaling. *Biochem. Biophys. Res. Commun.* **2010**, *402*, 186–189. [CrossRef] [PubMed]

140. Zhang, Y.; Wei, W.; Cheng, N.; Wang, K.; Li, B.; Jiang, X.; Sun, S. Hepatitis C Virus-induced upregulation of miR-155 promotes hepatocarcinogenesis by activating Wnt signaling. *Hepatology* **2012**, *56*, 1631–1640. [CrossRef] [PubMed]

141. Hu, W.; Ye, Y.; Zhang, W.; Wang, J.; Chen, A.; Guo, F. miR142-3p promotes osteoblast differentiation by modulating Wnt signaling. *Mol. Med. Rep.* **2013**, *7*, 689–693. [PubMed]

142. Li, M.; Tian, L.; Wang, L.; Yao, H.; Zhang, J.; Lu, J.; Sun, Y.; Gao, X.; Xiao, H.; Liu, M. Down-regulation of miR-129-5p inhibits growth and induces apoptosis in laryngeal squamous cell carcinoma by targeting APC. *PLoS ONE* **2013**, *8*, e77829. [CrossRef] [PubMed]

143. Shen, G.; Jia, H.; Tai, Q.; Li, Y.; Chen, D. miR-106b downregulates adenomatous polyposis coli and promotes cell proliferation in human hepatocellular carcinoma. *Carcinogenesis* **2013**, *34*, 211–219. [CrossRef] [PubMed]

144. Emmrich, S.; Rasche, M.; Schoning, J.; Reimer, C.; Keihani, S.; Maroz, A.; Xie, Y.; Li, Z.; Schambach, A.; Reinhardt, D.; *et al.* miR-99a/100~125b tricistrons regulate hematopoietic stem and progenitor cell homeostasis by shifting the balance between TGFβ and Wnt signaling. *Genes Dev.* **2014**, *28*, 858–874. [CrossRef] [PubMed]

145. Kim, J.S.; Park, M.G.; Lee, S.A.; Park, S.Y.; Kim, H.J.; Yu, S.K.; Kim, C.S.; Kim, S.G.; Oh, J.S.; You, J.S.; *et al.* Downregulation of adenomatous polyposis coli by microRNA-663 promotes odontogenic differentiation through activation of Wnt/β-catenin signaling. *Biochem. Biophys. Res. Commun.* **2014**, *446*, 894–900. [CrossRef] [PubMed]

146. Carraro, G.; Shrestha, A.; Rostkovius, J.; Contreras, A.; Chao, C.M.; El Agha, E.; Mackenzie, B.; Dilai, S.; Guidolin, D.; Taketo, M.M.; *et al.* miR-142-3p balances proliferation and differentiation of mesenchymal cells during lung development. *Development* **2014**, *141*, 1272–1281. [CrossRef] [PubMed]

147. Kapinas, K.; Kessler, C.; Ricks, T.; Gronowicz, G.; Delany, A.M. miR-29 modulates Wnt signaling in human osteoblasts through a positive feedback loop. *J. Biol. Chem.* **2010**, *285*, 25221–25231. [CrossRef] [PubMed]

148. Liu, Y.; Huang, T.; Zhao, X.; Cheng, L. MicroRNAs modulate the Wnt signaling pathway through targeting its inhibitors. *Biochem. Biophys. Res. Commun.* **2011**, *408*, 259–264. [CrossRef] [PubMed]

149. Zhou, B.; Wang, S.; Mayr, C.; Bartel, D.P.; Lodish, H.F. miR-150, a microRNA expressed in mature B and T cells, blocks early B cell development when expressed prematurely. *Proc. Natl. Acad. Sci. USA* **2007**, *104*, 7080–7085. [CrossRef] [PubMed]

150. Saydam, O.; Shen, Y.; Wurdinger, T.; Senol, O.; Boke, E.; James, M.F.; Tannous, B.A.; Stemmer-Rachamimov, A.O.; Yi, M.; Stephens, R.M.; *et al.* Downregulated microRNA-200a in meningiomas promotes tumor growth by reducing E-cadherin and activating the Wnt/β-catenin signaling pathway. *Mol. Cell Biol.* **2009**, *29*, 5923–5940. [CrossRef] [PubMed]

151. Abedi, N.; Mohammadi-Yeganeh, S.; Koochaki, A.; Karami, F.; Paryan, M. miR-141 as potential suppressor of β-catenin in breast cancer. *Tumour Biol.* **2015**. [CrossRef] [PubMed]

152. Kennell, J.A.; Gerin, I.; MacDougald, O.A.; Cadigan, K.M. The microRNA miR-8 is a conserved negative regulator of Wnt signaling. *Proc. Natl. Acad. Sci. USA* **2008**, *105*, 15417–15422. [CrossRef] [PubMed]

153. Deng, X.; Wu, B.; Xiao, K.; Kang, J.; Xie, J.; Zhang, X.; Fan, Y. miR-146b-5p promotes metastasis and induces epithelial-mesenchymal transition in thyroid cancer by targeting ZNRF3. *Cell. Physiol. Biochem.* **2015**, *35*, 71–82. [CrossRef] [PubMed]

154. De Lau, W.; Peng, W.C.; Gros, P.; Clevers, H. The R-spondin/Lgr5/Rnf43 module: Regulator of Wnt signal strength. *Genes Dev.* **2014**, *28*, 305–316. [CrossRef] [PubMed]

155. Hwang, W.L.; Jiang, J.K.; Yang, S.H.; Huang, T.S.; Lan, H.Y.; Teng, H.W.; Yang, C.Y.; Tsai, Y.P.; Lin, C.H.; Wang, H.W.; *et al.* MicroRNA-146a directs the symmetric division of Snail-dominant colorectal cancer stem cells. *Nat. Cell Biol.* **2014**, *16*, 268–280. [CrossRef] [PubMed]

156. Yook, J.I.; Li, X.Y.; Ota, I.; Hu, C.; Kim, H.S.; Kim, N.H.; Cha, S.Y.; Ryu, J.K.; Choi, Y.J.; Kim, J.; *et al.* A Wnt-Axin2-GSK3β cascade regulates Snail1 activity in breast cancer cells. *Nat. Cell Biol.* **2006**, *8*, 1398–1406. [CrossRef] [PubMed]

157. Mani, S.A.; Guo, W.; Liao, M.J.; Eaton, E.N.; Ayyanan, A.; Zhou, A.Y.; Brooks, M.; Reinhard, F.; Zhang, C.C.; Shipitsin, M.; *et al.* The epithelial-mesenchymal transition generates cells with properties of stem cells. *Cell* **2008**, *133*, 704–715. [CrossRef] [PubMed]

158. Davalos, V.; Moutinho, C.; Villanueva, A.; Boque, R.; Silva, P.; Carneiro, F.; Esteller, M. Dynamic epigenetic regulation of the microRNA-200 family mediates epithelial and mesenchymal transitions in human tumorigenesis. *Oncogene* **2012**, *31*, 2062–2074. [CrossRef] [PubMed]

159. Mongroo, P.S.; Rustgi, A.K. The role of the miR-200 family in epithelial-mesenchymal transition. *Cancer Biol. Ther.* **2010**, *10*, 219–222. [CrossRef] [PubMed]

160. Brabletz, S.; Brabletz, T. The ZEB/miR-200 feedback loop—A motor of cellular plasticity in development and cancer? *EMBO Rep.* **2010**, *11*, 670–677. [CrossRef] [PubMed]

161. Song, S.J.; Ito, K.; Ala, U.; Kats, L.; Webster, K.; Sun, S.M.; Jongen-Lavrencic, M.; Manova-Todorova, K.; Teruya-Feldstein, J.; Avigan, D.E.; *et al.* The oncogenic microRNA miR-22 targets the TET2 tumor suppressor to promote hematopoietic stem cell self-renewal and transformation. *Cell Stem Cell* **2013**, *13*, 87–101. [CrossRef] [PubMed]

162. Wels, C.; Joshi, S.; Koefinger, P.; Bergler, H.; Schaider, H. Transcriptional activation of ZEB1 by Slug leads to cooperative regulation of the epithelial-mesenchymal transition-like phenotype in melanoma. *J. Invest. Dermatol.* **2011**, *131*, 1877–1885. [CrossRef] [PubMed]

163. Ye, X.; Tam, W.L.; Shibue, T.; Kaygusuz, Y.; Reinhardt, F.; Ng Eaton, E.; Weinberg, R.A. Distinct EMT programs control normal mammary stem cells and tumour-initiating cells. *Nature* **2015**, *525*, 256–260. [CrossRef] [PubMed]

164. Suzuki, T.; Mizutani, K.; Minami, A.; Nobutani, K.; Kurita, S.; Nagino, M.; Shimono, Y.; Takai, Y. Suppression of the TGF-β1-induced protein expression of SNAI1 and N-cadherin by miR-199a. *Genes Cells* **2014**, *19*, 667–675. [CrossRef] [PubMed]

165. Qu, Y.; Li, W.C.; Hellem, M.R.; Rostad, K.; Popa, M.; McCormack, E.; Oyan, A.M.; Kalland, K.H.; Ke, X.S. miR-182 and miR-203 induce mesenchymal to epithelial transition and self-sufficiency of growth signals via repressing SNAI2 in prostate cells. *Int. J. Cancer* **2013**, *133*, 544–555. [CrossRef] [PubMed]

166. Dontu, G.; Jackson, K.W.; McNicholas, E.; Kawamura, M.J.; Abdallah, W.M.; Wicha, M.S. Role of Notch signaling in cell-fate determination of human mammary stem/progenitor cells. *Breast Cancer Res.* **2004**, *6*, R605–R615. [CrossRef] [PubMed]

167. Shi, W.; Harris, A.L. Notch signaling in breast cancer and tumor angiogenesis: Cross-talk and therapeutic potentials. *J. Mammary Gland Biol. Neoplasia* **2006**, *11*, 41–52. [CrossRef] [PubMed]

168. Gangopadhyay, S.; Nandy, A.; Hor, P.; Mukhopadhyay, A. Breast cancer stem cells: A novel therapeutic target. *Clin. Breast Cancer* **2013**, *13*, 7–15. [CrossRef] [PubMed]

169. Borggrefe, T.; Oswald, F. The Notch signaling pathway: Transcriptional regulation at Notch target genes. *Cell. Mol. Life Sci.* **2009**, *66*, 1631–1646. [CrossRef] [PubMed]

170. Brabletz, S.; Bajdak, K.; Meidhof, S.; Burk, U.; Niedermann, G.; Firat, E.; Wellner, U.; Dimmler, A.; Faller, G.; Schubert, J.; *et al.* The ZEB1/miR-200 feedback loop controls Notch signalling in cancer cells. *EMBO J.* **2011**, *30*, 770–782. [CrossRef] [PubMed]

171. Kuang, W.; Tan, J.; Duan, Y.; Duan, J.; Wang, W.; Jin, F.; Jin, Z.; Yuan, X.; Liu, Y. Cyclic stretch induced miR-146a upregulation delays C2C12 myogenic differentiation through inhibition of Numb. *Biochem. Biophys. Res. Commun.* **2009**, *378*, 259–263. [CrossRef] [PubMed]

172. Forloni, M.; Dogra, S.K.; Dong, Y.; Conte, D., Jr.; Ou, J.; Zhu, L.J.; Deng, A.; Mahalingam, M.; Green, M.R.; Wajapeyee, N. miR-146a promotes the initiation and progression of melanoma by activating Notch signaling. *eLife* **2014**, *3*, e01460. [CrossRef] [PubMed]

173. Lu, J.; Steeg, P.S.; Price, J.E.; Krishnamurthy, S.; Mani, S.A.; Reuben, J.; Cristofanilli, M.; Dontu, G.; Bidaut, L.; Valero, V.; *et al.* Breast cancer metastasis: Challenges and opportunities. *Cancer Res.* **2009**, *69*, 4951–4953. [CrossRef] [PubMed]

174. Liu, H.; Patel, M.R.; Prescher, J.A.; Patsialou, A.; Qian, D.; Lin, J.; Wen, S.; Chang, Y.F.; Bachmann, M.H.; Shimono, Y.; *et al.* Cancer stem cells from human breast tumors are involved in spontaneous metastases in orthotopic mouse models. *Proc. Natl. Acad. Sci. USA* **2010**, *107*, 18115–18120. [CrossRef] [PubMed]

175. Hermann, P.C.; Huber, S.L.; Herrler, T.; Aicher, A.; Ellwart, J.W.; Guba, M.; Bruns, C.J.; Heeschen, C. Distinct populations of cancer stem cells determine tumor growth and metastatic activity in human pancreatic cancer. *Cell Stem Cell* **2007**, *1*, 313–323. [CrossRef] [PubMed]

176. Pang, R.; Law, W.L.; Chu, A.C.; Poon, J.T.; Lam, C.S.; Chow, A.K.; Ng, L.; Cheung, L.W.; Lan, X.R.; Lan, H.Y.; *et al.* A subpopulation of CD26$^+$ cancer stem cells with metastatic capacity in human colorectal cancer. *Cell Stem Cell* **2010**, *6*, 603–615. [CrossRef] [PubMed]

177. Lawson, D.A.; Bhakta, N.R.; Kessenbrock, K.; Prummel, K.D.; Yu, Y.; Takai, K.; Zhou, A.; Eyob, H.; Balakrishnan, S.; Wang, C.Y.; *et al.* Single-cell analysis reveals a stem-cell program in human metastatic breast cancer cells. *Nature* **2015**, *526*, 131–135. [CrossRef] [PubMed]

178. DeRose, Y.S.; Wang, G.; Lin, Y.C.; Bernard, P.S.; Buys, S.S.; Ebbert, M.T.; Factor, R.; Matsen, C.; Milash, B.A.; Nelson, E.; *et al.* Tumor grafts derived from women with breast cancer authentically reflect tumor pathology, growth, metastasis and disease outcomes. *Nat. Med.* **2011**, *17*, 1514–1520. [CrossRef] [PubMed]

179. Bockhorn, J.; Prat, A.; Chang, Y.F.; Liu, X.; Huang, S.; Shang, M.; Nwachukwu, C.; Gomez-Vega, M.J.; Harrell, J.C.; Olopade, O.I.; *et al.* Differentiation and loss of malignant character of spontaneous pulmonary metastases in patient-derived breast cancer models. *Cancer Res.* **2014**, *74*, 7406–7417. [CrossRef] [PubMed]

180. Nobutani, K.; Shimono, Y.; Mizutani, K.; Ueda, Y.; Suzuki, T.; Kitayama, M.; Minami, A.; Momose, K.; Miyawaki, K.; Akashi, K.; *et al.* Downregulation of CXCR4 in metastasized breast cancer cells and implication in their dormancy. *PLoS ONE* **2015**, *10*, e0130032. [CrossRef] [PubMed]

181. Nobutani, K.; Shimono, Y.; Yoshida, M.; Mizutani, K.; Minami, A.; Kono, S.; Mukohara, T.; Yamasaki, T.; Itoh, T.; Takao, S.; *et al.* Absence of primary cilia in cell cycle-arrested human breast cancer cells. *Genes Cells* **2014**, *19*, 141–152. [CrossRef] [PubMed]

182. Lin, Y.; Liu, A.Y.; Fan, C.; Zheng, H.; Li, Y.; Zhang, C.; Wu, S.; Yu, D.; Huang, Z.; Liu, F.; *et al.* MicroRNA-33b inhibits breast cancer metastasis by targeting HMGA2, SALL4 and Twist1. *Sci. Rep.* **2015**, *5*, 9995. [CrossRef] [PubMed]

183. Cuiffo, B.G.; Campagne, A.; Bell, G.W.; Lembo, A.; Orso, F.; Lien, E.C.; Bhasin, M.K.; Raimo, M.; Hanson, S.E.; Marusyk, A.; *et al.* MSC-regulated microRNAs converge on the transcription factor FOXP2 and promote breast cancer metastasis. *Cell Stem Cell* **2014**, *15*, 762–774. [CrossRef] [PubMed]

184. Wang, B.; Wang, Q.; Wang, Z.; Jiang, J.; Yu, S.C.; Ping, Y.F.; Yang, J.; Xu, S.L.; Ye, X.Z.; Xu, C.; *et al.* Metastatic consequences of immune escape from NK cell cytotoxicity by human breast cancer stem cells. *Cancer Res.* **2014**, *74*, 5746–5757. [CrossRef] [PubMed]

185. Zhang, H.; Cai, K.; Wang, J.; Wang, X.; Cheng, K.; Shi, F.; Jiang, L.; Zhang, Y.; Dou, J. miR-7, inhibited indirectly by lincRNA HOTAIR, directly inhibits SETDB1 and reverses the EMT of breast cancer stem cells by downregulating the STAT3 pathway. *Stem Cells* **2014**, *32*, 2858–2868. [CrossRef] [PubMed]
186. Hou, P.; Zhao, Y.; Li, Z.; Yao, R.; Ma, M.; Gao, Y.; Zhao, L.; Zhang, Y.; Huang, B.; Lu, J. LincRNA-ROR induces epithelial-to-mesenchymal transition and contributes to breast cancer tumorigenesis and metastasis. *Cell Death Dis.* **2014**, *5*, e1287. [CrossRef] [PubMed]
187. Thery, C.; Zitvogel, L.; Amigorena, S. Exosomes: Composition, biogenesis and function. *Nat. Rev. Immunol.* **2002**, *2*, 569–579. [PubMed]
188. Falcone, G.; Felsani, A.; D'Agnano, I. Signaling by exosomal microRNAs in cancer. *J. Exp. Clin. Cancer Res.* **2015**, *34*, 32. [CrossRef] [PubMed]
189. Tominaga, N.; Kosaka, N.; Ono, M.; Katsuda, T.; Yoshioka, Y.; Tamura, K.; Lotvall, J.; Nakagama, H.; Ochiya, T. Brain metastatic cancer cells release microRNA-181c-containing extracellular vesicles capable of destructing blood-brain barrier. *Nat. Commun.* **2015**, *6*, 6716. [CrossRef] [PubMed]
190. Le, M.T.; Hamar, P.; Guo, C.; Basar, E.; Perdigao-Henriques, R.; Balaj, L.; Lieberman, J. miR-200-containing extracellular vesicles promote breast cancer cell metastasis. *J. Clin. Invest.* **2014**, *124*, 5109–5128. [CrossRef] [PubMed]
191. Rucci, N.; Teti, A. Osteomimicry: How tumor cells try to deceive the bone. *Front. Biosci. (Schol. Ed.)* **2010**, *2*, 907–915. [CrossRef] [PubMed]
192. Croset, M.; Kan, C.; Clezardin, P. Tumour-derived miRNAs and bone metastasis. *Bonekey Rep.* **2015**, *4*, 688. [CrossRef] [PubMed]
193. Ell, B.; Kang, Y. MicroRNAs as regulators of bone homeostasis and bone metastasis. *Bonekey Rep.* **2014**, *3*, 549. [CrossRef] [PubMed]
194. Hassan, M.Q.; Maeda, Y.; Taipaleenmaki, H.; Zhang, W.; Jafferji, M.; Gordon, J.A.; Li, Z.; Croce, C.M.; van Wijnen, A.J.; Stein, J.L.; *et al.* miR-218 directs a Wnt signaling circuit to promote differentiation of osteoblasts and osteomimicry of metastatic cancer cells. *J. Biol. Chem.* **2012**, *287*, 42084–42092. [CrossRef] [PubMed]
195. Dykxhoorn, D.M.; Wu, Y.; Xie, H.; Yu, F.; Lal, A.; Petrocca, F.; Martinvalet, D.; Song, E.; Lim, B.; Lieberman, J. miR-200 enhances mouse breast cancer cell colonization to form distant metastases. *PLoS ONE* **2009**, *4*, e7181. [CrossRef] [PubMed]
196. De Smet, M.D.; Meenken, C.J.; van den Horn, G.J. Fomivirsen—A phosphorothioate oligonucleotide for the treatment of CMV retinitis. *Ocul. Immunol. Inflamm.* **1999**, *7*, 189–198. [CrossRef] [PubMed]
197. Zhang, Y.; Wang, Z.; Gemeinhart, R.A. Progress in microRNA delivery. *J. Control Release* **2013**, *172*, 962–974. [CrossRef] [PubMed]
198. Bandiera, S.; Pfeffer, S.; Baumert, T.F.; Zeisel, M.B. miR-122—A key factor and therapeutic target in liver disease. *J. Hepatol.* **2015**, *62*, 448–457. [CrossRef] [PubMed]

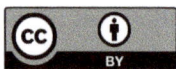

Journal of
*Clinical Medicine*

MDPI

*Review*

# microRNA-34a as a Therapeutic Agent against Human Cancer

**Yoshimasa Saito \*, Toshiaki Nakaoka and Hidetsugu Saito**

Division of Pharmacotherapeutics, Keio University Faculty of Pharmacy, 1-5-30 Shibakoen, Minato-ku, Tokyo 105-8512, Japan; toshiakinakaoka1116@gmail.com (T.N.); saito-hd@pha.keio.ac.jp (H.S.)

\* Author to whom correspondence should be addressed; saito-ys@pha.keio.ac.jp; Tel./Fax: +81-3-5400-2692.

Academic Editors: Takahiro Ochiya and Ryou-u Takahashi

Received: 20 October 2015; Accepted: 9 November 2015; Published: 16 November 2015

**Abstract:** microRNAs (miRNAs) are small non-coding RNAs that down-regulate expression of various target genes. Cancer-related miRNAs are aberrantly expressed and act as tumor suppressors or oncogenes during carcinogenesis. We and other researchers have demonstrated that important tumor suppressor miRNAs are silenced by epigenetic alterations, resulting in the activation of target oncogenes in cancer cells. miR-34a was identified as a target of p53 and induces a G1 cell cycle arrest, senescence and apoptosis in response to DNA damage. miR-34a is an important tumor suppressor whose expression is epigenetically silenced in various human cancers. Enforced expression of miR-34a induces cell cycle arrest, apoptosis, senescence, and suppression of epithelial-mesenchymal transition and inhibits cell proliferation of cancer stem cells. Epigenetic therapy with chromatin-modifying drugs such as inhibitors of DNA methylation and histone deacetylase has shown clinical promise for the treatment of malignancies. Restoring of miR-34a expression by epigenetic therapy and/or delivery of miR-34a mimics may be a promising therapeutic strategy against human cancer.

**Keywords:** microRNA; miR-34a; cancer; cancer stem cell; DNA methylation

## 1. Introduction

microRNAs (miRNAs) are 21–25 nucleotides non-coding RNAs that can post-transcriptionally down-regulate the expression of various target genes. Currently, ~2500 human miRNAs have been identified in the human genome, each of which potentially controls hundreds of target genes. miRNAs are expressed in a tissue-specific manner and play important roles in cell proliferation, apoptosis, and differentiation during mammalian development [1]. Links between miRNAs and the development of human malignancies have become apparent. Misexpression of cancer-related miRNAs leads to the initiation and progression of cancer by modulating their target oncogenes or tumor suppressor genes [2,3]. We have reported that some important tumor suppressor miRNAs are silenced by epigenetic alterations such as DNA methylation and histone modification in human cancer cells [4,5].

Accumulated evidence has clarified that cancer cells are heterogeneous with a hierarchy of "stemness" in solid cancer tissues [6]. Stem cells have the ability to perpetuate themselves through self-renewal and to generate mature cells of various tissues through differentiation. A subpopulation of cancer cells with distinct stem-like properties is responsible for tumor initiation, invasive growth, and metastasis formation, and these are defined as cancer stem cells (CSCs). As CSCs are considered to be resistant to conventional chemotherapies and radiation therapy, it would be desirable to develop a therapeutic strategy specifically targeting CSCs.

miR-34a was identified as a target of p53 and induces a G1 cell cycle arrest, senescence and apoptosis in response to DNA damage [7,8]. miR-34a is an important tumor suppressor whose expression is epigenetically silenced in various human cancers [9,10]. Enforced expression of miR-34a induces cell cycle arrest, apoptosis, senescence, suppression of epithelial-mesenchymal transition (EMT) and inhibits cell proliferation of CSCs [11]. Here we review about epigenetic silencing of miR-34a in human cancers and a therapeutic strategy targeting CSCs through up-regulating miR-34a expression.

## 2. Biogenesis and Target Genes of miR-34a

The miR-34a gene is located at the chromosome 1p36 locus. As shown in Figure 1, the miR-34a gene is transcribed from a transcription start site located in the CpG island by RNA polymerase II (pol II) to form primary transcript (pri-miR-34a). DNA hypermethylation of the CpG island promoter region is one of the most common reasons for silencing of miR-34a [9,10]. Pol II-transcribed pri-miR-34a is capped with 7-methylguanosine and is polyadenylated. The nuclear RNase III enzyme Drosha and its co-factor DGCR8 process pri-miR-34a into precursor miR-34a (pre-miR-34a), which forms an imperfect stem-loop structure. Pre-miR-34a is transported into the cytoplasm by exportin 5 and subsequently cleaved by Dicer into mature miR-34a, which is then loaded into the RNA-induced silencing complex (RISC). The miR-34a/RISC complex down-regulates specific gene products by translational repression via binding to partially complementary sequences in the 3′-untranslated regions (UTRs) of the target mRNAs such as CD44 or by directing mRNA degradation via binding to perfectly complementary sequences.

Identification of target genes of miR-34a is critical to determine its molecular function in cancer cells. A simple biochemical method to isolate mRNAs pulled down with a transfected, biotinylated miRNA was used to identify direct target genes of miR-34a [12]. Transcripts for 982 genes were enriched in the pull-down with miR-34a in K532 and HCT116 cancer cell lines, and most of them were validated as directly regulated by miR-34a. The transcripts pulled down with miR-34a were highly enriched for their roles in growth factor signaling and cell cycle progression. Thus, miR-34a is capable of regulating hundreds of genes associated with growth factor signal transduction and downstream pathways required for cell division.

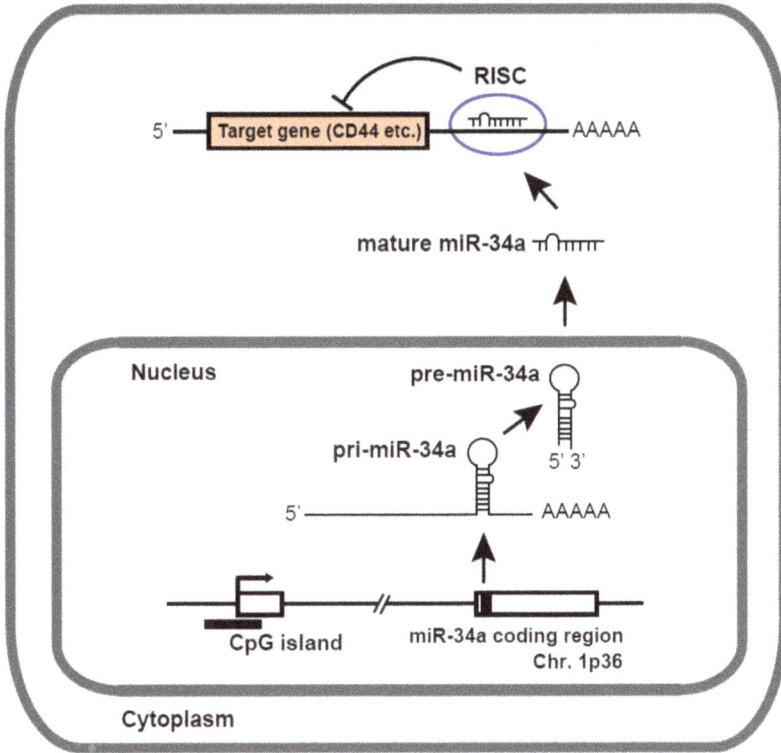

**Figure 1.** Biogenesis of miR-34a. miR-34a genes are transcribed from TSS by RNA pol II to form pri-miR-34a, which is capped with 7-methylguanosine and polyadenylated (AAAAA). Drosha and its co-factor DGCR8 process pri-miR-34a into pre-miR-34a. Pre-miR-34a is transported into the cytoplasm and subsequently cleaved by Dicer into mature miRNAs. Mature miR-34a is then loaded into RISC, where miR-34a down-regulates specific gene products by translational repression via binding to partially complementary sequences in the 3′UTR of the target mRNAs such as CD44 or by directing mRNA degradation via binding to perfectly complementary sequences.

Moreover, proteome analyses identified early targets of miR-34a that enhance tumor progression including signaling pathways such as TGF-β, WNT and mitogen-activated protein kinase (MAPK) in neuroblastoma [13]. Keller *et al.* [14] combined pulsed SILAC (Stable Isotope Labeling by Amino acids in Cell culture) and microarray analyses to identify alterations in protein and mRNA expression induced by miR-34a. This type of combined approach revealed that miR-34a plays important roles in multiple tumor-suppressive pathways by directly and indirectly suppressing the expression of numerous critical proteins.

### 3. Inactivation of miR-34a in Various Types of Cancers

miRNAs can have large-scale effects through regulation of a variety of target genes during carcinogenesis. Therefore, understanding the regulatory mechanisms controlling miRNA expression is very important. Many miRNAs are expressed in a tissue and tumor specific manner, implying that some miRNAs are under the epigenetic control. Since miR-34a is a direct target of p53, inactivating mutations of p53, increased expression of p53 inhibitors and genomic mutations at the p53-binding site in the miR-34a gene may cause loss of miR-34a expression. In addition, miR-34a resides on the chromosomal locus 1p36, which has been reported to be deleted in human malignancies. Thus, inactivation of the miR-34a gene is a common event during carcinogenesis. Recently, epigenetic inactivation of miR-34a was identified in various types of cancers. Epigenetics is an acquired modification of methylation and/or acetylation of chromatin DNA or histone proteins, which regulates downstream gene expression. Epigenetic alterations can be induced by aging, chronic inflammation, or viral infection, and aberrant DNA methylation and/or histone modification induces inactivation of tumor suppressor genes and play critical roles in the initiation and progression of human cancer [15].

We have shown that ~5% of human miRNAs are up-regulated more than three-fold by treatment of T24 bladder cancer cells with the DNA demethylating agent 5-aza-2′-deoxycytidine (5-Aza-CdR) and the histone deacetylase (HDAC) inhibitor 4-phenylbutyric acid (PBA). In particular, miR-127, which is embedded in a CpG island, is remarkably induced by a decrease in DNA methylation levels and an increase in active histone marks around the promoter region of the miR-127 gene. In addition, activation of miR-127 by epigenetic treatment induced down-regulation of its target oncogene BCL6 [4,5]. We have also demonstrated that treatment of gastric cancer cells with 5-Aza-CdR and PBA induces activation of miR-512-5p which is located at Alu repeats on chromosome 19. Activation of miR-512-5p by epigenetic treatment induces suppression of MCL1, resulting in apoptosis of gastric cancer cells [16]. These results indicate that chromatin remodeling by epigenetic therapy can directly activate miRNA expression and re-activation of silenced tumor suppressor miRNAs could be a novel therapeutic approach for human cancers.

A recent study has demonstrated that expression of the tumor suppressor miR-34a is silenced in breast, lung, colon, kidney, bladder and pancreatic cancers as well as melanoma due to aberrant CpG methylation of its promoter region [9]. Re-expression of miR-34a in cancer cell lines induced senescence and cell cycle arrest at least in part by targeting CDK6, indicating that miR-34a represents a tumor suppressor gene which is inactivated by CpG methylation in multiple types of cancer [9]. Epigenetic silencing of miR-34a via DNA hypermethylation of its promoter region is also observed in hematological malignancies such as non-Hodgikin's lymphoma [10]. The other miR-34 family members, miR-34b and miR-34c, are also reported to be silenced by aberrant CpG island methylation in colorectal cancer [17].

Long, non-coding RNAs (lncRNAs) are important new members of the non-coding RNA family that are greater than 200 nt without protein coding ability. The lncRNA HOX antisense intergenic RNA (HOTAIR) is overexpressed in various malignancies including colon, pancreatic and breast cancer. HOTAIR epigenetically silenced miR-34a expression by recruiting the polycomb repressive complex 2 (PRC2), which results in promotion of epithelial-mesenchymal transition (EMT) in gastric cancer cells [18].

## 4. Biological Effects of miR-34a in CSCs

Since miR-34a suppresses many oncogenes and cancer stem cell markers including CD44, CDK4, CDK6, c-Met, Notch-1, Notch-2, SIRT1 and DLL1 as its target genes [11,19–21], miR-34a plays important roles in cancer stem cells. The direct targets and biological effects of miR-34a in various CSCs are summarized in Figure 2.

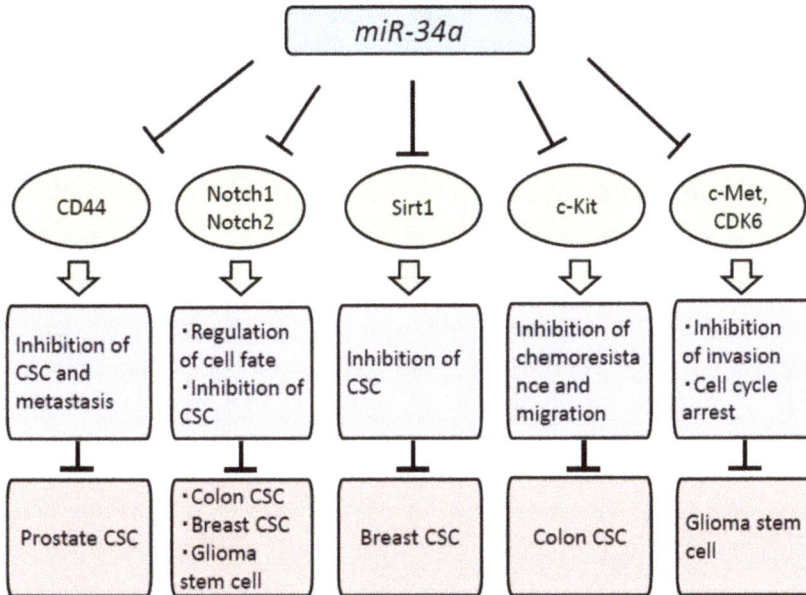

**Figure 2.** Biological effects of miR-34a in CSCs. The direct targets and biological effects of miR-34a in various CSCs are summarized; CSC; cancer stem cell.

CD44 is one of the important stem cell markers and was validated as a direct and functional target of miR-34a. Enforced expression of miR-34a inhibited prostate cancer stem cells and metastasis by directly repressing CD44, indicating that miR-34a is a key negative regulator of prostate CSCs and could be a novel therapeutic agent against prostate cancers [11]. Notch1 is also an important target of miR-34a and involved in the maintenance and self-renewal of CSCs. miR-34a plays as a cell-fate determinant in early-stage dividing colon CSCs [22] and inhibits breast CSCs and glioma stem cells by regulating Notch1 [23,24]. Gliomas are the most common tumors of central nervous system. The transformation to a glioma stem cell state is involved in aberrant expression of miRNAs including miR-34a. miR-34a suppresses cell proliferation and tumor growth of glioma stem cells by targeting Rictor through its effects on AKT/mTOR pathway and Wnt signaling [25].

Recent studies have revealed that enforced expression of miR-34a suppresses cell proliferation of lung CSCs, colon CSCs, malignant mesothelioma cells and breast CSCs by targeting Arhgap1, c-Kit, c-Met and Sirt1, respectively [26–29]. These findings indicate that miR-34a is a promising therapeutic agent targeting various CSCs through down-regulation of target oncogenes and stem cell markers.

### 5. miR-34a Is a Promising Therapeutic Agent against Human Cancer

Chromatin-modifying drugs such as DNA methylation inhibitors and HDAC inhibitors have shown clinical promise for cancer therapy [15,30]. The DNA methylation inhibitor 5-Aza-CdR, which is an analog of cytidine, has been widely studied and was recently approved for the treatment of myelodysplastic syndrome (MDS). The HDAC inhibitor suberoylanilide hydroxamic acid (SAHA) has been approved for patients with cutaneous T-cell lymphoma. Other inhibitors of DNA methylation and HDAC are also in clinical trials.

A promising option for cancer therapy is the use of epigenetic drugs which inhibit tumor growth via several mechanisms, including restoring the expression of epigenetically silenced miR-34a. Inhibitors of DNA methylation and histone deacetylation can work synergistically to suppress the growth of cancer cells. Many epigenetic drugs have shown promising results in clinical trials and recent advances in research suggest a new anticancer effect from this class of drugs. By inducing miR-34a expression, epigenetic therapy not only inhibits the growth of cancers, but may also inhibit the invasiveness and metastatic potential of CSCs. Re-expression of miR-34a by treatment with 5-Aza-CdR and SAHA strongly inhibited cell proliferation, cell cycle progression, self-renewal, EMT and invasion in pancreatic CSCs [31]. Further studies are necessary to develop chromatin-modifying drugs that specifically affect only the CpG island promoter region of miR-34a to reduce the side effects of epigenetic therapy.

Another option for restoring miR-34a expression is replacement therapy using miR-34a mimics. The concept of this therapy is to restore miR-34a expression in cancers to a comparable level to surrounding non-cancer tissues. A recent study has shown that systemic delivery of miR-34a mimics using a neutral lipid emulsion inhibits lung tumors in mice [32]. Mirna Therapeutics (http://www.mirnatherapeutics.com/) is developing MRX34, a mimic of naturally occurring miR-34a encapsulated in liposomal nanoparticle formulation. This has shown preliminary clinical evidence of anti-tumor activity in a Phase 1 clinical trial (NCT01829971). Tissue-specific delivery and cellular uptake of sufficient amounts of synthetic oligonucleotides to achieve sustained target inhibition are very important issues. In particular, biological instability of oligonucleotides in tissues and poor cellular uptake need to be resolved to make miRNA-based therapy successful. Since miRNAs have the ability to simultaneously regulate several cellular pathways, this multi-target property of miRNAs might potentially result in off-target side effects. We have to be careful about these potential side effects for future clinical applications of miRNA-based therapy.

## 6. Conclusions

The tumor suppressor miR-34a plays important roles in the initiation and progression of various types of human malignancies by down-regulating target oncogenes and CSC markers. Restoring of miR-34a expression through epigenetic therapy with inhibitors of DNA methylation and HDAC and/or delivery of miR-34a mimics could be a powerful cancer therapy targeting CSCs. Further studies are needed to develop chromatin-modifying drugs that specifically affect the miR-34a gene and miR-34a mimics that have anti-tumor activity with reduced side effects.

**Conflicts of Interest:** The authors declare no conflict of interest.

## References

1. He, L.; Hannon, G.J. microRNA: Small RNAs with a big role in gene regulation. *Nat. Rev. Genet.* **2004**, *5*, 522–531. [CrossRef] [PubMed]
2. Calin, G.A.; Croce, C.M. microRNA signatures in human cancers. *Nat. Rev. Cancer* **2006**, *6*, 857–866. [CrossRef] [PubMed]
3. Croce, C.M. Causes and consequences of microRNA dysregulation in cancer. *Nat. Rev. Genet.* **2009**, *10*, 704–714. [CrossRef] [PubMed]
4. Saito, Y.; Liang, G.; Egger, G.; Friedman, J.M.; Chuang, J.C.; Coetzee, G.A.; Jones, P.A. Specific activation of microRNA-127 with down regulation of the proto-oncogene BCL6 by chromatin-modifying drugs in human cancer cells. *Cancer Cell* **2006**, *9*, 435–443. [CrossRef] [PubMed]
5. Saito, Y.; Jones, P.A. Epigenetic activation of tumor suppressor microRNAs in human cancer cells. *Cell Cycle* **2006**, *5*, 2220–2222. [CrossRef] [PubMed]
6. Clevers, H. The cancer stem cell: Premises, promises and challenges. *Nat. Med.* **2011**, *17*, 313–319. [CrossRef] [PubMed]
7. Raver-Shapira, N.; Marciano, E.; Meiri, E.; Spector, Y.; Rosenfeld, N.; Moskovits, N.; Bentwich, Z.; Oren, M. Transcriptional activation of miR-34a contributes to p53-mediated apoptosis. *Mol. Cell* **2007**, *26*, 731–743. [CrossRef] [PubMed]
8. He, L.; He, X.; Lim, L.P.; de Stanchina, E.; Xuan, Z.; Liang, Y.; Xue, W.; Zender, L.; Magnus, J.; Ridzon, D.; *et al.* A microRNA component of the p53 tumour suppressor network. *Nature* **2007**, *447*, 1130–1134. [CrossRef] [PubMed]

9.  Lodygin, D.; Tarasov, V.; Epanchintsev, A.; Berking, C.; Knyazeva, T.; Korner, H.; Knyazev, P.; Diebold, J.; Hermeking, H. Inactivation of miR-34 by aberrant CpG methylation in multiple types of cancer. *Cell Cycle* **2008**, *7*, 2591–2600. [CrossRef] [PubMed]
10. Chim, C.S.; Wong, K.Y.; Qi, Y.; Loong, F.; Lam, W.L.; Wong, L.G.; Jin, D.Y.; Costello, J.F.; Liang, R. Epigenetic inactivation of the miR-34a in hematological malignancies. *Carcinogenesis* **2010**, *31*, 745–750. [CrossRef] [PubMed]
11. Liu, C.; Kelnar, K.; Liu, B.; Chen, X.; Calhoun-Davis, T.; Li, H.; Patrawala, L.; Yan, H.; Jeter, C.; Honorio, S.; *et al.* The microRNA miR-34a inhibits prostate cancer stem cells and metastasis by directly repressing cd44. *Nat. Med.* **2011**, *17*, 211–215. [CrossRef] [PubMed]
12. Lal, A.; Thomas, M.P.; Altschuler, G.; Navarro, F.; O'Day, E.; Li, X.L.; Concepcion, C.; Han, Y.C.; Thiery, J.; Rajani, D.K.; *et al.* Capture of microRNA-bound mRNAs identifies the tumor suppressor miR-34a as a regulator of growth factor signaling. *PLoS Genet.* **2011**, *7*, e1002363. [CrossRef] [PubMed]
13. De Antonellis, P.; Carotenuto, M.; Vandenbussche, J.; de Vita, G.; Ferrucci, V.; Medaglia, C.; Boffa, I.; Galiero, A.; di Somma, S.; Magliulo, D.; *et al.* Early targets of miR-34 in neuroblastoma. *Mol. Cell. Proteom.* **2014**, *13*, 2114–2131. [CrossRef] [PubMed]
14. Kaller, M.; Liffers, S.T.; Oeljeklaus, S.; Kuhlmann, K.; Roh, S.; Hoffmann, R.; Warscheid, B.; Hermeking, H. Genome-wide characterization of miR-34 induced changes in protein and mRNA expression by a combined pulsed SILAC and microarray analysis. *Mol. Cell. Proteom.* **2011**, *10*. [CrossRef] [PubMed]
15. Gal-Yam, E.N.; Saito, Y.; Egger, G.; Jones, P.A. Cancer epigenetics: Modifications, screening, and therapy. *Annu. Rev. Med.* **2008**, *59*, 267–280. [PubMed]
16. Saito, Y.; Suzuki, H.; Tsugawa, H.; Nakagawa, I.; Matsuzaki, J.; Kanai, Y.; Hibi, T. Chromatin remodeling at Alu repeats by epigenetic treatment activates silenced *microRNA-512-5p* with downregulation of *mcl-1* in human gastric cancer cells. *Oncogene* **2009**, *28*, 2738–2744. [CrossRef] [PubMed]
17. Toyota, M.; Suzuki, H.; Sasaki, Y.; Maruyama, R.; Imai, K.; Shinomura, Y.; Tokino, T. Epigenetic silencing of *microRNA-34b/c* and B-cell translocation *gene 4* is associated with CpG island methylation in colorectal cancer. *Cancer Res.* **2008**, *68*, 4123–4132. [CrossRef] [PubMed]
18. Liu, Y.W.; Sun, M.; Xia, R.; Zhang, E.B.; Liu, X.H.; Zhang, Z.H.; Xu, T.P.; De, W.; Liu, B.R.; Wang, Z.X. Linc*HOTAIR* epigenetically silences miR34a by binding to PRC2 to promote the epithelial-to-mesenchymal transition in human gastric cancer. *Cell Death Dis.* **2015**, *6*, e1802. [CrossRef] [PubMed]
19. Hermeking, H. The miR-34 family in cancer and apoptosis. *Cell Death Differ.* **2010**, *17*, 193–199. [CrossRef] [PubMed]
20. Chen, F.; Hu, S.J. Effect of microRNA-34a in cell cycle, differentiation, and apoptosis: A review. *J. Biochem. Mol. Toxicol.* **2012**, *26*, 79–86. [CrossRef] [PubMed]
21. De Antonellis, P.; Medaglia, C.; Cusanelli, E.; Andolfo, I.; Liguori, L.; De Vita, G.; Carotenuto, M.; Bello, A.; Formiggini, F.; Galeone, A.; *et al.* miR-34a targeting of notch ligand delta-like 1 impairs cd15+/cd133+ tumor-propagating cells and supports neural differentiation in medulloblastoma. *PLoS ONE* **2011**, *6*, e24584. [CrossRef] [PubMed]
22. Bu, P.; Chen, K.Y.; Chen, J.H.; Wang, L.; Walters, J.; Shin, Y.J.; Goerger, J.P.; Sun, J.; Witherspoon, M.; Rakhilin, N.; *et al.* A microRNA miR-34a-regulated bimodal switch targets notch in colon cancer stem cells. *Cell Stem Cell* **2013**, *12*, 602–615. [CrossRef] [PubMed]
23. Kang, L.; Mao, J.; Tao, Y.; Song, B.; Ma, W.; Lu, Y.; Zhao, L.; Li, J.; Yang, B.; Li, L. microRNA-34a suppresses the breast cancer stem cell-like characteristics by downregulating notch1 pathway. *Cancer Sci.* **2015**, *106*, 700–708. [CrossRef] [PubMed]
24. Li, Y.; Guessous, F.; Zhang, Y.; Dipierro, C.; Kefas, B.; Johnson, E.; Marcinkiewicz, L.; Jiang, J.; Yang, Y.; Schmittgen, T.D.; *et al.* MicroRNA-34a inhibits glioblastoma growth by targeting multiple oncogenes. *Cancer Res.* **2009**, *69*, 7569–7576. [CrossRef] [PubMed]
25. Rathod, S.S.; Rani, S.B.; Khan, M.; Muzumdar, D.; Shiras, A. Tumor suppressive miRNA-34a suppresses cell proliferation and tumor growth of glioma stem cells by targeting Akt and Wnt signaling pathways. *FEBS Open Bio.* **2014**, *4*, 485–495. [CrossRef] [PubMed]
26. Ahn, Y.H.; Gibbons, D.L.; Chakravarti, D.; Creighton, C.J.; Rizvi, Z.H.; Adams, H.P.; Pertsemlidis, A.; Gregory, P.A.; Wright, J.A.; Goodall, G.J.; *et al.* ZEB1 drives prometastatic actin cytoskeletal remodeling by downregulating miR-34a expression. *J. Clin. Invest.* **2012**, *122*, 3170–3183. [CrossRef] [PubMed]

27. Siemens, H.; Jackstadt, R.; Kaller, M.; Hermeking, H. Repression of c-kit by p53 is mediated by miR-34 and is associated with reduced chemoresistance, migration and stemness. *Oncotarget* **2013**, *4*, 1399–1415. [CrossRef] [PubMed]

28. Menges, C.W.; Kadariya, Y.; Altomare, D.; Talarchek, J.; Neumann-Domer, E.; Wu, Y.; Xiao, G.H.; Shapiro, I.M.; Kolev, V.N.; Pachter, J.A.; *et al.* Tumor suppressor alterations cooperate to drive aggressive mesotheliomas with enriched cancer stem cells via a p53-miR-34a-c-Met axis. *Cancer Res.* **2014**, *74*, 1261–1271. [CrossRef] [PubMed]

29. Ma, W.; Xiao, G.G.; Mao, J.; Lu, Y.; Song, B.; Wang, L.; Fan, S.; Fan, P.; Hou, Z.; Li, J.; *et al.* Dysregulation of the miR-34a-SIRT1 axis inhibits breast cancer stemness. *Oncotarget* **2015**, *6*, 10432–10444. [CrossRef] [PubMed]

30. Yoo, C.B.; Jones, P.A. Epigenetic therapy of cancer: Past, present and future. *Nat. Rev. Drug Discov.* **2006**, *5*, 37–50. [CrossRef] [PubMed]

31. Nalls, D.; Tang, S.N.; Rodova, M.; Srivastava, R.K.; Shankar, S. Targeting epigenetic regulation of mir-34a for treatment of pancreatic cancer by inhibition of pancreatic cancer stem cells. *PLoS ONE* **2011**, *6*, e24099. [CrossRef] [PubMed]

32. Trang, P.; Wiggins, J.F.; Daige, C.L.; Cho, C.; Omotola, M.; Brown, D.; Weidhaas, J.B.; Bader, A.G.; Slack, F.J. Systemic delivery of tumor suppressor microRNA mimics using a neutral lipid emulsion inhibits lung tumors in mice. *Mol. Therapy* **2011**, *19*, 1116–1122. [CrossRef] [PubMed]

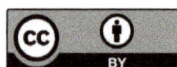

Journal of
*Clinical Medicine*

MDPI

*Review*

# Circulating microRNA Biomarkers as Liquid Biopsy for Cancer Patients: Pros and Cons of Current Assays

Shigeshi Ono, Stella Lam, Makoto Nagahara and Dave S. B. Hoon *

Department of Molecular Oncology, John Wayne Cancer Institute, Providence Saint John's Health Center, 2200 Santa Monica Blvd., Santa Monica, CA 90404, USA; onos@jwci.org (S.O.); lams@jwci.org (S.L.); Nagahara.srg2@tmd.ac.jp (M.N.)

* Author to whom correspondence should be addressed; hoond@jwci.org; Tel.: +1-310-449-5267.

Academic Editors: Takahiro Ochiya and Ryou-u Takahashi
Received: 7 July 2015; Accepted: 9 October 2015; Published: 23 October 2015

**Abstract:** An increasing number of studies have focused on circulating microRNAs (cmiRNA) in cancer patients' blood for their potential as minimally-invasive biomarkers. Studies have reported the utility of assessing specific miRNAs in blood as diagnostic/prognostic biomarkers; however, the methodologies are not validated or standardized across laboratories. Unfortunately, there is often minimum limited overlap in techniques between results reported even in similar type studies on the same cancer. This hampers interpretation and reliability of cmiRNA as potential cancer biomarkers. Blood collection and processing, cmiRNA extractions, quality and quantity control of assays, defined patient population assessment, reproducibility, and reference standards all affect the cmiRNA assay results. To date, there is no reported definitive method to assess cmiRNAs. Therefore, appropriate and reliable methodologies are highly necessary in order for cmiRNAs to be used in regulated clinical diagnostic laboratories. In this review, we summarize the developments made over the past decade towards cmiRNA detection and discuss the pros and cons of the assays.

**Keywords:** circulating microRNA; blood; cancer patients; diagnosis; prognosis; circulating nucleic acids; next-generation sequencing

## 1. Introduction

MicroRNAs (miRNAs) are small, single-stranded non-coding RNA sequences of about 18–22 nucleotides that interact with specific target mRNAs [1–5]. They are known to have important roles at post-transcriptional and translational levels. It is estimated that miRNAs regulate approximately one third of the human protein-coding genome [6].

One of the first reports suggesting a role of miRNAs in cancer was published in 2002 [7]. Takamizawa *et al.* later demonstrated the prognostic value of miRNAs by showing that let-7 expression was decreased in lung cancer and the direct correlation between low let-7 expression levels and poor survival in lung cancer patients [8]. In 2005, Calin *et al.* reported the first study showing the diagnostic/prognostic importance of miRNAs at the genome-wide level [9]. Croce *et al.* reported that certain tumor-associated miRNAs were expressed by cancer-related regions, exhibiting DNA amplification, deletion or translocation during tumor growth [10]. These pioneer studies suggest the potential of miRNA expression utilized as biomarkers for cancer diagnosis and prognosis in tissues [11].

Current techniques for cancer diagnosis commonly require a biopsy of the cancer tissue. In addition to the invasive nature of this procedure, it is not always clinically feasible and is also associated with morbidity; thus, several studies have focused on the search for molecular circulating cell-free nucleic acids as cancer-biomarkers in human body fluids, such as in plasma and serum [12]. The field of circulating cell-free tumor DNA (ctDNA) in cancer patients has grown over the past two decades [13] and certain assays have entered the clinic as CLIA assays [14]. Circulating tumor cells (CTCs) have also been promising as blood biomarkers [15]. Weber *et al.* reported miRNAs were present in all of the 12 body fluids assessed, including plasma, urine, saliva, peritoneal fluid, pleural fluid, seminal fluid, tears, amniotic fluid, breast milk, bronchial lavage, cerebrospinal fluid, and colostrum [16], although Watson *et al.* later reported major concerns about these results [17]. Nevertheless, since discovering the existence of circulating miRNA (cmiRNA) in body fluids, the non-invasive "liquid biopsy" has been featured as a promising blood biomarker assay in various cancers. The notable stability and simple handling of cmiRNAs may make this a more suitable biomarkers-detection technique, compared to other molecular blood biomarkers, mainly due to its stability in room temperature [18–20]. Recently, Montani *et al.* have reported the value of cmiRNA for detecting early lung cancer [21], which suggests the utility of cmiRNAs for predicting not only disease prognosis but also screening of healthy individuals. Generally, miRNA levels are non-specific and associated with a wide range of conditions and outcomes. Unfortunately, there are few overlapping reports amongst the findings of relatively similar studies of the same cancer. Methodological inconsistency has been thought to be one of the reasons for this irregularity [22,23]. As of now, there is no robust, consistent, and accurate approach for measuring cmiRNA expression in plasma and serum, rendering its clinical application difficult (Table 1). Optimizing the standardization of cmiRNA is essential for the assays to be informative in the clinic for patient decision making.

In this review, we summarize the application as well as the pros and cons of various detection methods and the quantification of cmiRNAs.

**Table 1.** Examples of various methodologies for circulating microRNAs (cmiRNA).

| Types of Cancer | Source | Anticoagulant | Volume (mL) | Isolation Method | Controls | Detection Method | References |
|---|---|---|---|---|---|---|---|
| Diffuse large B-cell lymphoma | Serum | N/A | 2 | TRIzol | miR-16 | RT-qPCR | [24] |
| Prostate | Serum/Plasma | EDTA | 10 | mirVana PARIS | Cel-miRs | RT-qPCR pre-amp | [18] |
| NSCLC* | Serum/Plasma | Heparin | 0.1 | Total RNA purification kit | Cel-miRs | RT-qPCR | [25] |
| NSCLC* | Serum | N/A | 0.5 | mirVana PARIS | dCt matrix | RT-qPCR | [26] |
| NSCLC* | Serum | N/A | 50 | TRIzol | Normalization to total RNA | RT-qPCR, sequencing | [27] |
| NSCLC* | Plasma EV | U | 3 | Dynabeads mirVana PARIS | miR-142-3p,-30b | RT-qPCR | [28] |
| Lung | Plasma | EDTA | 0.2 | mirVana PARIS | RNU-6B | Microarray; RT-qPCR | [29] |
| HCC** | Plasma | U | 0.25 | miRNeasy | U6 snRNA; cel-miR-39 | RT-qPCR TLDA cards A and B | [30] |
| Head and Neck | Plasma | EDTA | 0.3 | mirVana miRNA isolation kit | Cel-miR-39 | TaqMan Array RT-qPCR | [31] |
| Gastric | Plasma | N/A | N/A | miRNeasy Mini kit | Cel-miR-39 | RT-qPCR | [32] |
| HCC** | Plasma | N/A | N/A | N/A | miR-1228 | RT-qPCR microarrays | [33] |
| RCC*** | Serum | N/A | 0.4 | mirVana PARIS Kit | Cel-miR-39 | RT-qPCR | [34] |
| Breast | Serum | N/A | N/A | N/A | miR-16 | RT-qPCR-DS | [35] |
| Melanoma | Plasma | Sodium citrate | 0.01 | N/A | N/A | RT-qPCR-DP | [36] |
| Multiple myeloma | Serum | N/A | N/A | N/A | N/A | NanoString, RT-qPCR | [37] |

\* non-small cell lung cancer; ** hepatocellular carcinoma; *** renal cell carcinoma.

## 2. Blood Collection and Processing

Optimal conditions for collecting and processing blood specimens for cmiRNA assessment are yet to be determined. To prevent normal cell-derived miRNA contamination derived from the puncture site, discarding the first several ml of blood is important [38]. Blood must be processed within a few hours of collection to restrict contaminating levels of miRNA expression derived from lysed red blood cells, platelets, leukocytes, and circulating tumor cells in the cancer patients blood [39]. However, this is dependent on the type of blood collection tube used. Here we discuss the importance of utilization of appropriate blood collection tubes, which affects miRNA detection in both plasma and serum. Although previous approaches favored plasma for cmiRNA assessment, availability of newer types of blood collection tubes has made serum an alternative, albeit the more optimal fluid of the two remains a debatable topic. Nonetheless, serum contains more contaminating non-specific normal blood cell miRNA that may interfere with results' specificity and interpretations.

Blood collected for cmiRNA analysis is usually processed as plasma or serum. The debate over which type is the best, remains ongoing, however, serum is known to have more non-specific cmiRNA due to the presence of cell-secreted clotting factors. Plasma is collected in tubes containing standard blood anticoagulants, including heparin, EDTA, or sodium citrate followed by centrifugation. Serum collection is derived from blood tubes without anticoagulants. Based on previous reports, there is little difference in miRNA quantification through plasma *vs* serum [18,40,41]. However, higher concentrations of some miRNA were found in serum [42], while higher levels of other miRNA were detected in plasma collected in EDTA-containing tubes [43]. This may be due to assay specificity and sensitivity issues. Recently, contaminating platelets, which contain a wide spectrum of miRNAs, are also considered to contaminate cmiRNA detection [44,45]. Moreover, anti-platelet therapy is reported to affect cmiRNA expression derived from platelets [46]. Together, these reports necessitate the development of standard protocols for blood specimen collection and processing, as well as disclosure of detailed patients' clinical information in reports. Many of the discrepancies in results can be attributed to this early step in the process.

The duration and temperature conditions from the time of blood draw until the actual processing will influence miRNA levels. miRNA is more stable than DNA and mRNA, yet cryopreservation of plasma and serum must remain at −80 °C or below to prevent its potential degradation in long-term storage. Among the anticoagulant reagents for plasma, heparin is known to inhibit the reverse-transcriptase and polymerase enzymes used in PCR [47] and selectively affect the quantification of cmiRNAs in blood samples [48,49]. Heparinase treatment prior to reverse transcription quantitative-PCR (RT-qPCR) is effective, albeit its possible incomplete deactivation reduces RNA yield [50], therefore we believe the use of heparin must be avoided. Sodium citrate may also affect PCR result [51]; collection tubes containing EDTA were recommended over sodium citrate for miRNA assays by Fichtlschere *et al.* [52]; nonetheless, Kim *et al.* reported sodium citrate improved the sensitivity of miRNA detection compared with EDTA [50]. Currently, there is no single definitive reliable approach to processing blood for cmiRNA assays; to that end, detailed description of blood collection and processing methods in scientific publication must be reported. The Cell-Free DNA BCT® (Streck, Omaha, NE, USA) plasma collector tubes for cfDNA such as in the FDA approved prenatal testing maybe optimal as they have been quite reliable for blood cfNA tests.

## 3. RNA Extraction Methods: Quantity and Quality Assessment of cmiRNA

### 3.1. RNA Extraction

Phenol-chloroform based methods, such as Trizol, which contains phenol and guanidinium thiocyanate, are sufficient [53]. Due to the small size of the miRNA molecules, overnight precipitation is necessary to efficiently recover the miRNA [45]. Small RNA molecules with low GC frequency are known to be selectively lost when using Trizol, especially when a small amount of blood was analyzed [54]. Currently most RNA and miRNA extractions are performed using a phenol-chloroform

*J. Clin. Med.* **2015**, *4*, 1890–1907

based extraction technique that requires a large sample volume [55,56]. One major existing issue in RNA extraction from blood is the formation of a large aqueous phase, caused by the addition of Trizol and the subsequent centrifugation. The amount of the aqueous phase is dependent on the ratio of Trizol to sample, but reducing the ratio will result in denaturation of proteins. In addition to the plasma or serum volume processed, this is the most inconsistent step reported in protocols. Unfortunately, most studies do not report the yield of cmiRNA recovered from each specific condition, which makes determining the efficiency of these extraction protocols difficult. The most significant obstacle to cmiRNA extraction is its small size, hence easily lost during the extraction and purification procedures.

Moreover, cmiRNAs are not only present in exosomes [57], but are also bound to blood proteins and lipids [35,36]; this creates a problem in interpreting total cmiRNA yields and depending on the isolation method utilized, can cause variabilities in the yield. cmiRNAs associated to exosomes can be found in microvesicles, whereas cmiRNAs bound to protein like Ago2 can be found in serum/plasma [57]. These cmiRNAs are protected from RNases in vesicles. Differential ultracentrifugation helps purify the different types of extracellular vesicles and ribonucleoprotein complex in serum/plasma [44,58]. But establishing the size and morphology requires other methods such as electron microscopy or size exclusion chromatography. It is suggested that a large portion of cmiRNAs are associated to protein bound complexes such as Ago2 which helps prevent degradation [57]. cmiRNAs in vesicles possibly have a function in cell-to-cell communication. Proteases and detergents are often employed to release bound cmiRNA [35]. The inconsistency of retrieval levels of cmiRNA from plasma and serum is problematic in regards to the amount of cmiRNA bound and must be carefully addressed. Thus, when reporting total cmiRNA one has to be careful of the extraction procedure and bound miRNA actually obtained. This is a problem and not yet resolved in the actual reporting of cmiRNA using various assays. True comparative analyses have not been well analyzed.

Recently, several miRNA extraction kits have become commercially available for research (Table 2). The recovery rate from total RNA isolation is dependent on the optimized procedures and volumes. Several manufacturers have utilized their own specific strategies and proprietary reagents for this purpose. MiRCURY™ RNA Isolation Kit (Exiqon, Denmark) which indicates miRNA can be isolated from biofluids, including blood; however, *mir*Vana™ PARIS™ (Life Technologies, Grand Island, NY, USA) and miRNeasy® (Qiagen, Venlo, Limburg, Belgium) are more widely used for cmiRNA assays. Most studies do not mention the actual yield and quality of cmiRNA, which makes direct comparisons of these kits challenging. There are also several non-standard assays designed by individual laboratory groups and published, none have been validated. The accuracy of cmiRNA yields are important, since without it, identifying false negative results is virtually impossible. Therefore the yield of cmiRNA and quality need to be performed with accurate assays that are reproducible and robust. See below on various approaches to address this problem.

**Table 2.** Commercially available miRNA extraction kit.

| Kit | Company | Sample Type | Remarks |
|---|---|---|---|
| mirVana™ PARIS™ Kit | Life technologies (Carlsbad, CA, USA) | Tissues, Cells | Protein can be isolated from the same sample |
| miRNeasy® Mini Kit | QIAGEN (Venlo, Limburg, Blegium) | Tissues, Cells | |
| miRCURY™ RNA Isolation Kits | EXIQON (Vedbaek, Denmark) | *Biofluids*, Tissues, Cells, FFPE | Biofluids can be used as sources |
| mirPremier™ microRNA Isolation Kit | SIGMA-ALDRICH (St. Louis, MO, USA) | Tissues, Cells | No phenol and chloroform |
| miRNA Isolation Kit | FAVORGEN (Ping-Tung, Taiwan) | Tissues, Cells | No large RNA |
| MasterPure™ RNA Purification Kit | Epicenter (Madison, WI, USA) | Tissues, Cells | No spin column, No phenol and chloroform |
| microRNA Isolation Kit, Human Ago2 | Wako (Osaka, Japan) | Tissues, Cells | IP* with human anti-Ago2 Ab |
| miRNA Purification & Isolation Kit | Takara/Clontech (Shiga, Japan) | Tissues, Cells | Protein can be isolated from the same sample. |

Another existing challenge in clinical utility of cmiRNA is the sample size of both patients and healthy controls, which can invalidate assay result interpretations. A universal standardization of scientific data reporting is essential; by more clearly defining the parameters of the "Methods" section to implement particular requirements, such as the demographics details of the normal control samples to be compared, and the quantitation of the cmiRNA extracted. Scientific Journals can resolve the existing inconsistency in reporting and comparisons. Although many studies are reporting the presence of certain cmiRNA in cancer patients, it has been noted that several of these cmiRNAs are also elevated in healthy individuals and individuals with benign inflammatory diseases; since levels of cmiRNA vary based on gender, age, and health status (non-cancer), there has been much confusion in the literature that have reported particular cmiRNA as cancer blood biomarkers, although they are present in widely fluctuating levels in healthy individuals. The solution is to assess particular cmiRNAs used as cancer biomarkers in large normal control populations with well-defined representative demographics as mentioned above.

### 3.2. Quantity and Quality Assessment of miRNA

There are several methods for assessing the quality and quantity of extracted RNA, including spectrophotometric analysis; however, determination of the ratio of miRNA to total RNA is challenging, since the absorbance for extraction solutions can interfere with assessing the nucleic acids. This may lead to an over estimation of cmiRNA quantity. Thus, it is difficult to distinguish mature miRNA from other small RNAs, including precursor miRNAs. In this aspect, several studies recommend using a fixed volume of serum/plasma, rather than a fixed miRNA amount for RT-qPCR [18,59]. Measurement of miRNA concentration is cumbersome, thus fixed amount of serum/plasma may be more efficient to assess the miRNA expression. Recently, we have demonstrated the efficacy of employing a small amount of serum and plasma for a direct (no extraction from serum/plasma) cmiRNA assay (<50 μL) [36,60]. Additionally, in our preliminary findings, we showed that miR-107 in stage III melanoma patients' plasma is a biomarker for disease-free survival (DFS) (Figure 1A). We also assessed breast patients' serum of different AJCC stages, and showed miR-21, miR-29b and miR-210 to increase during tumor progression (Figure 1B–D). These methods eliminate the potential loss of cmiRNA during the extraction procedure, and the need to consider the miRNA ratio to total RNA. This approach also provides a more robust way to analyze cmiRNA analysis and easier to perform in a clinical laboratory routinely. In addition to cmiRNA loss prevention, this direct assay proves to reduce the complexity and increase the efficiency of cmiRNA assessment [36].

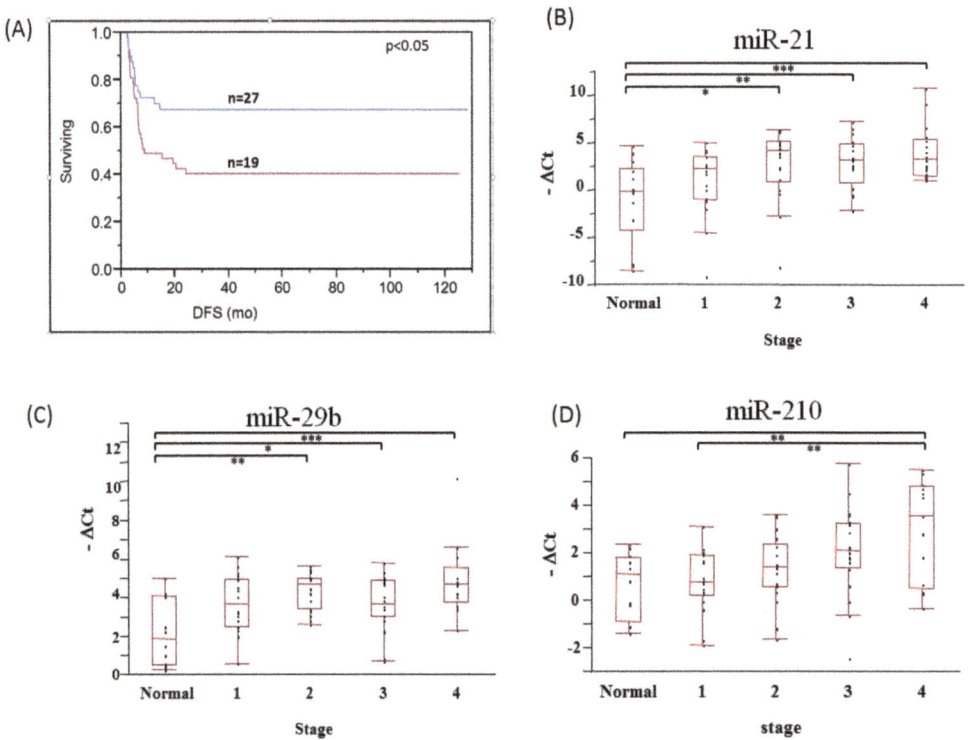

**Figure 1.** Direct cmiRNA assay of cancer patients (**A**) A level of miR-107 (50th percentile) in bleeds using direct cmRNA assay, taken at Day 0 significantly predict DFS. High levels predict worst prognosis; (**B–D**) Comparison of relative miRNA levels of breast cancer patients and normal samples in serum using a direct cmiRNA assay. The distribution chart shows each cmiRNA levels derived from normal samples *vs.* each AJCC stage.

As previously mentioned, quantitation of extracted cmiRNA can be difficult due to its low amounts. Agilent Technologies 2100 Bioanalyzer (Agilent, Santa Clara, CA, USA), which utilizes capillary electrophoresis, has been successful in assessing miRNA quantities [61]. This method provides RNA integrity number (RIN) to demonstrate miRNA quality; however, it still cannot discern precursor and mature miRNAs. A low RIN sample is considered not to be appropriate for microarray or NGS, but sufficient for RT-qPCR. RNA degradation is not as limiting for RT-qPCR as it is for NGSD and microarray analysis [62]. We consider a RIN below 8.0 to be too low for next-generation sequencing (NGS). To assess cfNA by NGS, one must perform deep sequencing to adequately assess majority of the miRNA, otherwise the sequencing results will be variable and not often representative of all cmiRNA. Currently employed traditional approaches of cmiRNA analysis by NGS are not very informative.

## 4. Methodological Variations of cmiRNA Detection Profiling

Currently, several methods have emerged to examine cmiRNA levels including RT-qPCR, microarrays and NGS. Each method has its pros and cons ranging from simplicity, quantification, and validity (Table 3). The sensitivity and specificity derived from these methods is often dependent on the type of samples and volumes of plasma or serum.

**Table 3.** Pros and cons of methodological variations.

|  | Sensitivity | Specificity | Accuracy | Analysis | Reproducibility | Discovery |
|---|---|---|---|---|---|---|
| RT-qPCR | ++++ | ++++ | ++++ | Easy | ++++ | Impossible |
| Affymetrix GeneChip miRNA Arrays 4.0 | + | + | + | Moderate | + | Impossible |
| Agilent oligonucleotides microarrays | + | + | + | Moderate | + | Impossible |
| Exiqon miRCURY LNA microRNA arrays | ++ | ++ | ++ | Moderate | + | Impossible |
| μParaflo®Microfluidic Biochip Technology | + | + | + | Moderate | + | Impossible |
| 3D-Gene® | +++ | +++ | +++ | Moderate | ++ | Impossible |
| Next-generation sequencing | ++ | ++ | ++ | Difficult | + | Possible |

Low to high: + to ++++. Utility scale.

## 4.1. RT-qPCR

Both the TaqMan® and SYBR® Green RT-qPCR assays are capable of analyzing the cmiRNA expression successfully. Each assay has specific reagents and protocols and is compatible with various PCR thermocyclers, thus introducing different quantitative and qualitative cmiRNA analysis.

Relative (comparative *Ct*) RT-qPCR is often used for cmiRNA analysis to measure the changes in gene expression of each sample to a suitable internal control. As of now, several internal controls have been used, including hsa-miR-16, hsa-miR-30b, and hsa-miR-142-3p, as well as the small RNA U6 and RNU-6B [24,28–30,35], though none of them are globally standard. For example, hsa-miR-16 has been most widely used as an internal control, but now it is known to be varied in several diseases and normal individuals [32,63–65]. Moreover, small RNA species such as RNU-6B is not native to human serum/plasma and is known to degrade during storage [66]. In addition, they are transcribed from a different RNA polymerase and may have different functions than from miRNA. This is problematic due to its presence in cancer patients, as well as normal individuals. Depending on the type of assay used, the resulting information may be false. U6 is recently reported to be an unsuitable internal control [67]. The stability of U6 expression is found to be less in serum especially after a number of freeze-thaw cycles. Some studies have suggested an external control to normalize the level of circulating miRNAs. The exogenous references are non-human mature miRNAs, including cel-miR-39, cel-miR-54, and cel-miR-238 [18,43,52,68]. These spike-in external controls are recommended as a measure of quality control for the RNA extraction and possibly RNA samples. However, it is difficult to control the amount of this artificial external control added into different samples. The artificial miRNAs are reconstituted in molecular biology grade or nuclease-free water at a set concentration followed by serial dilutions and stored in −80 °C. These artificial miRNAs are spiked-in to the samples at the lysis buffer step prior to RNA extraction. Precautions must be taken when adding these non-human external controls, because severe contamination can occur in samples. Baggish *et al.* used synthetic hsa-miR-422b, as it is minimally expressed in plasma [69]. As of now, we think exogenous references would be most useful, nevertheless further studies are needed to identify miRNAs that can serve as true universal miRNA controls. This is a major flaw of most assays reported. Standardization for cmiRNA quantification must be developed as for mRNA using similar approaches of MIQE guidelines [70,71]. Reproducible and comparable assay quantification are also issues in cfDNA analyses to date. Future cooperative studies are needed to define the parameters of cmiRNA quantification and reproducibility of assays reported.

On the other hand, absolute (standard curve) RT-qPCR may be used for analytical measurements of miRNA present in a given sample. One approach requires generating a standard curve for each miRNA, which is quite costly due to the amount of time and labor it requires. Furthermore, it is crucial that the stock sample used in generating these curves, to be accurately diluted each time with sufficient quantity to run multiple assays. The stability of the diluted standard curves must also be considered in regards to proper storage and freeze-thaw events prior to use. Alternatively, Droplet digital PCR (ddPCR) does not require a reference standard curve or an endogenous control. Instead the samples are divided and a ratio of positive (target molecule) to negative (no target) is used to count the number of target molecules in the sample, to allow accurate detection of low copy or rare allelic amplification. A study shows the potential use of ddPCR in miRNAs quantification and in this case in sputum for lung cancer diagnosis [72]. Additionally, pre-amplification may be necessary at times especially with low input sample or sample with low concentrations. However, it is important to consider that pre-amplification of the target samples may affect the PCR amplification and potentially produce bias in ddPCR results. The most significant drawback is the consumable costs and instrumental degree of specificity associated with ddPCR. There are different systems and instrument using ddPCR whereby, each have different sensitivities.

### 4.2. Microarray

Recently, microarray-based assays have also been widely applied to detect expression profiles of cmiRNAs (Table 4). The advantage of the microarray approach is its ability to assess genome-wide profiling of large numbers of cmiRNAs in blood and to identify candidate biomarkers for diagnostic and prognostic purposes in cancer patients. However, specific imaging systems and data analysis software are required to perform these methodologies. Depending on the manufacturers, they differ according to the reagents related to miRNA labeling, as well as methods and probe design used to immobilize the probes [22,73]. Direct and indirect miRNA labeling methods have been reported as follows [22,74,75]. For direct methods, T4 RNA ligase is used to directly add a fluorescent-modified nucleotide on the 3'-terminal of the miRNA. Another direct labeling method involves Poly-A tailing of the 3'-terminal. The latter overcomes the problem of circularization but might add various nucleotides in the tailing step, potentially altering hybridization properties [22]. On the other hand, for indirect labeling methods, RT is performed with amine-labeled dNTP mix, and the cDNA products are subsequently labeled with fluorescent dyes [75].

**Table 4.** Summary of microarrays for cmiRNA.

| Assay | Required Input (ng) | Probe Content |
| --- | --- | --- |
| Affymetrix GeneChip miRNA Arrays 4.0 | 130 | miRBase v.20 |
| Agilent oligonucleotides microarrays | 100 | miRBase v.21 |
| Exiqon miRCURY LNA microRNA arrays | 30 | miRBase v.19 |
| µParaflo®Microfluidic Biochip Technology | 1000 | miRBase v.21 |
| 3D-Gene® | 250 | miRBase v.21 |

As opposed to RT-qPCR, microarrays cannot be used for absolute quantification due to their lower sensitivity and specificity compared to RT-qPCR [22]. Moreover, arrays require a larger amount of total RNA and a pre-amplification step, which introduces risks of changing the original concentration of the cmiRNAs. Mestdagh *et al.* systematically compared 12 commercially available platforms for analysis of miRNA expression and determined each methods strengths and weaknesses [76]. They evaluated rates of miRNA detection in serum samples and determined RT-qPCR platforms provided higher sensitivity, accuracy, and reproducibility compared to microarray or sequencing platforms. They also concluded appropriate platforms should be chosen on the basis of the experimental setting. Chen *et al.* also quantified cmiRNA expression using both RT-qPCR and microarray and noted a weak correlation, implying the possibility of inaccuracies when using microarray-based methods [77,78]. In general microarray platforms for cmiRNA have not been very robust and have limited sensitivities as compared to PCR based assays. Recently, a highly sensitive 3D-Gene® (Toray, Tokyo, Japan) microarray was developed and reported in several publications [79–81]. It is not only sensitive but also has a high reproducibility that may contribute to the utility improvement of cmiRNA analysis.

### 4.3. Next-Generation Sequencing

Massive parallel sequencing (MPS) has been thought to be a current and promising technology for miRNA biomarker discovery. Knowledge of target miRNA and specific probes or primers is not necessary for this analysis, which enables investigators to assess unknown miRNAs.

In sample preparation, after total RNA extraction is followed by size fractionation of the small RNA population, RNAs are converted to cDNA. Adapter ligation and PCR amplification of cDNA is then performed according to the library preparation method appropriate for the respective MPS platform.

miRNA sequencing with library kits such as Illumina TruSeq Small RNA kit allows for direct sequencing and quantification of miRNA in samples and even extremely low expressing miRNAs can be detected. However, size selection is a tedious process, prone to human error and batch effect; library construction is also time consuming and requires a high input of high quality RNA.

Recently, the HTG EdgeSeq system (HTG molecular, Tuscon, AZ, USA) has developed a new approach of cmiRNA. This approach simplifies sample preparation for targeted sequencing of >2000 miRNAs [82]. This system does not require RNA extraction or manual library construction, and the fast and simplified protocol is highly automated with less user-related variation, reduced sample preparation and input requirements, and allows for detection of extremely low expressing miRNAs. The HTG EdgeSeq system relies on the specificity of the pre-designed probes and the *S1* enzyme digestion. Further validation is ongoing to determine its specificity and sensitivity in detecting cmiRNA.

As with all NGS assays, data analysis requires specific miRNA bioinformatics support. In addition, relative miRNA quantification is dependent on the sequencing read depth and appropriate normalization of the sequence reads. Other disadvantages of MPS assays are the required time and cost; MPS takes 1 week per run including sample preparation, which is longer compared to RT-qPCR. Although the cost is decreasing, it is still higher in comparison to RT-qPCR assays. However, the cost of individual miRNA detection is yet higher in PCR *vs.* microarray or NGS, implicating that an appropriate strategy must be carefully considered for each study design.

## 5. Discussion

Much progress has been made in methodological approach of cmiRNA detection profiling. However, given the significance of quality control in RT-qPCR microarray and MGS, the quality and quantity of the cmiRNA strongly affects the detection level of analysis. Traditional phenol-chloroform based RNA extraction techniques and several extraction kits are available; nevertheless, there is no gold standard for assessing cmiRNA. Since quality control is a major step in miRNA analysis prospective studies are highly necessary to reach a consensus on this important issue.

*J. Clin. Med.* **2015**, *4*, 1890–1907

In discussing the pros and cons of RT-qPCR, microarray, and NGS, we must compare the complexity, throughput, sensitivity/specificity, necessary time, required RNA input, and associated costs among them. RT-qPCR is the most useful for assessing several known specific miRNA because it is easily and quickly performed, in addition to having the highest sensitivity and quantification. Microarray and NGS are used for high-throughput or unknown targets, but accuracy, and cost have been a problem.

Despite the recent reduction in the cost of microarrays and NGS, and their improved computational accuracy, RT-qPCR remains the most widely used method in validating microarray and NGS results, likely because it exhibits the highest relative sensitivity and specificity. The search for useful diagnostic and prognostic cancer biomarkers obtained from "liquid biopsy" is in high demand. As highlighted throughout this review, employing microarrays and NGS for discovering novel cmiRNAs is quite promising. In addition, careful validation needs to be performed using RT-qPCR. In this phase, next crucial step is to define a robust standard methodology, including an endogenous control. While an abundance of studies report differential detection of miRNAs, the important procedural details have not been provided. Large scale, inter-laboratory reproducibility and assessment must be facilitated through methodological standardization. Many assays are available for tissue miRNA evaluation; however, adaptation to cmiRNA is not easily adaptable and reproducible. It is clear that more effort is needed in isolating and assessing cmiRNA more efficiently. Similar limitations exist in the analysis of circulating cell-free DNA in cancer patients.

cmiRNA biomarkers as liquid biopsy is most promising not only for cancer patients but also healthy individuals with benign diseases. Cancer screening, staging, and response to treatment may be assessed by evaluating specific miRNA expression levels in body fluids. As previously discussed, the technology of cmiRNA extraction and profiling has improved considerably. Translating basic molecular research into clinical biomarkers of relevance, calls for prospective multicenter studies to validate specific cmiRNAs using verified extraction and assay methodologies that have standardization qualities built in.

## 6. Conclusions

The methodology of assessing cmiRNAs still lacks consistency and standardization, which is causing discrepancies between the studies reported. Further efforts are required to establish standard result-reporting parameters for comparison verification of individual cmiRNA. Assessment of cmiRNAs as biomarkers has compelling potentials owed to their inherent properties. By developing more efficient assays, their clinical utility in cancer patients will be better demonstrated.

**Acknowledgments:** This study was supported in part by the ABC Foundation Beverly Hills CA (D.H.), The Leslie and Susan Gonda (Goldschmied) Foundation (D.H.), M. Peterson Foundation, and Ruth and Martin H. Weil Fund (D.H.).

**Author Contributions:** This study was designed by Shigeshi Ono, who also performed the literature search and authored the manuscript with Stella Lam, under Dave S.B. Hoon's review and supervision. Makoto Nagahara performed miR assays. We would like to thank Nousha Javanmardi for her critical editions.

**Conflicts of Interest:** The authors declare no conflict of interest.

## References

1. Kim, V.N. Microrna biogenesis: Coordinated cropping and dicing. *Nat. Rev. Mol. Cell Biol.* **2005**, *6*, 376–385. [PubMed]
2. Ambros, V. Micrornas: Tiny regulators with great potential. *Cell* **2001**, *107*, 823–826. [PubMed]
3. Bartel, D.P. Micrornas: Genomics, biogenesis, mechanism, and function. *Cell* **2004**, *116*, 281–297. [CrossRef]
4. Reinhart, B.J.; Slack, F.J.; Basson, M.; Pasquinelli, A.E.; Bettinger, J.C.; Rougvie, A.E.; Horvitz, H.R.; Ruvkun, G. The 21-nucleotide let-7 RNA regulates developmental timing in *Caenorhabditis elegans*. *Nature* **2000**, *403*, 901–906. [PubMed]

5.  Krek, A.; Grun, D.; Poy, M.N.; Wolf, R.; Rosenberg, L.; Epstein, E.J.; MacMenamin, P.; da Piedade, I.; Gunsalus, K.C.; Stoffel, M.; *et al.* Combinatorial microRNA target predictions. *Nat. Genet.* **2005**, *37*, 495–500. [CrossRef] [PubMed]
6.  Filipowicz, W.; Bhattacharyya, S.N.; Sonenberg, N. Mechanisms of post-transcriptional regulation by microRNAs: Are the answers in sight? *Nat. Rev. Genet.* **2008**, *9*, 102–114. [CrossRef] [PubMed]
7.  Calin, G.A.; Dumitru, C.D.; Shimizu, M.; Bichi, R.; Zupo, S.; Noch, E.; Aldler, H.; Rattan, S.; Keating, M.; Rai, K.; *et al.* Frequent deletions and down-regulation of micro-RNA genes miR15 and miR16 at 13q14 in chronic lymphocytic leukemia. *Proc. Natl. Acad. Sci. USA* **2002**, *99*, 15524–15529. [CrossRef] [PubMed]
8.  Takamizawa, J.; Konishi, H.; Yanagisawa, K.; Tomida, S.; Osada, H.; Endoh, H.; Harano, T.; Yatabe, Y.; Nagino, M.; Nimura, Y.; *et al.* Reduced expression of the let-7 microRNAs in human lung cancers in association with shortened postoperative survival. *Cancer Res.* **2004**, *64*, 3753–3756. [CrossRef] [PubMed]
9.  Calin, G.A.; Ferracin, M.; Cimmino, A.; Di Leva, G.; Shimizu, M.; Wojcik, S.E.; Iorio, M.V.; Visone, R.; Sever, N.I.; Fabbri, M.; *et al.* A microRNA signature associated with prognosis and progression in chronic lymphocytic leukemia. *N. Engl. J. Med.* **2005**, *353*, 1793–1801. [CrossRef] [PubMed]
10. Croce, C.M. Causes and consequences of microRNA dysregulation in cancer. *Nat. Rev. Genet.* **2009**, *10*, 704–714. [CrossRef] [PubMed]
11. Kasinski, A.L.; Slack, F.J. Epigenetics and genetics. MicroRNAs en route to the clinic: Progress in validating and targeting microRNAs for cancer therapy. *Nat. Rev. Cancer* **2011**, *11*, 849–864. [CrossRef] [PubMed]
12. Marzese, D.M.; Hirose, H.; Hoon, D.S. Diagnostic and prognostic value of circulating tumor-related DNA in cancer patients. *Expert Rev. Mol. Diagn.* **2013**, *13*, 827–844. [CrossRef] [PubMed]
13. Crowley, E.; Di Nicolantonio, F.; Loupakis, F.; Bardelli, A. Liquid biopsy: Monitoring cancer-genetics in the blood. *Nat. Rev. Clin. Oncol.* **2013**, *10*, 472–484. [CrossRef] [PubMed]
14. Clinical Laboratory Improvement Amendments (CLIA). Available online: http://www.fda.gov/medicaldevices/deviceregulationandguidance/ivdregulatoryassistance/ucm124105.htm (accessed on 1 August 2015).
15. Hoshimoto, S.; Shingai, T.; Morton, D.L.; Kuo, C.; Faries, M.B.; Chong, K.; Elashoff, D.; Wang, H.J.; Elashoff, R.M.; Hoon, D.S. Association between circulating tumor cells and prognosis in patients with stage III melanoma with sentinel lymph node metastasis in a phase III international multicenter trial. *J. Clin. Oncol.* **2012**, *30*, 3819–3826. [CrossRef] [PubMed]
16. Weber, J.A.; Baxter, D.H.; Zhang, S.; Huang, D.Y.; Huang, K.H.; Lee, M.J.; Galas, D.J.; Wang, K. The microRNA spectrum in 12 body fluids. *Clin. Chem.* **2010**, *56*, 1733–1741. [CrossRef] [PubMed]
17. Watson, A.K.; Witwer, K.W. Do platform-specific factors explain microRNA profiling disparities? *Clin. Chem.* **2012**, *58*, 472–474, author reply 474–475. [CrossRef] [PubMed]
18. Mitchell, P.S.; Parkin, R.K.; Kroh, E.M.; Fritz, B.R.; Wyman, S.K.; Pogosova-Agadjanyan, E.L.; Peterson, A.; Noteboom, J.; O'Briant, K.C.; Allen, A.; *et al.* Circulating microRNAs as stable blood-based markers for cancer detection. *Proc. Natl. Acad. Sci. USA* **2008**, *105*, 10513–10518. [CrossRef] [PubMed]
19. Schwarzenbach, H.; Hoon, D.S.; Pantel, K. Cell-free nucleic acids as biomarkers in cancer patients. *Nat. Rev. Cancer* **2011**, *11*, 426–437. [CrossRef] [PubMed]
20. Sourvinou, I.S.; Markou, A.; Lianidou, E.S. Quantification of circulating mirRNA in plasma: Effect of preanalytical and analytical parameters on their isolation and stability. *J. Mol. Diagn.* **2013**, *15*, 827–834. [CrossRef] [PubMed]
21. Montani, F.; Marzi, M.J.; Dezi, F.; Dama, E.; Carletti, R.M.; Bonizzi, G.; Bertolotti, R.; Bellomi, M.; Rampinelli, C.; Maisonneuve, P.; *et al.* MiR-test: A blood test for lung cancer early detection. *J. Natl. Cancer Inst.* **2015**, *107*, djv063. [CrossRef] [PubMed]
22. Pritchard, C.C.; Cheng, H.H.; Tewari, M. MicroRNA profiling: Approaches and considerations. *Nat. Rev. Genet.* **2012**, *13*, 358–369. [CrossRef] [PubMed]
23. Kirschner, M.B.; van Zandwijk, N.; Reid, G. Cell-free microRNAs: Potential biomarkers in need of standardized reporting. *Front. Genet.* **2013**, *4*, 56. [CrossRef] [PubMed]
24. Lawrie, C.H.; Gal, S.; Dunlop, H.M.; Pushkaran, B.; Liggins, A.P.; Pulford, K.; Banham, A.H.; Pezzella, F.; Boultwood, J.; Wainscoat, J.S.; *et al.* Detection of elevated levels of tumour-associated microRNAs in serum of patients with diffuse large b-cell lymphoma. *Br. J. Haematol.* **2008**, *141*, 672–675. [CrossRef] [PubMed]

25. Heegaard, N.H.; Schetter, A.J.; Welsh, J.A.; Yoneda, M.; Bowman, E.D.; Harris, C.C. Circulating micro-RNA expression profiles in early stage nonsmall cell lung cancer. *Int. J. Cancer* **2012**, *130*, 1378–1386. [CrossRef] [PubMed]

26. Hennessey, P.T.; Sanford, T.; Choudhary, A.; Mydlarz, W.W.; Brown, D.; Adai, A.T.; Ochs, M.F.; Ahrendt, S.A.; Mambo, E.; Califano, J.A. Serum microRNA biomarkers for detection of non-small cell lung cancer. *PLoS ONE* **2012**, *7*, e32307. [CrossRef] [PubMed]

27. Hu, Z.; Chen, X.; Zhao, Y.; Tian, T.; Jin, G.; Shu, Y.; Chen, Y.; Xu, L.; Zen, K.; Zhang, C.; *et al.* Serum microRNA signatures identified in a genome-wide serum microRNA expression profiling predict survival of non-small-cell lung cancer. *J. Clin. Oncol.* **2010**, *28*, 1721–1726. [CrossRef] [PubMed]

28. Silva, J.; Garcia, V.; Zaballos, A.; Provencio, M.; Lombardia, L.; Almonacid, L.; Garcia, J.M.; Dominguez, G.; Pena, C.; Diaz, R.; *et al.* Vesicle-related microRNAs in plasma of nonsmall cell lung cancer patients and correlation with survival. *Eur. Respir. J.* **2011**, *37*, 617–623. [CrossRef] [PubMed]

29. Shen, J.; Liu, Z.; Todd, N.W.; Zhang, H.; Liao, J.; Yu, L.; Guarnera, M.A.; Li, R.; Cai, L.; Zhan, M.; *et al.* Diagnosis of lung cancer in individuals with solitary pulmonary nodules by plasma microRNA biomarkers. *BMC Cancer* **2011**, *11*, 374. [CrossRef] [PubMed]

30. Shen, J.; Wang, A.; Wang, Q.; Gurvich, I.; Siegel, A.B.; Remotti, H.; Santella, R.M. Exploration of genome-wide circulating microRNA in hepatocellular carcinoma: MiR-483–5p as a potential biomarker. *Cancer Epidemiol. Biomark. Prev.* **2013**, *22*, 2364–2373. [CrossRef] [PubMed]

31. Summerer, I.; Niyazi, M.; Unger, K.; Pitea, A.; Zangen, V.; Hess, J.; Atkinson, M.J.; Belka, C.; Moertl, S.; Zitzelsberger, H. Changes in circulating microRNAs after radiochemotherapy in head and neck cancer patients. *Radiat. Oncol.* **2013**, *8*, 296. [CrossRef] [PubMed]

32. Zhu, C.; Ren, C.; Han, J.; Ding, Y.; Du, J.; Dai, N.; Dai, J.; Ma, H.; Hu, Z.; Shen, H.; *et al.* A five-microRNA panel in plasma was identified as potential biomarker for early detection of gastric cancer. *Br. J. Cancer* **2014**, *110*, 2291–2299. [CrossRef] [PubMed]

33. Zhou, J.; Yu, L.; Gao, X.; Hu, J.; Wang, J.; Dai, Z.; Wang, J.F.; Zhang, Z.; Lu, S.; Huang, X.; *et al.* Plasma microRNA panel to diagnose hepatitis b virus-related hepatocellular carcinoma. *J. Clin. Oncol.* **2011**, *29*, 4781–4788. [CrossRef] [PubMed]

34. Wulfken, L.M.; Moritz, R.; Ohlmann, C.; Holdenrieder, S.; Jung, V.; Becker, F.; Herrmann, E.; Walgenbach-Brunagel, G.; von Ruecker, A.; Muller, S.C.; *et al.* MicroRNAs in renal cell carcinoma: Diagnostic implications of serum mir-1233 levels. *PLoS ONE* **2011**, *6*, e25787. [CrossRef] [PubMed]

35. Asaga, S.; Kuo, C.; Nguyen, T.; Terpenning, M.; Giuliano, A.E.; Hoon, D.S. Direct serum assay for microRNA-21 concentrations in early and advanced breast cancer. *Clin. Chem.* **2011**, *57*, 84–91. [CrossRef] [PubMed]

36. Ono, S.; Oyama, T.; Lam, S.; Chong, K.; Foshag, L.J.; Hoon, D.S. A direct plasma assay of circulating microRNA-210 of hypoxia can identify early systemic metastasis recurrence in melanoma patients. *Oncotarget* **2015**, *6*, 7053–7064. [CrossRef] [PubMed]

37. Rocci, A.; Hofmeister, C.C.; Geyer, S.; Stiff, A.; Gambella, M.; Cascione, L.; Guan, J.; Benson, D.M.; Efebera, Y.A.; Talabere, T.; *et al.* Circulating mirna markers show promise as new prognosticators for multiple myeloma. *Leukemia* **2014**, *28*, 1922–1926. [CrossRef] [PubMed]

38. Witwer, K.W.; Buzas, E.I.; Bemis, L.T.; Bora, A.; Lasser, C.; Lotvall, J.; Nolte-'t Hoen, E.N.; Piper, M.G.; Sivaraman, S.; Skog, J.; *et al.* Standardization of sample collection, isolation and analysis methods in extracellular vesicle research. *J. Extracell. Vesicles* **2013**, *2*. [CrossRef] [PubMed]

39. Kannan, M.; Atreya, C. Differential profiling of human red blood cells during storage for 52 selected microrRNA. *Transfusion* **2010**, *50*, 1581–1588. [CrossRef] [PubMed]

40. Chen, X.; Ba, Y.; Ma, L.; Cai, X.; Yin, Y.; Wang, K.; Guo, J.; Zhang, Y.; Chen, J.; Guo, X.; *et al.* Characterization of microRNAs in serum: A novel class of biomarkers for diagnosis of cancer and other diseases. *Cell Res.* **2008**, *18*, 997–1006. [CrossRef] [PubMed]

41. D'Alessandra, Y.; Devanna, P.; Limana, F.; Straino, S.; Di Carlo, A.; Brambilla, P.G.; Rubino, M.; Carena, M.C.; Spazzafumo, L.; de Simone, M.; *et al.* Circulating microRNAs are new and sensitive biomarkers of myocardial infarction. *Eur. Heart J.* **2010**, *31*, 2765–2773. [CrossRef] [PubMed]

42. Wang, K.; Yuan, Y.; Cho, J.H.; McClarty, S.; Baxter, D.; Galas, D.J. Comparing the microRNA spectrum between serum and plasma. *PLoS ONE* **2012**, *7*, e41561. [CrossRef] [PubMed]

43. McDonald, J.S.; Milosevic, D.; Reddi, H.V.; Grebe, S.K.; Algeciras-Schimnich, A. Analysis of circulating microRNA: Preanalytical and analytical challenges. *Clin. Chem.* **2011**, *57*, 833–840. [CrossRef] [PubMed]

44. Cheng, H.H.; Yi, H.S.; Kim, Y.; Kroh, E.M.; Chien, J.W.; Eaton, K.D.; Goodman, M.T.; Tait, J.F.; Tewari, M.; Pritchard, C.C. Plasma processing conditions substantially influence circulating microRNA biomarker levels. *PLoS ONE* **2013**, *8*, e64795. [CrossRef] [PubMed]

45. Hunter, M.P.; Ismail, N.; Zhang, X.; Aguda, B.D.; Lee, E.J.; Yu, L.; Xiao, T.; Schafer, J.; Lee, M.L.; Schmittgen, T.D.; *et al.* Detection of microRNA expression in human peripheral blood microvesicles. *PLoS ONE* **2008**, *3*, e3694. [CrossRef] [PubMed]

46. Willeit, P.; Zampetaki, A.; Dudek, K.; Kaudewitz, D.; King, A.; Kirkby, N.S.; Crosby-Nwaobi, R.; Prokopi, M.; Drozdov, I.; Langley, S.R.; *et al.* Circulating microRNAs as novel biomarkers for platelet activation. *Circ. Res.* **2013**, *112*, 595–600. [CrossRef] [PubMed]

47. Al-Soud, W.A.; Radstrom, P. Purification and characterization of PCR-inhibitory components in blood cells. *J. Clin. Microbiol.* **2001**, *39*, 485–493. [CrossRef] [PubMed]

48. Boeckel, J.N.; Thome, C.E.; Leistner, D.; Zeiher, A.M.; Fichtlscherer, S.; Dimmeler, S. Heparin selectively affects the quantification of microRNAs in human blood samples. *Clin. Chem.* **2013**, *59*, 1125–1127. [CrossRef] [PubMed]

49. Kaudewitz, D.; Lee, R.; Willeit, P.; McGregor, R.; Markus, H.S.; Kiechl, S.; Zampetaki, A.; Storey, R.F.; Channon, K.M.; Mayr, M. Impact of intravenous heparin on quantification of circulating microRNAs in patients with coronary artery disease. *Thromb. Haemost.* **2013**, *110*, 609–615. [CrossRef] [PubMed]

50. Kim, D.J.; Linnstaedt, S.; Palma, J.; Park, J.C.; Ntrivalas, E.; Kwak-Kim, J.Y.; Gilman-Sachs, A.; Beaman, K.; Hastings, M.L.; Martin, J.N.; *et al.* Plasma components affect accuracy of circulating cancer-related microRNA quantitation. *J. Mol. Diagn.* **2012**, *14*, 71–80. [CrossRef] [PubMed]

51. Garcia, M.E.; Blanco, J.L.; Caballero, J.; Gargallo-Viola, D. Anticoagulants interfere with PCR used to diagnose invasive aspergillosis. *J. Clin. Microbiol.* **2002**, *40*, 1567–1568. [CrossRef] [PubMed]

52. Fichtlscherer, S.; De Rosa, S.; Fox, H.; Schwietz, T.; Fischer, A.; Liebetrau, C.; Weber, M.; Hamm, C.W.; Roxe, T.; Muller-Ardogan, M.; *et al.* Circulating microRNAs in patients with coronary artery disease. *Circ. Res.* **2010**, *107*, 677–684. [CrossRef] [PubMed]

53. Ma, W.; Wang, M.; Wang, Z.Q.; Sun, L.; Graber, D.; Matthews, J.; Champlin, R.; Yi, Q.; Orlowski, R.Z.; Kwak, L.W.; *et al.* Effect of long-term storage in TRIzol on microarray-based gene expression profiling. *Cancer Epidemiol. Biomarkers Prev.* **2010**, *19*, 2445–2452. [CrossRef] [PubMed]

54. Kim, Y.K.; Yeo, J.; Kim, B.; Ha, M.; Kim, V.N. Short structured RNAs with low GC content are selectively lost during extraction from a small number of cells. *Mol. Cell* **2012**, *46*, 893–895. [CrossRef] [PubMed]

55. Rio, D.C.; Ares, M., Jr.; Hannon, G.J.; Nilsen, T.W. Purification of RNA using TRIzol (TRI reagent). *Cold Spring Harb. Protoc.* **2010**, *2010*, pdb.prot5439. [CrossRef] [PubMed]

56. Rio, D.C.; Ares, M., Jr.; Hannon, G.J.; Nilsen, T.W. Guidelines for the use of RNA purification kits. *Cold Spring Harb. Protoc.* **2010**, *2010*, pdb.ip79. [CrossRef] [PubMed]

57. Tosar, J.P.; Gambaro, F.; Sanguinetti, J.; Bonilla, B.; Witwer, K.W.; Cayota, A. Assessment of small RNA sorting into different extracellular fractions revealed by high-throughput sequencing of breast cell lines. *Nucleic Acids Res.* **2015**, *43*, 5601–5616. [CrossRef] [PubMed]

58. Witwer, K.W. Circulating microRNA biomarker studies: Pitfalls and potential solutions. *Clin. Chem.* **2015**, *61*, 56–63. [CrossRef] [PubMed]

59. Kroh, E.M.; Parkin, R.K.; Mitchell, P.S.; Tewari, M. Analysis of circulating microRNA biomarkers in plasma and serum using quantitative reverse transcriptionPCR (qRT-PCR). *Methods* **2010**, *50*, 298–301. [CrossRef] [PubMed]

60. Asaga, S.; Hoon, D.S. Direct serum assay for microRNA in cancer patients. *Methods Mol. Biol.* **2013**, *1024*, 147–155. [PubMed]

61. Schroeder, A.; Mueller, O.; Stocker, S.; Salowsky, R.; Leiber, M.; Gassmann, M.; Lightfoot, S.; Menzel, W.; Granzow, M.; Ragg, T. The rin: An RNA integrity number for assigning integrity values to RNA measurements. *BMC Mol. Biol.* **2006**, *7*, 3. [CrossRef] [PubMed]

62. Jung, M.; Schaefer, A.; Steiner, I.; Kempkensteffen, C.; Stephan, C.; Erbersdobler, A.; Jung, K. Robust microRNA stability in degraded RNA preparations from human tissue and cell samples. *Clin. Chem.* **2010**, *56*, 998–1006. [CrossRef] [PubMed]

63. Aqeilan, R.I.; Calin, G.A.; Croce, C.M. MiR-15a and miR-16–1 in cancer: Discovery, function and future perspectives. *Cell Death Differ.* **2010**, *17*, 215–220. [CrossRef] [PubMed]

64. Wang, Y.; Gao, Y.; Shi, W.; Zhai, D.; Rao, Q.; Jia, X.; Liu, J.; Jiao, X.; Du, Z. Profiles of differential expression of circulating microrRNA in hepatitis b virus-positive small hepatocellular carcinoma. *Cancer Biomark. 201* **2015**, *15*, 171–180.

65. Filkova, M.; Aradi, B.; Senolt, L.; Ospelt, C.; Vettori, S.; Mann, H.; Filer, A.; Raza, K.; Buckley, C.D.; Snow, M.; *et al.* Association of circulating miR-223 and miR-16 with disease activity in patients with early rheumatoid arthritis. *Ann. Rheum. Dis.* **2014**, *73*, 1898–1904. [CrossRef] [PubMed]

66. Haider, B.A.; Baras, A.S.; McCall, M.N.; Hertel, J.A.; Cornish, T.C.; Halushka, M.K. A critical evaluation of microRNA biomarkers in non-neoplastic disease. *PLoS ONE* **2014**, *9*, e89565. [CrossRef] [PubMed]

67. Xiang, M.; Zeng, Y.; Yang, R.; Xu, H.; Chen, Z.; Zhong, J.; Xie, H.; Xu, Y.; Zeng, X. U6 is not a suitable endogenous control for the quantification of circulating microrRNA. *Biochem. Biophys. Res. Commun.* **2014**, *454*, 210–214. [CrossRef] [PubMed]

68. Zeng, X.; Xiang, J.; Wu, M.; Xiong, W.; Tang, H.; Deng, M.; Li, X.; Liao, Q.; Su, B.; Luo, Z.; *et al.* Circulating miR-17, miR-20a, miR-29c, and miR-223 combined as non-invasive biomarkers in nasopharyngeal carcinoma. *PLoS ONE* **2012**, *7*, e46367. [CrossRef] [PubMed]

69. Baggish, A.L.; Hale, A.; Weiner, R.B.; Lewis, G.D.; Systrom, D.; Wang, F.; Wang, T.J.; Chan, S.Y. Dynamic regulation of circulating microrna during acute exhaustive exercise and sustained aerobic exercise training. *J. Physiol.* **2011**, *589*, 3983–3994. [CrossRef] [PubMed]

70. Bustin, S.A.; Benes, V.; Garson, J.A.; Hellemans, J.; Huggett, J.; Kubista, M.; Mueller, R.; Nolan, T.; Pfaffl, M.W.; Shipley, G.L.; *et al.* The miqe guidelines: Minimum information for publication of quantitative real-time PCR experiments. *Clin. Chem.* **2009**, *55*, 611–622. [CrossRef] [PubMed]

71. Huggett, J.F.; Foy, C.A.; Benes, V.; Emslie, K.; Garson, J.A.; Haynes, R.; Hellemans, J.; Kubista, M.; Mueller, R.D.; Nolan, T.; *et al.* The digital MIQE guidelines: Minimum information for publication of quantitative digital PCR experiments. *Clin. Chem.* **2013**, *59*, 892–902. [CrossRef] [PubMed]

72. Li, N.; Ma, J.; Guarnera, M.A.; Fang, H.; Cai, L.; Jiang, F. Digital PCR quantification of mirRNA in sputum for diagnosis of lung cancer. *J. Cancer Res. Clin. Oncol.* **2014**, *140*, 145–150. [CrossRef] [PubMed]

73. Moldovan, L.; Batte, K.; Wang, Y.; Wisler, J.; Piper, M. Analyzing the circulating microRNAs in exosomes/extracellular vesicles from serum or plasma by qRT-PCR. *Methods Mol. Biol.* **2013**, *1024*, 129–145. [PubMed]

74. Git, A.; Dvinge, H.; Salmon-Divon, M.; Osborne, M.; Kutter, C.; Hadfield, J.; Bertone, P.; Caldas, C. Systematic comparison of microarray profiling, real-time PCR, and next-generation sequencing technologies for measuring differential microrna expression. *RNA* **2010**, *16*, 991–1006. [CrossRef] [PubMed]

75. Li, W.; Ruan, K. MicroRNA detection by microarray. *Anal. Bioanal. Chem.* **2009**, *394*, 1117–1124. [CrossRef] [PubMed]

76. Mestdagh, P.; Hartmann, N.; Baeriswyl, L.; Andreasen, D.; Bernard, N.; Chen, C.; Cheo, D.; D'Andrade, P.; DeMayo, M.; Dennis, L.; *et al.* Evaluation of quantitative miRNA expression platforms in the microRNA quality control (miRQC) study. *Nat. Methods* **2014**, *11*, 809–815. [CrossRef] [PubMed]

77. Chen, Y.; Gelfond, J.A.; McManus, L.M.; Shireman, P.K. Reproducibility of quantitative RT-PCR array in miRNA expression profiling and comparison with microarray analysis. *BMC Genom.* **2009**, *10*, 407. [CrossRef] [PubMed]

78. Hansen, T.F.; Carlsen, A.L.; Heegaard, N.H.; Sorensen, F.B.; Jakobsen, A. Changes in circulating microRNA-126 during treatment with chemotherapy and bevacizumab predicts treatment response in patients with metastatic colorectal cancer. *Br. J. Cancer* **2015**, *112*, 624–629. [CrossRef] [PubMed]

79. Komatsu, S.; Ichikawa, D.; Hirajima, S.; Kawaguchi, T.; Miyamae, M.; Okajima, W.; Ohashi, T.; Arita, T.; Konishi, H.; Shiozaki, A.; *et al.* Plasma microrna profiles: Identification of miR-25 as a novel diagnostic and monitoring biomarker in oesophageal squamous cell carcinoma. *Br. J. Cancer* **2014**, *111*, 1614–1624. [CrossRef] [PubMed]

80. Tanaka, Y.; Tsuda, S.; Kunikata, H.; Sato, J.; Kokubun, T.; Yasuda, M.; Nishiguchi, K.M.; Inada, T.; Nakazawa, T. Profiles of extracellular mirnas in the aqueous humor of glaucoma patients assessed with a microarray system. *Sci. Rep.* **2014**, *4*, 5089. [CrossRef] [PubMed]

*J. Clin. Med.* **2015**, *4*, 1890–1907

81. Ono, M.; Kosaka, N.; Tominaga, N.; Yoshioka, Y.; Takeshita, F.; Takahashi, R.U.; Yoshida, M.; Tsuda, H.; Tamura, K.; Ochiya, T. Exosomes from bone marrow mesenchymal stem cells contain a microRNA that promotes dormancy in metastatic breast cancer cells. *Sci. Signal.* **2014**, *7*, ra63. [CrossRef] [PubMed]

82. Thompson, D.; Botros, I.; Rounseville, M.; Liu, Q.; Wang, E.; Harrison, H.; Roche, P. Automated High Fidelity RNA Expression Profiling Using Nuclease Protection Coupled with next Generation Sequencing. Available online: http://www.htgmolecular.com/sites/default/files/Merck%20poster%2030-Apr-2014.pdf (accessed on 20 October 2015).

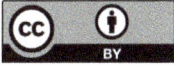

Journal of
*Clinical Medicine*

MDPI

*Review*

# MicroRNAs and Osteolytic Bone Metastasis: The Roles of MicroRNAs in Tumor-Induced Osteoclast Differentiation

**Tadayoshi Kagiya**

Division of Functional Morphology, Department of Anatomy, Iwate Medical University, 2-1-1 Nishitokuta, Yahaba-cho, Iwate, 028-3694, Japan; tkagiya@iwate-med.ac.jp; Tel.: +81-19-651-5111; Fax: +81-19-908-8010.

Academic Editors: Takahiro Ochiya and Ryou-u Takahashi
Received: 1 July 2015; Accepted: 24 August 2015; Published: 28 August 2015

**Abstract:** Osteolytic bone metastasis frequently occurs in the later stages of breast, lung, and several other cancers. Osteoclasts, the only cells that resorb bone, are hijacked by tumor cells, which break down bone remodeling systems. As a result, osteolysis occurs and may cause patients to suffer bone fractures, pain, and hypercalcemia. It is important to understand the mechanism of bone metastasis to establish new cancer therapies. MicroRNAs are small, noncoding RNAs that are involved in various biological processes, including cellular differentiation, proliferation, apoptosis, and tumorigenesis. MicroRNAs have significant clinical potential, including their use as new therapeutic targets and disease-specific biomarkers. Recent studies have revealed that microRNAs are involved in osteoclast differentiation and osteolytic bone metastasis. In this review focusing on microRNAs, the author discusses the roles of microRNAs in osteoclastogenesis and osteolytic bone metastasis.

**Keywords:** Bone Metastasis; Osteoclasts; MicroRNAs; Exosomes; Extracellular Vesicles

## 1. Introduction

Cancer is one of the most common causes of death, and bone is the third most common cancer metastatic site following the lung and liver [1]. Patients with metastasis to bone often present with lesions that can be osteoblastic, osteolytic, or a mixture of the two [2]. These lesions result from an imbalance between osteoblastic bone formation and osteoclastic bone resorption. Osteoblastic bone metastasis is caused by excessive osteoblast activity relative to osteoclast activity, a characteristic of prostate cancer [2]. In contrast, osteolytic bone metastasis is caused by excessive osteoclast activity relative to osteoblast activity [2]. Osteolytic bone metastasis frequently occurs in the later stages of breast, lung, and several other cancers [2,3]. Osteoclasts are hijacked by tumor cells, which break down bone remodeling systems [3,4]. As a result, osteolysis occurs and may cause patients to suffer bone fractures, pain, and hypercalcemia [3,4]. Thus, the quality of life of patients is negatively affected.

Osteoclasts are the only cells that resorb bone [5]. Osteoclasts are tartrate-resistant acid phosphatase (TRAP)-positive multinucleated giant cells [5–7], and are formed by the fusion of hematopoietic cells of the monocyte/macrophage lineage. Although osteoclastogenesis is regulated by a variety of hormones, growth factors, and cytokines, macrophage colony-stimulating factor (M-CSF) and receptor activator of nuclear factor κB ligand (RANKL), which are expressed in stromal cells and osteoblasts, are essential for osteoclast differentiation [5,6]. The binding of M-CSF to its receptor, c-Fms, induces the transcription factor c-Fos, whereas the binding of RANKL to its receptor, receptor activator of nuclear factor κB (RANK), leads to the recruitment of TNF-receptor-associated factor 6 (TRAF6), the main adapter molecule of RANK. TRAF6 activates nuclear factor κB (NF-κB) and mitogen-activated kinases, including c-Jun N-terminal kinase (JNK). JNK in turn activates the transcription factor c-Jun [8]. RANKL/RANK also induces c-Fos to form activator protein-1 (AP-1), a heterodimeric transcription factor, with c-Jun. AP-1 and NF-κB then induce nuclear factor of activated T cell cytoplasmic 1 (NFATc1), a master transcription factor that regulates osteoclast differentiation. NFATc1 works together with other transcription factors such as AP-1, PU.1, and microphthalmia-associated transcription factor (MITF) to induce various osteoclast-specific genes [8]. Thus, M-CSF and RANKL signaling pathways are crucial for osteoclastogenesis. In contrast, the RANK–RANKL interaction is inhibited by the decoy receptor osteoprotegerin (OPG), a soluble member of the TNF receptor superfamily expressed by stromal cells and osteoblasts [9,10] (Figure 1). Thus, osteoclastogenesis is appropriately regulated in normal physiological conditions.

## 2. Bone Metastasis

Metastasis to bone is mainly blood-borne [1,9,11,12]. Tumor cells first detach from the primary lesion and invade the blood vessels. Once in the bloodstream, tumor cells are attracted to preferred sites of metastasis through site-specific interactions between tumor cells and cells in the target organ [1,11]. To metastasize, a tumor cell must gain access to the vasculature from the primary tumor, survive the circulation, escape immune surveillance, and localize in the vasculature of the target organ [1,13]. Most single or clustered tumor cells are thought to expire in the circulation and fail to metastasize because of either anoikis, mechanical trauma, or attack and clearance by the host defense system [13]. Although circulating tumor cells have been hypothesized to persist as single cells or small cell clusters, there is another pathway of blood-borne metastasis [13–16]. Tumor nets are enveloped by vascular endothelial cells and enter the circulation, and tumor emboli may form [13–15]. Tumor emboli are composed of multicellular tumor nets that are sufficiently large enough to arrest in the target organ, where they thrive and create expansive secondary tumors [13–15]. In patients with hepatocellular carcinoma, the tumor emboli conserve elements of their primary tumor tissue organization, and are associated with the basement membrane and vascular endothelial cells on the surface [13]. This architecture can provide an integrated ecosystem that protects the tumor cells from anoikis, mechanical trauma, and immunological engagement during dissemination [13]. Whether this "invasion-independent metastasis" is involved in bone metastasis is unknown and, considering the abundance of blood in bone tissue, there is a possibility of invasion-independent bone metastasis.

Once tumor cells that metastasize to the skeleton reach the bone marrow, they interact with anatomical entities in contact with the bone called niches. Two different niches exist: the endosteal niche, where stem cells are closely associated with stromal cells and osteoblasts, and the vascular niche, where hematopoietic cells are located [12].

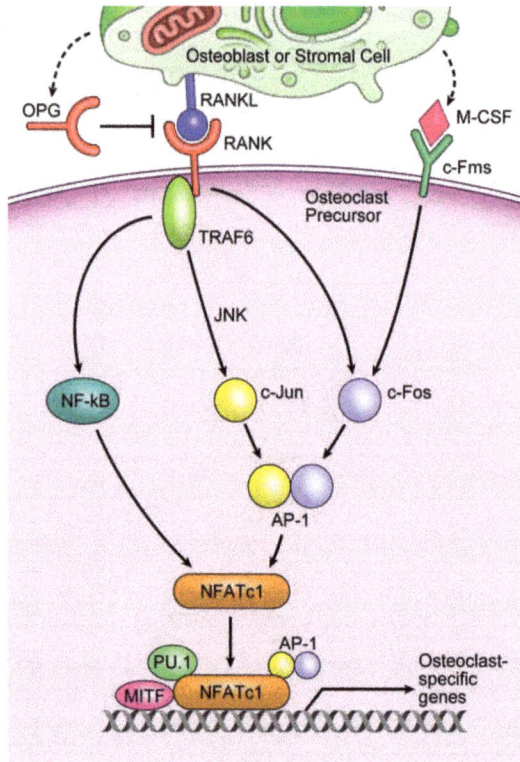

**Figure 1.** An important signaling cascade of osteoclastogenesis. The binding of M-CSF to its receptor, c-Fms, induces the transcription factor c-Fos, whereas the binding of RANKL to its receptor, RANK, leads to the recruitment of TRAF6, the main adapter molecule of RANK. TRAF6 activates NF-κB and mitogen-activated kinases including JNK. JNK in turn activates the transcription factor c-Jun. RANKL/RANK also induces c-Fos to form AP-1, a heterodimeric transcription factor, with c-Jun. AP-1 and NF-κB then induce NFATc1, a master transcription factor that regulates osteoclast differentiation. NFATc1 works together with other transcription factors such as AP-1, PU.1, and MITF to induce various osteoclast-specific genes. Thus, M-CSF and RANKL signaling pathways are crucial for osteoclastogenesis. On the other hand, the RANK–RANKL interaction is inhibited by the decoy receptor OPG expressed by stromal cells and osteoblasts.

## 3. Microenvironment of Osteolytic Lesions

### 3.1. Growth Factors in the Microenvironment of Osteolytic Lesions

The bone microenvironment comprises osteoblasts, stromal cells, osteoclasts, mineralized bone matrix, hematopoietic cells, and many other cell types [11]. Bone matrix contains a variety of growth factors, such as insulin-like growth factors (IGFs), transforming growth factor β (TGF-β), fibroblast growth factors, platelet-derived growth factors, and bone morphogenetic proteins [1,2,9,11,12,17,18]. These bone-derived growth factors are released by osteoclastic bone resorption, and colonization of tumor cells in bone is under the influence of these growth factors. For example, TGF-β is one of the most abundant growth factors in bone matrix [11]. TGF-β released from bone matrix inhibits T-cell proliferation and activity and the function of natural killer cells, thereby suppressing the immune system [17]. In addition, TGF-β promotes tumor cell proliferation and survival [1]. In breast cancer,

TGF-β released from the matrix as a result of increased bone resorption can cause tumor cells to produce growth factors such as parathyroid hormone-related protein (PTHrP) and interleukin 11 (IL-11) that can perturb the RANKL/OPG balance, resulting in further osteoclastogenesis and perpetuation of osteolytic disease [2] (Figure 2).

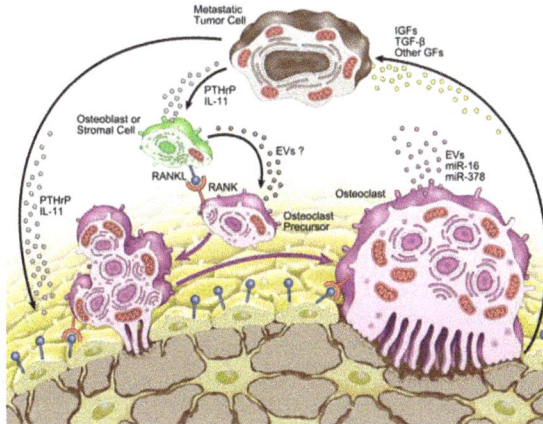

**Figure 2.** Schematic view of tumor-induced osteoclast formation. Bone-derived growth factors (IGFs, TGF-β and other growth factors) are released by osteoclastic bone resorption. These factors promote tumor cell proliferation and survival. TGF-β acts on tumor cells to produce growth factors, such as PTHrP and IL-11. PTHrP acts on osteoblasts and stromal cells and promotes the expression of RANKL, resulting in the enhancement of osteoclastogenesis and destruction of bone. Osteoclasts secrete extracellular vesicles (EVs) containing specific microRNAs, such as miR-21, miR-210, and miR-378. miR-16 and miR-378 are secreted biomarkers for osteolytic bone metastasis.

PTHrP is one of the most important mediators of osteoclast activation [1,2,9,11,12,17–19]. More than 90% of patients with breast cancer that has metastasized to bone overexpress PTHrP [17,19]. In addition, PTHrP expression has been determined to be a risk factor for predicting bone metastasis in patients with breast cancer [2]. In the bone microenvironment, PTHrP is produced by osteoblasts, stromal cells, and cancer cells [1,2,9,11,12,17–19]. PTHrP acts on osteoblasts and stromal cells and promotes cellular expression of RANKL, resulting in enhancement of osteoclastogenesis and destruction of bone [2,9,11,17–19]. Consequently, growth factors are further released from resorbing bone and promote colonization of metastatic tumor cells in bone [1,2,9,11,17–19]. This represents a "vicious circle" between metastatic tumor cells and bone cells (Figure 2).

### 3.2. Involvement of microRNAs in Tumor-Induced Osteoclast Differentiation

It was recently revealed that microRNAs (miRNAs) play important roles in tumorigenesis and tumor progression [20]. miRNAs are small, endogenous, noncoding RNAs of approximately 20 to 22 nucleotides in length [3,5,6,20]. Although the biological functions of most miRNAs are not yet fully understood, they participate in the regulation of cellular differentiation, proliferation, apoptosis, and cancer development [5,6,20]. Transcription of miRNA genes yields noncoding transcripts that are subsequently processed through sequential digestion by the RNase III enzymes Drosha and Dicer [5,6,20]. The resulting single-stranded mature miRNAs are finally incorporated into an RNA-induced silencing complex (RISC) that contains argonaute (Ago) family proteins [5,6,20]. The Ago proteins recruit miRNAs specific to the target mRNAs, and the RISC inhibits the translation of target mRNAs and/or degrades target mRNAs. Thus, miRNAs are involved in post-transcriptional regulation of mRNA function [5,6,20].

*J. Clin. Med.* **2015**, *4*, 1741–1752

Recent studies have revealed that miRNAs play critical roles in osteoclastogenesis. We reported that the expression of 52 mature miRNAs differed more than two-fold between untreated cells and cells treated with RANKL during osteoclastogenesis [5]. As a key factor in osteoclast differentiation, miR-223 regulates nuclear factor I-A and M-CSF receptor levels [21,22]. miR-124 regulates osteoclastogenesis by suppressing NFATc1, a master transcription factor of osteoclast differentiation [23]. RANKL-induced c-Fos upregulates miR-21, which downregulates the expression of programmed cell death 4 (PDCD4), a negative regulator of osteoclastogenesis [24]. Overexpression of miR-155 blocks osteoclast differentiation by repressing MITF and PU.1, which are crucial transcription factors for osteoclast differentiation [25]. These reports are based on murine cell experiments; recent work has begun to uncover the roles of miRNAs in human osteoclast differentiation and function. miR-29b negatively regulates human osteoclastic cell differentiation and function by suppressing c-Fos [26]. The expression level of miR-503, which directly targets RANK, is markedly lower in progenitors of osteoclasts from postmenopausal women with osteoporosis than in those from postmenopausal healthy women [27]. The repressive effects on monocyte-specific genes by let-7e/miR-99b/125a/132/212 are crucial for human osteoclast differentiation. These miRNAs are activated directly by NF-κB and exhibit rapid upregulation during osteoclast differentiation. Their inhibition impairs osteoclastogenesis [28].

It was recently revealed that miRNAs are involved in tumor-induced osteoclast differentiation (Table 1). Ell *et al.* [3] reported that five miRNAs (miR-33a, miR-133a, miR-141, miR-190, and miR-219) are significantly downregulated during osteoclastogenesis in both normal physiological conditions and pathophysiological cancer conditions. Ectopic expression of miR-133a, miR-141, and miR-219 strongly inhibited osteoclast differentiation and bone resorption by directly targeting *Mitf/Mmp14*, *Mitf/Calcr*, and *Mitf/Traf6*, respectively. Remarkably, miR-141 and miR-219 administered systemically led to a significant decrease in the number of osteoclasts *in vivo*, and also reduced the metastatic tumor burden in an experimental breast cancer model [3]. Krzezinski *et al.* [29] reported that miR-34a blocks osteoporosis and bone metastasis by inhibiting osteoclastogenesis. The expression level of miR-34a decreases during osteoclastogenesis, and knockdown of miR-34a promotes osteoclast differentiation, while ectopic miR-34a inhibits this differentiation. They also identified transforming growth factor β-induced factor 2 (Tgif2), which is induced by NFATc1 and AP-1 during osteoclast differentiation, as a direct target of miR-34a. miR-34a plays important roles in osteoblast and osteoclast differentiation. Osteoblast differentiation is reduced in miR-34a knockout mice but increased in osteoblastic miR-34a conditional transgenic mice [29].

The involvement of miRNAs in growth factors of osteolytic lesions has also been shown. TGF-β is released from bone matrix during osteoclastic bone resorption and induces cancer cells to produce osteolytic factors such as IL-11 [30]. Three miRNAs (miR-204, miR-211, and miR-379) inhibit TGF-β-induced IL-11 production in bone metastatic breast cancer cells [30]. Kuo *et al.* [31] reported that miR-33a functions as a bone metastasis suppressor in lung cancer by targeting *PTHrP*. miR-33a is downregulated in lung cancer cells, which express high levels of PTHrP. PTHrP enhances osteoclastogenesis by altering the ratio of osteoclastogenesis activator (M-CSF and RANKL)/inhibitor (OPG) produced by osteoblasts. Ectopic miR-33a decreases the induction of lung cancer cells in the production of M-CSF and RANKL in osteoblasts and increases that of OPG in osteoblasts by suppressing PTHrP [31].

Collectively, specific miRNAs play critical roles in osteoclastogenesis under normal physiological conditions and in tumor-induced osteoclast differentiation.

## 4. Involvement of Extracellular Vesicles in Osteolytic Bone Metastasis

miRNAs were recently reported to be present in exosomes [41], a kind of extracellular vesicle (EV), and to function in other cells [37,42]. EVs are lipid bilayered vesicles that exist outside of cells. There are three main types of EVs: apoptotic bodies, microvesicles, and exosomes. Apoptotic bodies are 800 to 5000 nm in diameter and are released by apoptotic cells. Microvesicles are 50 to 1000 nm in diameter and are formed by budding directly from the plasma membrane. Exosomes are 40 to 100 nm in diameter and are derived from multivesicular bodies [43–45]. Two principal methods of collecting EVs are currently used: with and without ultracentrifugation [6,45]. However, the techniques are inadequate for collecting each type of EV [44,45]. Considering this fact and that the nomenclature of exosomes is confusing [46], this paper does not use the term "exosomes," but rather "EVs". EVs have an important role in cell-to-cell communication via the transfer of miRNAs, mRNAs, proteins, and bioactive lipids to target cells [6,37,41,42,44,47]. The secretion of EVs containing miRNAs depends on the cell type, biological condition, and types of miRNAs the cells contain [6,47].

**Table 1.** Selected miRNAs important for progression of osteolytic metastasis.

| miRNA | Function(s) | Reference(s) |
|---|---|---|
| miR-16 | Potential circulating biomarker for bone metastasis | [3] |
| miR-21 | Functions as an oncogene | [32] |
|  | Highly expressed during osteoclastogenesis | [24] |
|  | Highly detected in osteoclast EVs | [6] |
| miR-31 | Inhibits breast cancer metastasis | [33] |
|  | Promotes ring-shaped mature osteoclast formation | [34] |
| miR-33a | Inhibits bone metastasis by targeting *PTHrP* | [31] |
|  | Downregulated during osteoclastogenesis | [3] |
| miR-34a | Inhibits osteoclast differentiation by targeting *Tgif2* | [29] |
|  | Attenuates bone metastasis | [29] |
| miR-125a | Tumor suppressor in breast cancer | [32] |
|  | Upregulated during osteoclastogenesis | [28] |
|  | Inhibits osteoclast differentiation by targeting *TRAF6* | [35] |
| miR-133a | Inhibits osteoclast differentiation by targeting *Mitf* and *Mmp14* | [3] |
| miR-141 | Inhibits osteoclast differentiation by targeting *Mitf* and *Calcr* | [3] |
| miR-155 | Highly expressed in invasive tumors | [32] |
|  | Inhibits osteoclastogenesis by repressing MITF and PU.1 | [25] |
|  | Deficiency promotes tumor growth *in vivo* | [36] |
| miR-190 | Inhibits osteoclast differentiation by targeting *Calcr* | [3] |
| miR-192 | Inhibits angiogenesis and decreases bone metastasis | [37] |
| miR-219 | Inhibits osteoclast differentiation by targeting *Mitf* and *Traf6* | [3] |
| miR-223 | Inhibits murine osteoclast differentiation | [21,22] |
|  | Decreases breast cancer cell proliferation | [38] |
| miR-326 | Potential circulating biomarker for bone metastasis | [39] |
| miR-378 | Potential circulating biomarker for bone metastasis | [3] |
|  | Highly detected in osteoclast EVs | [6] |
|  | Promotes cell survival, tumor growth, and angiogenesis | [40] |
| miR-204/211/379 | Inhibits TGF-β-induced IL-11 production | [30] |

Although osteoclasts play important roles in osteolytic bone metastasis, whether osteoclasts secrete EVs containing miRNAs was unknown until recently. Therefore, we investigated eight miRNAs in the EVs deemed important for osteoclastogenesis in our previous study: let-7e, miR-21, miR-33, miR-155, miR-210, miR-223, miR-378, and miR-1224 [6]. Of these, the expression levels of miR-378, miR-21, and miR-210 were very high, while no significant expression of miR-33 or miR-1224 was detected [6]. These results suggest that osteoclasts secrete EVs containing specific miRNAs, but that they do not contain the entire set of intracellular miRNAs. miR-16 and miR-378 are reportedly higher in serum from mice with highly metastatic breast cancer cells and in serum from patients with breast cancer metastasis to bone than in healthy female donors [3]. miRNAs in serum and plasma are divided into two populations: a vesicle-associated membrane-bound form and a ribonucleoprotein-associated non-membrane-bound form [48]. Considering that most miR-16 in human serum is present in the ribonucleoprotein-associated non-membrane-bound form [48], increased levels of miR-16 in the serum of patients with bone metastasis may be of the ribonucleoprotein-associated non-membrane-bound form. Valencia *et al.* [39] reported that serum miR-326 could potentially serve as a novel biochemical marker for monitoring bone metastasis from lung cancer. They reported that the level of miR-326 may not only reflect tumor-autonomous release, but also host-derived factors acting on tumor cells, because

*J. Clin. Med.* **2015**, *4*, 1741–1752

miR-326 has been implicated in lymphocytic differentiation, chemoresistance, and tumor-suppressive activities [39].

While these reports are important, the function of miRNAs and EVs was not mentioned. Several reports suggest the involvement of EVs in osteolytic bone metastasis. One suggests that forced expression of miR-192 in EVs of highly metastatic lung cancer cells decreases osteolytic lesions in a mouse model. miR-192 in the EVs is transferred to endothelial cells and inhibits angiogenesis [37]. A second study showed that EVs from multiple myeloma cells increase CXC-chemokine receptor 4 expression in pre-osteoclasts and modulate cell migration. EVs derived from the serum of patients with multiple myeloma promote osteoclast differentiation [49]. A third report showed that EVs from parathyroid hormone (PTH)-treated UAMS-32P cells from a stromal/osteoblastic cell line promote osteoclast differentiation. The EVs containing RANK, RANKL receptor, and RANKL antibody treatment inhibited osteoclastogenesis [50]. Thus, EVs from PTH-treated osteoblastic cells promote osteoclast differentiation via RANK/RANKL signaling. Given that both PTH and PTHrP bind to the same receptor, the PTH/PTHrP receptor, PTHrP from tumor cells may stimulate stromal/osteoblastic cells to secrete EVs, and thus the EVs may induce osteoclast differentiation (Figure 2).

## 5. Conclusions

Bone metastasis is a highly complicated process, and the bone microenvironment contains numerous physical factors. Although a single miRNA generally represses the production of hundreds of proteins, the repression is typically mild [51]. Considering this mild effect, it may be necessary to combine miRNA-based and traditional routine therapies to successfully treat bone metastasis. For example, combination treatments with miRNAs and currently approved osteoclast-targeting agents, such as bisphosphonates and the anti-RANKL antibody denosumab, might provide enhanced clinical efficiency. Although it may be a long way to the use of miRNAs as therapeutic agents, we anticipate that this new therapeutic target for bone metastasis opens another door to cancer treatment.

**Acknowledgments:** This work was supported, in part, by the grant from the Scientific Research (C) (No. 26462853) from the Ministry of Education, Culture, Sports, Science and Technology, Japan.

**Conflicts of Interest:** The author declares no conflict of interest.

## References

1. Krzeszinski, J.Y.; Wan, Y. New therapeutic targets for cancer bone metastasis. *Trends Pharmacol. Sci.* **2015**, *36*, 360–373. [CrossRef] [PubMed]
2. Browne, G.; Taipaleenmaki, H.; Stein, G.S.; Stein, J.L.; Lian, J.B. MicroRNAs in the control of metastatic bone disease. *Trends Endocrinol. Metab.* **2014**, *25*, 320–327. [CrossRef] [PubMed]
3. Ell, B.; Mercatali, L.; Ibrahim, T.; Campbell, N.; Schwarzenbach, H.; Pantel, K.; Amadori, D.; Kang, Y. Tumor-induced osteoclast miRNA changes as regulators and biomarkers of osteolytic bone metastasis. *Cancer Cell* **2013**, *24*, 542–556. [CrossRef] [PubMed]
4. Waning, D.L.; Mohammad, K.S.; Guise, T.A. Cancer-associated osteoclast differentiation takes a good look in the miR(NA)ror. *Cancer Cell* **2013**, *24*, 407–409. [CrossRef] [PubMed]
5. Kagiya, T.; Nakamura, S. Expression profiling of microRNAs in RAW264.7 cells treated with a combination of tumor necrosis factor alpha and RANKL during osteoclast differentiation. *J. Periodontal Res.* **2013**, *48*, 373–385. [CrossRef] [PubMed]
6. Kagiya, T.; Taira, M. Expression of MicroRNAs in the Extracellular Microvesicles of Murine Osteoclasts. *J. Oral Tissue Engin.* **2013**, *10*, 142–150.
7. Itzstein, C.; Coxon, F.P.; Rogers, M.J. The regulation of osteoclast function and bone resorption by small GTPases. *Small GTPases* **2011**, *2*, 117–130. [CrossRef] [PubMed]
8. Nakashima, T.; Takayanagi, H. Osteoclasts and the immune system. *J. Bone Miner. Metab.* **2009**, *27*, 519–529. [CrossRef] [PubMed]
9. Weilbaecher, K.N.; Guise, T.A.; McCauley, L.K. Cancer to bone: a fatal attraction. *Nat. Rev. Cancer* **2011**, *11*, 411–425. [CrossRef] [PubMed]

*J. Clin. Med.* **2015**, *4*, 1741–1752

10. Jones, D.H.; Nakashima, T.; Sanchez, O.H.; Kozieradzki, I.; Komarova, S.V.; Sarosi, I.; Morony, S.; Rubin, E.; Sarao, R.; Hojilla, C.V.; *et al.* Regulation of cancer cell migration and bone metastasis by RANKL. *Nature* **2006**, *440*, 692–696. [CrossRef] [PubMed]

11. Kingsley, L.A.; Fournier, P.G.; Chirgwin, J.M.; Guise, T.A. Molecular biology of bone metastasis. *Mol. Cancer Ther.* **2007**, *6*, 2609–2617. [CrossRef] [PubMed]

12. Croset, M.; Santini, D.; Iuliani, M.; Fioramonti, M.; Zoccoli, A.; Vincenzi, B.; Tonini, G.; Pantano, F. MicroRNAs and bone metastasis: a new challenge. *Molecules* **2014**, *19*, 10115–10128. [CrossRef] [PubMed]

13. Sugino, T.; Yamaguchi, T.; Hoshi, N.; Kusakabe, T.; Ogura, G.; Goodison, S.; Suzuki, T. Sinusoidal tumor angiogenesis is a key component in hepatocellular carcinoma metastasis. *Clin. Exp. Metastasis* **2008**, *25*, 835–841. [CrossRef] [PubMed]

14. Sugino, T.; Kusakabe, T.; Hoshi, N.; Yamaguchi, T.; Kawaguchi, T.; Goodison, S.; Sekimata, M.; Homma, Y.; Suzuki, T. An invasion-independent pathway of blood-borne metastasis: a new murine mammary tumor model. *Am. J. Pathol.* **2002**, *160*, 1973–1980. [CrossRef]

15. Kats-Ugurlu, G.; Roodink, I.; de Weijert, M.; Tiemessen, D.; Maass, C.; Verrijp, K.; van der Laak, J.; de Waal, R.; Mulders, P.; Oosterwijk, E.; *et al.* Circulating tumour tissue fragments in patients with pulmonary metastasis of clear cell renal cell carcinoma. *J. Pathol.* **2009**, *219*, 287–293. [CrossRef] [PubMed]

16. Al-Mehdi, A.B.; Tozawa, K.; Fisher, A.B.; Shientag, L.; Lee, A.; Muschel, R.J. Intravascular origin of metastasis from the proliferation of endothelium-attached tumor cells: a new model for metastasis. *Nat. Med.* **2000**, *6*, 100–102. [PubMed]

17. Suva, L.J.; Washam, C.; Nicholas, R.W.; Griffin, R.J. Bone metastasis: mechanisms and therapeutic opportunities. *Nat. Rev. Endocrinol.* **2011**, *7*, 208–218. [CrossRef] [PubMed]

18. Hiraga, T.; Myoui, A.; Hashimoto, N.; Sasaki, A.; Hata, K.; Morita, Y.; Yoshikawa, H.; Rosen, C.J.; Mundy, G.R.; Yoneda, T. Bone-derived IGF mediates crosstalk between bone and breast cancer cells in bony metastases. *Cancer Res.* **2012**, *72*, 4238–4249. [CrossRef] [PubMed]

19. Martin, T.J. Manipulating the environment of cancer cells in bone: a novel therapeutic approach. *J. Clin. Invest.* **2002**, *110*, 1399–1401. [CrossRef] [PubMed]

20. Takahashi, R.U.; Miyazaki, H.; Ochiya, T. The Roles of MicroRNAs in Breast Cancer. *Cancers* **2015**, *7*, 598–616. [CrossRef] [PubMed]

21. Sugatani, T.; Hruska, K.A. MicroRNA-223 is a key factor in osteoclast differentiation. *J. Cell Biochem.* **2007**, *101*, 996–999. [CrossRef] [PubMed]

22. Sugatani, T.; Hruska, K.A. Impaired micro-RNA pathways diminish osteoclast differentiation and function. *J. Biol. Chem.* **2009**, *284*, 4667–4678. [CrossRef] [PubMed]

23. Lee, Y.; Kim, H.J.; Park, C.K.; Kim, Y.G.; Lee, H.J.; Kim, J.Y.; Kim, H.H. MicroRNA-124 regulates osteoclast differentiation. *Bone* **2013**, *56*, 383–389. [CrossRef] [PubMed]

24. Sugatani, T.; Vacher, J.; Hruska, K.A. A microRNA expression signature of osteoclastogenesis. *Blood* **2011**, *117*, 3648–3657. [CrossRef] [PubMed]

25. Mann, M.; Barad, O.; Agami, R.; Geiger, B.; Hornstein, E. miRNA-based mechanism for the commitment of multipotent progenitors to a single cellular fate. *Proc. Natl. Acad. Sci. USA* **2010**, *107*, 15804–15809. [CrossRef] [PubMed]

26. Rossi, M.; Pitari, M.R.; Amodio, N.; Di Martino, M.T.; Conforti, F.; Leone, E.; Botta, C.; Paolino, F.M.; Del Giudice, T.; Iuliano, E.; *et al.* miR-29b negatively regulates human osteoclastic cell differentiation and function: implications for the treatment of multiple myeloma-related bone disease. *J. Cell Physiol.* **2013**, *228*, 1506–1515. [CrossRef] [PubMed]

27. Chen, C.; Cheng, P.; Xie, H.; Zhou, H.D.; Wu, X.P.; Liao, E.Y.; Luo, X.H. MiR-503 regulates osteoclastogenesis via targeting RANK. *J. Bone Miner. Res.* **2014**, *29*, 338–347. [CrossRef] [PubMed]

28. De la Rica, L.; Garcia-Gomez, A.; Comet, N.R.; Rodriguez-Ubreva, J.; Ciudad, L.; Vento-Tormo, R.; Company, C.; Alvarez-Errico, D.; Garcia, M.; Gomez-Vaquero, C.; *et al.* NF-kappaB-direct activation of microRNAs with repressive effects on monocyte-specific genes is critical for osteoclast differentiation. *Genome Biol.* **2015**, *16*, 2. [CrossRef] [PubMed]

29. Krzeszinski, J.Y.; Wei, W.; Huynh, H.; Jin, Z.; Wang, X.; Chang, T.C.; Xie, X.J.; He, L.; Mangala, L.S.; Lopez-Berestein, G.; *et al.* miR-34a blocks osteoporosis and bone metastasis by inhibiting osteoclastogenesis and Tgif2. *Nature* **2014**, *512*, 431–435. [CrossRef] [PubMed]

30. Pollari, S.; Leivonen, S.K.; Perala, M.; Fey, V.; Kakonen, S.M.; Kallioniemi, O. Identification of microRNAs inhibiting TGF-beta-induced IL-11 production in bone metastatic breast cancer cells. *PLoS One* **2012**, *7*, e37361. [CrossRef] [PubMed]

31. Kuo, P.L.; Liao, S.H.; Hung, J.Y.; Huang, M.S.; Hsu, Y.L. MicroRNA-33a functions as a bone metastasis suppressor in lung cancer by targeting parathyroid hormone related protein. *Biochim. Biophys. Acta.* **2013**, *1830*, 3756–3766. [CrossRef] [PubMed]

32. O'Day, E.; Lal, A. MicroRNAs and their target gene networks in breast cancer. *Breast Cancer Res.* **2010**, *12*, 201. [CrossRef] [PubMed]

33. Valastyan, S.; Weinberg, R.A. miR-31: a crucial overseer of tumor metastasis and other emerging roles. *Cell Cycle* **2010**, *9*, 2124–2129. [CrossRef] [PubMed]

34. Mizoguchi, F.; Murakami, Y.; Saito, T.; Miyasaka, N.; Kohsaka, H. miR-31 controls osteoclast formation and bone resorption by targeting RhoA. *Arthritis Res. Ther.* **2013**, *15*, R102. [CrossRef] [PubMed]

35. Guo, L.J.; Liao, L.; Yang, L.; Li, Y.; Jiang, T.J. MiR-125a TNF receptor-associated factor 6 to inhibit osteoclastogenesis. *Exp. Cell Res.* **2014**, *321*, 142–152. [CrossRef] [PubMed]

36. Wang, J.; Yu, F.; Jia, X.; Iwanowycz, S.; Wang, Y.; Huang, S.; Ai, W.; Fan, D. MicroRNA-155 deficiency enhances the recruitment and functions of myeloid-derived suppressor cells in tumor microenvironment and promotes solid tumor growth. *Int. J. Cancer* **2015**, *136*, E602–E613. [CrossRef] [PubMed]

37. Valencia, K.; Luis-Ravelo, D.; Bovy, N.; Anton, I.; Martinez-Canarias, S.; Zandueta, C.; Ormazabal, C.; Struman, I.; Tabruyn, S.; Rebmann, V.; *et al.* miRNA cargo within exosome-like vesicle transfer influences metastatic bone colonization. *Mol. Oncol.* **2014**, *8*, 689–703. [CrossRef] [PubMed]

38. Lim, P.K.; Bliss, S.A.; Patel, S.A.; Taborga, M.; Dave, M.A.; Gregory, L.A.; Greco, S.J.; Bryan, M.; Patel, P.S.; Rameshwar, P. Gap junction-mediated import of microRNA from bone marrow stromal cells can elicit cell cycle quiescence in breast cancer cells. *Cancer Res.* **2011**, *71*, 1550–1560. [CrossRef] [PubMed]

39. Valencia, K.; Martin-Fernandez, M.; Zandueta, C.; Ormazabal, C.; Martinez-Canarias, S.; Bandres, E.; de la Piedra, C.; Lecanda, F. miR-326 associates with biochemical markers of bone turnover in lung cancer bone metastasis. *Bone* **2013**, *52*, 532–539. [CrossRef] [PubMed]

40. Lee, D.Y.; Deng, Z.; Wang, C.H.; Yang, B.B. MicroRNA-378 promotes cell survival, tumor growth, and angiogenesis by targeting SuFu and Fus-1 expression. *Proc. Natl Acad Sci USA* **2007**, *104*, 20350–20355. [CrossRef] [PubMed]

41. Valadi, H.; Ekstrom, K.; Bossios, A.; Sjostrand, M.; Lee, J.J.; Lotvall, J.O. Exosome-mediated transfer of mRNAs and microRNAs is a novel mechanism of genetic exchange between cells. *Nat. Cell. Biol.* **2007**, *9*, 654–659. [CrossRef] [PubMed]

42. Kosaka, N.; Iguchi, H.; Yoshioka, Y.; Takeshita, F.; Matsuki, Y.; Ochiya, T. Secretory mechanisms and intercellular transfer of microRNAs in living cells. *J. Biol. Chem.* **2010**, *285*, 17442–17452. [CrossRef] [PubMed]

43. Carandini, T.; Colombo, F.; Finardi, A.; Casella, G.; Garzetti, L.; Verderio, C.; Furlan, R. Microvesicles: What is the Role in Multiple Sclerosis? *Front Neurol.* **2015**, *6*, 111. [CrossRef] [PubMed]

44. Nishida-Aoki, N.; Ochiya, T. Interactions between cancer cells and normal cells via miRNAs in extracellular vesicles. *Cell. Mol. Life Sci.* **2015**, *72*, 1849–1861. [CrossRef] [PubMed]

45. Crescitelli, R.; Lasser, C.; Szabo, T.G.; Kittel, A.; Eldh, M.; Dianzani, I.; Buzas, E.I.; Lotvall, J. Distinct RNA profiles in subpopulations of extracellular vesicles: apoptotic bodies, microvesicles and exosomes. *J. Extracell Vesicles* **2013**, *2*, 20677. [CrossRef] [PubMed]

46. Gould, S.J.; Raposo, G. As we wait: coping with an imperfect nomenclature for extracellular vesicles. *J. Extracell Vesicles* **2013**, *2*, 20389. [CrossRef] [PubMed]

47. Kagiya, T.; Taira, M. A New Application for Microarrays: Analysis of Global MicroRNA Expression Profiles in the Extracellular Microvesicles of Human Macrophage-like Cells. In *Microarrays: Principles, Applications and Technologies*; Rogers, J.V., Ed.; Nova Science Publishers: New York, NY, USA, 2014; pp. 69–80.

48. Arroyo, J.D.; Chevillet, J.R.; Kroh, E.M.; Ruf, I.K.; Pritchard, C.C.; Gibson, D.F.; Mitchell, P.S.; Bennett, C.F.; Pogosova-Agadjanyan, E.L.; Stirewalt, D.L.; *et al.* Argonaute2 complexes carry a population of circulating microRNAs independent of vesicles in human plasma. *Proc. Natl. Acad. Sci. USA* **2011**, *108*, 5003–5008. [CrossRef] [PubMed]

49. Raimondi, L.; De Luca, A.; Amodio, N.; Manno, M.; Raccosta, S.; Taverna, S.; Bellavia, D.; Naselli, F.; Fontana, S.; Schillaci, O.; *et al.* Involvement of multiple myeloma cell-derived exosomes in osteoclast differentiation. *Oncotarget* **2015**, *6*, 13772–13789. [PubMed]
50. Deng, L.; Wang, Y.; Peng, Y.; Wu, Y.; Ding, Y.; Jiang, Y.; Shen, Z.; Fu, Q. Osteoblast-derived microvesicles: A novel mechanism for communication between osteoblasts and osteoclasts. *Bone* **2015**, *79*, 37–42. [CrossRef] [PubMed]
51. Selbach, M.; Schwanhausser, B.; Thierfelder, N.; Fang, Z.; Khanin, R.; Rajewsky, N. Widespread changes in protein synthesis induced by microRNAs. *Nature* **2008**, *455*, 58–63. [CrossRef] [PubMed]

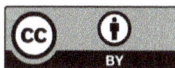

Journal of
*Clinical Medicine*

MDPI

*Review*

# Clinical Potential of microRNA-7 in Cancer

Jessica L. Horsham [1,2], Felicity C. Kalinowski [1], Michael R. Epis [1], Clarissa Ganda [1], Rikki A. M. Brown [1] and Peter J. Leedman [1,2,*]

[1] Laboratory for Cancer Medicine, Harry Perkins Institute of Medical Research, The University of Western Australia Centre for Medical Research, Perth, WA 6000, Australia; jessica.horsham@perkins.uwa.edu.au (J.L.H.); felicity.kalinowski@perkins.uwa.edu.au (F.C.K.); michael.epis@perkins.uwa.edu.au (M.R.E.); clarissa.ganda@perkins.uwa.edu.au (C.G.); rikki.brown@perkins.uwa.edu.au (R.A.M.B.)

[2] School of Medicine and Pharmacology, University of Western Australia, Nedlands, WA 6009, Australia

[*] Author to whom correspondence should be addressed; peter.leedman@perkins.uwa.edu.au; Tel.: +61-8-6151-0704; Fax: +61-8-6151-0701.

Academic Editors: Takahiro Ochiya and Ryou-u Takahashi
Received: 30 June 2015; Accepted: 17 August 2015; Published: 25 August 2015

**Abstract:** microRNAs (miRNAs) are a family of short, non-coding RNA molecules that drive a complex network of post-transcriptional gene regulation by enhancing target mRNA decay and/or inhibiting protein synthesis from mRNA transcripts. They regulate genes involved in key aspects of normal cell growth, development and the maintenance of body homeostasis and have been closely linked to the development and progression of human disease, in particular cancer. Over recent years there has been much interest regarding their potential as biomarkers and as therapeutic agents or targets. microRNA-7 (miR-7) is a 23 nucleotide (nt) miRNA known primarily to act as a tumour suppressor. miR-7 directly inhibits a number of oncogenic targets and impedes various aspects of cancer progression *in vitro* and *in vivo*, however, some studies have also implicated miR-7 in oncogenic roles. This review summarises the role of miR-7 in cancer, its potential in miRNA-based replacement therapy and its capacity as both a diagnostic and prognostic biomarker.

**Keywords:** microRNA-7; microRNA replacement therapy; biomarker; cancer; tumour suppressor

## 1. Introduction

microRNAs (miRNAs) are a class of short (~22 nt), non-coding RNA molecules which play a central role, together with the RNA-induced silencing complex (RISC), in sequence specific post-transcriptional gene attenuation. miRNAs are generally evolutionarily conserved and their endogenous expression is tightly regulated [1]. Genes under the post-transcriptional control of miRNAs are manifold and consequently, miRNAs modulate the expression of proteins involved in various pathways essential for cell function, proliferation, differentiation, survival and development. The link between deregulated miRNA expression and cancer development and progression has been firmly established. Depending on their mRNA targets, miRNAs may act as oncogenes (oncomiRs) or tumour suppressors. microRNA-7 (miR-7) is considered to be a tumour suppressor miRNA in a number of malignancies such as breast [2], brain [3], head and neck [4], liver [5], colon [6] and melanoma [7]. However, there is also evidence to the contrary with a number conflicting reports suggesting both a tumour suppressive and oncogenic role for miR-7, particularly in lung cancers [8–11]. This review is focused on miR-7 and its clinical potential in cancer, as a therapeutic molecule in itself or as a target for overexpression. In addition we examine its potential as a prognostic and diagnostic biomarker.

*J. Clin. Med.* **2015**, *4*, 1668–1687

## 2. microRNA-7 Expression and Regulation

### 2.1. Biogenesis

Expression of miR-7 stems from three loci in humans, *MIR7-1*, *MIR7-2* and *MIR7-3*. *MIR7-1* is located in the last intron of the widely expressed heterogeneous nuclear ribonucleoprotein K (*hnRNPK*) gene on chromosome 9 and is believed to be the most highly expressed source of mature miR-7 [12]. *MIR7-2* is found in an intergenic region of chromosome 15, and *MIR7-3* is located intronically within the pituitary gland specific factor 1 (*PGSF1*) gene on chromosome 19 [13]. Each miR-7 gene gives rise to three unique primary miRNA transcripts termed pri-miR-7-1, pri-miR-7-2 and pri-miR-7-3. Primary miRNA transcripts are commonly >1000 nt in length and contain stem-loop structures [1]. They are subsequently cleaved by Drosha to generate hairpin precursor miRNAs termed pre-miR-7-1, pre-miR-7-2 and pre-miR-7-3. Following Drosha cleavage, the resulting precursor miRNAs which are ~110 nt in length are transported to the cytoplasm where the terminal loop is removed by Dicer, creating a short duplex mature miRNA consisting of a miR-7-5p and miR-7-3p strand. To date, the majority of studies have concentrated on miR-7-5p which is commonly referred to simply as "miR-7". One strand, termed the "guide strand" or "leading strand" becomes associated with RISC. The guide strand may be either the -5p or the -3p strand and is determined in part by the relative stability of the 5′ end and excess of purine *versus* pyrimidine composition [14]. The passenger strand, referred to as miRNA*, is considered inactive and is typically degraded. The miRNA subsequently guides RISC to target mRNA via sequence-specific recognition, providing an interface for interaction with the corresponding mRNA. Binding typically occurs at the 3′ untranslated region (3′-UTR) of mRNA transcripts, although examples exist of binding sites within the 5′ untranslated region (5′-UTR) or mapped coding regions. Complementarity is often imperfect and central bulging results in translational repression of the mRNA, however, in the event of complete complementarity, mRNA cleavage ensues with accelerated mRNA decay. Target site recognition is dependent on perfect base pairing at nucleotides 2–8 of the miRNA known as the "seed" region. miRNAs generally exert only modest repression on their targets and so their action is more akin to "fine-tuning" gene expression [15,16]. An in-depth discussion of miRNA biogenesis can be found in a recent review by Ha and Kim (2014) [1].

All three miR-7 loci give rise to the same mature miR-7 sequence which is evolutionarily conserved. However, it should be noted that alternative sequences of miRNAs termed isomiRs have been identified in RNA-seq studies and may have biological significance. These isomiRs potentially arise from AGO2 cleavage independent of Dicer, producing base substitutions and size variations and are thought to be functionally relevant, possibly cooperating with canonical miRNAs to target common molecules and pathways [17]. Although miR-7 is expressed widely at low levels, it is enriched in various regions of the brain, particularly the pituitary [18] (noting the location of *MIR7-3* in the intron of pituitary-specific *PGSF1*), hypothalamus [19] and pancreatic islets [20,21]. Studies suggest miR-7 may have a key role in pancreatic beta cell development and maturation and accordingly is postulated to be a therapeutic target in diabetes [22,23]. The complete role of miR-7 in the brain is yet to be fully elucidated, however recent studies suggest it has roles in brain and neuronal cell development [24]. The lack of miR-7 expression in non-neuronal tissues, despite the widespread expression of the miR-7 host gene *hnRNPK*, is thought to be governed at the processing rather than at the transcriptional level [25]. Expression of intronic miRNAs may also stem from their own promoter regions [26], as has been shown for *MIR7-1* [2,8].

### 2.2. Transcriptional and Post-Transcriptional Regulation

The regulation of mature miR-7 expression occurs at the transcriptional level as well as at various stages throughout the miRNA maturation process, and there are many examples. At the transcriptional level, miR-7 expression has been shown to be promoted by epidermal growth factor receptor (EGFR) signaling in lung cancer via Rat sarcoma (Ras)/extracellular signal-regulated kinase (ERK)/v-Myc avian myelocytomatosis viral oncogene homolog (c-Myc) and phosphoinositide 3-kinase (PI3K)/v-Akt murine thymoma viral oncogene homolog (Akt) pathways. Whilst the exact mechanism of miR-7 stimulation via the PI3K/Akt pathway is yet to be identified, the transcription factor c-Myc was found to directly bind and stimulate expression from the *MIR7-1* promoter [8]. This finding is supported by an earlier study which also found miR-7 upregulation as a result of c-Myc expression in lymphoma [27]. Other transcription factors have similarly been involved in promoting miR-7 expression via directly interacting with the promoter regions of miR-7 genes including homeobox D10 (HOXD10) via the *MIR7-1* promoter region in breast cancer [2] and Hepatocyte Nuclear Factor 4 alpha (HNF4α) via the *MIR7-2* promoter in hepatocellular carcinoma (HCC). HNF4α was identified as part of a feedback loop also involving miR-124, miR-21 and nuclear factor-kappa B (NF-κB) [5]. Binding of these proteins to *MIR7-1* and *MIR7-2* promotor regions is illustrated in Figure 1. The transcription factor Forkhead box P3 (FOXP3) which also positively regulates miR-7 expression in breast cancer [28] has been found to have potential binding regions in the locality of *MIR7-1* and *MIR7-2* genes [29]. miR-7 expression is further promoted by hepatitis B virus X protein (HBx) in hepatitis B virus-associated HCC. The transduction of signals between HBx and miR-7 activation is postulated to involve nuclear I kappa B kinase alpha (IKKα) and I kappa B kinase (IKK)/NF-κB signaling pathways, however, this relationship is yet to be elucidated [30]. A recent study in gastric cancer found miR-7 to be involved in a negative feeback loop with IKKε and v-Rel avian reticuloendotheliosis viral oncogene homolog A (RELA). miR-7 targets and inhibits IKKε and RELA expression, and IKKε and RELA were found to suppress pri-miR-7 expression. Direct binding of RELA to both *MIR7-1* and *MIR7-2* promoter regions was confirmed [31]. Further, ubiquitin-specific peptidase 18 (Usp18) negatively regulates miR-7 expression. Knockdown of Usp18 was found to increase expression of miR-7 host genes and intergenic pri-miR-7-2 and subsequently mature miR-7 [32]. miR-7 expression is further negatively regulated by the oncogenic long non-coding RNA, Hox transcriptase antisense RNA (HOTAIR). HOTAIR indirectly inhibits miR-7 expression via HOXD10 suppression. Downregulated HOTAIR showed an anti-correlative relationship with both HOXD10 and miR-7 in MDA-MB-231 breast cancer cells and miR-7 was inversely correlated with HOTAIR expression in breast cancer patients [33].

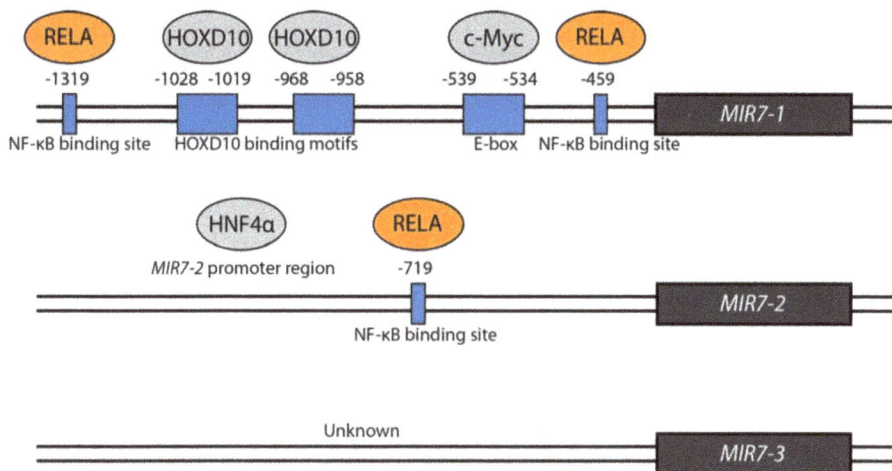

**Figure 1.** Transcriptional regulation of miR-7 by proteins confirmed to bind to *MIR7* promoter regions. Those shown in grey positively regulate miR-7 expression while those shown in orange negatively regulate miR-7 expression. The transcription factors HOXD10 and c-Myc bind to and stimulate expression from the *MIR7-1* promoter. HOXD10 may bind to two binding motifs −1019 to −1028 bp and −958 to −968 bp upstream of the *MIR7-1* transcription initiation site [2]. C-Myc has been found to bind to an E-box motif at positions −534 to −539 bp upstream of *MIR7-1* [8]. HNF4α similarly binds and stimulates expression from the *MIR7-2* promotor region. The exact location is not described [5]. RELA binds to three predicted NF-κB binding sites at −459 and −1391 bp in the *MIR7-1* and −719 bp *MIR7-2* promoters [31]. Proteins which bind and stimulate or inhibit expression from a *MIR7-3* promoter are currently unknown.

Post-transcriptional regulation of miR-7 is promoted by serine/arginine-rich splicing factor 1 (SRSF1, also known as SF2/ASF) in a splicing-independent fashion. SRSF1 promotes maturation of many miRNAs including miR-7 via enhancing Drosha cleavage of the primary transcript. miR-7 in turn targets and inhibits translation of SRSF1 via its 3′UTR, completing a negative feedback loop [34]. Conversely, the RNA binding protein, Human antigen R (HuR), negatively affects miR-7 maturation. Lebedeva *et al.* (2011) showed HuR knockdown to be negatively correlated to the specific and substantial upregulation of miR-7 [35]. Li *et al.* (2013) similarly found miR-7 expression to be impeded by toll like receptor 9 (TLR9)-induced HuR upregulation in lung cancer cells [36]. Furthermore, Musashi homolog 2 (MSI2) was found to bind to the terminal loop of the pri-miR-7 transcript in an HuR-dependent manner in non-neural cells resulting in failure of the pri-miR-7-1 transcript to mature [25]. Quaking homologs, KH domain RNA binding 5 and 6 (QKI-5 and QKI-6), have also been implicated in the failure of miR-7-1 to be processed into mature miR-7 and exported to the cytoplasm in glioblastoma. QKI binding sites were found in pri-miR-7-1 and pri-miR-7-2 but not pri-miR-7-3. QKI-5 and QKI-6 are speculated to increase association of miR-7-1 with Drosha [37].

A circular RNA (circRNA) sponge for miR-7 termed "ciRS-7" (also referred to as CDR1NAT, CDR1-AS and CDR1as) has been recently identified [38,39]. ciRS-7 is derived from the antisense transcript of the coding CDR1 gene [38] and is highly and stably expressed in human and mouse brain [38]. ciRS-7 is suggested to act as a competing endogenous RNA or miRNA "sponge" in neuronal tissues and contains >70 seed-matched miR-7 binding sites. The pattern of ciRS-7 expression in the mouse brain closely aligns with that of miR-7, especially in the hippocampus and neocortex [39] and in the developing brain of mouse embryos [40]. Whilst ciRS-7 is able to considerably attenuate miR-7 activity and thereby reduce repression of miR-7 targets [39], the biological function of ciRS-7 is yet to be defined. It is suggested that ciRS-7 may act as a buffer of miR-7 activity by competing with miR-7 targets, thereby reducing the availability of miR-7 for low-affinity target mRNAs. To add an additional level of regulation, miR-671 via near-perfect complementarity has been shown to cause RISC-induced endonucleolytic ciRS-7 degradation [38]. It is speculated that upon ciRS-7 degradation, sequestered miR-7 is released. Therefore, miR-671 could possibly be considered a positive regulator of miR-7 either by release of ciRS-7 bound miR-7 or by reducing the number of available ciRS-7 molecules for miR-7 sequestration [12]. In summary, circRNAs that act as miRNA sponges are only beginning to be understood and their role in cellular homeostasis is yet to be elucidated. A summary of molecules involved in miR-7 regulation can be found in Table 1.

**Table 1.** Summary of miR-7 regulatory molecules and their effect on miR-7 expression in cancer cell lines.

| Regulatory Molecule/Pathway | miR-7 Up-(↑)/Down-(↓) Regulation | Action | Direct/Indirect Interaction | Cancer Type | Reference |
|---|---|---|---|---|---|
| EGFR signaling | ↑ | Via Ras/ERK/Myc and additionally by PI3K/Akt pathways | Indirect | Lung | Chou *et al.* (2010) [8] |
| c-Myc | ↑ | Binds and stimulates expression from the *MIR7-1* promoter | Direct | Lung | Chou *et al.* (2010) [8] |
| HOXD10 | ↑ | Binds and stimulates expression from the *MIR7-1* promoter | Direct | Breast | Reddy *et al.* (2008) [2] |
| HNF4α | ↑ | Interacts with *MIR7-2* promoter | Direct | Liver | Ning *et al.* (2014) [5] |
| FOXP3 | ↑ | Predicted binding regions in proximity to *MIR7-1* and *MIR7-2* loci | Not confirmed | Breast | McInnes *et al.* (2012) [28] |
| HBx | ↑ | Postulated to involve IKKα and IKK/NF-κB signaling | Indirect | Liver | Chen *et al.* (2013) [30] |
| RELA | ↓ | Binds to *MIR7-1* and *MIR7-2* promoter regions | Direct | Gastric | Zhao *et al.* (2015) [31] |
| Usp18 | ↓ | Mechanism not identified | Not confirmed | Cervical, Head and neck, Brain | Duex *et al.* (2011) [32] |
| HOTAIR | ↓ | Via inhibiting HOXD10 | Indirect | Breast | Zhang *et al.* (2014) [33] |
| SF2/ASF | ↑ | Binds to pri-miR-7 and promotes maturation via enhancing Drosha cleavage | Direct | Cervical | Wu *et al.* (2010) [34] |
| HuR | ↓ | Hypothesised to represses miR-7-1 processing which may involve HuR binding in the intron of *hnRNPK* which hosts the *MIR7-1* gene | Not confirmed | Cervical, Lung | Lebedeva *et al.* (2011) [35], Li *et al.* (2013) [36] |
| TLR9 signaling | ↓ | Via HuR upregulation which is suggested to involve the PI3K/Akt pathway | Indirect | Lung | Li *et al.* (2013) [36] |
| MSI2 | ↓ | Binds to the terminal loop of the pri-miR-7 transcript in an HuR-dependent manner resulting in failure of the pri-miR-7-1 transcript to mature | Direct | Cervical, Brain | Choudhury *et al.* (2013) [25] |
| QKI 5 and QKI 6 | ↓ | Bind to QKI response elements in pri-miR-7-1 resulting in processing failure (binding sites also identified in pri-miR-7-2) | Direct | Brain | Wang *et al.* 2013 [37] |
| ciRS-7 | ↓ | Contains >70 seed-matched miR-7 binding sites that can sequester miR-7 | Direct | Proof of concept demonstrated in HeLa and HEK293 cells | Hansen *et al.* 2013 [39], Memczak *et al.* 2013 [40] |

## 3. The Role of microRNA-7 in Cancer

*3.1. miR-7 is a Tumour Suppressor*

Key molecular targets of miR-7 in various tumourigenic processes and pathways have been systematically and extensively reviewed recently by Kalinowski *et al.* (2014) and by Gu *et al.* (2015) [41,42]. Expression profiling data from our own group and others suggests that miR-7 targets ~100–200 mRNAs in cancer cells, many of those targets containing putative miR-7 binding sites, so that there is significant enrichment of miR-7 activity [4,43]. One of the additional remarkable features of miRNAs such as miR-7, is that they have the potential to target multiple parts of a signaling pathway simultaneously (e.g., EGFR) which can produce a more profound inhibition of signaling compared to targeting a single site of the pathway, with a tyrosine kinase inhibitor, such as erlotinib.

The significance of miR-7 in cancer is well-documented having been shown to directly target and inhibit key oncogenic signaling molecules involved in cell cycle, proliferation, invasion and metastasis. For example, Proteasome Activator Subunit 3 (PA28γ) which promotes cell cycle progression has been shown to be directly targeted by miR-7 in the hamster ovarian cell line CHO, non-small cell lung cancer (NSCLC) and breast cancer via its 3′-UTR [44–46]. Shi *et al.* (2015) reported that miR-7 suppresses cell proliferation and induces G0/G1 phase arrest and apoptosis in breast cancer in part, via its interaction with PA28γ [46]. Moreover, miR-7 was also shown to cause cell cycle arrest in G1 phase by directly targeting cyclin E1 (CCNE1) in HCC [47].

miR-7 has also been shown to inhibit proliferation *in vitro* and importantly, tumour growth *in vivo*, with regulation of EGFR commonly being attributed to this effect [4,48,49]. EGFR is a well described target of miR-7, is a prominent regulator of normal cell differentiation, development and proliferation, and is commonly targeted for therapy in cancer [3,10,32,43,50–52]. Additionally, miR-7 affects the activity of multiple oncogenic molecules in the EGFR signaling cascade such as Akt and ERK1/2 [4,53], V-Raf-1 murine leukemia viral oncogene homolog (RAF1) [4,10,43,53], P21 protein (Cdc42/Rac)-activated kinase 1 (PAK1) [2,51], activated CDC42 kinase 1 (ACK1) [51], phosphatidylinositol-4,5-bisphosphate 3-kinase, catalytic subunit delta (PIK3CD), mammalian target of rapamycin (mTOR), phosphoprotein 70 ribosomal protein S6 kinase (p70S6K) [54] and PI3K [53] across several cancer types, demonstrating broad regulatory control over this signaling network.

miR-7 also targets key regulators of migration, invasion and epithelial-mesenchymal transition (EMT). Molecules such as focal adhesion kinase (FAK) [55,56], kruppel-like factor 4 (KLF4) [57], insulin-like growth factor-1 receptor (IGF1R) [58], insulin receptor substrate 1 (IRS-1) [2], insulin receptor substrate 2 (IRS-2) [7] and SET domain bifurcated 1 (SETDB1) [33] are all attributed to these processes. An example of this is SETDB1, which is involved in maintaining stem cell state, and is downregulated by miR-7 leading to partial reversal of EMT and inhibition of invasion and metastasis in breast cancer stem cells isolated from the MDA-MB-231 cell line. This effect can be explained by reduced activation of Signal transducer and activator of transcription 3 (STAT3) as a result of SETDB1 downregulation. SETDB1 was found to bind directly to the promoter of STAT3 and induce its expression. In contrast, knockdown of SETDB1 using RNA interference resulted in decreased STAT3 expression and activation [33]. Similarly, in an earlier study, Wang *et al.* (2013) showed that miR-7 transfected into glioma cells reduced the active phosphorylated form of STAT3 [59]. In addition, Ning *et al.* (2014) have reported miR-7 can inhibit metastasis in HCC through perturbation of NF-κB signaling by way of directly targeting and decreasing RELA and subsequently NF-κB activation [5]. Other *in vivo* studies have reported miR-7 to inhibit angiogenesis in glioblastoma xenografts [60], suppress tumour progression in gastric cancer [61] and play a role in the de-repression of epigenetically silenced tumour suppressor genes, which result in decreased colony formation and cell cycle progression in breast cancer [62].

193

*3.2. miR-7: The Oncogene?*

Whilst miR-7 expression has frequently been reported to be downregulated in several malignancies [6,7,10,33,41,43,45,54,58], increased levels have been associated with tumour aggressiveness, most notably in oestrogen receptor positive/lymph node negative (ER+/LNN) breast cancer [63], urothelial carcinoma [64] and in Human papillomavirus (HPV) infected cervical cancer patients [65]. Additionally, viral oncogene E6/E7 expression in the HPV-positive HeLa cell line was associated with upregulated miR-7 [66]. In colorectal cancer (CRC), miR-7 was found to be upregulated in advanced cancers and in selected cell lines (SW480, DLD-1, and COLO201) compared to normal mucosa. In addition, transfection with anti-miR-7 was shown to suppress cell growth in DLD-1 and COLO201 [67]. miR-7 was also reported to be increased in the stool of CRC patients, giving rise to the notion of a screening method for CRC [68]. In contrast to these examples, many reports suggest a tumour suppressive role for miR-7 in CRC. Zhang *et al.* (2013) reported miR-7 to be downregulated in CRC tumours and in six out of seven CRC cell lines when compared to normal colon tissue (these cell lines included SW480 and DLD-1) [6]. In addition, Suto *et al.* (2015) found low miR-7 expression to be associated with poor prognosis in CRC and showed miR-7 could inhibit proliferation in SW480 cells [48]. Zhang *et al.* (2013) found miR-7 overexpression resulted in reduced proliferation and induced G1 phase arrest and apoptosis via targeting yin yang 1 transcription factor (YY1) in CRC [6] and Xu *et al.* (2014) showed miR-7 targets the protein X-ray repair complementing defective repair in Chinese hamster cells 2 (XRCC2) to inhibit proliferation and induce apoptosis [69].

Conflicting reports have also emerged regarding the role of miR-7 in lung cancer. Chou *et al.* (2010) reported miR-7 to be induced via EGFR/Ras/ERK/Myc signaling and subsequently promote cell proliferation and tumour formation. However, miR-7 overexpression was also shown to attenuate EGFR expression in lung adenocarcinoma CLI-5 cells [8], suggesting the existence of an EGFR/miR-7 regulatory loop. Studies carried out in the epithelial NSCLC cell line A549 have demonstrated varied roles for miR-7. The findings of Chou *et al.* (2010) are supported by an earlier study which found that inhibiting miR-7 downregulated A549 cell growth [70]. Meza-sosa *et al.* (2014) showed that miR-7 induced proliferation and migration in A549 cells stably overexpressing miR-7, suggesting miR-7 may act as an oncomiR in an epithelial context. To strengthen this argument, naturally immortalised skin cells HaCaT also exhibited enhanced proliferation upon stable miR-7 overexpression. This was found to be due to direct downregulation of KLF4, a transcription factor which mediates diverse cellular processes including proliferation, by miR-7 [9]. In contrast, Rai *et al.* (2011) overexpressed miR-7 episomally and reported no significant growth inhibition in A549 cells, but showed suppressed growth in EGFR-addicted cell lines such as the NSCLC cell lines PC-9, H3255 and H1975. They did however observe much higher miR-7 levels in EGFR-addicted cells compared to non-addicted cells, suggesting an EGFR-mediated activation of miR-7 consistent with the findings of Chou *et al.* (2010) [10]. In work by Xiong *et al.* (2011), transient miR-7 overexpression inhibited migration, proliferation and induced apoptosis in A549 cells through targeting the anti-apoptotic molecule B-cell lymphoma 2 (BCL-2) [11]. We have found miR-7 to inhibit EGFR expression and signaling in A549 cells, consistent with it having a tumour suppressive effect [43]. In summary, clearly the role of miR-7 in lung cancer is more complex than initially envisaged, and may be particularly cell type specific and possibly dependent on the method of influencing miR-7 expression experimentally.

*3.3. Genetic Influence on the Role of miR-7*

The regulatory capacity of miR-7 is complex, given the numerous targets reported across many cell types. KLF4, a known target of miR-7 [9,57], elicits context-dependent oncogenic and tumour suppressive responses [71] and indeed, oncogenesis has been reported as a result of KLF4 suppression by miR-7 [9], as well as the opposite [57]. Similarly, with respect to the mutational profile of the cell, STAT3 (an indirect target of miR-7) can either promote or suppress tumourigenesis depending on biochemical and genetic factors [72,73]. Hence, the role/s of miR-7 may be adversely affected by the cells mutational background. Rai *et al.* (2011) suggest that the level of EGFR-addiction will play an important role in the effect of miR-7 [10]. Also, as observed in the studies conducted in A549 cells mentioned above [9–11,43,70] the experimental approach could be responsible for conflicting observations [41], which include scenarios whereby miR-7 is over- or under- expressed, the degree of miR-7 overexpression within the cell or whether miR-7 overexpression is sustained.

Given miR-7 is demonstrated to participate in feedback and "feedforward" loops, as well as regulating several transcription factors, changes in miR-7 expression may result in a "ripple" effect; that is, the indirect regulation of the expression of other genes, and even miRNAs. To emphasise this point, a study investigating miR-7 transient overexpression in ovarian cancer cells reported a change in the expression of hundreds of genes in diverse pathways; however, only ~20% of the regulated genes were predicted to be direct targets, concluding that the majority of the observed changes to gene expression are an indirect consequence of miR-7 expression and effect [74].

## 4. microRNA-7 Has Biomarker Potential

miRNAs have great potential as predictive, diagnostic and prognostic biomarkers both for cancer and other diseases, such as schizophrenia [75]. Reports indicate that free circulating miRNAs stably exist in body fluids such as blood serum, saliva [76] and urine [77]. It is hypothesised that these miRNAs have been secreted by cells in exosomes allowing for their inherent stability and resistance to RNase activity, which would otherwise degrade exogenous sources of miRNA [78,79]. Exosome secreted miRNAs found in blood and other body fluids are thought to act in cell-to-cell communication [79]. Microvesicle-free miRNA in body fluids may also exist stably associated with argonaute RISC catalytic component 2 (AGO2) [80] or high-density lipoprotein (HDL) [81]. These miRNAs provide a readily accessible and minimally invasive source for biomarker testing. miRNAs identified as potential biomarkers for cancers have also been measured in urine [82–84], saliva [85], and stool [86,87] and can be found in most body fluids [88]. Alternatively, miRNA expression may also be profiled directly from tumours and tissues or from circulating tumour cells (CTCs). CTCs represent the most preferable option as they offer a more reliable representation of the tumour miRNA profile than cell-free miRNAs and can be isolated relatively non-invasively, however, their isolation from the leukocyte background is currently challenging [89,90]. Biomarker miRNAs may not only be useful in diagnosis, especially for asymptomatic cancers such as pancreatic cancer which have no early detectable signs/symptoms, but particularly in patient stratification and even for identifying tumour origin from secondary lesions based on similarities in miRNA signatures [91].

In a study conducted by Wang *et al.* (2015), miR-7 was identified as one of three miRNAs (along with miR-93 and miR-409-3p) from an array of 723 human miRNAs, which were found to be powerful predictors of CRC. This panel of miRNAs could be used to distinguish CRC patients from healthy patients, as well as early stage CRC (nonmetastatic) and late stage CRC (metastatic) from healthy patients with great accuracy. The miRNAs were isolated from blood plasma, potentially preventing healthy patients from having to undergo uncomfortable and unnecessary colonoscopies [92]. A small proof-of-concept study by Ahmed *et al.* (2013), also conducted in CRC, found miR-7, among eleven other miRNAs, to be increased in stool samples from a small cohort of CRC patients when compared with healthy controls. This finding highlights the availability of miRNAs from stool samples which may be useful biomarkers for CRC [68]. Kitano *et al.* (2012) found miR-7 to be a useful biomarker for the prediction of benign thyroid tumours from malignant thyroid cancer, specifically in those cases where diagnosis is difficult to ascertain from fine-needle aspiration biopsies. The model was highly sensitive with a negative prediction value of 100%. Therefore, the model could correctly identify benign tumours, but lacked adequate positive prediction (identification of malignant lesions) [93]. This highlights the potential clinical usefulness of miRNA biomarkers and also the need for further investigation to achieve greater specificity and sensitivity in diagnostic assays.

In many cancer types, high or low levels of miR-7 have been associated with poor or more promising prognoses and may be harnessed for biomarker profiling. In a study identifying miRNA biomarkers involved in the progression of hormone-sensitive prostate cancer to castrate-resistant prostate cancer (CRPC), Santos *et al.* (2014) identified miR-7 levels in peripheral whole blood as a useful prognostic biomarker for CRPC development. Higher miR-7 levels in peripheral whole-blood in combination with high-Gleason score tumours was correlated with significantly earlier progression to castrate resistance and further trended toward lower overall survival of patients [94]. In contrast, in another cancer phenotype, Okuda *et al.* (2013) have suggested that low levels of miR-7 and inversely high KLF4 expression may be useful as prognostic biomarkers for predicting brain metastasis of breast cancer [57]. Thus, further evaluation of miR-7 expression in carefully selected clinical cohorts will be required to refine the potential application as a biomarker.

## 5. Potential for microRNA-7 in Cancer Therapy

### 5.1. miR-7 Replacement Therapy Alone and in Combination with Current Therapeutic Agents

miRNAs present themselves as attractive potential therapies, either in the context of replacement of tumour suppressors or suppression of oncomiR activity. miRNA therapy can be broadly assigned into two categories, replacement and inhibition. As the overwhelming majority of reports suggest miR-7 acts as a tumour suppressor, there is increasing focus on replacement therapy. One strategy is systemic administration and delivery of miR-7. Two methods have been used to successfully deliver miR-7 *in vivo* to treat cancer. In a study developed by Babae *et al.* (2014), a miR-7 mimic was systemically delivered using clinically viable, biodegradable, targeted polyamide nanoparticles. This achieved successful inhibition of tumour growth and vascularisation in a glioblastoma xenograft [60]. In an earlier study, Wang *et al.* (2013) was able to inhibit glioma xenograft growth and metastasis using a plasmid based miR-7 vector systemically delivered by encapsulation in a cationic liposome formulation [59].

miRNA-based replacement therapy is most likely to be given as a tumour suppressive miRNA in combination with other therapeutic agents, such as tyrosine kinase inhibitors. It has been suggested that miR-7 may enhance the effect of current therapeutic drugs. A number of studies have demonstrated restored therapeutic sensitivity to targeted treatments as a result of miR-7 expression *in vitro*. Results from our laboratory showed miR-7 was able to increase the sensitivity of erlotinib-resistant head and neck cancer cells to erlotinib [4]. An earlier study by Pogribny *et al.* (2010) reported miR-7 expression directly targeted and significantly inhibited multidrug resistance-associated protein 1 (MPR1) which increased sensitivity to cisplatin in cisplatin-resistant breast cancer [95]. An *in vitro* study by Suto *et al.* (2015) showed miR-7 overexpression increased sensitivity to cetuximab in HCT-116 and SW480 cetuximab-resistant CRC cells harbouring a Kirsten rat sarcoma viral oncogene homolog (KRAS) mutation. However, miR-7 was ineffective in the CRC cell line HT-29 which expresses a v-Raf murine sarcoma viral oncogene homolog B (BRAF) mutation. This was reportedly due to miR-7 targeting of not only EGFR but also RAF-1 which plays an key role in mutant KRAS signaling, but not in BRAF mutants [48]. Additionally, miR-7 was found to increase sensitivity of NSCLC to paclitaxel (PTX) by promoting PTX-induced apoptosis [96]. Results from microarray and qPCR analyses in gefitinib resistant A549 cells compared to the parental A549 cell line found miR-7 to be downregulated which suggests possible involvement in the development of gefitinib resistance, however further study is required to identify whether miR-7 has the potential to improve gefitinib sensitivity [97]. Acquired resistance to chemotherapy is common in many patients and presents a real clinical challenge. miRNAs that increase the sensitivity of cancers to current therapies offer potential for use in combinational therapy. miRNAs as therapeutics have the added advantage of concurrently regulating multiple molecules and members of various pathways which may reduce the chance of acquired resistance developing such as often the case with inhibitors that target single molecules or pathways.

### 5.2. Potential for Small Molecule Activation of microRNA-7

As previously discussed, there is the potential to regulate miRNAs at both the transcriptional and processing level. High-throughput screens have identified compounds with demonstrated potential

*J. Clin. Med.* **2015**, *4*, 1668–1687

to both promote and inhibit miRNA transcription. One example of this is curcumin, which has been shown to upregulate a number of miRNAs, including miR-7, in pancreatic cancer [98]. Also, the antibacterial enoxacin was observed to increase the processing of certain miRNAs, including miR-7, from the precursor form to the mature form in RKO and HCT-116 CRC cell lines [99] while in another study, the histone deacetylase inhibitor Thichostatin A (TSA) was found to induce miR-7 in MDA-MB-231 breast cancer cells resulting in inhibition of EGFR expression [100]. Experimentally validated relationships between small molecules and miRNA expression in various species are compiled and accessible in the SM2miR database [101]. Whilst this highlights the potential for small molecule mediated miRNA regulation, it must be emphasised that the action of these small molecules is often nonspecific, which raises the possibility of significant "off target" effects.

## 6. Conclusions

Whilst the broad coordinated simultaneous downregulation of multiple gene networks with miRNAs is an attractive therapeutic option, the potential for off-target effects is still to be well defined and requires further investigation. Nonetheless, miRNA therapy may offer clinical practice the ability to treat diseases at a network level rather than targeting a single gene. In the interim, methods to achieve effective systemic administration of miRNAs are being actively pursued; however there are several hurdles to overcome before miRNA replacement therapy becomes routinely clinically achievable for diseases beyond the liver. Alternatively, several publications have highlighted the potential for small molecules to affect and regulate miR-7 expression, opening up further therapeutic possibilities. Whilst the topic of miR-7 in cancer is the subject of a small number of reports suggesting an oncomiR-phenotype, the vast majority of literature indicates miR-7 is a tumour suppressor with many prominent oncogenic targets. In addition, several studies have demonstrated the clinical potential of miR-7 as a biomarker in diagnosis and prognosis of disease. One of miR-7's key clinical applications may relate to its capacity to sensitise tumours that are resistant to other targeted therapies (e.g., erlotinib). In summary, the accumulating *in vitro* and *in vivo* preclinical data continues to build a strong case for the use of miR-7 replacement therapy in specific cancers, especially HCC and head and neck cancer. It will be of great interest in the next few years to see if this prediction comes to fruition.

**Acknowledgments:** The authors gratefully acknowledge funding from the National Health and Medical Research Council (NHMRC) of Australia, the Cancer Council of Western Australia (CCWA), the Royal Perth Hospital Medical Research Foundation, and the Harry Perkins Institute of Medical Research.

**Author Contributions:** Jessica L. Horsham wrote the manuscript in conjunction with coauthors who edited and approved the final version of the manuscript.

**Conflicts of Interest:** The authors declare no conflict of interest.

## References

1. Ha, M.; Kim, V.N. Regulation of microrna biogenesis. *Nat. Rev. Mol. Cell Biol.* **2014**, *15*, 509–524. [CrossRef] [PubMed]
2. Reddy, S.D.; Ohshiro, K.; Rayala, S.K.; Kumar, R. Microrna-7, a homeobox d10 target, inhibits p21-activated kinase 1 and regulates its functions. *Cancer Res.* **2008**, *68*, 8195–8200. [CrossRef] [PubMed]
3. Kefas, B.; Godlewski, J.; Comeau, L.; Li, Y.; Abounader, R.; Hawkinson, M.; Lee, J.; Fine, H.; Chiocca, E.A.; Lawler, S.; *et al.* Microrna-7 inhibits the epidermal growth factor receptor and the akt pathway and is down-regulated in glioblastoma. *Cancer Res.* **2008**, *68*, 3566–3572. [CrossRef] [PubMed]
4. Kalinowski, F.C.; Giles, K.M.; Candy, P.A.; Ali, A.; Ganda, C.; Epis, M.R.; Webster, R.J.; Leedman, P.J. Regulation of epidermal growth factor receptor signaling and erlotinib sensitivity in head and neck cancer cells by mir-7. *PLoS One* **2012**, *7*, e47067. [CrossRef] [PubMed]
5. Ning, B.F.; Ding, J.; Liu, J.; Yin, C.; Xu, W.P.; Cong, W.M.; Zhang, Q.; Chen, F.; Han, T.; Deng, X.; *et al.* Hepatocyte nuclear factor 4alpha-nuclear factor-kappab feedback circuit modulates liver cancer progression. *Hepatology* **2014**, *60*, 1607–1619. [CrossRef]

6.   Zhang, N.; Li, X.; Wu, C.W.; Dong, Y.; Cai, M.; Mok, M.T.; Wang, H.; Chen, J.; Ng, S.S.; Chen, M.; *et al.* Microrna-7 is a novel inhibitor of yy1 contributing to colorectal tumorigenesis. *Oncogene* **2013**, *32*, 5078–5088. [CrossRef] [PubMed]

7.   Giles, K.M.; Brown, R.A.; Epis, M.R.; Kalinowski, F.C.; Leedman, P.J. Mirna-7-5p inhibits melanoma cell migration and invasion. *Biochem. Biophys. Res. Commun.* **2013**, *430*, 706–710. [CrossRef] [PubMed]

8.   Chou, Y.T.; Lin, H.H.; Lien, Y.C.; Wang, Y.H.; Hong, C.F.; Kao, Y.R.; Lin, S.C.; Chang, Y.C.; Lin, S.Y.; Chen, S.J.; *et al.* Egfr promotes lung tumorigenesis by activating mir-7 through a ras/erk/myc pathway that targets the ets2 transcriptional repressor erf. *Cancer Res.* **2010**, *70*, 8822–8831. [CrossRef] [PubMed]

9.   Meza-Sosa, K.F.; Perez-Garcia, E.I.; Camacho-Concha, N.; Lopez-Gutierrez, O.; Pedraza-Alva, G.; Perez-Martinez, L. Mir-7 promotes epithelial cell transformation by targeting the tumor suppressor klf4. *PLoS One* **2014**, *9*, e103987. [CrossRef] [PubMed]

10.  Rai, K.; Takigawa, N.; Ito, S.; Kashihara, H.; Ichihara, E.; Yasuda, T.; Shimizu, K.; Tanimoto, M.; Kiura, K. Liposomal delivery of microrna-7-expressing plasmid overcomes epidermal growth factor receptor tyrosine kinase inhibitor-resistance in lung cancer cells. *Mol. Cancer Ther.* **2011**, *10*, 1720–1727. [CrossRef] [PubMed]

11.  Xiong, S.; Zheng, Y.; Jiang, P.; Liu, R.; Liu, X.; Chu, Y. Microrna-7 inhibits the growth of human non-small cell lung cancer a549 cells through targeting bcl-2. *Int. J. Biol. Sci.* **2011**, *7*, 805–814. [CrossRef] [PubMed]

12.  Hansen, T.B.; Kjems, J.; Damgaard, C.K. Circular rna and mir-7 in cancer. *Cancer Res.* **2013**, *73*, 5609–5612. [CrossRef] [PubMed]

13.  Ncbi Database, Gene. Available online: http://www.ncbi.nlm.nih.gov/gene/?term=hsa-miR-7 (accessed on 11 June 2015).

14.  Meijer, H.A.; Smith, E.M.; Bushell, M. Regulation of mirna strand selection: Follow the leader? *Biochem. Soc. Trans.* **2014**, *42*, 1135–1140. [CrossRef] [PubMed]

15.  Baek, D.; Villen, J.; Shin, C.; Camargo, F.D.; Gygi, S.P.; Bartel, D.P. The impact of micrornas on protein output. *Nature* **2008**, *455*, 64–71. [CrossRef] [PubMed]

16.  Ebert, M.S.; Sharp, P.A. Roles for micrornas in conferring robustness to biological processes. *Cell* **2012**, *149*, 515–524. [CrossRef] [PubMed]

17.  Cloonan, N.; Wani, S.; Xu, Q.; Gu, J.; Lea, K.; Heater, S.; Barbacioru, C.; Steptoe, A.L.; Martin, H.C.; Nourbakhsh, E.; *et al.* Micrornas and their isomirs function cooperatively to target common biological pathways. *Genome Biol.* **2011**, *12*. [CrossRef] [PubMed]

18.  Landgraf, P.; Rusu, M.; Sheridan, R.; Sewer, A.; Iovino, N.; Aravin, A.; Pfeffer, S.; Rice, A.; Kamphorst, A.O.; Landthaler, M.; *et al.* A mammalian microrna expression atlas based on small rna library sequencing. *Cell* **2007**, *129*, 1401–1414. [CrossRef] [PubMed]

19.  Farh, K.K.; Grimson, A.; Jan, C.; Lewis, B.P.; Johnston, W.K.; Lim, L.P.; Burge, C.B.; Bartel, D.P. The widespread impact of mammalian micrornas on mrna repression and evolution. *Science* **2005**, *310*, 1817–1821. [CrossRef] [PubMed]

20.  Bravo-Egana, V.; Rosero, S.; Molano, R.D.; Pileggi, A.; Ricordi, C.; Dominguez-Bendala, J.; Pastori, R.L. Quantitative differential expression analysis reveals mir-7 as major islet microrna. *Biochem. Biophys. Res. Commun.* **2008**, *366*, 922–926. [CrossRef] [PubMed]

21.  Correa-Medina, M.; Bravo-Egana, V.; Rosero, S.; Ricordi, C.; Edlund, H.; Diez, J.; Pastori, R.L. Microrna mir-7 is preferentially expressed in endocrine cells of the developing and adult human pancreas. *Gene Expr. Patterns GEP* **2009**, *9*, 193–199. [CrossRef] [PubMed]

22.  Wang, Y.; Liu, J.; Liu, C.; Naji, A.; Stoffers, D.A. Microrna-7 regulates the mtor pathway and proliferation in adult pancreatic beta-cells. *Diabetes* **2013**, *62*, 887–895. [CrossRef] [PubMed]

23.  Latreille, M.; Hausser, J.; Stutzer, I.; Zhang, Q.; Hastoy, B.; Gargani, S.; Kerr-Conte, J.; Pattou, F.; Zavolan, M.; Esguerra, J.L.; *et al.* Microrna-7a regulates pancreatic beta cell function. *J. Clin. Investig.* **2014**, *124*, 2722–2735. [CrossRef] [PubMed]

24.  Chen, H.; Shalom-Feuerstein, R.; Riley, J.; Zhang, S.D.; Tucci, P.; Agostini, M.; Aberdam, D.; Knight, R.A.; Genchi, G.; Nicotera, P.; *et al.* Mir-7 and mir-214 are specifically expressed during neuroblastoma differentiation, cortical development and embryonic stem cells differentiation, and control neurite outgrowth *in vitro*. *Biochem. Biophys. Res. Commun.* **2010**, *394*, 921–927. [CrossRef]

25.  Choudhury, N.R.; de Lima Alves, F.; de Andres-Aguayo, L.; Graf, T.; Caceres, J.F.; Rappsilber, J.; Michlewski, G. Tissue-specific control of brain-enriched mir-7 biogenesis. *Genes Dev.* **2013**, *27*, 24–38. [CrossRef] [PubMed]

26. Ozsolak, F.; Poling, L.L.; Wang, Z.; Liu, H.; Liu, X.S.; Roeder, R.G.; Zhang, X.; Song, J.S.; Fisher, D.E. Chromatin structure analyses identify mirna promoters. *Genes Dev.* **2008**, *22*, 3172–3183. [CrossRef] [PubMed]

27. Chang, T.C.; Yu, D.; Lee, Y.S.; Wentzel, E.A.; Arking, D.E.; West, K.M.; Dang, C.V.; Thomas-Tikhonenko, A.; Mendell, J.T. Widespread microrna repression by myc contributes to tumorigenesis. *Nat. Genet.* **2008**, *40*, 43–50. [CrossRef] [PubMed]

28. McInnes, N.; Sadlon, T.J.; Brown, C.Y.; Pederson, S.; Beyer, M.; Schultze, J.L.; McColl, S.; Goodall, G.J.; Barry, S.C. Foxp3 and foxp3-regulated micrornas suppress satb1 in breast cancer cells. *Oncogene* **2012**, *31*, 1045–1054. [CrossRef] [PubMed]

29. Sadlon, T.J.; Wilkinson, B.G.; Pederson, S.; Brown, C.Y.; Bresatz, S.; Gargett, T.; Melville, E.L.; Peng, K.; D'Andrea, R.J.; Glonek, G.G.; *et al.* Genome-wide identification of human foxp3 target genes in natural regulatory t cells. *J. Immunol.* **2010**, *185*, 1071–1081. [CrossRef] [PubMed]

30. Chen, Y.J.; Chien, P.H.; Chen, W.S.; Chien, Y.F.; Hsu, Y.Y.; Wang, L.Y.; Chen, J.Y.; Lin, C.W.; Huang, T.C.; Yu, Y.L.; *et al.* Hepatitis b virus-encoded x protein downregulates egfr expression via inducing microrna-7 in hepatocellular carcinoma cells. *Evid.-Based Complement. Altern. Med. eCAM* **2013**, *2013*. [CrossRef] [PubMed]

31. Zhao, X.-D.; Lu, Y.-Y.; Guo, H.; Xie, H.-H.; He, L.-J.; Shen, G.-F.; Zhou, J.-F.; Li, T.; Hu, S.-J.; Zhou, L.; *et al.* Microrna-7/nf-κb signaling regulatory feedback circuit regulates gastric carcinogenesis. *J. Cell Biol.* **2015**, *210*, 613–627. [CrossRef]

32. Duex, J.E.; Comeau, L.; Sorkin, A.; Purow, B.; Kefas, B. Usp18 regulates epidermal growth factor (egf) receptor expression and cancer cell survival via microrna-7. *J. Biol. Chem.* **2011**, *286*, 25377–25386. [CrossRef] [PubMed]

33. Zhang, H.; Cai, K.; Wang, J.; Wang, X.; Cheng, K.; Shi, F.; Jiang, L.; Zhang, Y.; Dou, J. Mir-7, inhibited indirectly by lincrna hotair, directly inhibits setdb1 and reverses the emt of breast cancer stem cells by downregulating the stat3 pathway. *Stem Cells* **2014**, *32*, 2858–2868. [CrossRef] [PubMed]

34. Wu, H.; Sun, S.; Tu, K.; Gao, Y.; Xie, B.; Krainer, A.R.; Zhu, J. A splicing-independent function of sf2/asf in microrna processing. *Mol. Cell* **2010**, *38*, 67–77. [CrossRef] [PubMed]

35. Lebedeva, S.; Jens, M.; Theil, K.; Schwanhausser, B.; Selbach, M.; Landthaler, M.; Rajewsky, N. Transcriptome-wide analysis of regulatory interactions of the rna-binding protein hur. *Mol. Cell* **2011**, *43*, 340–352. [CrossRef] [PubMed]

36. Li, Y.J.; Wang, C.H.; Zhou, Y.; Liao, Z.Y.; Zhu, S.F.; Hu, Y.; Chen, C.; Luo, J.M.; Wen, Z.K.; Xu, L.; *et al.* Tlr9 signaling repressed tumor suppressor mir-7 expression through up-regulation of hur in human lung cancer cells. *Cancer Cell Int.* **2013**, *13*. [CrossRef] [PubMed]

37. Wang, Y.; Vogel, G.; Yu, Z.; Richard, S. The qki-5 and qki-6 rna binding proteins regulate the expression of microrna 7 in glial cells. *Mol. Cell. Biol.* **2013**, *33*, 1233–1243. [CrossRef] [PubMed]

38. Hansen, T.B.; Wiklund, E.D.; Bramsen, J.B.; Villadsen, S.B.; Statham, A.L.; Clark, S.J.; Kjems, J. Mirna-dependent gene silencing involving ago2-mediated cleavage of a circular antisense rna. *EMBO J.* **2011**, *30*, 4414–4422. [CrossRef] [PubMed]

39. Hansen, T.B.; Jensen, T.I.; Clausen, B.H.; Bramsen, J.B.; Finsen, B.; Damgaard, C.K.; Kjems, J. Natural rna circles function as efficient microrna sponges. *Nature* **2013**, *495*, 384–388. [CrossRef] [PubMed]

40. Memczak, S.; Jens, M.; Elefsinioti, A.; Torti, F.; Krueger, J.; Rybak, A.; Maier, L.; Mackowiak, S.D.; Gregersen, L.H.; Munschauer, M.; *et al.* Circular rnas are a large class of animal rnas with regulatory potency. *Nature* **2013**, *495*, 333–338. [CrossRef] [PubMed]

41. Kalinowski, F.C.; Brown, R.A.; Ganda, C.; Giles, K.M.; Epis, M.R.; Horsham, J.; Leedman, P.J. Microrna-7: A tumor suppressor mirna with therapeutic potential. *Int. J. Biochem. Cell Biol.* **2014**, *54*, 312–317. [CrossRef] [PubMed]

42. Gu, D.N.; Huang, Q.; Tian, L. The molecular mechanisms and therapeutic potential of microrna-7 in cancer. *Expert opin. Ther. Targets* **2015**, *19*, 415–426. [CrossRef] [PubMed]

43. Webster, R.J.; Giles, K.M.; Price, K.J.; Zhang, P.M.; Mattick, J.S.; Leedman, P.J. Regulation of epidermal growth factor receptor signaling in human cancer cells by microrna-7. *J. Biol. Chem.* **2009**, *284*, 5731–5741. [CrossRef] [PubMed]

44. Sanchez, N.; Gallagher, M.; Lao, N.; Gallagher, C.; Clarke, C.; Doolan, P.; Aherne, S.; Blanco, A.; Meleady, P.; Clynes, M.; *et al.* Mir-7 triggers cell cycle arrest at the g1/s transition by targeting multiple genes including skp2 and psme3. *PLoS ONE* **2013**, *8*, e65671. [CrossRef] [PubMed]

45. Xiong, S.; Zheng, Y.; Jiang, P.; Liu, R.; Liu, X.; Qian, J.; Gu, J.; Chang, L.; Ge, D.; Chu, Y.; *et al.* Pa28gamma emerges as a novel functional target of tumour suppressor microrna-7 in non-small-cell lung cancer. *Br. J. Cancer* **2014**, *110*, 353–362. [CrossRef] [PubMed]

46. Shi, Y.; Luo, X.; Li, P.; Tan, J.; Wang, X.; Xiang, T.; Ren, G. Mir-7-5p suppresses cell proliferation and induces apoptosis of breast cancer cells mainly by targeting reggamma. *Cancer Lett.* **2015**, *358*, 27–36. [CrossRef] [PubMed]

47. Zhang, X.; Hu, S.; Zhang, X.; Wang, L.; Zhang, X.; Yan, B.; Zhao, J.; Yang, A.; Zhang, R. Microrna-7 arrests cell cycle in g1 phase by directly targeting ccne1 in human hepatocellular carcinoma cells. *Biochem. Biophys. Res. Commun.* **2014**, *443*, 1078–1084. [CrossRef] [PubMed]

48. Suto, T.; Yokobori, T.; Yajima, R.; Morita, H.; Fujii, T.; Yamaguchi, S.; Altan, B.; Tsutsumi, S.; Asao, T.; Kuwano, H.; *et al.* Microrna-7 expression in colorectal cancer is associated with poor prognosis and regulates cetuximab sensitivity via egfr regulation. *Carcinogenesis* **2015**, *36*, 338–345. [CrossRef] [PubMed]

49. Li, J.; Zheng, Y.; Sun, G.; Xiong, S. Restoration of mir-7 expression suppresses the growth of lewis lung cancer cells by modulating epidermal growth factor receptor signaling. *Oncol. Rep.* **2014**, *32*, 2511–2516. [CrossRef] [PubMed]

50. Lee, K.M.; Choi, E.J.; Kim, I.A. Microrna-7 increases radiosensitivity of human cancer cells with activated egfr-associated signaling. *Radiother. Oncol.* **2011**, *101*, 171–176. [CrossRef] [PubMed]

51. Saydam, O.; Senol, O.; Wurdinger, T.; Mizrak, A.; Ozdener, G.B.; Stemmer-Rachamimov, A.O.; Yi, M.; Stephens, R.M.; Krichevsky, A.M.; Saydam, N.; *et al.* Mirna-7 attenuation in schwannoma tumors stimulates growth by upregulating three oncogenic signaling pathways. *Cancer Res.* **2011**, *71*, 852–861. [CrossRef] [PubMed]

52. Xie, J.; Chen, M.; Zhou, J.; Mo, M.S.; Zhu, L.H.; Liu, Y.P.; Gui, Q.J.; Zhang, L.; Li, G.Q. Mir-7 inhibits the invasion and metastasis of gastric cancer cells by suppressing epidermal growth factor receptor expression. *Oncol. Rep.* **2014**, *31*, 1715–1722. [CrossRef] [PubMed]

53. Liu, Z.; Jiang, Z.; Huang, J.; Huang, S.; Li, Y.; Yu, S.; Yu, S.; Liu, X. Mir-7 inhibits glioblastoma growth by simultaneously interfering with the pi3k/atk and raf/mek/erk pathways. *Int. J. Oncol.* **2014**, *44*, 1571–1580. [CrossRef] [PubMed]

54. Fang, Y.; Xue, J.L.; Shen, Q.; Chen, J.; Tian, L. Microrna-7 inhibits tumor growth and metastasis by targeting the phosphoinositide 3-kinase/akt pathway in hepatocellular carcinoma. *Hepatology* **2012**, *55*, 1852–1862. [CrossRef] [PubMed]

55. Wu, D.G.; Wang, Y.Y.; Fan, L.G.; Luo, H.; Han, B.; Sun, L.H.; Wang, X.F.; Zhang, J.X.; Cao, L.; Wang, X.R.; *et al.* Microrna-7 regulates glioblastoma cell invasion via targeting focal adhesion kinase expression. *Chin. Med. J.* **2011**, *124*, 2616–2621. [PubMed]

56. Kong, X.; Li, G.; Yuan, Y.; He, Y.; Wu, X.; Zhang, W.; Wu, Z.; Chen, T.; Wu, W.; Lobie, P.E.; *et al.* Microrna-7 inhibits epithelial-to-mesenchymal transition and metastasis of breast cancer cells via targeting fak expression. *PLoS ONE* **2012**, *7*, e41523. [CrossRef] [PubMed]

57. Okuda, H.; Xing, F.; Pandey, P.R.; Sharma, S.; Watabe, M.; Pai, S.K.; Mo, Y.Y.; Iiizumi-Gairani, M.; Hirota, S.; Liu, Y.; *et al.* Mir-7 suppresses brain metastasis of breast cancer stem-like cells by modulating klf4. *Cancer Res.* **2013**, *73*, 1434–1444. [CrossRef] [PubMed]

58. Zhao, X.; Dou, W.; He, L.; Liang, S.; Tie, J.; Liu, C.; Li, T.; Lu, Y.; Mo, P.; Shi, Y.; *et al.* Microrna-7 functions as an anti-metastatic microrna in gastric cancer by targeting insulin-like growth factor-1 receptor. *Oncogene* **2013**, *32*, 1363–1372. [CrossRef] [PubMed]

59. Wang, W.; Dai, L.X.; Zhang, S.; Yang, Y.; Yan, N.; Fan, P.; Dai, L.; Tian, H.W.; Cheng, L.; Zhang, X.M.; *et al.* Regulation of epidermal growth factor receptor signaling by plasmid-based microrna-7 inhibits human malignant gliomas growth and metastasis *in vivo*. *Neoplasma* **2013**, *60*, 274–283. [CrossRef] [PubMed]

60. Babae, N.; Bourajjaj, M.; Liu, Y.; van Beijnum, J.R.; Cerisoli, F.; Scaria, P.V.; Verheul, M.; van Berkel, M.P.; Pieters, E.H.; van Haastert, R.J.; *et al.* Systemic mirna-7 delivery inhibits tumor angiogenesis and growth in murine xenograft glioblastoma. *Oncotarget* **2014**, *5*, 6687–6700. [PubMed]

61. Cao, D.; Jiang, J.; Tsukamoto, T.; Liu, R.; Ma, L.; Jia, Z.; Kong, F.; Oshima, M.; Cao, X. Canolol inhibits gastric tumors initiation and progression through cox-2/pge2 pathway in k19-c2me transgenic mice. *PLoS ONE* **2015**, *10*, e0120938. [CrossRef] [PubMed]

62. Li, Q.; Zhu, F.; Chen, P. Mir-7 and mir-218 epigenetically control tumor suppressor genes rassf1a and claudin-6 by targeting hoxb3 in breast cancer. *Biochem. Biophys. Res. Commun.* **2012**, *424*, 28–33. [CrossRef] [PubMed]

63. Foekens, J.A.; Sieuwerts, A.M.; Smid, M.; Look, M.P.; de Weerd, V.; Boersma, A.W.; Klijn, J.G.; Wiemer, E.A.; Martens, J.W. Four mirnas associated with aggressiveness of lymph node-negative, estrogen receptor-positive human breast cancer. *Proc. Natl. Acad. Sci. USA* **2008**, *105*, 13021–13026. [CrossRef] [PubMed]

64. Veerla, S.; Lindgren, D.; Kvist, A.; Frigyesi, A.; Staaf, J.; Persson, H.; Liedberg, F.; Chebil, G.; Gudjonsson, S.; Borg, A.; *et al.* Mirna expression in urothelial carcinomas: Important roles of mir-10a, mir-222, mir-125b, mir-7 and mir-452 for tumor stage and metastasis, and frequent homozygous losses of mir-31. *Int. J. Cancer* **2009**, *124*, 2236–2242. [CrossRef] [PubMed]

65. Rao, Q.; Shen, Q.; Zhou, H.; Peng, Y.; Li, J.; Lin, Z. Aberrant microrna expression in human cervical carcinomas. *Med. Oncol.* **2012**, *29*, 1242–1248. [CrossRef] [PubMed]

66. Honegger, A.; Schilling, D.; Bastian, S.; Sponagel, J.; Kuryshev, V.; Sultmann, H.; Scheffner, M.; Hoppe-Seyler, K.; Hoppe-Seyler, F. Dependence of intracellular and exosomal micrornas on viral e6/e7 oncogene expression in hpv-positive tumor cells. *PLoS Pathog.* **2015**, *11*, e1004712. [CrossRef] [PubMed]

67. Nakagawa, Y.; Akao, Y.; Taniguchi, K.; Kamatani, A.; Tahara, T.; Kamano, T.; Nakano, N.; Komura, N.; Ikuno, H.; Ohmori, T.; *et al.* Relationship between expression of onco-related mirnas and the endoscopic appearance of colorectal tumors. *Int. J. Mol. Sci.* **2015**, *16*, 1526–1543. [CrossRef] [PubMed]

68. Ahmed, F.E.; Ahmed, N.C.; Vos, P.W.; Bonnerup, C.; Atkins, J.N.; Casey, M.; Nuovo, G.J.; Naziri, W.; Wiley, J.E.; Mota, H.; *et al.* Diagnostic microrna markers to screen for sporadic human colon cancer in stool: I. Proof of principle. *Cancer Genom. Proteom.* **2013**, *10*, 93–113.

69. Xu, K.; Chen, Z.; Qin, C.; Song, X. Mir-7 inhibits colorectal cancer cell proliferation and induces apoptosis by targeting xrcc2. *OncoTargets Ther.* **2014**, *7*, 325–332. [CrossRef] [PubMed]

70. Cheng, A.M.; Byrom, M.W.; Shelton, J.; Ford, L.P. Antisense inhibition of human mirnas and indications for an involvement of mirna in cell growth and apoptosis. *Nucleic Acids Res.* **2005**, *33*, 1290–1297. [CrossRef] [PubMed]

71. Rowland, B.D.; Peeper, D.S. Klf4, p21 and context-dependent opposing forces in cancer. *Nat. Rev. Cancer* **2006**, *6*, 11–23. [CrossRef] [PubMed]

72. De la Iglesia, N.; Konopka, G.; Puram, S.V.; Chan, J.A.; Bachoo, R.M.; You, M.J.; Levy, D.E.; Depinho, R.A.; Bonni, A. Identification of a pten-regulated stat3 brain tumor suppressor pathway. *Genes Dev.* **2008**, *22*, 449–462. [CrossRef] [PubMed]

73. Zhang, H.F.; Lai, R. Stat3 in cancer-friend or foe? *Cancers* **2014**, *6*, 1408–1440. [CrossRef] [PubMed]

74. Shahab, S.W.; Matyunina, L.V.; Hill, C.G.; Wang, L.; Mezencev, R.; Walker, L.D.; McDonald, J.F. The effects of microrna transfections on global patterns of gene expression in ovarian cancer cells are functionally coordinated. *BMC Med. Genom.* **2012**, *5*. [CrossRef] [PubMed]

75. Sun, X.Y.; Zhang, J.; Niu, W.; Guo, W.; Song, H.T.; Li, H.Y.; Fan, H.M.; Zhao, L.; Zhong, A.F.; Dai, Y.H.; *et al.* A preliminary analysis of microrna as potential clinical biomarker for schizophrenia. *Am. J. Med. Genet. Part B Neuropsychiatr. Genet.* **2015**, *163B*, 170–178. [CrossRef] [PubMed]

76. Gallo, A.; Tandon, M.; Alevizos, I.; Illei, G.G. The majority of micrornas detectable in serum and saliva is concentrated in exosomes. *PLoS ONE* **2012**, *7*, e30679. [CrossRef] [PubMed]

77. Lv, L.L.; Cao, Y.; Liu, D.; Xu, M.; Liu, H.; Tang, R.N.; Ma, K.L.; Liu, B.C. Isolation and quantification of micrornas from urinary exosomes/microvesicles for biomarker discovery. *Int. J. Biol. Sci.* **2013**, *9*, 1021–1031. [CrossRef] [PubMed]

78. Mitchell, P.S.; Parkin, R.K.; Kroh, E.M.; Fritz, B.R.; Wyman, S.K.; Pogosova-Agadjanyan, E.L.; Peterson, A.; Noteboom, J.; O'Briant, K.C.; Allen, A.; *et al.* Circulating micrornas as stable blood-based markers for cancer detection. *Proc. Natl. Acad. Sci. USA* **2008**, *105*, 10513–10518. [CrossRef] [PubMed]

79. Zhang, J.; Li, S.; Li, L.; Li, M.; Guo, C.; Yao, J.; Mi, S. Exosome and exosomal microrna: Trafficking, sorting, and function. *Genom. Proteom. Bioinform.* **2015**, *13*, 17–24. [CrossRef] [PubMed]

80. Arroyo, J.D.; Chevillet, J.R.; Kroh, E.M.; Ruf, I.K.; Pritchard, C.C.; Gibson, D.F.; Mitchell, P.S.; Bennett, C.F.; Pogosova-Agadjanyan, E.L.; Stirewalt, D.L.; *et al.* Argonaute2 complexes carry a population of circulating micrornas independent of vesicles in human plasma. *Proc. Natl. Acad. Sci. USA* **2011**, *108*, 5003–5008. [CrossRef] [PubMed]

81. Vickers, K.C.; Palmisano, B.T.; Shoucri, B.M.; Shamburek, R.D.; Remaley, A.T. Micrornas are transported in plasma and delivered to recipient cells by high-density lipoproteins. *Nat. Cell Biol.* **2011**, *13*, 423–433. [CrossRef] [PubMed]

82. Abdalla, M.A.; Haj-Ahmad, Y. Promising candidate urinary microrna biomarkers for the early detection of hepatocellular carcinoma among high-risk hepatitis c virus egyptian patients. *J. Cancer* **2012**, *3*, 19–31. [CrossRef] [PubMed]

83. Haj-Ahmad, T.A.; Abdalla, M.A.; Haj-Ahmad, Y. Potential urinary mirna biomarker candidates for the accurate detection of prostate cancer among benign prostatic hyperplasia patients. *J. Cancer* **2014**, *5*, 182–191. [CrossRef] [PubMed]

84. Erbes, T.; Hirschfeld, M.; Rucker, G.; Jaeger, M.; Boas, J.; Iborra, S.; Mayer, S.; Gitsch, G.; Stickeler, E. Feasibility of urinary microrna detection in breast cancer patients and its potential as an innovative non-invasive biomarker. *BMC Cancer* **2015**, *15*. [CrossRef] [PubMed]

85. Salazar, C.; Nagadia, R.; Pandit, P.; Cooper-White, J.; Banerjee, N.; Dimitrova, N.; Coman, W.B.; Punyadeera, C. A novel saliva-based microrna biomarker panel to detect head and neck cancers. *Cell. Oncol.* **2014**, *37*, 331–338. [CrossRef] [PubMed]

86. Yau, T.O.; Wu, C.W.; Dong, Y.; Tang, C.M.; Ng, S.S.; Chan, F.K.; Sung, J.J.; Yu, J. Microrna-221 and microrna-18a identification in stool as potential biomarkers for the non-invasive diagnosis of colorectal carcinoma. *Br. J. Cancer* **2014**, *111*, 1765–1771. [CrossRef] [PubMed]

87. Wu, C.W.; Ng, S.C.; Dong, Y.; Tian, L.; Ng, S.S.; Leung, W.W.; Law, W.T.; Yau, T.O.; Chan, F.K.; Sung, J.J.; et al. Identification of microrna-135b in stool as a potential noninvasive biomarker for colorectal cancer and adenoma. *Clin. Cancer Res.* **2014**, *20*, 2994–3002. [CrossRef] [PubMed]

88. Weber, J.A.; Baxter, D.H.; Zhang, S.; Huang, D.Y.; Huang, K.H.; Lee, M.J.; Galas, D.J.; Wang, K. The microrna spectrum in 12 body fluids. *Clin. Chem.* **2010**, *56*, 1733–1741. [CrossRef] [PubMed]

89. Sieuwerts, A.M.; Mostert, B.; Bolt-de Vries, J.; Peeters, D.; de Jongh, F.E.; Stouthard, J.M.; Dirix, L.Y.; van Dam, P.A.; van Galen, A.; de Weerd, V.; et al. Mrna and microrna expression profiles in circulating tumor cells and primary tumors of metastatic breast cancer patients. *Clin. Cancer Res.* **2011**, *17*, 3600–3618. [CrossRef] [PubMed]

90. Mostert, B.; Sieuwerts, A.M.; Martens, J.W.; Sleijfer, S. Diagnostic applications of cell-free and circulating tumor cell-associated mirnas in cancer patients. *Expert Rev. Mol. Diagn.* **2011**, *11*, 259–275. [PubMed]

91. Rosenfeld, N.; Aharonov, R.; Meiri, E.; Rosenwald, S.; Spector, Y.; Zepeniuk, M.; Benjamin, H.; Shabes, N.; Tabak, S.; Levy, A.; et al. Micrornas accurately identify cancer tissue origin. *Nat. Biotechnol.* **2008**, *26*, 462–469. [CrossRef] [PubMed]

92. Wang, S.; Xiang, J.; Li, Z.; Lu, S.; Hu, J.; Gao, X.; Yu, L.; Wang, L.; Wang, J.; Wu, Y.; et al. A plasma microrna panel for early detection of colorectal cancer. *Int. J. Cancer* **2015**, *136*, 152–161. [CrossRef] [PubMed]

93. Kitano, M.; Rahbari, R.; Patterson, E.E.; Steinberg, S.M.; Prasad, N.B.; Wang, Y.; Zeiger, M.A.; Kebebew, E. Evaluation of candidate diagnostic micrornas in thyroid fine-needle aspiration biopsy samples. *Thyroid* **2012**, *22*, 285–291. [CrossRef] [PubMed]

94. Santos, J.I.; Teixeira, A.L.; Dias, F.; Mauricio, J.; Lobo, F.; Morais, A.; Medeiros, R. Influence of peripheral whole-blood microrna-7 and microrna-221 high expression levels on the acquisition of castration-resistant prostate cancer: Evidences from *in vitro* and *in vivo* studies. *Tumour Biol.* **2014**, *35*, 7105–7113. [CrossRef] [PubMed]

95. Pogribny, I.P.; Filkowski, J.N.; Tryndyak, V.P.; Golubov, A.; Shpyleva, S.I.; Kovalchuk, O. Alterations of micrornas and their targets are associated with acquired resistance of mcf-7 breast cancer cells to cisplatin. *Int. J. Cancer.* **2010**, *127*, 1785–1794. [CrossRef] [PubMed]

96. Liu, R.; Liu, X.; Zheng, Y.; Gu, J.; Xiong, S.; Jiang, P.; Jiang, X.; Huang, E.; Yang, Y.; Ge, D.; et al. Microrna-7 sensitizes non-small cell lung cancer cells to paclitaxel. *Oncol. Lett.* **2014**, *8*, 2193–2200. [CrossRef] [PubMed]

97. Ge, X.; Zheng, L.; Huang, M.; Wang, Y.; Bi, F. Microrna expression profiles associated with acquired gefitinib-resistance in human lung adenocarcinoma cells. *Mol. Med. Rep.* **2015**, *11*, 333–340. [CrossRef] [PubMed]

98. Ma, J.; Fang, B.; Zeng, F.; Pang, H.; Zhang, J.; Shi, Y.; Wu, X.; Cheng, L.; Ma, C.; Xia, J.; et al. Curcumin inhibits cell growth and invasion through up-regulation of mir-7 in pancreatic cancer cells. *Toxicol. Lett.* **2014**, *231*, 82–91. [CrossRef] [PubMed]

99. Melo, S.; Villanueva, A.; Moutinho, C.; Davalos, V.; Spizzo, R.; Ivan, C.; Rossi, S.; Setien, F.; Casanovas, O.; Simo-Riudalbas, L.; *et al.* Small molecule enoxacin is a cancer-specific growth inhibitor that acts by enhancing tar rna-binding protein 2-mediated microrna processing. *Proc. Natl. Acad. Sci. USA* **2011**, *108*, 4394–4399. [CrossRef] [PubMed]

100. Tu, C.Y.; Chen, C.H.; Hsia, T.C.; Hsu, M.H.; Wei, Y.L.; Yu, M.C.; Chen, W.S.; Hsu, K.W.; Yeh, M.H.; Liu, L.C.; *et al.* Trichostatin a suppresses egfr expression through induction of microrna-7 in an hdac-independent manner in lapatinib-treated cells. *BioMed Res. Int.* **2014**, *2014*. [CrossRef] [PubMed]

101. Liu, X.; Wang, S.; Meng, F.; Wang, J.; Zhang, Y.; Dai, E.; Yu, X.; Li, X.; Jiang, W. Sm2mir: A database of the experimentally validated small molecules' effects on microrna expression. *Bioinformatics* **2013**, *29*, 409–411. [CrossRef] [PubMed]

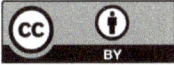

Journal of
*Clinical Medicine*

MDPI

*Review*

# MicroRNA Processing and Human Cancer

Masahisa Ohtsuka [1], Hui Ling [1], Yuichiro Doki [2], Masaki Mori [2] and George Adrian Calin [1,*]

[1] Department of Experimental Therapeutics, The University of Texas, MD Anderson Cancer Center, 1881 East Road, Unit 1950, APT 1125, Houston, TX 77030, USA; MOhtsuka@mdanderson.org (M.O.); HLing@mdanderson.org (H.L.);

[2] Department of Gastroenterological Surgery, Osaka University Graduate School of Medicine, Yamadaoka 2-2, Suita, Osaka 565-0871, Japan; ydoki@gesurg.med.osaka-u.ac.jp (Y.D.); mmori@gesurg.med.osaka-u.ac.jp (M.M.)

* Author to whom correspondence should be addressed; gcalin@mdanderson.org; Tel.: +1-713-792-5461; Fax: +1-713-745-4528.

Academic Editors: Takahiro Ochiya and Ryou-u Takahashi
Received: 30 June 2015; Accepted: 12 August 2015; Published: 21 August 2015

**Abstract:** MicroRNAs (miRNAs) are short non-coding RNAs of 20 to 25 nucleotides that regulate gene expression post-transcriptionally mainly by binding to a specific sequence of the 3′ end of the untranslated region (3′UTR) of target genes. Since the first report on the clinical relevance of miRNAs in cancer, many miRNAs have been demonstrated to act as oncogenes, whereas others function as tumor suppressors. Furthermore, global miRNA dysregulation, due to alterations in miRNA processing factors, has been observed in a large variety of human cancer types. As previous studies have shown, the sequential miRNA processing can be divided into three steps: processing by RNAse in the nucleus; transportation by Exportin-5 (XPO5) from the nucleus; and processing by the RNA-induced silencing complex (RISC) in the cytoplasm. Alteration in miRNA processing genes, by genomic mutations, aberrant expression or other means, could significantly affect cancer initiation, progression and metastasis. In this review, we focus on the biogenesis of miRNAs with emphasis on the potential of miRNA processing factors in human cancers.

**Keywords:** MicroRNAs; biogenesis; cancer

## 1. Introduction

MiRNAs are small non-coding RNAs of 20 to 25 nucleotides that do not code for proteins, but regulate their expression levels via post-transcriptional regulation. The canonical mechanism of miRNA action is through interaction with 3′UTR based on sequence complementarity. Recent studies suggest a much diverse mechanism of miRNA action mechanisms, including binding to the 5′UTR or the coding region with functional consequences [1]. Nonetheless, the interaction between miRNAs and their target genes changes protein output by either affecting mRNA stability or affecting protein translation. Importantly, absolute sequence complementarity between the miRNAs and their target messenger RNAs (mRNAs) is not necessary; this flexibility implies that each miRNA could bind and regulate numerous mRNAs [2,3]. It has been estimated that miRNAs regulate about 50% of all protein coding genes in mammals [4–6].

The first miRNA, lin-4, was discovered in *Caenorhabditis elegans* in 1993 [7]. However, the connection of miRNA to human cancer was not appreciated until 2002, when George Calin and Carlo Croce revealed that the deletion miR-15a/16-1 in chromosome 13q14 is associated with chronic lymphocytic leukemia (CLL) [8]. Subsequently, a huge number of miRNAs have been reported as "oncomiRs" or "tumor suppressive miRNAs". For instance, the miR-17–92 cluster was identified as an oncomiR that is overexpressed in several types of B-cell lymphomas and accelerates tumor development in a c-myc-driven murine model [9,10]. On the contrary, the let-7 family is reported to have tumor suppressive effects. For example, ectopic ovderexpression of let-7 in pancreatic cancer cells with low let-7 expression blocked phosphorylation and activation of STAT3, and reduced the growth and migration of the cancer cells [11].

Dysregulation of miRNAs has been found in almost all human cancer types, and the aberrant miRNA expression can be caused by genomic deletion, transcription regulation, and miRNA processing. While factors such as genomic deletion and transcription regulation tend to change single or a small group of miRNAs, defects in miRNA processing machinery usually lead to broad changes at a larger scale. Early in 2006, Lu *et al.* performed miRNA profiling of 217 mammalian miRNAs and reported a general down-regulation of miRNAs in cancer, indicating a possible defect in miRNA processing [12]. Several other reports showed processing defects in the step from pre-miRNAs to mature miRNAs for several miRNAs, including miR-125b and miR-26b in human thyroid anaplastic carcinoma [13–16]. Additionally, several reports have shown that the main regulators of miRNA maturation are aberrant expressed in cancer [17–19]. More recently, Wegert *et al.* and Walz *et al.* demonstrated the essential role of DGCR8 (DiGeorge syndrome critical region 8) and Drosha, two key factors in miRNA processing, in carcinogenesis of Wilms tumors [20,21]. Thus, it is of particular importance to understand the involvement of miRNA biogenesis defects in human cancer for exploring novel cancer biomarkers and novel anticancer targets.

The research on miRNA processing is rapidly evolving. In this review, we focus on factors and mechanisms that regulate miRNA biogenesis, and discuss the relevance of such alterations in human cancer.

## 2. MicroRNA Processing Machinery

The processing of miRNAs includes multiple steps that initiate in the nucleus and complete in the cytoplasm. First, miRNAs are transcribed from the genome by RNA polymerase II (RNAP II) into primary transcripts (pri-miRNA) that contain a stem-loop structure [22]. Second, pri-miRNAs are cleaved into precursor miRNAs (pre-miRNAs) with hairpin structures by the ribonuclease (RNAase) III family enzyme Drosha, which forms a micro-processor complex with the DNA-binding protein DGCR8 [23]. Previous research showed that the double-stranded stem structure and the unpaired flanking regions of pri-miRNAs are essential for binding and cleavage by DGCR8 and Drosha. DGCR8 binds to pri-miRNAs and the central part of the Drosha protein, ensuring a correct assembling. Drosha has two RNAase III domains (RIIIDs), which cleave the 3'- and 5'-strand of the stem-loop structure of miRNAs, respectively to create pre-miRNAs [24,25]. Third, pre-miRNAs are exported to the cytoplasm by a Ran-GTP-dependent dsRNA-binding protein, XPO5 [26,27]. Fourth, Dicer, an RNAase III-type endonuclease, together with transactivating response RNA-binding protein (TRBP) and Kinase R-activating protein (PACT), cleaves pre-miRNAs in the cytoplasm. The cleavage by Dicer generates a 20–25 nucleotide miRNA duplex consisting of a guide (referred to as miRNA) and passenger (referred to as miRNA*) strand [28,29]. The guide miRNA generated by Dicer is loaded onto RISC, consisting of Dicer, TRBP and PACT, Argonaute 2 (AGO2) and GW182/TNRC6 [28,30]. The RISC-miRNA complex (named miRISC) functions as a guide to detect the 3'UTR of target genes [31]. This process induces degradation or translational inhibition of the target mRNA, depending on the degree of complementarity between miRNA and its mRNA targets [32]. Generally, miRNA from the passive strand (miRNA*) is degraded and exhibits no effect on gene regulation. However, recent studies have shown that miRNA*s can also associate with the RISC complex and subsequently repress target mRNAs with biological effects similar to that of mature miRNAs [33]. Therefore, biogenesis of miRNAs is tightly controlled at multiple levels, and any defects in such processes could have important biological effects in cancer (Figure 1).

## 3. Pri- to Pre-miRNA Processing in Cancer

The genes encoding microRNAs are first transcribed by RNAP II into pri-miRNAs, which are further processed by the micro-processor complex including Drosha and DGCR8 to generate pre-miRNAs. Dysregulation of DGCR8 and Drosha have been reported to play significant roles in cancer. Deletion of DGCR8 causes DiGeorge syndrome, also known as 22q11.2 deletion syndrome, the symptoms of which include hypokalemia (due to hypoparathyroidism), immune dysfunction (due to thymic hypoplasia) and congenital heart disease [34]. In mice, deletion of DGCR8 blocks stem cell development in its early stage and decreases cell proliferation [35]. Aberrantly high expression of DGCR8 is also observed in cancer. Kim *et al.* revealed that DGCR8 mRNA expression is significantly increased in colorectal cancer compared with adjacent, histological normal tissue [36]. Conversely, down-regulation of DGCR8 enhances cellular transformation and tumor growth in lung cancer [19]. Indeed, both upregulation and downregulation of Drosha have been reported in human cancers [19,37–40]. Because the expression pattern of DGCR8 and Drosha in cancer is still controversial, further studies are necessary to elucidate the mechanisms whereby their expression patterns influence cancer pathways related to miRNA processing in the nucleus.

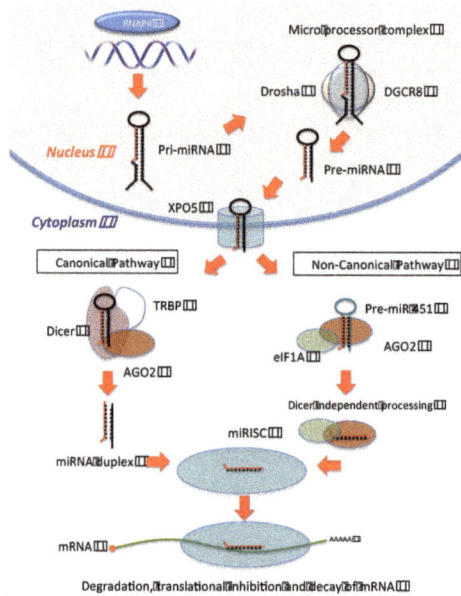

**Figure 1.** MiRNAs Biogenesis Pathway; Canonical Pathway; First, miRNAs are transcribed from the genome by RNA polymerase II (RNAP II) into primary transcripts (pri-miRNA) in the nucleus. Second, pri-miRNAs are cleaved into precursor miRNAs (pre-miRNAs) by the ribonuclease (RNAase) III family enzyme Drosha, which forms a micro-processor complex with the DNA-binding protein DGCR8. Third, miRNA precursors (pre-miRNAs) are exported to the cytoplasm by a Ran-GTP-dependent dsRNA-binding protein, Exportin-5 (XPO5). Fourth, Dicer, an RNAase III-type endonuclease, together with transactivating response RNA-binding protein (TRBP) and Kinase R-activating protein (PACT), cleaves pre-miRNAs in the cytoplasm. Finally, the guide miRNA generated by Dicer is loaded onto the RNA-induced silencing complex (RISC) consisting of Dicer, TRBP and PACT and Argonaute 2 (AGO2) and consequently binds to the 3′UTR of target genes, inducing degradation or translational inhibition of the target mRNA. Non-canonical Pathway (Dicer independent); Following transportation from nucleus to cytoplasm, pre-miR-451 is directly assembled onto AGO2-eIF1A complex. Consequently, the pre-miR-451 hairpin structure is cleaved by the Argonaute RNAase H-like motif to form the single strand mature miR-451. The generated mature miR-451 binds to the 3′UTR, and regulate expression of target genes.

The recognition of the stem-loop structure of pri-miRNAs by DGCR8 is the first step in miRNA biogenesis and Alarcon *et al.* contributed immensely to our knowledge of this process [41]. They focused on RNA methyltransferase-like3 (METTL3), as it is enriched in pri-miRNA sequence in contradiction to pre-miRNA sequence. METTL3 methylates pri-miRNAs (m$^6$A), which marks them for recognition and processing by DGCR8. This indicates that METTL3 might influence the expression of oncomiRs and tumor suppressive miRNAs.

RNA-binding proteins (RBPs) are closely associated with miRNA biogenesis, because they regulate each step of miRNA processing, localization and degradation. For instance, p68 (DEAD-box5 (DDX5)) and p72 (DDX72) are well known RBPs that are highly expressed in several types of human cancer [42,43]. In the nucleus, both p68 and p72 are essential for miRNA processing by Drosha, as knocking out either of these decreases the efficiency of miRNAs processing [44]. Furthermore, the Drosha complex associates with p68, which promotes conversion of pri-miRNAs to pre-miRNAs. Meanwhile p68 is related to the well-known tumor suppressor p53 and inactive p53 mutants interfere with functional assembly between the Drosha complex and p68, thereby inhibiting miRNA processing [45,46]. MiR-21, a well known oncomiR, is one of the miRNAs regulated by p68 through transforming growth factor-β (TGFβ) and bone morphogenetic protein (BMP)-specific SMAD signaling. Once p68 is down-regulated, pre-miR-21 and mature miR-21 expression is abolished, although pri-miR21 expression does not change significantly, indicating that p68 has a crucial role in miR-21 biogenesis in its TGF-β/BMP-regulated synthesis. Similarly, SMAD binds directly to the stem region of TGFβ/BMP-regulated miRNAs, thereby indirectly regulating gene expression via its regulation of miRNA maturation [47,48]. Furthermore, SMAD nuclear interacting protein 1 (SNIP1), a human forkhead-associated domain-containing protein and inhibits SMAD4, is revealed to directly combine with Drosha and regulate miRNAs processing in the nucleus by immnoprecipitation [49].

Recent studies revealed that KH-type splicing regulatory protein (KSRP) plays an important role in miRNAs biogenesis by regulating Drosha. Zhang and colleagues studied the association between this regulation system and DNA-damage response. They revealed that ATM, a regulator of DNA double-strand breaks [50–52], binds and phosphorylates KSRP directly as a DNA damage response, which promotes the interaction of KSRP and pri-miRNAs. Consequently, the processing of pri-miRNAs by Drosha is increased, suggesting that DNA damage pathway is associated with miRNAs biogenesis [53]. Similarly, they reported DDX1, one of the Drosha associated polypeptides, promotes pri-miRNAs maturation in ovarian cancer. After DNA damage, the ATM phosphorylation reinforces the connection of DDX1 and DDX dependent pri-miRNAs (miR-200a, miR-29c, miR-141 and miR-101), inducing cleavage of these pri-miRNAs by Drosha. These miRNAs were reported to be related to a mesenchymal feature in serous ovarian cancer [54], suggesting that DDX1 might regulate the progression of ovarian cancer [55]. As described above, DNA damage response affects multidirectionally miRNAs maturation by Drosha.

Most recently, two study groups showed that mutations in DGCR8, Drosha, together with mutations in SIX1/2, are associated with blastemal type Wilms tumors (WT) [20,21]. Walz *et al.* reported decreased expression of mature let-7 in tumors with mutations or copy number loss of the microRNA processing genes (miRNAPGs) DGCR8 and Drosha, although the expression of primary let-7a was higher in the miRNAPG mutant group compared with the non-mutant group. This decrease in let-7a is consistent with previous reports that associate let-7a deletion with WT development through the regulation of LIN28, an RBP [56,57]. Interestingly, the miR-200 family (miR-200a, -200b, -141 and -429), which is associated with Mesenchymal-Epithelial Transition (MET) and stem cell maintenance is also decreased following mutations in miRNAPGs. MET induces renal structural formation during early development and blocking MET by down-regulation of the miR-200 family is thought to increase undifferentiated cells, consequently promoting WT development [21]. Wegert *et al.* also mentioned that all miRNAs evaluated by the microarray are significantly decreased in the mutant Drosha group, although there is no clear study showing that Drosha mutation induces global miRNAs dysregulation in WT [20]. These studies substantiate the importance of DGCR and Drosha in miRNAs processing in cancer (Table 1).

### 4. MiRNA Transportation and Cancer

The transporter protein XPO5 transfers pre-miRNAs from the nucleus to the cytoplasm via the small GTPase Ran. In the nucleus, XPO5 and pre-miRNAs bind to RanGTP and this complex is then transported to the cytoplasm where pre-miRNAs are released by the RanGAP-induced hydrolysis of RanGTP to RanGDP.

In cancer, this transportation process can be disrupted by several factors. Melo *et al.* reported that XPO5 mutation constrains pre-miRNAs to the nucleus, thereby preventing miRNA maturation. In XPO5-mutant cancer cells, XPO5 transfection increases expression of the miR-200 family, let-7a and miR-26a (recognized tumor-suppressors), indicating that XPO5 has tumor-suppressive features [58]. Additionally, mutant XPO5 lacks the C-terminal region that facilitates binding of pre-miRNAs to XPO5 and RanGTP, which leads to accumulation of pre-miRNAs in the nucleus [59]. Interestingly, Li *et al.* showed that miR-138 regulates XPO5 stability by regulating required for meiotic nuclear division the expression of 5 homolog A (RMND5A). MiR-138 is associated with tumor progression, metastasis and cell differentiation in Hela cells. Additionally, in neck squamous cell carcinoma, miR-138 decreases the downstream E-cadherin gene (CDH1) and influences EMT by altering expression of EZH2, VIM and ZEB2 [60]. As expected, miR-138 is also processed by XPO5, but miR-138 represses the stability of XPO5 and decreases miRNA processing, indicating the existence of a feedback loop in the miR-138/RMND5A/XPO5 pathway [61]. In contrast, DNA damage accelerates miRNA processing through the ATM-AKT pathway. During the DNA damage response, ATM phosphorylates effector proteins and induces DNA-damage signaling. Once AKT is phosphorylated and activated by ATM, Nup153 (a nucleopore) is phosphorylated and binds to XPO5, which induces nuclear export of pre-miRNAs [62] (Table 1).

### 5. Pre-miR to Mature MiRNA Processing and Cancer

Dicer belongs to the Ribonuclease III family of nucleases and contains Piwi/Argonaute/Zwille (PAZ) domains that bind the 2-nt $3'$ overhang of dsRNA, inducing shortening of the dsRNA strand. Dicer has been well studied and is thought to be essential for miRNA as well as siRNA biogenesis [63,64].

Aberrant expression of Dicer has been reported in several types of cancer. For example, Merritt *et al.* reported that high levels of Dicer expression are associated with good prognosis in ovarian cancer, as well as lung and breast cancer [39]. In contrast, in colorectal and prostate cancer, increased expression of Dicer is associated with poor prognosis [65–67]. Down-regulation of Dicer is associated with poor prognosis in CLL, where unfavorable cytogenetic aberrations are more frequently found in patients with lower levels of Dicer [68]. Because of the variation in Dicer expression by cancer type, using Dicer as a biomarker in cancer remains controversial.

**Table 1.** Dysregulation of MiRNAs Biogenesis in Cancers.

| Location | MiRNAs Processing Related Factors | Clinical Relevance | Referrence |
|---|---|---|---|
| Nucleus | DGCR8 | Deletion of DGCR8 induces DiGeorge syndrome (22q.2 deletion syndrome). | [34] |
| | | Deletion of DGCR8 reduces stem cell development and cell proliferation in mice. | [35] |
| | | In colorectal cancer, DGCR8 expression is increased in tumors compared with normal tissue. | [36] |
| | | Down-regulation of DGCR8 enhances cellular transformation and tumor gurowth in lung cancer. | [19] |
| | Drosha | Up-regulation of Drosha regulates cell proliferation; associated with poor prognosis of esophageal cancer and non-small cell lung cancer. | [37,38] |
| | | Low expression of Drosha is associated with poor prognosis of ovarian cancer and neurobastoma. | [39,40] |
| | Mutations of DGCR8 and Drosha | Together with the mutations in SIX1/2, mutations of DGCR8 and Drosha are associated with Wilms tumor. | [20,21] |
| | METTL3 | METTL3 regulates the recognition of stem-loop structure of pri-miRNAs by DGCR8. | [41] |
| | P68 and P72; RBPs | p68 and p72 are highly expressed in cancer and associated with miRNAs processing by Drosha. | [42–46] |
| | SMAD and SNIP1 | By regulating Drosha, SMAD and SNIP1 block the maturation of oncomiRs. | [47–49] |
| | KSRP, DDX1; DNA damage | ATM phosphorylation regulates the binding of KSRP and DDX1 to Drosha. | [53–55] |
| Trans Nuclear Membrane | XP05 | XP05 increases the expression levels of tumor-suppressor miRNAs, indicating that XP05 has tumor-suppressive features. | [58,59] |
| | RMND5A | RMNDA5A regulates XP05 stability together with miR-138. | [60,61] |
| | AKM-AKT signal; DNA damage | The activation of ATM-AKT signal after DNA damage, Nup153 binds to XP05, which induces nuclear export of pre-miRNAs. | [62] |
| Cytoplasm | Dicer | High levels of Dicer expression are associated with god prognosis in ovarian cancer, breast cancer and CLL. | [39] |
| | | Up-regulation of Dicer is associated with poor progonosis in colorectal and prostate cancer. | [65–67] |
| | Mutation of Dicer | Dicer mutation incue a Dicer-related disorders including PPB. | [69,70] |
| | TRBP and TARBP2 | TRBP and TARBP2 destabilize Dicer, impairing miRNAs processing in human cancer. | [74,75] |
| | AG02 | AG02 regulates Dicer independent miRNA-451 through the non-canonical pathway. | [88,89] |
| | EGFR | In hypoxic condition, EGFR binds to AG02 and blocks miRNAs maturation. | [90,91] |

Dicer mutations influence cancer initiation and/or development. The first report of a Dicer mutation in cancer was in pleuropulmonary blastoma (PPB), a rare childhood malignancy of the lung or pleural cavity [69]. This study found loss-of-function mutations in Dicer1 in eleven PPB-affected families by DNA sequencing. They showed that this mutation induced aberrant expression of miRNAs, which promoted mesenchymal cell proliferation. Since this first report, Dicer1 mutation has been reported in several tumors, such as Sertoli-Leydig cell tumors, embryonal rhabdomyosarcoma and multinodular goiter; these disorders are now widely recognized as Dicer1-related disorders [70] (Table 1).

## 6. RISC-Related Defects in Cancer

The RISC proteins include, but limited to Dicer, TRBP, PACT and AGO2. The double-stranded RNA (dsRNA)-binding proteins TRBP and PACT, associate with Dicer and regulate its function of miRNA biogenesis [71]. Lee *et al.* revealed that PACT is essential for accumulation of mature miRNAs, because depletion of PACT promotes miRNA maturation [72]. Although TRBP and PACT both possess dsRNA-binding domains (dsRBDs), TRBP and PACT have different roles in Dicer-related miRNA processing. DsRBD 1 and 2 (the two *N*-terminal dsRBDs of each protein) are essential for the interaction between Dicer and TRBP or PACT; differences in these domains (between TRBP and PACT) alters Dicer-dependent dsRNA substrate recognition and processing, affecting both substrate and cleavage specificity during miRNA and siRNA production [73].

Decreased expression of TRBP (induced by mutation of TAR RNA-binding protein 2 (TARBP2)) is related to a destabilization of Dicer, which impairs miRNA processing in human cancer cell lines and sporadic and heredity carcinomas with microsatellite instability [74]. Furthermore, TARBP2-dependent miRNAs, miRNA-143 and miRNA-145, restrict development and tumor growth in cancer stem cells of Ewing sarcoma family tumor [75]. These data show that TRBP acts as a tumor suppressor through its role in miRNA processing.

Finally, AGO2 is an important component of miRISC. Argonaute protein was initially discovered in plants and is now recognized as a highly conserved protein between all species [76–78]. Agonaute proteins have four domains (*N*-terminal domain, PAZ domain, MID domain and PIWI domain) with two linker structures (L1 and L2) [79]. The PAZ domain binds to the 3′ end of small RNAs including miRNAs, whereas the MID domain binds to the 5′ end [80,81]. The PIWI domain plays a role in cleaving small RNAs, as this domain has an RNase-H like structure [82,83]. Of the four Argonaute proteins (AGO1–4), only AGO2 has endonucleolytic and consequent gene silencing activity against mRNAs [84,85]. Furthermore, AGO2 increases the level of mature miRNAs independently from its RNAse activity, suggesting that AGO2 also affects miRNAs maturation [86,87]. However, it has recently been reported that AGO2 affects miR-451 maturation mainly through the non-canonical pathway of miRNA biogenesis [88]. Instead of being processed by Dicer, pre-miR-451 is loaded onto AGO2 [89]; eukaryotic translation initiation factor (eIF1A) binds to the MID domain of AGO2 to form an eIF1A-AGO2 complex, promoting miR-451 maturation through the non-canonical pathway [88]. Since Dicer-independent miR-451 is an important cancer biomarker, AGO2-dependent miRNA biogenesis requires further investigation (Figure 1).

Furthermore, epidermal growth factor receptor (EGFR), a well-known oncogene, regulates miRNAs biogenesis in hypoxic condition associated with AGO2. Shen *et al.* revealed that hypoxia enhances the connection between EGFR and AGO2, which induces specific AGO-2 phosphorylaiton (AGO2-Y393 phosphorylation). As a consequence, the binding of AGO2 to Dicer is diminished, blocking miRNAs maturation in cytoplasm [90]. Conversely, Hypoxia is reported to promote miRNAs by hydroxylation of AGO2, which enhances its endonuclease activity [91]. Hence, the regulation mechanism of AGO2 is still controversial and needs further studies (Table 1).

## 7. Conclusions

Since the first discovery of miRNAs, an enormous amount of studies have focused on uncovering the clinical importance of these small RNAs. There are currently several clinical trials targeting miRNAs or using miRNA mimics [92]. Miravirsen, a locked nucleic acid-modified DNA phosphorothioate oligonucleotide complementary to miR-122, binds to two adjacent target sites in 5′UTR region of hepatitis C virus (HCV) RNA that is essential for its RNA replication [93]. Consequently, this drug decreases the expression of HCV RNA in a dose-dependent manner in the patients with HCV-induced cirrhosis [94]. In the cancer field, tumor suppressors miR-34 and let-7 have been explored as possible

*J. Clin. Med.* **2015**, *4*, 1651–1667

therapeutic agents. The clinical trial of miR-34 mimics (MRX34) against hepatocellular carcinoma and metastatic liver cancer is now in phase I (ClinicalTrials.gov Identifier: NCT01829971). Thus, miRNA-targeted therapeutics is likely to be a promising treatment option against several diseases, including cancer. Although miRNA-targeted therapy has certain obstacles challenging effective and precise conveyance to the tumor sites, with the advancement on the nucleotide delivery system, we are optimal that miRNA therapies will likely be used in treating cancer patients in the near future. Furthermore, circulating miRNAs are remarkably stable even in human body fluids, and thus have been extensively explored as cancer biomarkers. Some studies suggest that the stability of circulating miRNAs are due to membrane-bound vesicles, which envelope miRNAs and prevent degradation from RNAase [95–97]. Interestingly, recent study reported that exsomes (one of membrane-bound vesicles) derived from cancer tissue contains not only miRNAs, but also RISC complex which induce maturation of oncogenin miRNAs [98]. These findings indicate that circulating exosomal microRNA biogenesis factors might affect carcinogenesis and tumor progression, and thus represent unique candidates of novel cancer biomarkers.

Conversely, mechanisms of miRNA biogenesis disregulation are relatively less well studied compared with miRNAs themselves. However, Dicer-substrate siRNAs (DsiRNAs), Dicer related gene knocking down system, are of current interest as new therapeutic tools in cancer [99–102]. Conventionally, small interfering RNAs (siRNAs) are designed as 21mer RNA duplexes and the active strand silences gene expression post-transcriptionally by binding of short strands of homologous RNA to target mRNA. On the other hand, 27mer dsiRNAs are cleaved by Dicer into 21mer siRNAs and perform better silencing than canonical siRNAs. Since siRNAs cleaved from dsiRNAs are directly connected to RISC complex, this system is thought to enhance gene knockdown efficacy [99]. Currently, two clinical trials are ongoing using DCR-MYC, which is the first MYC-targeting siRNA to enter clinical trials. A phase 1 clinical trial of DCR-MYC is being conducted in patients with solid tumors, multiple myeloma or lymphoma, and a phase 1b/2 trial in patients with hepatocellular carcinoma (ClinicalTrials.gov Identifier: NCT02110563 and NCT02314052). Thus, the new treatments related to microRNAs biogenesis factors have just started. The success of this technique indicates that the efficacy of miRNAs mimics (Double-stranded RNA oligonucleotides) could improve with similar strategy.

As numerous miRNAs are regulated by miRNA-processing-related factors, this multiplicity indicates the difficulty of applying them in a clinical setting and meanwhile includes additional potential opportunities to develop these factors as possible biomarkers and therapeutic targets. Hence, further research is necessary to unveil the comprehensive miRNA biogenesis network, which will undoubtedly lead to novel discoveries relevant to the diagnosis and treatment of cancer.

**Acknowledgments:** GAC is The Alan M. Gewirtz Leukemia and Lymphoma Society Scholar. Work in GAC laboratory is supported in part by the NIH/NCI grants 1UH2TR00943-01 and 1 R01 CA182905-01, the UT MD Anderson Cancer Center SPORE in Melanoma grant from NCI (P50 CA093459), Aim at Melanoma Foundation and the Miriam and Jim Mulva research funds, the Brain SPORE (2P50CA127001), the Center for radiation Oncology Research Project, the Center for Cancer Epigenetics Pilot project, a 2014 Knowledge GAP MDACC grant, a CLL Moonshot pilot project, the UT MD Anderson Cancer Center Duncan Family Institute for Cancer Prevention and Risk Assessment, an SINF grant in colon cancer, the Laura and John Arnold Foundation, the RGK Foundation and the Estate of C. G. Johnson, Jr.

**Author Contributions:** Masahisa Ohtsuka and Hui Ling wrote the paper. Yuichiro Doki, Masaki Mori and George Adrian Calin conceived and designed this review manuscript.

**Conflicts of Interest:** The authors declare no conflict of interest.

## References

1. Orom, U.A.; Nielsen, F.C.; Lund, A.H. Microrna-10a binds the 5'utr of ribosomal protein mRNAs and enhances their translation. *Mol. Cell* **2008**, *30*, 460–471. [CrossRef] [PubMed]
2. Baek, D.; Villen, J.; Shin, C.; Camargo, F.D.; Gygi, S.P.; Bartel, D.P. The impact of MicroRNAs on protein output. *Nature* **2008**, *455*, 64–71. [CrossRef] [PubMed]

*J. Clin. Med.* **2015**, *4*, 1651–1667

3. Selbach, M.; Schwanhausser, B.; Thierfelder, N.; Fang, Z.; Khanin, R.; Rajewsky, N. Widespread changes in protein synthesis induced by MicroRNAs. *Nature* **2008**, *455*, 58–63. [CrossRef] [PubMed]
4. Kozomara, A.; Griffiths-Jones, S. Mirbase: Annotating high confidence MicroRNAs using deep sequencing data. *Nucleic Acids Res.* **2014**, *42*, D68–D73. [CrossRef] [PubMed]
5. Krol, J.; Loedige, I.; Filipowicz, W. The widespread regulation of MicroRNA biogenesis, function and decay. *Nat. Rev. Genet.* **2010**, *11*, 597–610. [CrossRef] [PubMed]
6. Huang, Y.; Shen, X.J.; Zou, Q.; Wang, S.P.; Tang, S.M.; Zhang, G.Z. Biological functions of MicroRNAs: A review. *J. Physiol. Biochem.* **2011**, *67*, 129–139. [CrossRef] [PubMed]
7. Reinhart, B.J.; Slack, F.J.; Basson, M.; Pasquinelli, A.E.; Bettinger, J.C.; Rougvie, A.E.; Horvitz, H.R.; Ruvkun, G. The 21-nucleotide let-7 RNA regulates developmental timing in *Caenorhabditis elegans*. *Nature* **2000**, *403*, 901–906. [PubMed]
8. Calin, G.A.; Dumitru, C.D.; Shimizu, M.; Bichi, R.; Zupo, S.; Noch, E.; Aldler, H.; Rattan, S.; Keating, M.; Rai, K.; *et al.* Frequent deletions and down-regulation of micro- RNA genes mir15 and mir16 at 13q14 in chronic lymphocytic leukemia. *Proc. Natl. Acad. Sci. USA* **2002**, *99*, 15524–15529. [CrossRef] [PubMed]
9. Ota, A.; Tagawa, H.; Karnan, S.; Tsuzuki, S.; Karpas, A.; Kira, S.; Yoshida, Y.; Seto, M. Identification and characterization of a novel gene, c13orf25, as a target for 13q31-q32 amplification in malignant lymphoma. *Cancer Res.* **2004**, *64*, 3087–3095. [CrossRef] [PubMed]
10. He, L.; Thomson, J.M.; Hemann, M.T.; Hernando-Monge, E.; Mu, D.; Goodson, S.; Powers, S.; Cordon-Cardo, C.; Lowe, S.W.; Hannon, G.J.; *et al.* A MicroRNA polycistron as a potential human oncogene. *Nature* **2005**, *435*, 828–833. [CrossRef] [PubMed]
11. Patel, K.; Kollory, A.; Takashima, A.; Sarkar, S.; Faller, D.V.; Ghosh, S.K. MicroRNA let-7 downregulates stat3 phosphorylation in pancreatic cancer cells by increasing socs3 expression. *Cancer Lett.* **2014**, *347*, 54–64. [CrossRef] [PubMed]
12. Lu, J.; Getz, G.; Miska, E.A.; Alvarez-Saavedra, E.; Lamb, J.; Peck, D.; Sweet-Cordero, A.; Ebert, B.L.; Mak, R.H.; Ferrando, A.A.; *et al.* MicroRNA expression profiles classify human cancers. *Nature* **2005**, *435*, 834–838. [CrossRef] [PubMed]
13. Lee, E.J.; Baek, M.; Gusev, Y.; Brackett, D.J.; Nuovo, G.J.; Schmittgen, T.D. Systematic evaluation of MicroRNA processing patterns in tissues, cell lines, and tumors. *RNA* **2008**, *14*, 35–42. [CrossRef] [PubMed]
14. Michael, M.Z.; SM, O.C.; van Holst Pellekaan, N.G.; Young, G.P.; James, R.J. Reduced accumulation of specific MicroRNAs in colorectal neoplasia. *Mol. Cancer Res.* **2003**, *1*, 882–891. [PubMed]
15. Gaur, A.; Jewell, D.A.; Liang, Y.; Ridzon, D.; Moore, J.H.; Chen, C.; Ambros, V.R.; Israel, M.A. Characterization of MicroRNA expression levels and their biological correlates in human cancer cell lines. *Cancer Res.* **2007**, *67*, 2456–2468. [CrossRef] [PubMed]
16. Visone, R.; Pallante, P.; Vecchione, A.; Cirombella, R.; Ferracin, M.; Ferraro, A.; Volinia, S.; Coluzzi, S.; Leone, V.; Borbone, E.; *et al.* Specific MicroRNAs are downregulated in human thyroid anaplastic carcinomas. *Oncogene* **2007**, *26*, 7590–7595. [CrossRef] [PubMed]
17. Kim, M.S.; Oh, J.E.; Kim, Y.R.; Park, S.W.; Kang, M.R.; Kim, S.S.; Ahn, C.H.; Yoo, N.J.; Lee, S.H. Somatic mutations and losses of expression of MicroRNA regulation-related genes ago2 and tnrc6a in gastric and colorectal cancers. *J. Pathol.* **2010**, *221*, 139–146. [CrossRef] [PubMed]
18. Zhang, L.; Huang, J.; Yang, N.; Greshock, J.; Megraw, M.S.; Giannakakis, A.; Liang, S.; Naylor, T.L.; Barchetti, A.; Ward, M.R.; *et al.* MicroRNAs exhibit high frequency genomic alterations in human cancer. *Proc. Natl. Acad. Sci. USA* **2006**, *103*, 9136–9141. [CrossRef] [PubMed]
19. Kumar, M.S.; Lu, J.; Mercer, K.L.; Golub, T.R.; Jacks, T. Impaired MicroRNA processing enhances cellular transformation and tumorigenesis. *Nat. Genet.* **2007**, *39*, 673–677. [CrossRef] [PubMed]
20. Wegert, J.; Ishaque, N.; Vardapour, R.; Georg, C.; Gu, Z.; Bieg, M.; Ziegler, B.; Bausenwein, S.; Nourkami, N.; Ludwig, N.; *et al.* Mutations in the six1/2 pathway and the drosha/dgcr8 miRNA microprocessor complex underlie high-risk blastemal type wilms tumors. *Cancer Cell* **2015**, *27*, 298–311. [CrossRef] [PubMed]
21. Walz, A.L.; Ooms, A.; Gadd, S.; Gerhard, D.S.; Smith, M.A.; Guidry Auvil, J.M.; Meerzaman, D.; Chen, Q.R.; Hsu, C.H.; Yan, C.; *et al.* Recurrent dgcr8, drosha, and six homeodomain mutations in favorable histology wilms tumors. *Cancer Cell* **2015**, *27*, 286–297. [CrossRef] [PubMed]
22. Bartel, D.P. MicroRNAs: Genomics, biogenesis, mechanism, and function. *Cell* **2004**, *116*, 281–297. [CrossRef]
23. Kim, V.N. MicroRNA biogenesis: Coordinated cropping and dicing. *Nat. Rev. Mol. Cell Biol.* **2005**, *6*, 376–385. [CrossRef] [PubMed]

24. Han, J.; Lee, Y.; Yeom, K.H.; Kim, Y.K.; Jin, H.; Kim, V.N. The drosha-dgcr8 complex in primary MicroRNA processing. *Genes Dev.* **2004**, *18*, 3016–3027. [CrossRef] [PubMed]
25. Grund, S.E.; Polycarpou-Schwarz, M.; Luo, C.; Eichmuller, S.B.; Diederichs, S. Rare drosha splice variants are deficient in MicroRNA processing but do not affect general MicroRNA expression in cancer cells. *Neoplasia* **2012**, *14*, 238–248. [CrossRef] [PubMed]
26. Yi, R.; Qin, Y.; Macara, I.G.; Cullen, B.R. Exportin-5 mediates the nuclear export of pre-MicroRNAs and short hairpin RNAs. *Genes Dev.* **2003**, *17*, 3011–3016. [CrossRef] [PubMed]
27. Zeng, Y.; Cullen, B.R. Structural requirements for pre-MicroRNA binding and nuclear export by exportin 5. *Nucleic Acids Res.* **2004**, *32*, 4776–4785. [CrossRef] [PubMed]
28. Chendrimada, T.P.; Gregory, R.I.; Kumaraswamy, E.; Norman, J.; Cooch, N.; Nishikura, K.; Shiekhattar, R. Trbp recruits the dicer complex to ago2 for MicroRNA processing and gene silencing. *Nature* **2005**, *436*, 740–744. [CrossRef] [PubMed]
29. Feng, Y.; Zhang, X.; Graves, P.; Zeng, Y. A comprehensive analysis of precursor MicroRNA cleavage by human dicer. *RNA* **2012**, *18*, 2083–2092. [CrossRef] [PubMed]
30. Maniataki, E.; Mourelatos, Z. A human, atp-independent, risc assembly machine fueled by pre-miRNA. *Genes Dev.* **2005**, *19*, 2979–2990. [CrossRef] [PubMed]
31. Ghildiyal, M.; Zamore, P.D. Small silencing RNAs: An expanding universe. *Nat. Rev. Genet.* **2009**, *10*, 94–108. [CrossRef] [PubMed]
32. Filipowicz, W.; Bhattacharyya, S.N.; Sonenberg, N. Mechanisms of post-transcriptional regulation by MicroRNAs: Are the answers in sight? *Nat. Rev. Genet.* **2008**, *9*, 102–114. [CrossRef] [PubMed]
33. Marco, A.; Macpherson, J.I.; Ronshaugen, M.; Griffiths-Jones, S. MicroRNAs from the same precursor have different targeting properties. *Silence* **2012**, *3*, 8. [CrossRef] [PubMed]
34. Shiohama, A.; Sasaki, T.; Noda, S.; Minoshima, S.; Shimizu, N. Molecular cloning and expression analysis of a novel gene dgcr8 located in the digeorge syndrome chromosomal region. *Biochem. Biophys. Res. Commun.* **2003**, *304*, 184–190. [CrossRef]
35. Wang, Y.; Medvid, R.; Melton, C.; Jaenisch, R.; Blelloch, R. Dgcr8 is essential for MicroRNA biogenesis and silencing of embryonic stem cell self-renewal. *Nat. Genet.* **2007**, *39*, 380–385. [CrossRef] [PubMed]
36. Kim, B.; Lee, J.H.; Park, J.W.; Kwon, T.K.; Baek, S.K.; Hwang, I.; Kim, S. An essential MicroRNA maturing microprocessor complex component dgcr8 is up-regulated in colorectal carcinomas. *Clin. Exp. Med.* **2014**, *14*, 331–336. [CrossRef] [PubMed]
37. Sugito, N.; Ishiguro, H.; Kuwabara, Y.; Kimura, M.; Mitsui, A.; Kurehara, H.; Ando, T.; Mori, R.; Takashima, N.; Ogawa, R.; *et al.* Rnasen regulates cell proliferation and affects survival in esophageal cancer patients. *Clin. Cancer Res.* **2006**, *12*, 7322–7328. [CrossRef] [PubMed]
38. Diaz-Garcia, C.V.; Agudo-Lopez, A.; Perez, C.; Lopez-Martin, J.A.; Rodriguez-Peralto, J.L.; de Castro, J.; Cortijo, A.; Martinez-Villanueva, M.; Iglesias, L.; Garcia-Carbonero, R.; *et al.* Dicer1, drosha and miRNAs in patients with non-small cell lung cancer: Implications for outcomes and histologic classification. *Carcinogenesis* **2013**, *34*, 1031–1038. [CrossRef] [PubMed]
39. Merritt, W.M.; Lin, Y.G.; Han, L.Y.; Kamat, A.A.; Spannuth, W.A.; Schmandt, R.; Urbauer, D.; Pennacchio, L.A.; Cheng, J.F.; Nick, A.M.; *et al.* Dicer, drosha, and outcomes in patients with ovarian cancer. *N. Engl. J. Med.* **2008**, *359*, 2641–2650. [CrossRef] [PubMed]
40. Lin, R.J.; Lin, Y.C.; Chen, J.; Kuo, H.H.; Chen, Y.Y.; Diccianni, M.B.; London, W.B.; Chang, C.H.; Yu, A.L. Microrna signature and expression of dicer and drosha can predict prognosis and delineate risk groups in neuroblastoma. *Cancer Res.* **2010**, *70*, 7841–7850. [CrossRef] [PubMed]
41. Alarcon, C.R.; Lee, H.; Goodarzi, H.; Halberg, N.; Tavazoie, S.F. N6-methyladenosine marks primary MicroRNAs for processing. *Nature* **2015**, *519*, 482–485. [CrossRef] [PubMed]
42. Shiohama, A.; Sasaki, T.; Noda, S.; Minoshima, S.; Shimizu, N. Nucleolar localization of dgcr8 and identification of eleven dgcr8-associated proteins. *Exp. Cell Res.* **2007**, *313*, 4196–4207. [CrossRef] [PubMed]
43. Fuller-Pace, F.V.; Moore, H.C. RNA helicases p68 and p72: Multifunctional proteins with important implications for cancer development. *Future Oncol.* **2011**, *7*, 239–251. [CrossRef] [PubMed]
44. Gregory, R.I.; Yan, K.P.; Amuthan, G.; Chendrimada, T.; Doratotaj, B.; Cooch, N.; Shiekhattar, R. The microprocessor complex mediates the genesis of MicroRNAs. *Nature* **2004**, *432*, 235–240. [CrossRef] [PubMed]

45. Van Kouwenhove, M.; Kedde, M.; Agami, R. MicroRNA regulation by RNA-binding proteins and its implications for cancer. *Nat. Rev. Cancer* **2011**, *11*, 644–656. [CrossRef] [PubMed]

46. Suzuki, H.I.; Yamagata, K.; Sugimoto, K.; Iwamoto, T.; Kato, S.; Miyazono, K. Modulation of MicroRNA processing by p53. *Nature* **2009**, *460*, 529–533. [CrossRef] [PubMed]

47. Davis, B.N.; Hilyard, A.C.; Lagna, G.; Hata, A. Smad proteins control drosha-mediated MicroRNA maturation. *Nature* **2008**, *454*, 56–61. [CrossRef] [PubMed]

48. Davis, B.N.; Hilyard, A.C.; Nguyen, P.H.; Lagna, G.; Hata, A. Smad proteins bind a conserved RNA sequence to promote MicroRNA maturation by drosha. *Mol. Cell* **2010**, *39*, 373–384. [CrossRef] [PubMed]

49. Yu, B.; Bi, L.; Zheng, B.; Ji, L.; Chevalier, D.; Agarwal, M.; Ramachandran, V.; Li, W.; Lagrange, T.; Walker, J.C.; *et al.* The FHA domain proteins dawdle in arabidopsis and snip1 in humans act in small RNA biogenesis. *Proc. Natl. Acad. Sci. USA* **2008**, *105*, 10073–10078. [CrossRef] [PubMed]

50. Diaz-Moreno, I.; Hollingworth, D.; Frenkiel, T.A.; Kelly, G.; Martin, S.; Howell, S.; Garcia-Mayoral, M.; Gherzi, R.; Briata, P.; Ramos, A. Phosphorylation-mediated unfolding of a KH domain regulates KSRP localization via 14-3-3 binding. *Nat. Struct. Mol. Boil.* **2009**, *16*, 238–246. [CrossRef] [PubMed]

51. Banin, S.; Moyal, L.; Shieh, S.; Taya, Y.; Anderson, C.W.; Chessa, L.; Smorodinsky, N.I.; Prives, C.; Reiss, Y.; Shiloh, Y.; *et al.* Enhanced phosphorylation of p53 by atm in response to DNA damage. *Science* **1998**, *281*, 1674–1677. [CrossRef] [PubMed]

52. Garcia-Mayoral, M.F.; Hollingworth, D.; Masino, L.; Diaz-Moreno, I.; Kelly, G.; Gherzi, R.; Chou, C.F.; Chen, C.Y.; Ramos, A. The structure of the C-terminal KH domains of KSRP reveals a noncanonical motif important for MRNA degradation. *Structure* **2007**, *15*, 485–498. [CrossRef] [PubMed]

53. Zhang, X.; Wan, G.; Berger, F.G.; He, X.; Lu, X. The ATM kinase induces MicroRNA biogenesis in the DNA damage response. *Mol. Cell* **2011**, *41*, 371–383. [CrossRef] [PubMed]

54. Yang, D.; Sun, Y.; Hu, L.; Zheng, H.; Ji, P.; Pecot, C.V.; Zhao, Y.; Reynolds, S.; Cheng, H.; Rupaimoole, R.; *et al.* Integrated analyses identify a master MicroRNA regulatory network for the mesenchymal subtype in serous ovarian cancer. *Cancer Cell* **2013**, *23*, 186–199. [CrossRef] [PubMed]

55. Han, C.; Liu, Y.; Wan, G.; Choi, H.J.; Zhao, L.; Ivan, C.; He, X.; Sood, A.K.; Zhang, X.; Lu, X. The RNA-binding protein ddx1 promotes primary MicroRNA maturation and inhibits ovarian tumor progression. *Cell Rep.* **2014**, *8*, 1447–1460. [CrossRef] [PubMed]

56. Urbach, A.; Yermalovich, A.; Zhang, J.; Spina, C.S.; Zhu, H.; Perez-Atayde, A.R.; Shukrun, R.; Charlton, J.; Sebire, N.; Mifsud, W.; *et al.* Lin28 sustains early renal progenitors and induces wilms tumor. *Genes Dev.* **2014**, *28*, 971–982. [CrossRef] [PubMed]

57. Viswanathan, S.R.; Powers, J.T.; Einhorn, W.; Hoshida, Y.; Ng, T.L.; Toffanin, S.; O'Sullivan, M.; Lu, J.; Phillips, L.A.; Lockhart, V.L.; *et al.* Lin28 promotes transformation and is associated with advanced human malignancies. *Nat. Genet.* **2009**, *41*, 843–848. [CrossRef] [PubMed]

58. Melo, S.A.; Moutinho, C.; Ropero, S.; Calin, G.A.; Rossi, S.; Spizzo, R.; Fernandez, A.F.; Davalos, V.; Villanueva, A.; Montoya, G.; *et al.* A genetic defect in exportin-5 traps precursor MicroRNAs in the nucleus of cancer cells. *Cancer Cell* **2010**, *18*, 303–315. [CrossRef] [PubMed]

59. Melo, S.A.; Esteller, M. A precursor MicroRNA in a cancer cell nucleus: Get me out of here! *Cell Cycle* **2011**, *10*, 922–925. [CrossRef] [PubMed]

60. Liu, X.; Wang, C.; Chen, Z.; Jin, Y.; Wang, Y.; Kolokythas, A.; Dai, Y.; Zhou, X. Microrna-138 suppresses epithelial-mesenchymal transition in squamous cell carcinoma cell lines. *Biochem. J.* **2011**, *440*, 23–31. [CrossRef] [PubMed]

61. Li, J.; Chen, Y.; Qin, X.; Wen, J.; Ding, H.; Xia, W.; Li, S.; Su, X.; Wang, W.; Li, H.; *et al.* Mir-138 downregulates miRNA processing in hela cells by targeting rmnd5a and decreasing exportin-5 stability. *Nucleic Acids Res.* **2014**, *42*, 458–474. [CrossRef] [PubMed]

62. Wan, G.; Zhang, X.; Langley, R.R.; Liu, Y.; Hu, X.; Han, C.; Peng, G.; Ellis, L.M.; Jones, S.N.; Lu, X. DNA-damage-induced nuclear export of precursor MicroRNAs is regulated by the atm-akt pathway. *Cell Rep.* **2013**, *3*, 2100–2112. [CrossRef] [PubMed]

63. Bernstein, E.; Caudy, A.A.; Hammond, S.M.; Hannon, G.J. Role for a bidentate ribonuclease in the initiation step of RNA interference. *Nature* **2001**, *409*, 363–366. [CrossRef] [PubMed]

64. Hutvagner, G.; McLachlan, J.; Pasquinelli, A.E.; Balint, E.; Tuschl, T.; Zamore, P.D. A cellular function for the RNA-interference enzyme dicer in the maturation of the let-7 small temporal RNA. *Science* **2001**, *293*, 834–838. [CrossRef] [PubMed]

65. Chiosea, S.; Jelezcova, E.; Chandran, U.; Acquafondata, M.; McHale, T.; Sobol, R.W.; Dhir, R. Up-regulation of dicer, a component of the MicroRNA machinery, in prostate adenocarcinoma. *Am. J. Pathol.* **2006**, *169*, 1812–1820. [CrossRef] [PubMed]

66. Faber, C.; Horst, D.; Hlubek, F.; Kirchner, T. Overexpression of dicer predicts poor survival in colorectal cancer. *Eur. J. Cancer* **2011**, *47*, 1414–1419. [CrossRef] [PubMed]

67. Stratmann, J.; Wang, C.J.; Gnosa, S.; Wallin, A.; Hinselwood, D.; Sun, X.F.; Zhang, H. Dicer and mirna in relation to clinicopathological variables in colorectal cancer patients. *BMC Cancer* **2011**, *11*, 345. [CrossRef] [PubMed]

68. Zhu, D.X.; Fan, L.; Lu, R.N.; Fang, C.; Shen, W.Y.; Zou, Z.J.; Wang, Y.H.; Zhu, H.Y.; Miao, K.R.; Liu, P.; et al. Downregulated dicer expression predicts poor prognosis in chronic lymphocytic leukemia. *Cancer Sci.* **2012**, *103*, 875–881. [CrossRef] [PubMed]

69. Hill, D.A.; Ivanovich, J.; Priest, J.R.; Gurnett, C.A.; Dehner, L.P.; Desruisseau, D.; Jarzembowski, J.A.; Wikenheiser-Brokamp, K.A.; Suarez, B.K.; Whelan, A.J.; et al. Dicer1 mutations in familial pleuropulmonary blastoma. *Science* **2009**, *325*, 965. [CrossRef] [PubMed]

70. Doros, L.; Schultz, K.A.; Stewart, D.R.; Bauer, A.J.; Williams, G.; Rossi, C.T.; Carr, A.; Yang, J.; Dehner, L.P.; Messinger, Y.; et al. Dicer1-related disorders. *GeneReviews®* **2014**, 1993–2015.

71. Heyam, A.; Lagos, D.; Plevin, M. Dissecting the roles of TRBP and pact in double-stranded RNA recognition and processing of noncoding RNAs. *Wiley Interdisc. Rev. RNA* **2015**, *6*, 271–289. [CrossRef] [PubMed]

72. Lee, Y.; Hur, I.; Park, S.Y.; Kim, Y.K.; Suh, M.R.; Kim, V.N. The role of pact in the RNA silencing pathway. *EMBO J.* **2006**, *25*, 522–532. [CrossRef] [PubMed]

73. Lee, H.Y.; Zhou, K.; Smith, A.M.; Noland, C.L.; Doudna, J.A. Differential roles of human dicer-binding proteins TRBP and pact in small RNA processing. *Nucleic Acids Res.* **2013**, *41*, 6568–6576. [CrossRef] [PubMed]

74. Melo, S.A.; Ropero, S.; Moutinho, C.; Aaltonen, L.A.; Yamamoto, H.; Calin, G.A.; Rossi, S.; Fernandez, A.F.; Carneiro, F.; Oliveira, C.; et al. A tarbp2 mutation in human cancer impairs microrna processing and dicer1 function. *Nat. Genet.* **2009**, *41*, 365–370. [CrossRef] [PubMed]

75. De Vito, C.; Riggi, N.; Cornaz, S.; Suva, M.L.; Baumer, K.; Provero, P.; Stamenkovic, I. A tarbp2-dependent miRNA expression profile underlies cancer stem cell properties and provides candidate therapeutic reagents in ewing sarcoma. *Cancer Cell* **2012**, *21*, 807–821. [CrossRef] [PubMed]

76. Bohmert, K.; Camus, I.; Bellini, C.; Bouchez, D.; Caboche, M.; Benning, C. Ago1 defines a novel locus of arabidopsis controlling leaf development. *EMBO J.* **1998**, *17*, 170–180. [CrossRef] [PubMed]

77. Van Grootheest, D.S.; van den Berg, S.M.; Cath, D.C.; Willemsen, G.; Boomsma, D.I. Marital resemblance for obsessive-compulsive, anxious and depressive symptoms in a population-based sample. *Psychol. Med.* **2008**, *38*, 1731–1740. [CrossRef] [PubMed]

78. Hutvagner, G.; Simard, M.J. Argonaute proteins: Key players in RNA silencing. *Nat. Rev. Mol. Cell Biol.* **2008**, *9*, 22–32. [CrossRef] [PubMed]

79. Song, J.J.; Smith, S.K.; Hannon, G.J.; Joshua-Tor, L. Crystal structure of argonaute and its implications for risc slicer activity. *Science* **2004**, *305*, 1434–1437. [CrossRef] [PubMed]

80. Frank, F.; Sonenberg, N.; Nagar, B. Structural basis for 5′-nucleotide base-specific recognition of guide RNA by human ago2. *Nature* **2010**, *465*, 818–822. [CrossRef] [PubMed]

81. Yan, K.S.; Yan, S.; Farooq, A.; Han, A.; Zeng, L.; Zhou, M.M. Structure and conserved RNA binding of the Paz domain. *Nature* **2003**, *426*, 468–474. [CrossRef] [PubMed]

82. Parker, J.S.; Roe, S.M.; Barford, D. Structural insights into MRNA recognition from a piwi domain-siRNA guide complex. *Nature* **2005**, *434*, 663–666. [CrossRef] [PubMed]

83. Ma, J.B.; Yuan, Y.R.; Meister, G.; Pei, Y.; Tuschl, T.; Patel, D.J. Structural basis for 5′-end-specific recognition of guide RNA by the a. Fulgidus piwi protein. *Nature* **2005**, *434*, 666–670. [CrossRef] [PubMed]

84. Liu, J.; Carmell, M.A.; Rivas, F.V.; Marsden, C.G.; Thomson, J.M.; Song, J.J.; Hammond, S.M.; Joshua-Tor, L.; Hannon, G.J. Argonaute2 is the catalytic engine of mammalian RNAI. *Science* **2004**, *305*, 1437–1441. [CrossRef] [PubMed]

85. Meister, G.; Landthaler, M.; Patkaniowska, A.; Dorsett, Y.; Teng, G.; Tuschl, T. Human argonaute2 mediates RNA cleavage targeted by miRNAs and siRNAs. *Mol. Cell* **2004**, *15*, 185–197. [CrossRef] [PubMed]

86. Diederichs, S.; Haber, D.A. Dual role for argonautes in MicroRNA processing and posttranscriptional regulation of MicroRNA expression. *Cell* **2007**, *131*, 1097–1108. [CrossRef] [PubMed]

87. Winter, J.; Diederichs, S. Argonaute proteins regulate microrna stability: Increased MicroRNA abundance by argonaute proteins is due to MicroRNA stabilization. *RNA Biol.* **2011**, *8*, 1149–1157. [CrossRef] [PubMed]

88. Yi, T.; Arthanari, H.; Akabayov, B.; Song, H.; Papadopoulos, E.; Qi, H.H.; Jedrychowski, M.; Guttler, T.; Guo, C.; Luna, R.E.; *et al.* Eif1a augments ago2-mediated dicer-independent miRNA biogenesis and RNA interference. *Nat. Commun.* **2015**, *6*, 7194. [CrossRef] [PubMed]

89. Yang, J.S.; Lai, E.C. Alternative miRNA biogenesis pathways and the interpretation of core miRNA pathway mutants. *Mol. Cell* **2011**, *43*, 892–903. [CrossRef] [PubMed]

90. Shen, J.; Xia, W.; Khotskaya, Y.B.; Huo, L.; Nakanishi, K.; Lim, S.O.; Du, Y.; Wang, Y.; Chang, W.C.; Chen, C.H.; *et al.* Egfr modulates MicroRNA maturation in response to hypoxia through phosphorylation of ago2. *Nature* **2013**, *497*, 383–387. [CrossRef] [PubMed]

91. Wu, C.; So, J.; Davis-Dusenbery, B.N.; Qi, H.H.; Bloch, D.B.; Shi, Y.; Lagna, G.; Hata, A. Hypoxia potentiates MicroRNA-mediated gene silencing through posttranslational modification of argonaute2. *Mol. Cell. Biol.* **2011**, *31*, 4760–4774. [CrossRef] [PubMed]

92. Ling, H.; Fabbri, M.; Calin, G.A. MicroRNAs and other non-coding RNAs as targets for anticancer drug development. *Nat. Rev. Drug Discov.* **2013**, *12*, 847–865. [CrossRef] [PubMed]

93. Machlin, E.S.; Sarnow, P.; Sagan, S.M. Masking the 5' terminal nucleotides of the hepatitis C virus genome by an unconventional MicroRNA-target RNA complex. *Proc. Natl. Acad. Sci. USA* **2011**, *108*, 3193–3198. [CrossRef] [PubMed]

94. Janssen, H.L.; Reesink, H.W.; Lawitz, E.J.; Zeuzem, S.; Rodriguez-Torres, M.; Patel, K.; van der Meer, A.J.; Patick, A.K.; Chen, A.; Zhou, Y.; *et al.* Treatment of HCV infection by targeting MicroRNA. *N. Engl. J. Med.* **2013**, *368*, 1685–1694. [CrossRef] [PubMed]

95. Valadi, H.; Ekstrom, K.; Bossios, A.; Sjostrand, M.; Lee, J.J.; Lotvall, J.O. Exosome-mediated transfer of mRNAs and MicroRNAs is a novel mechanism of genetic exchange between cells. *Nat. Cell Biol.* **2007**, *9*, 654–659. [CrossRef] [PubMed]

96. Fleischhacker, M.; Schmidt, B. Circulating nucleic acids (cnas) and cancer—A survey. *Biochim. Biophys. Acta* **2007**, *1775*, 181–232. [CrossRef] [PubMed]

97. Skog, J.; Wurdinger, T.; van Rijn, S.; Meijer, D.H.; Gainche, L.; Sena-Esteves, M.; Curry, W.T., Jr.; Carter, B.S.; Krichevsky, A.M.; Breakefield, X.O. Glioblastoma microvesicles transport rna and proteins that promote tumour growth and provide diagnostic biomarkers. *Nat. Cell Biol.* **2008**, *10*, 1470–1476. [CrossRef] [PubMed]

98. Melo, S.A.; Sugimoto, H.; O'Connell, J.T.; Kato, N.; Villanueva, A.; Vidal, A.; Qiu, L.; Vitkin, E.; Perelman, L.T.; Melo, C.A.; *et al.* Cancer exosomes perform cell-independent microrna biogenesis and promote tumorigenesis. *Cancer Cell* **2014**, *26*, 707–721. [CrossRef] [PubMed]

99. Kim, D.H.; Behlke, M.A.; Rose, S.D.; Chang, M.S.; Choi, S.; Rossi, J.J. Synthetic dsrna dicer substrates enhance rnai potency and efficacy. *Nat. Biotechnol.* **2005**, *23*, 222–226. [CrossRef] [PubMed]

100. Amarzguioui, M.; Lundberg, P.; Cantin, E.; Hagstrom, J.; Behlke, M.A.; Rossi, J.J. Rational design and *in vitro* and *in vivo* delivery of dicer substrate siRNA. *Nat. Protoc.* **2006**, *1*, 508–517. [CrossRef] [PubMed]

101. Dore-Savard, L.; Roussy, G.; Dansereau, M.A.; Collingwood, M.A.; Lennox, K.A.; Rose, S.D.; Beaudet, N.; Behlke, M.A.; Sarret, P. Central delivery of dicer-substrate sirna: A direct application for pain research. *Mol. Ther.* **2008**, *16*, 1331–1339. [CrossRef] [PubMed]

102. Dudek, H.; Wong, D.H.; Arvan, R.; Shah, A.; Wortham, K.; Ying, B.; Diwanji, R.; Zhou, W.; Holmes, B.; Yang, H.; *et al.* Knockdown of beta-catenin with dicer-substrate siRNAs reduces liver tumor burden *in vivo*. *Mol. Ther.* **2014**, *22*, 92–101.

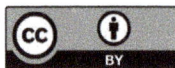

Journal of
*Clinical Medicine*

MDPI

*Review*

# Exploring miRNA-Associated Signatures with Diagnostic Relevance in Glioblastoma Multiforme and Breast Cancer Patients

Véronique C. LeBlanc and Pier Jr Morin *

Department of Chemistry and Biochemistry, Université de Moncton, 18 Antonine-Maillet avenue, Moncton, NB E1A 3E9, Canada; evl6741@umoncton.ca

* Author to whom correspondence should be addressed; pier.morin@umoncton.ca; Tel.: +506-858-4355; Fax: +506-858-4541.

Academic Editors: Takahiro Ochiya and Ryou-u Takahashi

Received: 30 June 2015; Accepted: 4 August 2015; Published: 14 August 2015

**Abstract:** The growing attention that non-coding RNAs have attracted in the field of cancer research in recent years is undeniable. Whether investigated as prospective therapeutic targets or prognostic indicators or diagnostic biomarkers, the clinical relevance of these molecules is starting to emerge. In addition, identification of non-coding RNAs in a plethora of body fluids has further positioned these molecules as attractive non-invasive biomarkers. This review will first provide an overview of the synthetic cascade that leads to the production of the small non-coding RNAs microRNAs (miRNAs) and presents their strengths as biomarkers of disease. Our interest will next be directed at exploring the diagnostic utility of miRNAs in two types of cancer: the brain tumor glioblastoma multiforme (GBM) and breast cancer. Finally, we will discuss additional clinical implications associated with miRNA detection as well as introduce other non-coding RNAs that have generated recent interest in the cancer research community.

**Keywords:** microRNAs; glioma; glioblastoma multiforme; breast cancer; cancer diagnosis; cancer therapeutics; non-coding RNAs; long non-coding RNAs

## 1. Introduction

Tremendous effort has been dedicated in recent years to elucidating the underlying functions of non-coding RNAs, including the small microRNAs (miRNAs), in numerous types of cancer. Several studies have characterized the roles played by miRNAs in primary tumors and have positioned these molecules as significant drivers of malignancy [1–3]. Importantly, such work has put the light on miRNAs as appealing cancer biomarkers, notably due to their significant stability and their ability to reveal crucial information on tumor grade and treatment response [4–6]. With an emphasis on *in vivo* human studies, this review first presents the potential advantages associated with miRNAs as cancer biomarkers and subsequently discusses studies that have identified miRNAs with diagnostic relevance in two types of cancers: glioblastoma multiforme and breast carcinomas. Finally, we introduce examples of work that have assessed the usefulness of miRNAs in other, non-diagnostic, clinical applications as well as present additional non-coding RNAs with diagnostic relevance to cancer.

## 2. MiRNAs: An Overview

MiRNA biogenesis usually starts with the transcription of miRNA genes by RNA polymerase II to generate a primary miRNA transcript termed pri-miRNA [7,8]. This capped and polyadenylated structure is further processed in the nucleus by the microprocessor complex comprised of the RNase III enzyme Drosha and the cofactor DiGeorge syndrome critical region gene 8 (DGCR8) to generate a pre-miRNA that is subsequently exported to the cytoplasm via Exportin-5 [7,9–12]. The RNase III enzyme Dicer performs pre-miRNA cleavage to yield a 20–24 nucleotide duplex miRNA from which the mature miRNA sequence will associate with Argonaute and other proteins to form the miRNA-induced silencing complex (miRISC) [13,14]. MiRISC can interact, via imperfect base pairing, with the 3′-untranslated region (3′-UTR) of transcript targets and alter their expression via translational repression or mRNA destabilization. Complementarity between the seed region of the miRNAs (nucleotides 2–8) and nucleotides of the target mRNA plays a pivotal role in target recognition and silencing [15]. Recent evidences suggest that miRNA/transcript target interaction can also occur in the 5′-UTR or within the coding region of some mRNAs [16,17].

There are multiple arguments that support the investigation of miRNAs as biomarkers for diseases. MiRNAs can notably be packaged into exosomes, small bioactive reservoirs secreted by cells, and subsequently regulate transcript targets of recipient cells [18]. Previous work has demonstrated that miRNAs secreted by cancer cells can have various effects such as increased drug resistance and transformation of target cells [19,20]. Isolation and characterization of the molecules present in exosomes for diagnostic and prognostic purposes have been performed in different types of cancer including gliomas and breast cancer [21,22], the focus of the current review. Accordingly, miRNAs are thus present in various body fluids including serum, urine and saliva, making them collectable and quantifiable via non-invasive methods [23–25]. Furthermore, miRNAs are significantly stable in a variety of biological specimens such as blood, urine and postmortem formalin-fixed paraffin-embedded (FFPE) tissues [26–28]. MiRNA isolation from these sources is thoroughly documented and their subsequent quantification can be performed with a variety of techniques such as quantitative reverse transcription polymerase chain reaction (qRT-PCR), miRNA microarrays or next-generation sequencing to name a few [29–31]. Finally, miRNA levels, in primary tissues and in circulating samples, have also been associated with different clinical parameters in cancer such as metastatic progression and response to chemotherapeutic agents [32,33]. MiRNAs thus possess a number of criteria that position them as appealing cancer biomarkers, and the subsequent sections will focus on the diagnostic potential of miRNAs in two types of cancer.

## 3. Glioblastoma Multiforme and MiRNAs

Glioblastoma multiforme (GBM) is the most aggressive and frequently diagnosed primary brain tumor [34]. This grade IV glioma is highly malignant and the prognosis for patients diagnosed with a GBM remains poor with a median survival rate between 12 to 15 months [35,36]. Standard of care consists of surgical resection of the tumor followed by a combination of radiotherapy and chemotherapy [37]. At the molecular level, GBMs can be divided into four subtypes based on the following gene signatures: classical, mesenchymal, neural and proneural [38]. Amplification of the epidermal growth factor receptor (*EGFR*) gene is a frequent occurrence in primary GBMs as well as mutations of phosphatase and tensin homolog (*PTEN*) tumor suppressor gene [39,40]. Interestingly, selected biomarker status is progressively being considered in the clinical assessment and management of certain subtypes of brain tumors such as the evaluation of O6-methylguanine-DNA methyltransferase (*MGMT*) promoter methylation status in elderly patients diagnosed with a GBM [41].

MiRNAs are appealing therapeutic targets and potential biomarkers of GBMs [42]. Deregulation of these molecules, capable of impacting several processes including cell proliferation, cell cycle regulation and angiogenesis, underlie GBM pathogenesis [43]. Not surprisingly, numerous miRNAs are differentially expressed in primary GBM tumors with targets that notably include transcript coding for proteins with oncogenic or tumor suppressive functions. Early work that assessed miRNA expression via microarray in tissue samples obtained from nine primary GBM patients and ten GBM cell lines notably revealed elevated miR-221 levels in this tumor [44]. It was subsequently demonstrated that the tumor suppressor p27(Kip1), which displays reduced protein levels in GBMs, was a direct miR-221 target [45]. Two additional tumor suppressors, CDKN1A (p21) and CDKN2A (p16), were shown to be direct targets of miR-10b, a miRNA significantly upregulated in malignant gliomas [46]. MiR-21 and miR-26a are also overexpressed in primary GBM tumors and can alter PTEN expression [47,48]. MiR-21 has been associated with GBM cell proliferation and response to cisplatin by targeting FOXO1 [49]. MiR-21 can also impact GBM cell proliferation by regulating Fas ligand (FASLG) protein expression [50]. Interestingly, miR-21 downregulation significantly reduces the oncogenic potential of GBM cell lines independently of PTEN status and affects Akt activity as well as EGFR levels [48]. Expression of the latter is also regulated, directly or indirectly, in GBMs by miRNAs such as miR-7, miR-34a, miR-146b-5p and miR-219-5p [51–54]. The strong invasiveness observed in GBMs is also mediated by differential expression of miRNAs including miR-218, a miRNA that directly targets LEF1 and affects MMP-9 protein levels [55], as well as miR-491-5p and miR-491-3p, which notably target CDK6 and other molecular players linked with GBM cell invasion [56].

While examples abound of modulated miRNAs in primary GBM tumors, miRNAs are also released by GBMs and can be subsequently isolated and quantified in various body fluid samples, thus positioning these molecules as circulating biomarkers of malignancy. A study revealed significant miR-128 upregulation and miR-342-3p downregulation in blood samples of GBM patients when compared with healthy individuals [57]. Subsequent work confirmed altered miR-128 and miR-342-3p levels in plasma samples of GBM patients and showed that these miRNAs positively correlated with histopathological grades of glioma [58]. It is important to mention that miR-128 levels, as opposed to circulating samples, are reduced in primary GBM specimens which positions this miRNA as an interesting therapeutic target for this malignancy [59,60]. Monitoring miRNAs in pre-operative plasma samples also revealed increased miR-21 levels in GBMs [61]. MiR-21 was also identified as significantly upregulated in extra-cellular vesicles (EVs) isolated from cerebrospinal fluid (CSF) of GBM patients when compared with EVs from healthy subjects further supporting the diagnostic relevance of miR-21 [62]. A similar study investigated the miRNA content of serum microvesicles collected from 25 GBM patients and notably highlighted a correlation between miR-320 and miR-574-3p levels and GBM diagnosis [63]. Overall, these studies provide a glimpse of the potential associated with miRNAs as non-invasive biomarkers for GBM diagnosis.

## 4. Breast Cancer and MiRNAs

Breast cancer, unlike GBM, is at the opposite end of the cancer incidence being the most frequent carcinoma observed in women in the United States. It is also the cancer that ranks second on the list of estimated deaths per cancer types for the same gender [64]. As for other types of cancer, early breast cancer detection is of crucial importance to improve the chance of patient survival. Substantial profiling of primary breast tumors has highlighted a variety of subtypes, such as luminal A, luminal B, HER2-enriched and basal-like, with different molecular background and clinical outcomes [65]. The latter subtype also includes triple-negative breast cancer, which lacks immunohistochemical detection of estrogen receptor (ER), progesterone receptor (PR) and human epithelial growth factor receptor-2 (HER-2) [66]. Mutations of the *BRCA1* gene, besides conferring a significant lifetime risk of breast cancer diagnosis [67], are also frequently observed in the triple-negative phenotype [68].

Pioneering work performed in tumor samples collected from a cohort of 344 patients diagnosed with primary breast cancer revealed strong miR-21 expression [69]. MiR-21 was correlated with limited disease-free survival in early stage patients. Subsequent work further positioned miR-21 as an important miRNA underlying breast cancer as it displayed strong expression in triple-negative primary breast cancers as well as in breast cancer patients with short disease-free survival [70,71]. Interestingly, and as previously observed in GBMs, miR-21 can target the tumor suppressor protein programmed cell death 4 (PDCD4) in human breast cancer cells [72]. This miRNA can also target, as in GBMs, PTEN in breast cancer and impact the response to chemotherapeutic agents [73]. An overview of the principal miR-21 validated targets in GBMs and breast cancer is presented in Figure 1.

The former study also demonstrated elevated miR-221 and miR-222 expression in the triple-negative specimens. MiR-221/222 is upregulated in HER2-positive primary human breast cancer tissues and has been linked with tamoxifen resistance [74]. MiR-221/222 deregulation leads to modulation of p53 upregulated modulator of apoptosis (PUMA), a pro-apoptotic protein, in human gliomas and breast cancer cells [75,76]. Interestingly, miR-221 can regulate the expression of the tumor suppressor proteins p27 and PTEN in GBMs and breast cancer models [45,77,78]. An overview of the principal miR-221/222 validated targets in GBMs and breast cancer is shown in Figure 2.

MiR-155 is also one of the first miRNAs to be reported as significantly deregulated in primary breast tumors [79]. Several subsequent studies confirmed miR-155 overexpression in breast cancer tissues [80–82] and recent work presented the tumor protein p53-induced nuclear protein 1 (TP53INP1) as a miR-155 target in MCF-7 cells [83]. MiR-10b is another example of a miRNA with oncogenic properties that is differentially expressed in primary breast cancer. MiR-10b levels in primary breast carcinomas correlate with several clinical parameters including tumor size, pathological grading, clinical staging and lymph node metastasis [84,85]. While these oncogenic miRNAs are only the tip of the iceberg when it comes to deregulated miRNAs in breast cancer, it is important to mention that several deregulated miRNAs with tumor suppressive functions have also been identified. Examples include miR-125b, a miRNA that directly targets the ETS1 proto-oncogene in breast cancer [86], which exhibits differential expression between primary and metastatic breast tumors [87] and was most recently reported to impact breast cancer chemoresistance in blood serum samples of breast cancer patients [88]. Downregulation of miR-205, a direct regulator of HER3 receptor expression in breast cancer [89], was observed in primary tumor tissues *versus* adjacent benign breast tissue [90] and subsequent work in FFPE tissues of patients with early breast cancer further demonstrated that differential expression of this miRNA could impact overall survival [91]. MiR-206 levels were measured in cancer tissues of 128 breast cancer patients via qRT-PCR and revealed reduced expression when compared with normal adjacent tissues [92]. The tumor suppressive properties of miR-206 are likely explained via modulation of its validated target Cyclin D1 [93]. Interestingly, Cyclin D1 is a well-characterized occurrence in primary breast cancer [94] and this further highlights the potential importance of the miR-206-Cyclin D1 axis in this malignancy.

As for GBMs, miRNAs have also been identified in circulating samples of breast cancer patients and have been investigated further for their diagnostic potential [95]. Early work revealed elevated miR-195 levels in blood samples collected from pre-operative breast cancer patients when compared with samples processed from matched controls [96]. The same study also revealed circulating miR-155 overexpression in multiple types of cancer. MiR-155 serum levels were subsequently reported to identify healthy subjects from breast cancer patients further strengthening its diagnostic potential [97,98]. As in primary breast cancer tissues, differential expression of miR-21 in circulating samples has been demonstrated in numerous studies. MiR-21 levels measured by qRT-PCR in serum samples collected from 102 breast cancer patients and 20 healthy female donors highlighted the capacity of this miRNA to discriminate between the two groups [99]. Subsequent work in different cohorts of breast cancer patients further reported miR-21 differential expression between circulating samples collected from patients and samples obtained from healthy individuals [100,101]. Novel studies have revealed signatures of multiple miRNAs associated with breast cancer [102,103] and validation of such footprints in other cohorts of breast cancer patients is foreseen to better decipher their clinical relevance.

## 5. MiRNAs as Biomarkers: Beyond Diagnostic

Several miRNAs with diagnostic potential in GBMs and in breast cancer have been presented up to this point and a list of commonly deregulated miRNAs in these two types of cancer is presented in Table 1.

In addition and as alluded in this article, the clinical usefulness of miRNAs reach beyond their capabilities of diagnosing malignancy. Indeed, miRNAs have also been investigated as prognostic markers. Specific examples in brain tumors include miR-328 which is strongly expressed in glioma cells *in vivo* and is associated with poor overall patient survival [104] as well as elevated miR-210 levels in serum samples of GBM patients which correlate with poor survival [105]. In breast cancer, miRNA expression by qRT-PCR was performed in blood samples collected from patients and healthy individuals and revealed that miR-200c and miR-141 levels correlated with overall survival [106]. A signature comprising of miR-18b, miR-103, miR-107 and miR-652 efficiently predicted overall survival in serum samples obtained from a cohort of 60 triple-negative breast cancer patients [107]. Examples of miRNAs as potential biomarkers of therapeutic response also exist. In GBMs, elevated MGMT levels confer resistance to the alkylating agent temozolomide (TMZ) [108]. MiR-181d was shown to act as a suitable predictor of TMZ response in GBM cases and to directly regulate MGMT expression [109]. Other examples of miRNAs capable of modulating MGMT expression include miR-221, miR-222, miR-603, miR-648 and miR-767-3p, further supporting the underlying importance of these non-coding RNAs in TMZ response in GBMs [110–112]. MiRNAs such as let-7i, miR-93, miR-130a, miR151-3p, miR-423-5p, miR-938, miR-1238, and miR-1280 have also been correlated with TMZ response in GBMs independently of MGMT status [113,114]. In breast cancer, elevated miR-125b levels were detected in blood serum samples collected from 56 patients and were associated with poor chemotherapeutic response [86]. A study in plasma samples of breast cancer patients also linked circulating miR-210 levels with trastuzumab resistance [115]. While this review has focused on the diagnostic potential of miRNAs, there is clear evidence that these molecules also possess additional clinical properties.

## 6. Conclusions

In addition to miRNAs, it is important to mention that other non-coding RNAs such as long non-coding RNAs (lncRNAs) are appealing molecules to investigate for their diagnostic potential in different types of cancer. While the information available regarding lncRNAs as potential cancer biomarkers in human *in vivo* models is not as vast as for the miRNAs, interesting work is starting to emerge in this research area. Two studies notably reported elevated HOX antisense intergenic RNA (HOTAIR) lncRNA levels in blood samples collected from cervical and colorectal cancer patients and correlated this observation with poor prognosis [116,117]. In gliomas, the identification of subtypes based on lncRNA expression provided pioneering work for the clinical relevance of lncRNAs in brain tumors [118]. MEG3, an lncRNA with tumor-suppressive functions, displayed significant downregulation in glioma tissue samples when compared with adjacent normal tissues and its overexpression in two GBM cell lines promoted apoptosis [119]. Early work in breast cancer FFPE tissues notably showed that strong HOTAIR expression was linked with ER and PR expression [120] and a recent study observed elevated lncRNA RP11-445H22.4 levels in serum samples collected from a cohort of 136 breast cancer patients [121].

In conclusion, whether to monitor treatment response in GBMs or for early breast cancer detection, several examples exist that illustrate non-coding RNAs with diagnostic, prognostic and therapeutic response assessment potential. Deciphering the circulating miRNA footprint associated with these malignancies is undoubtedly of great clinical interest and tremendous progress has been made in this research area in recent years. Nevertheless, challenges remain before non-coding RNAs are leveraged as bona fide biomarkers in the two types of cancer explored in this review and further investigation is needed in this research field to unveil clinically relevant miRNA-based signatures.

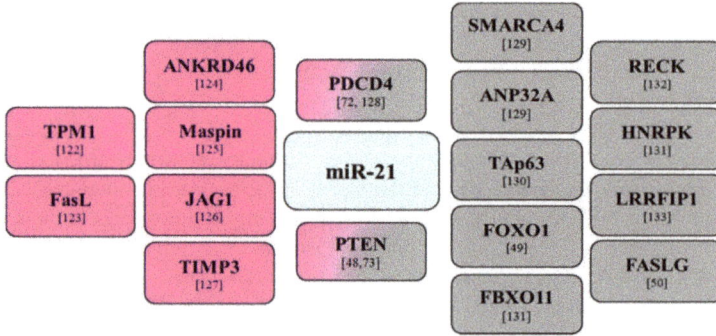

**Figure 1.** MiR-21 validated targets in glioblastoma multiforme and breast cancer studies. Targets in breast cancer are shown in pink and targets in glioblastoma multiforme are shown in gray.

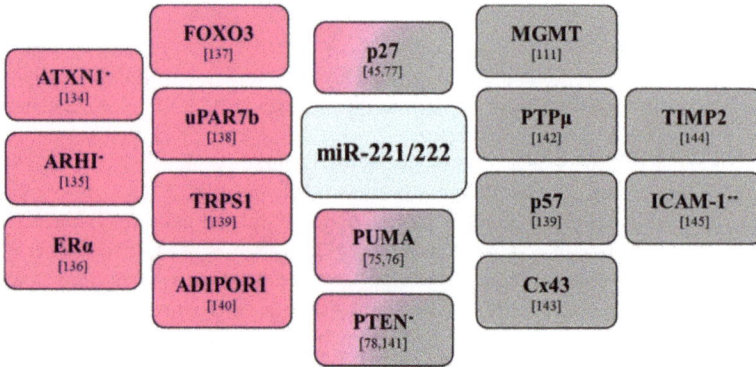

**Figure 2.** MiR-221/222 validated targets in glioblastoma multiforme and breast cancer studies. Targets in breast cancer are shown in pink and targets in glioblastoma multiforme are shown in gray. * Targets regulated by miR-221 alone. ** Target regulated by miR-222 alone.

**Table 1.** Commonly deregulated microRNAs (miRNAs) in primary and circulating glioblastoma multiforme (GBM) and breast cancer (BC) samples. BC: Differential expression of miRNA only reported in breast cancer.

| miRNA | Differential expression | Sample type | References |
|---|---|---|---|
| miR-7-5p | Downregulated | Primary tumors | [146,147] |
| miR-10b | Upregulated | Primary tumors Serum (BC) | [148–151] |
| miR-17/92 | Upregulated | Primary tumors | [152,153] |
| miR-21 | Upregulated | Primary tumors Plasma | [61,69,154,155] |
| miR-155 | Upregulated | Primary tumors Serum (BC) | [79,150,156] |
| miR-182 | Upregulated | Primary tumors | [157,158] |
| miR-221 | Upregulated | Primary tumors | [44,70] |
| miR-222 | Upregulated | Primary tumors | [44,74] |

**Acknowledgments:** Pier Jr Morin is supported by the Beatrice Hunter Cancer Research Institute (BHCRI), the New Brunswick Health Research Foundation (NBHRF), the New Brunswick Innovation Foundation (NBIF) and the Université de Moncton. Véronique C. LeBlanc would also like to thank the BHCRI and the NBHRF for funding.

*J. Clin. Med.* **2015**, *4*, 1612–1630

**Author Contributions:** Véronique C. LeBlanc wrote parts of the manuscript and created the table and figures. Pier Jr Morin wrote parts of the manuscript and edited the document.

**Conflicts of Interest:** The authors declare no conflict of interest.

## References

1.  Leivonen, S.K.; Sahlberg, K.K.; Mäkelä, R.; Due, E.U.; Kallioniemi, O.; Børresen-Dale, A.L.; Perälä, M. High-throughput screens identify microRNAs essential for HER2 positive breast cancer cell growth. *Mol. Oncol.* **2014**, *8*, 93–104. [CrossRef] [PubMed]
2.  Rupaimoole, R.; Wu, S.Y.; Pradeep, S.; Ivan, C.; Pecot, C.V.; Gharpure, K.M.; Nagaraja, A.S.; Armaiz-Pena, G.N.; McGuire, M.; Zand, B.; *et al.* Hypoxia-mediated downregulation of miRNA biogenesis promotes tumour progression. *Nat. Commun.* **2014**, *5*. [CrossRef] [PubMed]
3.  Valeri, N.; Braconi, C.; Gasparini, P.; Murgia, C.; Lampis, A.; Paulus-Hock, V.; Hart, J.R.; Ueno, L.; Grivennikov, S.I.; Lovat, F.; *et al.* MicroRNA-135b promotes cancer progression by acting as a downstream effector of oncogenic pathways in colon cancer. *Cancer Cell* **2014**, *25*, 469–483. [CrossRef] [PubMed]
4.  Chen, X.; Ba, Y.; Ma, L.; Cai, X.; Yin, Y.; Wang, K.; Guo, J.; Zhang, Y.; Chen, J.; Guo, X.; *et al.* Characterization of microRNAs in serum: A novel class of biomarkers for diagnosis of cancer and other diseases. *Cell Res.* **2008**, *18*, 997–1006. [CrossRef] [PubMed]
5.  Kodahl, A.R.; Lyng, M.B.; Binder, H.; Cold, S.; Gravgaard, K.; Knoop, A.S.; Ditzel, H.J. Novel circulating microRNA signature as a potential non-invasive multi-marker test in ER-positive early-stage breast cancer: A case control study. *Mol. Oncol.* **2014**, *8*, 874–883. [CrossRef] [PubMed]
6.  Hansen, T.F.; Carlsen, A.L.; Heegaard, N.H.; Sørensen, F.B.; Jakobsen, A. Changes in circulating microRNA-126 during treatment with chemotherapy and bevacizumab predicts treatment response in patients with metastatic colorectal cancer. *Br. J. Cancer* **2015**, *112*, 624–629. [CrossRef] [PubMed]
7.  Lee, L.; Kim, M.; Han, J.; Yeom, K.H.; Lee, S.; Baek, S.H.; Kim, V.N. MicroRNA genes are transcribed by RNA polymerase II. *EMBO J.* **2004**, *23*, 4051–4060. [CrossRef] [PubMed]
8.  Borchert, G.M.; Lanier, W.; Davidson, B.L. RNA polymerase III transcribes human microRNAs. *Nat. Struct. Mol. Biol.* **2006**, *13*, 1097–1101. [CrossRef] [PubMed]
9.  Lee, Y.; Jeon, K.; Lee, J.T.; Kim, S.; Kim, V.N. MicroRNA maturation: Stepwise processing and subcellular localization. *EMBO J.* **2002**, *21*, 4663–4670. [CrossRef] [PubMed]
10. Yi, R.; Qin, Y.; Macara, I.G.; Cullen, B.R. Exportin-5 mediates the nuclear export of pre-microRNAs and short hairpin RNAs. *Genes Dev.* **2003**, *17*, 3011–3016. [CrossRef] [PubMed]
11. Cai, X.; Hagedorn, C.H.; Cullen, B.R. Human microRNAs are processed from capped, polyadenylated transcripts that can also function as mRNAs. *RNA* **2004**, *10*, 1957–1966. [CrossRef] [PubMed]
12. Landthaler, M.; Yalcin, A.; Tuschl, T. The human DiGeorge syndrome critical region gene 8 and its D. melanogaster homolog are required for miRNA biogenesis. *Curr. Biol.* **2004**, *14*, 2162–2167. [CrossRef] [PubMed]
13. Bernstein, E.; Caudy, A.A.; Hammond, S.M.; Hannon, G.J. Role for a bidentate ribonuclease in the initiation step of RNA interference. *Nature* **2001**, *409*, 363–366. [CrossRef] [PubMed]
14. Meister, G.; Landthaler, M.; Patkaniowska, A.; Dorsett, Y.; Teng, G.; Tuschl, T. Human Argonaute2 mediates RNA cleavage targeted by miRNAs and siRNAs. *Mol. Cell* **2004**, *15*, 185–197. [CrossRef] [PubMed]
15. Lewis, B.P.; Shih, I.H.; Jones-Rhoades, M.W.; Bartel, D.P.; Burge, C.B. Prediction of mammalian microRNA targets. *Cell* **2003**, *115*, 787–798. [CrossRef]
16. Lee, I.; Ajay, S.S.; Yook, J.I.; Kim, H.S.; Hong, S.H.; Kim, N.H.; Dhanasekaran, S.M.; Chinnaiyan, A.M.; Athey, B.D. New class of microRNA targets containing simultaneous 5-UTR and 3-UTR interaction site. *Genome Res.* **2009**, *19*, 1175–1183. [CrossRef] [PubMed]
17. Brümmer, A.; Hausser, J. MicroRNA binding sites in the coding region of mRNAs: Extending the repertoire of post-transcriptional gene regulation. *Bioessays* **2014**, *36*, 617–626. [CrossRef] [PubMed]
18. Valadi, H.; Ekström, K.; Bossios, A.; Sjöstrand, M.; Lee, J.J.; Lötvall, J.O. Exosome-mediated transfer of mRNAs and microRNAs is a novel mechanism of genetic exchange between cells. *Nat. Cell Biol.* **2007**, *9*, 654–659. [CrossRef] [PubMed]

19. Ohshima, K.; Inoue, K.; Fujiwara, A.; Hatakeyama, K.; Kanto, K.; Watanabe, Y.; Muramatsu, K.; Fukuda, Y.; Ogura, S.; Yamaguchi, K.; *et al.* Let-7 microRNA family is selectively secreted into the extracellular environment via exosomes in a metastatic gastric cancer cell line. *PLoS ONE* **2010**, *5*, e13247. [CrossRef] [PubMed]

20. Wei, Y.; Lai, X.; Yu, S.; Chen, S.; Ma, Y.; Zhang, Y.; Li, H.; Zhu, X.; Yao, L.; Zhang, J. Exosomal miR-221/222 enhances tamoxifen resistance in recipient ER-positive breast cancer cells. *Breast Cancer Res. Treat.* **2014**, *147*, 423–431. [CrossRef] [PubMed]

21. Friel, A.M.; Corcoran, C.; Crown, J.; O'Driscoll, L. Relevance of circulating tumor cells, extracellular nucleic acids, and exosomes in breast cancer. *Breast Cancer Res. Treat.* **2010**, *123*, 613–625. [CrossRef] [PubMed]

22. Santiago-Dieppa, D.R.; Steinberg, J.; Gonda, D.; Cheung, V.J.; Carter, B.S.; Chen, C.C. Extracellular vesicles as a platform for "liquid biopsy" in glioblastoma patients. *Expert Rev. Mol. Diagn.* **2014**, *14*, 819–825. [CrossRef] [PubMed]

23. Lawrie, C.H.; Gal, S.; Dunlop, H.M.; Pushkaran, B.; Liggins, A.P.; Pulford, K.; Banham, A.H.; Pezzella, F.; Boultwood, J.; Wainscoat, J.S.; *et al.* Detection of elevated levels of tumour-associated microRNAs in serum of patients with diffuse large B-cell lymphoma. *Br. J. Haematol.* **2008**, *141*, 672–675. [CrossRef] [PubMed]

24. Park, N.J.; Zhou, H.; Elashoff, D.; Hemson, B.S.; Kastratovic, D.A.; Abemayor, E.; Wong, D.T. Salivary microRNA: Discovery, characterization, and clinical utility for oral cancer detection. *Clin. Cancer Res.* **2009**, *15*, 5473–5477. [CrossRef] [PubMed]

25. Hanke, M.; Hoefig, K.; Merz, H.; Feller, A.C.; Kausch, I.; Jocham, D.; Warnecke, J.M.; Sczakiel, G. A robust methodology to study urine microRNA as tumor marker: microRNA-126 and microRNA-182 are related to urinary bladder cancer. *Urol. Oncol.* **2010**, *28*, 655–661. [CrossRef] [PubMed]

26. Mitchell, P.S.; Parkin, R.K.; Kroh, E.M.; Fritz, B.R.; Wyman, S.K.; Pogosova-Agadjanyan, E.L.; Peterson, A.; Noteboom, J.; O'Briant, K.C.; Allen, A.; *et al.* Circulating microRNAs as stable blood-based markers for cancer detection. *Proc. Natl. Acad. Sci. USA* **2008**, *105*, 10513–10518. [CrossRef] [PubMed]

27. Mall, C.; Rocke, D.M.; Durbin-Johnson, B.; Weiss, R.H. Stability of miRNA in human urine supports its biomarker potential. *Biomark. Med.* **2013**, *7*, 623–631. [CrossRef] [PubMed]

28. Kakimoto, Y.; Kamiguchi, H.; Ochiai, E.; Satoh, F.; Osawa, M. MicroRNA Stability in Postmortem FFPE Tissues: Quantitative Analysis Using Autoptic Samples from Acute Myocardial Infarction Patients. *PLoS ONE* **2015**, *10*, e0129338. [CrossRef] [PubMed]

29. Lodes, M.J.; Caraballo, M.; Suciu, D.; Munro, S.; Kumar, A.; Anderson, B. Detection of cancer with serum miRNAs on an oligonucleotide microarray. *PLoS ONE* **2009**, *4*, 1–12. [CrossRef] [PubMed]

30. Kroh, E.M.; Parkin, R.K.; Mitchell, P.S.; Tewari, M. Analysis of circulating microRNA biomarkers in plasma and serum using quantitative reverse transcription-PCR (qRT-PCR). *Methods* **2010**, *50*, 298–301. [CrossRef] [PubMed]

31. Dedeoğlu, B.G. High-throughput approaches for microRNA expression analysis. *Methods Mol. Biol.* **2014**, *1107*, 91–103. [PubMed]

32. Schetter, A.J.; Leung, S.Y.; Sohn, J.J.; Zanetti, K.A.; Bowman, E.D.; Yanaihara, N.; Yuen, S.T.; Chan, T.L.; Kwong, D.L.; Au, G.K.; *et al.* MicroRNA expression profiles associated with prognosis and therapeutic outcome in colonadenocarcinoma. *JAMA* **2008**, *299*, 425–436. [CrossRef] [PubMed]

33. Zhou, W.; Fong, M.Y.; Min, Y.; Somlo, G.; Liu, L.; Palomares, M.R.; Yu, Y.; Chow, A.; O'Connor, S.T.; Chin, A.R.; *et al.* Cancer-secreted miR-105 destroys vascular endothelial barriers to promote metastasis. *Cancer Cell* **2014**, *25*, 501–515. [CrossRef] [PubMed]

34. Davis, F.G.; McCarthy, B.J. Current epidemiological trends and surveillance issues in brain tumors. *Expert Rev. Anticancer Ther.* **2001**, *1*, 395–401. [CrossRef] [PubMed]

35. Louis, D.N.; Ohgaki, H.; Wiestler, O.D.; Cavenee, W.K.; Burger, P.C.; Jouvet, A.; Scheithauer, B.W.; Kleihues, P. The 2007 WHO classification of tumours of the central nervous system. *Acta Neuropathol.* **2007**, *114*, 97–109. [CrossRef] [PubMed]

36. Huse, J.T.; Holland, E.C. Targeting brain cancer: Advances in the molecular pathology of malignant glioma and medulloblastoma. *Nat. Rev. Cancer* **2010**, *10*, 319–331. [CrossRef] [PubMed]

37. Stupp, R.; Mason, W.P.; van den Bent, M.J.; Weller, M.; Fisher, B.; Taphoorn, M.J.B.; Belanger, K.; Brandes, A.A.; Marosi, C.; Bogdahn, U.; *et al.* Radiotherapy plus concomitant and adjuvant temozolomide for glioblastoma. *N. Engl. J. Med.* **2005**, *352*, 987–996. [CrossRef] [PubMed]

38. Verhaak, R.G.; Hoadley, K.A.; Purdom, E.; Wang, V.; Qi, Y.; Wilkerson, M.D.; Miller, C.R.; Ding, L.; Golub, T.; Mesirov, J.P.; *et al.* Cancer Genome Atlas Research Network. Integrated genomic analysis identifies clinically relevant subtypes of glioblastoma characterized by abnormalities in PDGFRA, IDH1, EGFR, and NF1. *Cancer Cell* **2010**, *17*, 98–110. [CrossRef] [PubMed]

39. Wong, A.J.; Bigner, S.H.; Bigner, D.D.; Kinzler, K.W.; Hamilton, S.R.; Vogelstein, B. Increased expression of the epidermal growth factor receptor gene in malignant gliomas is invariably associated with gene amplification. *Proc. Natl. Acad. Sci. USA* **1987**, *84*, 6899–6903. [CrossRef] [PubMed]

40. Wang, S.I.; Puc, J.; Li, J.; Bruce, J.N.; Cairns, P.; Sidransky, D.; Parsons, R. Somatic mutations of PTEN in glioblastoma multiforme. *Cancer Res.* **1997**, *57*, 4183–4186. [PubMed]

41. Weller, M.; Pfister, S.M.; Wick, W.; Hegi, M.E.; Reifenberger, G.; Stupp, R. Molecular neuro-oncology in clinical practice: A new horizon. *Lancet Oncol.* **2013**, *14*, e370–e379. [CrossRef]

42. Hummel, R.; Maurer, J.; Haier, J. MicroRNAs in brain tumors: A new diagnostic and therapeutic perspective. *Mol. Neurobiol.* **2011**, *44*, 223–234. [CrossRef] [PubMed]

43. Novakova, J.; Slaby, O.; Vyzula, R.; Michalek, J. MicroRNA involvement in glioblastoma pathogenesis. *Biochem. Biophys. Res. Commun.* **2009**, *386*, 1–5. [CrossRef] [PubMed]

44. Ciafrè, S.A.; Galardi, S.; Mangiola, A.; Ferracin, M.; Liu, C.G.; Sabatino, G.; Negrini, M.; Maira, G.; Croce, C.M.; Farace, M.G. Extensive modulation of a set of microRNAs in primary glioblastoma. *Biochem. Biophys. Res. Commun.* **2005**, *334*, 1351–1358. [CrossRef] [PubMed]

45. Gillies, J.K.; Lorimer, I.A. Regulation of p27Kip1 by miRNA 221/222 in glioblastoma. *Cell Cycle* **2007**, *6*, 2005–2009. [CrossRef] [PubMed]

46. Gabriely, G.; Yi, M.; Narayan, R.S.; Niers, J.M.; Wurdinger, T.; Imitola, J.; Ligon, K.L.; Kesari, S.; Esau, C.; Stephens, R.M.; *et al.* Human glioma growth is controlled by microRNA-10b. *Cancer Res.* **2011**, *71*, 3563–3572. [CrossRef] [PubMed]

47. Kim, H.; Huang, W.; Jiang, X.; Pennicooke, B.; Park, P.J.; Johnson, M.D. Integrative genome analysis reveals an oncomir/oncogene cluster regulating glioblastoma survivorship. *Proc. Natl. Acad. Sci. USA* **2010**, *107*, 2183–2188. [CrossRef] [PubMed]

48. Zhou, X.; Ren, Y.; Moore, L.; Mei, M.; You, Y.; Xu, P.; Wang, B.; Wang, G.; Jia, Z.; Pu, P.; *et al.* Downregulation of miR-21 inhibits EGFR pathway and suppresses the growth of human glioblastoma cells independent of PTEN status. *Lab. Investig.* **2010**, *90*, 144–155. [CrossRef] [PubMed]

49. Lei, B.X.; Liu, Z.H.; Li, Z.J.; Li, C.; Deng, Y.F. miR-21 induces cell proliferation and suppresses the chemosensitivity in glioblastoma cells via downregulation of FOXO1. *Int. J. Clin. Exp. Med.* **2014**, *7*, 2060–2066. [PubMed]

50. Shang, C.; Guo, Y.; Hong, Y.; Liu, Y.H.; Xue, Y.X. MiR-21 up-regulation mediates glioblastoma cancer stem cells apoptosis and proliferation by targeting FASLG. *Mol. Biol. Rep.* **2015**, *42*, 721–727. [CrossRef] [PubMed]

51. Kefas, B.; Godlewski, J.; Comeau, L.; Li, Y.; Abounader, R.; Hawkinson, M.; Lee, J.; Fine, H.; Chiocca, E.A.; Lawler, S.; *et al.* MicroRNA-7 inhibits the epidermal growth factor receptor and the Akt pathway and is down-regulated in glioblastoma. *Cancer Res.* **2008**, *68*, 3566–3572. [CrossRef] [PubMed]

52. Katakowski, M.; Zheng, X.; Jiang, F.; Rogers, T.; Szalad, A.; Chopp, M. MiR-146b-5p suppresses EGFR expression and reduces *in vitro* migration and invasion of glioma. *Cancer Investig.* **2010**, *28*, 1024–1030. [CrossRef] [PubMed]

53. Rao, S.A.; Arimappamagan, A.; Pandey, P.; Santosh, V.; Hegde, A.S.; Chandramouli, B.A.; Somasundaram, K. miR-219-5p inhibits receptor tyrosine kinase pathway by targeting EGFR in glioblastoma. *PLoS ONE* **2013**, *8*, e63164. [CrossRef] [PubMed]

54. Yin, D.; Ogawa, S.; Kawamata, N.; Leiter, A.; Ham, M.; Li, D.; Doan, N.B.; Said, J.W.; Black, K.L.; Phillip Koeffler, H. miR-34a functions as a tumor suppressor modulating EGFR in glioblastoma multiforme. *Oncogene* **2013**, *32*, 1155–1163. [CrossRef] [PubMed]

55. Liu, Y.; Yan, W.; Zhang, W.; Chen, L.; You, G.; Bao, Z.; Wang, Y.; Wang, H.; Kang, C.; Jiang, T. MiR-218 reverses high invasiveness of glioblastoma cells by targeting the oncogenic transcription factor LEF1. *Oncol. Rep.* **2012**, *28*, 1013–1021. [PubMed]

56. Li, X.; Liu, Y.; Granberg, K.J.; Wang, Q.; Moore, L.M.; Ji, P.; Gumin, J.; Sulman, E.P.; Calin, G.A.; Haapasalo, H.; *et al.* Two mature products of MIR-491 coordinate to suppress key cancer hallmarks in glioblastoma. *Oncogene* **2015**, *34*, 1619–1628. [CrossRef] [PubMed]

57. Roth, P.; Wischhusen, J.; Happold, C.; Chandran, P.A.; Hofer, S.; Eisele, G.; Weller, M.; Keller, A. A specific miRNA signature in the peripheral blood of glioblastoma patients. *J. Neurochem.* **2011**, *118*, 449–457. [CrossRef] [PubMed]

58. Wang, Q.; Li, P.; Li, A.; Jiang, W.; Wang, H.; Wang, J.; Xie, K. Plasma specific miRNAs as predictive biomarkers for diagnosis and prognosis of glioma. *J. Exp. Clin. Cancer Res.* **2012**, *31*. [CrossRef] [PubMed]

59. Godlewski, J.; Nowicki, M.O.; Bronisz, A.; Williams, S.; Otsuki, A.; Nuovo, G.; Raychaudhury, A.; Newton, H.B.; Chiocca, E.A.; Lawler, S. Targeting of the Bmi-1 oncogene/stem cell renewal factor by microRNA-128 inhibits glioma proliferation and self-renewal. *Cancer Res.* **2008**, *68*, 9125–9130. [CrossRef] [PubMed]

60. Papagiannakopoulos, T.; Friedmann-Morvinski, D.; Neveu, P.; Dugas, J.C.; Gill, R.M.; Huillard, E.; Liu, C.; Zong, H.; Rowitch, D.H.; Barres, B.A.; *et al.* Pro-neural miR-128 is a glioma tumor suppressor that targets mitogenic kinases. *Oncogene* **2012**, *31*, 1884–1895. [CrossRef] [PubMed]

61. Ilhan-Mutlu, A.; Wagner, L.; Wöhrer, A.; Furtner, J.; Widhalm, G.; Marosi, C.; Preusser, M. Plasma MicroRNA-21 concentration may be a useful biomarker in glioblastoma patients. *Cancer Investig.* **2012**, *30*, 615–621. [CrossRef] [PubMed]

62. Akers, J.C.; Ramakrishnan, V.; Kim, R.; Skog, J.; Nakano, I.; Pingle, S.; Kalinina, J.; Hua, W.; Kesari, S.; Mao, Y.; *et al.* MiR-21 in the extracellular vesicles (EVs) of cerebrospinal fluid (CSF): A platform for glioblastoma biomarker development. *PLoS ONE* **2013**, *8*, e78115. [CrossRef] [PubMed]

63. Manterola, L.; Guruceaga, E.; Gállego Pérez-Larraya, J.; González-Huarriz, M.; Jauregui, P.; Tejada, S.; Diez-Valle, R.; Segura, V.; Samprón, N.; Barrena, C.; *et al.* A small noncoding RNA signature found in exosomes of GBM patient serum as a diagnostic tool. *Neuro-Oncology* **2014**, *16*, 520–527. [CrossRef] [PubMed]

64. Jemal, A.; Siegel, R.; Xu, J.; Ward, E. Cancer statistics, 2010. *CA Cancer J. Clin.* **2010**, *60*, 277–300. [CrossRef] [PubMed]

65. Curtis, C.; Shah, S.P.; Chin, S.F.; Turashvili, G.; Rueda, O.M.; Dunning, M.J.; Speed, D.; Lynch, A.G.; Samarajiwa, S.; Yuan, Y.; *et al.* The genomic and transcriptomic architecture of 2000 breast tumours reveals novel subgroups. *Nature* **2012**, *486*, 346–352. [PubMed]

66. Livasy, C.A.; Karaca, G.; Nanda, R.; Tretiakova, M.S.; Olopade, O.I.; Moore, D.T.; Perou, C.M. Phenotypic evaluation of the basal-like subtype of invasive breast carcinoma. *Modern Pathol.* **2006**, *19*, 264–271. [CrossRef] [PubMed]

67. Narod, S.A.; Foulkes, W.D. BRCA1 and BRCA2: 1994 and beyond. *Nat. Rev. Cancer* **2004**, *4*, 665–676. [CrossRef] [PubMed]

68. Arnes, J.B.; Brunet, J.S.; Stefansson, I.; Bégin, L.R.; Wong, N.; Chappuis, P.O.; Akslen, L.A.; Foulkes, W.D. Placental cadherin and the basal epithelial phenotype of BRCA1-related breast cancer. *Clin. Cancer Res.* **2005**, *11*, 4003–4011. [CrossRef] [PubMed]

69. Qian, B.; Katsaros, D.; Lu, L.; Preti, M.; Durando, A.; Arisio, R.; Mu, L.; Yu, H. High miR-21 expression in breast cancer associated with poor disease-free survival in early stage disease and high TGF-beta1. *Breast Cancer Res. Treat.* **2009**, *117*, 131–140. [CrossRef] [PubMed]

70. Radojicic, J.; Zaravinos, A.; Vrekoussis, T.; Kafousi, M.; Spandidos, D.A.; Stathopoulos, E.N. MicroRNA expression analysis in triple-negative (ER, PR and Her2/neu) breast cancer. *Cell Cycle* **2011**, *10*, 507–517. [CrossRef] [PubMed]

71. Ozgün, A.; Karagoz, B.; Bilgi, O.; Tuncel, T.; Baloglu, H.; Kandemir, E.G. MicroRNA-21 as an indicator of aggressive phenotype in breast cancer. *Onkologie* **2013**, *36*, 115–118. [CrossRef] [PubMed]

72. Sun, X.; Luo, S.; He, Y.; Shao, Y.; Liu, C.; Chen, Q.; Cui, S.; Liu, H. Screening of the miRNAs related to breast cancer and identification of its target genes. *Eur. J. Gynaecol. Oncol.* **2014**, *35*, 696–700. [PubMed]

73. Wang, Z.X.; Lu, B.B.; Wang, H.; Cheng, Z.X.; Yin, Y.M. MicroRNA-21 modulates chemosensitivity of breast cancer cells to doxorubicin by targeting PTEN. *Arch. Med. Res.* **2011**, *42*, 281–290. [CrossRef] [PubMed]

74. Miller, T.E.; Ghoshal, K.; Ramaswamy, B.; Roy, S.; Datta, J.; Shapiro, C.L.; Jacob, S.; Majumder, S. MicroRNA-221/222 confers tamoxifen resistance in breast cancer by targeting p27Kip1. *J. Biol. Chem.* **2008**, *283*, 29897–29903. [CrossRef] [PubMed]

75. Zhang, C.Z.; Zhang, J.X.; Zhang, A.L.; Shi, Z.D.; Han, L.; Jia, Z.F.; Yang, W.D.; Wang, G.X.; Jiang, T.; You, Y.P.; *et al.* MiR-221 and miR-222 target PUMA to induce cell survival in glioblastoma. *Mol. Cancer* **2010**, *9*, 229. [CrossRef] [PubMed]

76.  Zhang, C.; Zhang, J.; Zhang, A.; Wang, Y.; Han, L.; You, Y.; Pu, P.; Kang, C. PUMA is a novel target of miR-221/222 in human epithelial cancers. *Int. J. Oncol.* **2010**, *37*, 1621–1626. [PubMed]

77.  Medina, R.; Zaidi, S.K.; Liu, C.G.; Stein, J.L.; van Wijnen, A.J.; Croce, C.M.; Stein, G.S. MicroRNAs 221 and 222 bypass quiescence and compromise cell survival. *Cancer Res.* **2008**, *68*, 2773–2780. [CrossRef] [PubMed]

78.  Ye, X.; Bai, W.; Zhu, H.; Zhang, X.; Chen, Y.; Wang, L.; Yang, A.; Zhao, J.; Jia, L. MiR-221 promotes trastuzumab-resistance and metastasis in HER2-positive breast cancers by targeting PTEN. *BMB Rep.* **2014**, *47*, 268–273. [CrossRef] [PubMed]

79.  Iorio, M.V.; Ferracin, M.; Liu, C.G.; Veronese, A.; Spizzo, R.; Sabbioni, S.; Magri, E.; Pedriali, M.; Fabbri, M.; Campiglio, M.; *et al.* MicroRNA gene expression deregulation in human breast cancer. *Cancer Res.* **2005**, *65*, 7065–7070. [CrossRef] [PubMed]

80.  Jiang, S.; Zhang, H.W.; Lu, M.H.; He, X.H.; Li, Y.; Gu, H.; Liu, M.F.; Wang, E.D. MicroRNA-155 functions as an OncomiR in breast cancer by targeting the suppressor of cytokine signaling 1 gene. *Cancer Res.* **2010**, *70*, 3119–3127. [CrossRef] [PubMed]

81.  Kong, W.; He, L.; Coppola, M.; Guo, J.; Esposito, N.N.; Coppola, D.; Cheng, J.Q. MicroRNA-155 regulates cell survival, growth, and chemosensitivity by targeting FOXO3a in breast cancer. *J. Biol. Chem.* **2010**, *285*, 17869–17879. [CrossRef] [PubMed]

82.  Ouyang, M.; Li, Y.; Ye, S.; Ma, J.; Lu, L.; Lv, W.; Chang, G.; Li, X.; Li, Q.; Wang, S.; *et al.* MicroRNA profiling implies new markers of chemoresistance of triple-negative breast cancer. *PLoS ONE* **2014**, *9*, e96228. [CrossRef] [PubMed]

83.  Zhang, C.M.; Zhao, J.; Deng, H.Y. MiR-155 promotes proliferation of human breast cancer MCF-7 cells through targeting tumor protein 53-induced nuclear protein 1. *J. Biomed. Sci.* **2013**, *20*, 79. [CrossRef] [PubMed]

84.  Ma, L.; Teruya-Feldstein, J.; Weinberg, R.A. Tumour invasion and metastasis initiated by microRNA-10b in breast cancer. *Nature* **2007**, *449*, 682–688. [CrossRef] [PubMed]

85.  Liu, Y.; Zhao, J.; Zhang, P.Y.; Zhang, Y.; Sun, S.Y.; Yu, S.Y.; Xi, Q.S. MicroRNA-10b targets E-cadherin and modulates breast cancer metastasis. *Med. Sci. Monitor* **2012**, *18*, BR299–BR308. [CrossRef]

86.  Zhang, Y.; Yan, L.X.; Wu, Q.N.; Du, Z.M.; Chen, J.; Liao, D.Z.; Huang, M.Y.; Hou, J.H.; Wu, Q.L.; Zeng, M.S.; *et al.* miR-125b is methylated and functions as a tumor suppressor by regulating the ETS1 proto-oncogene in human invasive breast cancer. *Cancer Res.* **2011**, *71*, 3552–3562. [CrossRef] [PubMed]

87.  Baffa, R.; Fassan, M.; Volinia, S.; O'Hara, B.; Liu, C.G.; Palazzo, J.P.; Gardiman, M.; Rugge, M.; Gomella, L.G.; Croce, C.M.; *et al.* MicroRNA expression profiling of human metastatic cancers identifies cancer gene targets. *J. Pathol.* **2009**, *219*, 214–221. [CrossRef] [PubMed]

88.  Wang, H.; Tan, G.; Dong, L.; Cheng, L.; Li, K.; Wang, Z.; Luo, H. Circulating MiR-125b as a marker predicting chemoresistance in breast cancer. *PLoS ONE* **2012**, *7*, e34210. [CrossRef] [PubMed]

89.  Iorio, M.V.; Casalini, P.; Piovan, C.; Di Leva, G.; Merlo, A.; Triulzi, T.; Ménard, S.; Croce, C.M.; Tagliabue, E. microRNA-205 regulates HER3 in human breast cancer. *Cancer Res.* **2009**, *69*, 2195–2200. [CrossRef] [PubMed]

90.  Elgamal, O.A.; Park, J.K.; Gusev, Y.; Azevedo-Pouly, A.C.; Jiang, J.; Roopra, A.; Schmittgen, T.D. Tumor suppressive function of mir-205 in breast cancer is linked to HMGB3 regulation. *PLoS ONE* **2013**, *8*, e76402. [CrossRef] [PubMed]

91.  Markou, A.; Yousef, G.M.; Stathopoulos, E.; Georgoulias, V.; Lianidou, E. Prognostic significance of metastasis-related microRNAs in early breast cancer patients with a long follow-up. *Clin. Chem.* **2014**, *60*, 197–205. [CrossRef] [PubMed]

92.  Li, Y.; Hong, F.; Yu, Z. Decreased expression of microRNA-206 in breast cancer and its association with disease characteristics and patient survival. *J. Int. Med. Res.* **2013**, *41*, 596–602. [CrossRef] [PubMed]

93.  Elliman, S.J.; Howley, B.V.; Mehta, D.S.; Fearnhead, H.O.; Kemp, D.M.; Barkley, L.R. Selective repression of the oncogene cyclin D1 by the tumor suppressor miR-206 in cancers. *Oncogenesis* **2014**, *3*, e113. [CrossRef] [PubMed]

94.  Elsheikh, S.; Green, A.R.; Aleskandarany, M.A.; Grainge, M.; Paish, C.E.; Lambros, M.B.; Reis-Filho, J.S.; Ellis, I.O. CCND1 amplification and cyclin D1 expression in breast cancer and their relation with proteomic subgroups and patient outcome. *Breast Cancer Res. Treat.* **2008**, *109*, 325–335. [CrossRef] [PubMed]

95.  Schwarzenbach, H. Circulating nucleic acids as biomarkers in breast cancer. *Breast Cancer Res.* **2013**, *15*, 211. [CrossRef] [PubMed]

96. Heneghan, H.M.; Miller, N.; Kelly, R.; Newell, J.; Kerin, M.J. Systemic miRNA-195 differentiates breast cancer from other malignancies and is a potential biomarker for detecting noninvasive and early stage disease. *Oncologist* **2010**, *15*, 673–682. [CrossRef] [PubMed]

97. Roth, C.; Rack, B.; Müller, V.; Janni, W.; Pantel, K.; Schwarzenbach, H. Circulating microRNAs as blood-based markers for patients with primary and metastatic breast cancer. *Breast Cancer Res.* **2010**, *12*, R90. [CrossRef] [PubMed]

98. Sun, Y.; Wang, M.; Lin, G.; Sun, S.; Li, X.; Qi, J.; Li, J. Serum microRNA-155 as a potential biomarker to track disease in breast cancer. *PLoS ONE* **2012**, *7*, e47003. [CrossRef] [PubMed]

99. Asaga, S.; Kuo, C.; Nguyen, T.; Terpenning, M.; Giuliano, A.E.; Hoon, D.S. Direct serum assay for microRNA-21 concentrations in early and advanced breast cancer. *Clin. Chem.* **2011**, *57*, 84–91. [CrossRef] [PubMed]

100. Chan, M.; Liaw, C.S.; Ji, S.M.; Tan, H.H.; Wong, C.Y.; Thike, A.A.; Tan, P.H.; Ho, G.H.; Lee, A.S. Identification of circulating microRNA signatures for breast cancer detection. *Clin. Cancer Res.* **2013**, *19*, 4477–4487. [CrossRef] [PubMed]

101. Kumar, S.; Keerthana, R.; Pazhanimuthu, A.; Perumal, P. Overexpression of circulating miRNA-21 and miRNA-146a in plasma samples of breast cancer patients. *Indian J. Biochem. Biophys.* **2013**, *50*, 210–214. [PubMed]

102. Matamala, N.; Vargas, M.T.; González-Cámpora, R.; Miñambres, R.; Arias, J.I.; Menéndez, P.; Andrés-León, E.; Gómez-López, G.; Yanowsky, K.; Calvete-Candenas, J.; *et al.* Tumor MicroRNA Expression Profiling Identifies Circulating MicroRNAs for Early Breast Cancer Detection. *Clin. Chem.* **2015**, *61*, 1098–1106. [CrossRef] [PubMed]

103. Shin, V.Y.; Siu, J.M.; Cheuk, I.; Ng, E.K.; Kwong, A. Circulating cell-free miRNAs as biomarker for triple-negative breast cancer. *Br. J. Cancer* **2015**, *112*, 1751–1759. [CrossRef] [PubMed]

104. Delic, S.; Lottmann, N.; Stelzl, A.; Liesenberg, F.; Wolter, M.; Götze, S.; Zapatka, M.; Shiio, Y.; Sabel, M.C.; Felsberg, J.; *et al.* MiR-328 promotes glioma cell invasion via SFRP1-dependent Wnt-signaling activation. *Neuro-Oncology* **2014**, *16*, 179–190. [CrossRef] [PubMed]

105. Lai, N.S.; Wu, D.G.; Fang, X.G.; Lin, Y.C.; Chen, S.S.; Li, Z.B.; Xu, S.S. Serum microRNA-210 as potential noninvasive biomarker for the diagnosis and prognosis of glioma. *Br. J. Cancer* **2015**, *112*, 1241–1246. [CrossRef] [PubMed]

106. Antolín, S.; Calvo, L.; Blanco-Calvo, M.; Santiago, M.P.; Lorenzo-Patiño, M.J.; Haz-Conde, M.; Santamarina, I.; Figueroa, A.; Antón-Aparicio, L.M.; Valladares-Ayerbes, M. Circulating miR-200c and miR-141 and outcomes in patients with breast cancer. *BMC Cancer* **2015**, *15*. [CrossRef] [PubMed]

107. Kleivi Sahlberg, K.; Bottai, G.; Naume, B.; Burwinkel, B.; Calin, G.A.; Børresen-Dale, A.L.; Santarpia, L. A serum microRNA signature predicts tumor relapse and survival in triple-negative breast cancer patients. *Clin. Cancer Res.* **2015**, *21*, 1207–1214. [CrossRef] [PubMed]

108. Bocangel, D.B.; Finkelstein, S.; Schold, S.C.; Bhakat, K.K.; Mitra, S.; Kokkinakis, D.M. Mulfaceted resistance of gliomas to temozolomide. *Clin. Cancer Res.* **2002**, *8*, 2725–2734. [PubMed]

109. Zhang, W.; Zhang, J.; Hoadley, K.; Kushwaha, D.; Ramakrishnan, V.; Li, S.; Kang, C.; You, Y.; Jiang, C.; Song, S.W.; *et al.* miR-181d: A predictive glioblastoma biomarker that downregulates MGMT expression. *Neuro-Oncology* **2012**, *14*, 712–719. [CrossRef] [PubMed]

110. Kreth, S.; Limbeck, E.; Hinske, L.C.; Schütz, S.V.; Thon, N.; Hoefig, K.; Egensperger, R.; Kreth, F.W. In human glioblastomas transcript elongation by alternative polyadenylation and miRNA targeting is a potent mechanism of MGMT silencing. *Acta Neuropathol.* **2013**, *125*, 671–681. [CrossRef] [PubMed]

111. Quintavalle, C.; Mangani, D.; Roscigno, G.; Romano, G.; Diaz-Lagares, A.; Iaboni, M.; Donnarumma, E.; Fiore, D.; de Marinis, P.; Soini, Y.; *et al.* MiR-221/222 target the DNA methyltransferase MGMT in glioma cells. *PLoS ONE* **2013**, *8*, e74466. [CrossRef] [PubMed]

112. Kushwaha, D.; Ramakrishnan, V.; Ng, K.; Steed, T.; Nguyen, T.; Futalan, D.; Akers, J.C.; Sarkaria, J.; Jiang, T.; Chowdhury, D.; *et al.* A genome-wide miRNA screen revealed miR-603 as a MGMT- regulating miRNA in glioblastomas. *Oncotarget* **2014**, *5*, 4026–4039. [CrossRef] [PubMed]

113. Chen, H.; Li, X.; Li, W.; Zheng, H. miR-130a can predict response to temozolomide in patients with glioblastoma multiforme, independently of O6-methylguanine-DNA methyltransferase. *J. Transl. Med.* **2015**, *13*. [CrossRef] [PubMed]

114. Yan, W.; Liu, Y.; Yang, P.; Whang, Z.; You, Y.; Jiang, T. MicroRNA profiling of Chinese primary glioblastoma reveals a temozolomide-chemoresistant subtype. *Oncotarget* **2015**, *6*, 11676–11682. [PubMed]
115. Jung, E.J.; Santarpia, L.; Kim, J.; Esteva, F.J.; Moretti, E.; Buzdar, A.U.; Di Leo, A.; Le, X.F.; Bast, R.C., Jr.; Park, S.T.; *et al.* Plasma microRNA 210 levels correlate with sensitivity to trastuzumab and tumor presence in breast cancer patients. *Cancer* **2012**, *118*, 2603–2614. [CrossRef] [PubMed]
116. Svoboda, M.; Slyskova, J.; Schneiderova, M.; Makovicky, P.; Bielik, L.; Levy, M.; Lipska, L.; Hemmelova, B.; Kala, Z.; Protivankova, M.; *et al.* HOTAIR long non-coding RNA is a negative prognostic factor not only in primary tumors, but also in the blood of colorectal cancer patients. *Carcinogenesis* **2014**, *35*, 1510–1515. [CrossRef] [PubMed]
117. Li, J.; Wang, Y.; Yu, J.; Dong, R.; Qiu, H. A high level of circulating HOTAIR is associated with progression and poor prognosis of cervical cancer. *Tumour Biol.* **2015**, *36*, 1661–1665. [CrossRef] [PubMed]
118. Li, R.; Qian, J.; Wang, Y.Y.; Zhang, J.X.; You, Y.P. Long noncoding RNA profiles reveal three molecular subtypes in glioma. *CNS Neurosci. Ther.* **2014**, *20*, 339–343. [CrossRef] [PubMed]
119. Wang, P.; Ren, Z.; Sun, P. Overexpression of the long non-coding RNA MEG3 impairs *in vitro* glioma cell proliferation. *J. Cell. Biochem.* **2012**, *113*, 1868–1874. [CrossRef] [PubMed]
120. Chisholm, K.M.; Wan, Y.; Li, R.; Montgomery, K.D.; Chang, H.Y.; West, R.B. Detection of long non-coding RNA in archival tissue: Correlation with polycomb protein expression in primary and metastatic breast carcinoma. *PLoS ONE* **2012**, *7*, e47998. [CrossRef] [PubMed]
121. Xu, N.; Chen, F.; Wang, F.; Lu, X.; Wang, X.; Lv, M.; Lu, C. Clinical significance of high expression of circulating serum lncRNA RP11–445H22.4 in breast cancer patients: A Chinese population-based study. *Tumour Biol.* **2015**. [CrossRef] [PubMed]
122. Zhu, S.; Si, M.L.; Wu, H.; Mo, Y.Y. MicroRNA-21 targets the tumor suppressor gene tropomyosin 1 (TPM1). *J. Biol. Chem.* **2007**, *282*, 14328–14336. [CrossRef] [PubMed]
123. Wu, M.F.; Yang, J.; Xiang, T.; Shi, Y.Y.; Liu, L.J. miR-21 targets Fas ligand-mediated apoptosis in breast cancer cell line MCF-7. *J. Huazhong Univ. Sci. Technologie Med. Sci.* **2014**, *34*, 190–194. [CrossRef] [PubMed]
124. Yan, L.X.; Wu, Q.N.; Zhang, Y.; Li, Y.Y.; Liao, D.Z.; Hou, J.H.; Fu, J.; Zeng, M.S.; Yun, J.P.; Wu, Q.L.; *et al.* Knockdown of miR-21 in human breast cancer cell lines inhibits proliferation, *in vitro* migration and *in vivo* tumor growth. *Breast Cancer Res.* **2011**, *13*, R2. [CrossRef] [PubMed]
125. Zhu, S.; Wu, H.; Wu, F.; Nie, D.; Sheng, S.; Mo, Y.Y. MicroRNA-21 targets tumor suppressor genes in invasion and metastasis. *Cell Res.* **2008**, *18*, 350–359. [CrossRef] [PubMed]
126. Selcuklu, S.D.; Donoghue, M.T.; Kerin, M.J.; Spillane, C. Regulatory interplay between miR-21, JAG1 and 17beta-estradiol (E2) in breast cancer cells. *Biochem. Biophys. Res. Commun.* **2012**, *423*, 234–239. [CrossRef] [PubMed]
127. Song, B.; Wang, C.; Liu, J.; Wang, X.; Lv, L.; Wei, L.; Xie, L.; Zheng, Y.; Song, X. MicroRNA-21 regulates breast cancer invasion partly by targeting tissue inhibitor of metalloproteinase 3 expression. *J. Exp. Clin. Cancer Res.* **2010**, *29*. [CrossRef] [PubMed]
128. Chen, Y.; Liu, W.; Chao, T.; Zhang, Y.; Yan, X.; Gong, Y.; Qiang, B.; Yuan, J.; Sun, M.; Peng, X. MicroRNA-21 down-regulates the expression of tumor suppressor PDCD4 in human glioblastoma cell T98G. *Cancer Lett.* **2008**, *272*, 197–205. [CrossRef] [PubMed]
129. Schramedei, K.; Mörbt, N.; Pfeifer, G.; Läuter, J.; Rosolowski, M.; Tomm, J.M.; von Bergen, M.; Horn, F.; Brocke-Heidrich, K. MicroRNA-21 targets tumor suppressor genes ANP32A and SMARCA4. *Oncogene* **2011**, *30*, 2975–2985. [CrossRef] [PubMed]
130. Papagiannakopoulos, T.; Shapiro, A.; Kosik, K.S. MicroRNA- 21 targets a network of key tumor-suppressive pathways in glioblastoma cells. *Cancer Res.* **2008**, *68*, 8164–8172. [CrossRef] [PubMed]
131. Yang, C.H.; Pfeffer, S.R.; Sims, M.; Yue, J.; Wang, Y.; Linga, V.G.; Paulus, E.; Davidoff, A.M.; Pfeffer, L.M. The oncogenic microRNA-21 inhibits the tumor suppressive activity of FBXO11 to promote tumorigenesis. *J. Biol. Chem.* **2015**, *290*, 6037–6046. [CrossRef] [PubMed]
132. Gabriely, G.; Würdinger, T.; Kesari, S.; Esau, C.C.; Burchard, J.; Linsley, P.S.; Krichevsky, A.M. MicroRNA 21 promotes glioma invasion by targeting matrix metalloproteinase regulators. *Mol. Cell Biol.* **2008**, *28*, 5369–5380. [CrossRef] [PubMed]
133. Li, Y.; Li, W.; Yang, Y.; Lu, Y.; He, C.; Hu, G.; Liu, H.; Chen, J.; He, J.; Yu, H. MicroRNA-21 targets LRRFIP1 and contributes to VM-26 resistance in glioblastoma multiforme. *Brain Res.* **2009**, *1286*, 13–18. [CrossRef] [PubMed]

134. Ke, J.; Zhao, Z.; Hong, S.H.; Bai, S.; He, Z.; Malik, F.; Xu, J.; Zhou, L.; Chen, W.; Wu, X.; *et al.* Role of microRNA221 in regulating normal mammary epithelial hierarchy and breast cancer stem-like cells. *Oncotarget* **2015**, *6*, 3709–3721. [PubMed]

135. Li, Y.; Liu, M.; Zhang, Y.; Han, C.; You, J.; Yang, J.; Cao, C.; Jiao, S. Effects of ARHI on breast cancer cell biological behavior regulated by microRNA-221. *Tumour Biol.* **2013**, *34*, 3545–3554. [CrossRef] [PubMed]

136. Zhao, J.J.; Lin, J.; Yang, H.; Kong, W.; He, L.; Ma, X.; Coppola, D.; Cheng, J.Q. MicroRNA-221/222 negatively regulates estrogen receptor alpha and is associated with tamoxifen resistance in breast cancer. *J. Biol. Chem.* **2008**, *283*, 31079–31086. [CrossRef] [PubMed]

137. Di Leva, G.; Gasparini, P.; Piovan, C.; Ngankeu, A.; Garofalo, M.; Taccioli, C.; Iorio, M.V.; Li, M.; Volinia, S.; Alder, H.; *et al.* MicroRNA cluster 221–222 and estrogen receptor alpha interactions in breastcancer. *J. Natl. Cancer Inst.* **2010**, *102*, 706–721. [CrossRef] [PubMed]

138. Falkenberg, N.; Anastasov, N.; Schaub, A.; Radulovic, V.; Schmitt, M.; Magdolen, V.; Aubele, M. Secreted uPAR isoform 2 (uPAR7b) is a novel direct target of miR-221. *Oncotarget* **2015**, *6*, 8103–8114. [PubMed]

139. Stinson, S.; Lackner, M.R.; Adai, A.T.; Yu, N.; Kim, H.J.; O'Brien, C.; Spoerke, J.; Jhunjhunwala, S.; Boyd, Z.; Januario, T.; *et al.* TRPS1 targeting by miR-221/222 promotes the epithelial-to-mesenchymal transition in breast cancer. *Sci. Signal.* **2011**, *4*, ra41. [PubMed]

140. Hwang, M.S.; Yu, N.; Stinson, S.Y.; Yue, P.; Newman, R.J.; Allan, B.B.; Dornan, D. miR-221/222 targets adiponectin receptor 1 to promote the epithelial-to-mesenchymal transition in breast cancer. *PLoS ONE* **2013**, *8*, e66502. [CrossRef] [PubMed]

141. Xie, Q.; Yan, Y.; Huang, Z.; Zhong, X.; Huang, L. MicroRNA-221 targeting PI3-K/Akt signaling axis induces cell proliferation and BCNU resistance in human glioblastoma. *Neuropathology* **2014**, *34*, 455–464. [CrossRef] [PubMed]

142. Quintavalle, C.; Garofalo, M.; Zanca, C.; Romano, G.; Iaboni, M.; del Basso De Caro, M.; Martinez-Montero, J.C.; Incoronato, M.; Nuovo, G.; Croce, C.M.; *et al.* miR-221/222 overexpression in human glioblastoma increases invasiveness by targeting the protein phosphate PTPμ. *Oncogene* **2011**, *31*, 858–868. [CrossRef] [PubMed]

143. Hao, J.; Zhang, C.; Zhang, A.; Wang, K.; Jia, Z.; Wang, G.; Han, L.; Kang, C.; Pu, P. miR-221/222 is the regulator of Cx43 expression in human glioblastoma cells. *Oncol. Rep.* **2012**, *27*, 1504–1510. [PubMed]

144. Yang, F.; Wang, W.; Zhou, C.; Xi, W.; Yuan, L.; Chen, X.; Li, Y.; Yang, A.; Zhang, J.; Wang, T. MiR-221/222 promote human glioma cell invasion and angiogenesis by targeting TIMP2. *Tumour Biol.* **2015**, *36*, 3763–3773. [CrossRef] [PubMed]

145. Ueda, R.; Kohanbash, G.; Sasaki, K.; Fujita, M.; Zhu, X.; Kastenhuber, E.R.; McDonald, H.A.; Potter, D.M.; Hamilton, R.L.; Lotze, M.T.; *et al.* Dicer-regulated microRNAs 222 and 339 promote resistance of cancer cells to cytotoxic T-lymphocytes by down-regulation of ICAM-1. *Proc. Natl. Acad. Sci. USA* **2009**, *106*, 10746–10751. [CrossRef] [PubMed]

146. Shi, Y.; Luo, X.; Li, P.; Tan, J.; Wang, X.; Xiang, T.; Ren, G. miR-7-5p suppresses cell proliferation and induces apoptosis of breast cancer cells mainly by targeting REGγ. *Cancer Lett.* **2015**, *358*, 27–36. [CrossRef] [PubMed]

147. Liu, Z.; Liu, Y.; Li, L.; Xu, Z.; Bi, B.; Wang, Y.; Li, J.Y. MiR-7-5p is frequently downregulated in glioblastoma microvasculature and inhibits vascular endothelial cell proliferation by targeting RAF1. *Tumour Biol.* **2014**, *35*, 10177–10184. [CrossRef] [PubMed]

148. Sasayama, T.; Nishihara, M.; Kondoh, T.; Hosoda, K.; Kohmura, E. MicroRNA-10b is overexpressed in malignant glioma and associated with tumor invasive factors, uPAR and RhoC. *Int. J. Cancer* **2009**, *125*, 1407–1413. [CrossRef] [PubMed]

149. Sun, L.; Yan, W.; Wang, Y.; Sun, G.; Luo, H.; Zhang, J.; Wang, X.; You, Y.; Yang, Z.; Liu, N. MicroRNA-10b induces glioma cell invasion by modulating MMP-14 and uPAR expression via HOXD10. *Brain Res.* **2011**, *1389*, 9–18. [CrossRef] [PubMed]

150. Mar-Aguilar, F.; Mendoza-Ramírez, J.A.; Malagón-Santiago, I.; Espino-Silva, P.K.; Ruiz-Flores, P.; Santuario-Facio, S.K.; Rodríguez-Padilla, C.; Reséndez-Pérez, D. Serum circulating microRNA profiling for identification of potential breast cancer biomarkers. *Dis. Markers* **2013**, *34*, 163–169. [CrossRef] [PubMed]

151. Ahmad, A.; Sethi, S.; Chen, W.; Ali-Fehmi, R.; Mittal, S.; Sarkar, F.H. Up-regulation of microRNA-10b is associated with the development of breast cancer brain metastasis. *Am. J. Transl. Res.* **2014**, *6*, 384–390. [PubMed]

152. Ernst, A.; Campos, B.; Meier, J.; Devens, F.; Liesenberg, F.; Wolter, M.; Reifenberger, G.; Herold-Mende, C.; Lichter, P.; Radlwimmer, B. De-repression of CTGF via the miR-17-92 cluster upon differentiation of human glioblastoma spheroid cultures. *Oncogene* **2010**, *29*, 3411–3422. [CrossRef] [PubMed]

153. Leung, C.M.; Chen, T.W.; Li, S.C.; Ho, M.R.; Hu, L.Y.; Liu, W.S.; Wu, T.T.; Hsu, P.C.; Chang, H.T.; Tsai, K.W. MicroRNA expression profiles in human breast cancer cells after multifraction and single-dose radiation treatment. *Oncol. Rep.* **2014**, *31*, 2147–2156. [CrossRef] [PubMed]

154. Chan, J.A.; Krichevsky, A.M.; Kosik, K.S. MicroRNA-21 is an antiapoptotic factor in human glioblastoma cells. *Cancer Res.* **2005**, *65*, 6029–6033. [CrossRef] [PubMed]

155. Ng, E.K.; Li, R.; Shin, V.Y.; Jin, H.C.; Leung, C.P.; Ma, E.S.; Pang, R.; Chua, D.; Chu, K.M.; Law, W.L.; *et al.* Circulating microRNAs as specific biomarkers for breast cancer detection. *PLoS ONE* **2013**, *8*, e53141. [CrossRef] [PubMed]

156. D'Urso, P.I.; D'Urso, O.F.; Storelli, C.; Mallardo, M.; Gianfreda, C.D.; Montinaro, A.; Cimmino, A.; Pietro, C.; Marsigliante, S. miR-155 is up-regulated in primary and secondary glioblastoma and promotes tumour growth by inhibiting GABA receptors. *Int. J. Oncol.* **2012**, *41*, 228–234. [PubMed]

157. Jiang, L.; Mao, P.; Song, L.; Wu, J.; Huang, J.; Lin, C.; Yuan, J.; Qu, L.; Cheng, S.Y.; Li, J. miR-182 as a prognostic marker for glioma progression and patient survival. *Am. J. Pathol.* **2010**, *177*, 29–38. [CrossRef] [PubMed]

158. Chiang, C.H.; Hou, M.F.; Hung, W.C. Up-regulation of miR-182 by β-catenin in breast cancer increases tumorigenicity and invasiveness by targeting the matrix metalloproteinase inhibitor RECK. *Biochim. Biophys. Acta* **2013**, *1830*, 3067–3076. [CrossRef] [PubMed]

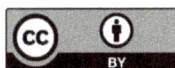

Journal of
*Clinical Medicine*

MDPI

*Review*

# MicroRNAs and Growth Factors: An Alliance Propelling Tumor Progression

**Merav Kedmi [†], Aldema Sas-Chen and Yosef Yarden \***

Department of Biological Regulation, Weizmann Institute of Science, Rehovot 76100, Israel;
meravk@tlvmc.gov.il (M.K.); aldema.sas@weizmann.ac.il (A.S.-C.)
\* Author to whom correspondence should be addressed; yosef.yarden@weizmann.ac.il;
  Tel.: +972-8-934-3974; Fax: +972-8-934-2488.
† Current Address: Genetic Institute, Tel Aviv Medical Centre, Tel Aviv 64239, Israel.

Academic Editors: Takahiro Ochiya and Ryou-u Takahashi
Received: 2 July 2015; Accepted: 31 July 2015; Published: 13 August 2015

**Abstract:** Tumor progression requires cancer cell proliferation, migration, invasion, and attraction of blood and lymph vessels. These processes are tightly regulated by growth factors and their intracellular signaling pathways, which culminate in transcriptional programs. Hence, oncogenic mutations often capture growth factor signaling, and drugs able to intercept the underlying biochemical routes might retard cancer spread. Along with messenger RNAs, microRNAs play regulatory roles in growth factor signaling and in tumor progression. Because growth factors regulate abundance of certain microRNAs and the latter modulate the abundance of proteins necessary for growth factor signaling, the two classes of molecules form a dense web of interactions, which are dominated by a few recurring modules. We review specific examples of the alliance formed by growth factors and microRNAs and refer primarily to the epidermal growth factor (EGF) pathway. Clinical applications of the crosstalk between microRNAs and growth factors are described, including relevance to cancer therapy and to emergence of resistance to specific drugs.

**Keywords:** cancer therapy; carcinoma; epidermal growth factor (EGF); metastasis; network; receptor tyrosine kinase; signal transduction; transcription

## 1. Introduction

Somatic mutations encompassing single base mutations, inter- and intrachromosomal rearrangements, as well as copy number changes are major initiators of the multistep process leading to malignancy. Germ line mutations, such as loss of tumor suppressor functions and the induction of oncogene functions facilitate somatic mutations [1,2], but the major driver of genetic aberrations is likely replication stress imposed by rapid divisions of stem cells and their immediate progenies [3,4]. The number of oncogenic (driver) mutations per common adult epithelial cancer is thought to exceed four aberrations [5], but fewer events are required in hematological cancers. On the way to become a metastatic tumor, the single initiated cancer cell must undergo rapid cell divisions, which fixate the oncogenic mutations, attract blood and lymph vessels that supply oxygen and nutrients, and invade the surrounding extracellular matrix and vessels, which permits dissemination and colonization in distant sites. This train of events is controlled by a plethora of tissue-specific growth factors [6]. For example, the 11 members of the epidermal growth factor (EGF) family act as both mitogens and motogens of epithelial cells, the precursors of carcinomas. The receptors for EGF family ligands and for other growth factors are typically transmembrane proteins sharing a tyrosine kinase catalytic function (called receptor tyrosine kinases, RTKs). Although growth factors are essential for progression of many solid tumors, accrual of specific oncogenic mutations might free cancer cells from their reliance on growth factors. This explains why a relatively large fraction of the genes undergoing recurrent somatic mutations in cancer affect protein kinases and other signaling proteins placed downstream of RTKs [7], such as B-RAF (in melanoma), RAS (in pancreatic cancer) ERBB2/HER2 (in breast cancer), and EGFR (in brain cancer). While the majority of tumors are characterized by enhanced secretion of growth factors (termed autocrine secretion [8]), driver mutations directly affecting growth factor genes are relatively rare. One example entails a platelet-derived growth factor gene fused to collagen, which is often found in dermatofibrosarcoma protuberans [9,10].

Importantly, growth factors and their downstream signaling pathways propel not only tumor progression, but also survival of cancer cells under the intense stress imposed by chemotherapy and radiotherapy [6,11]. This broad spectrum of cellular outcomes is enabled by a cascade of biochemical events that transmit growth factor signals from an activated RTK, which undergoes rapid conformational alterations, followed by autophosphorylation [12] and recruitment of upstream adaptors, such as GRB2, SHC and IRS. Each adaptor instigates a vertical biochemical cascade. In the case of EGFR and its co-receptors, HER2, HER3, and HER4 (also called ERBB2 through ERBB4), the major cascades are the ERK mitogen-activated protein kinase (MAPK) pathway and the phosphatidylinositide 3-kinase (PI3K) route, leading to activation of the AKT kinase (see Figure 1). In addition to their cytoplasmic actions, the cascades initiated by RTKs lead to regulation of transcription of specific genes in the nucleus. This is often associated with movement of proteins into or out of the nucleus. For instance some MAPK substrates, including the E26 transformation specific (ETS) family member ERF, depart from the nucleus upon phosphorylation [13]. Similarly the FoxO family transcription factors, which are substrates for AKT, also leave the nucleus and therefore become inactive as transcription factors [14]. The first genes activated by a growth factor are typically seen to accumulate beginning approximately 20 min after the stimulus [15,16]. These early genes, called immediate early genes or IEGs, usually rise rapidly and then shortly after rising they quickly fall. Following the wave of IEGs, another set of genes, called the delayed early genes (or DEGs), some are negative regulators such as transcription repressors and MAPK phosphatases, are activated and like the IEGs they also rise and fall. Finally, approximately 2.5 h after stimulation, a third set of genes, termed late response genes, or LRGs, begins to rise. Unlike the IEGs and the DEGs, the LRGs do not drop in expression as long as the stimulus is maintained, but instead reach a steady state level of expression between 4 and 8 h after the stimulus [17].

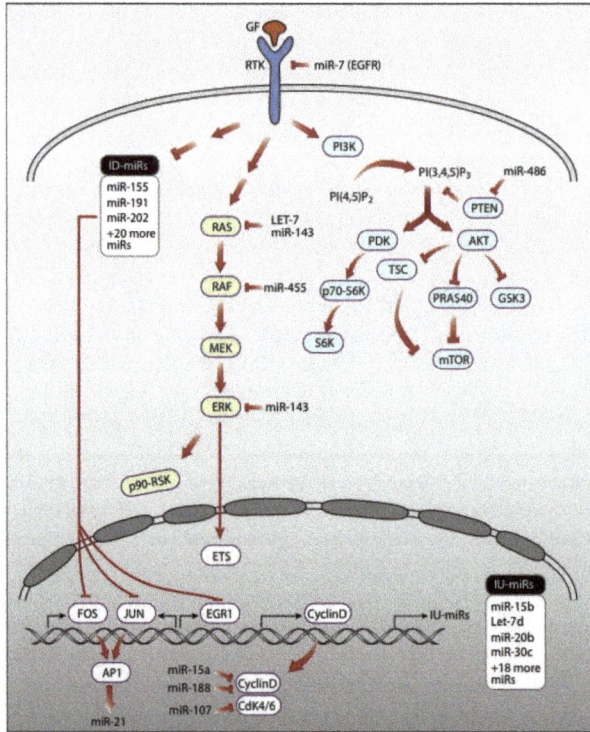

**Figure 1.** Schematic representation of RTK signaling pathways and representative regulatory microRNAs. Several biochemical signaling pathways are simultaneously activated upon binding of a growth factor (GF) to a receptor tyrosine kinase (RTK). Shown are two major cascades of protein kinases: the RAS-ERK pathway, which culminates in translocation of active ERK molecules to the nucleus, and the PI3K-to-AKT pathway, which requires phosphorylation of the inositol ring of phosphatitylinosated 4,5 bisphosphate at carbon position number 5. Both pathways regulate transcription factors, such as AP1, which comprises dimers of JUN and FOS. Note that many components of the signaling pathways are modulated at the mRNA level by microRNAs. Likewise, several microRNAs are induced or inhibited by RTK signals. They include a large group of microRNA molecules that undergo immediate down-regulation upon activation of EGFR (termed: ID-miRs) and several groups of microRNAs that are up-regulated immediately following RTK activation. For example, the group of IU-miRs is induced as early as 20 min after stimulation of EGFR.

Similarly complex, wave-like patterns of expression might relate to microRNAs (miRNAs or miRs). miRNAs are distinguished by their size of 19–22 nucleotides, and a step-wise biogenesis pathway (see Figure 2). These relatively short RNA molecules are transcribed by RNA polymerase II as large primary transcripts (pri-miRs) that are processed by Drosha to yield 60–110 nucleotide long hairpins containing precursor miRNAs (pre-miRs) [18]. Following transport of the pre-miRs to the cytoplasm, mature miRNAs are excised from the pre-miRs by RNaseIII enzyme called Dicer [19] and loaded into the RNA-induced silencing complex (RISC) [20]. Once completed their maturation, miRNA molecules become competent to target mRNAs for decay or for translational arrest [21,22]. Targeting of an mRNA by a miRNA is mediated by base-pairing between nucleotides 2–8 of the miRNA and a target element in the transcript's 3′ un-translated region (UTR) [23]. Because miRNAs are negative regulators of gene expression [24], and because each miRNA targets several hundreds of distinct mRNAs molecules [25], they greatly impact cellular processes involving de novo synthesis of proteins, such as tumor progression. This review highlights the cooperative interactions of miRNAs, their mRNA targets and growth factor signaling, in the context of tumor progression.

## 2. Occurrence and Biogenesis of microRNAs and Their Relevance to Cancer

According to the latest release of the miRBase database (release 21; June 2014), there are at least 2588 mature human microRNAs. miRNAs play profound roles in cancer progression, including metastasis. They can act both as oncogenes, namely, oncomiRs, and as tumor suppressor miRNAs. Changes in the abundance of specific miRNAs were demonstrated in many types of cancer, and their expression levels influence cell migration, invasion and proliferation [26]. Most of the miRNAs in cancer cells show down-regulated abundance compared to normal cells, however, several miRNAs are specifically up-regulated in cancer. In line with global alterations, it has been shown that malignant processes involve dysregulation or dysfunction of the miRNA biogenesis machinery due to mutations or epigenetic events (reviewed by [27] and by [28]). For example, expression of Drosha and/or Dicer is decreased in some tumor types, including neuroblastoma, liposarcoma, lung, breast, and ovarian cancers [29–31]. Growth factor signaling pathways, such as the epidermal growth factor receptor (EGFR) and the transforming growth factor beta (TGF-β) pathways, might affect general processing of miRNAs. EGFR restrains the maturation of specific tumor suppressor miRNAs, such as miR-31, -192, and miR-193a-5p, by phosphorylation of Argonaute 2 (AGO2) at Tyr393. This phosphorylation reduces the ability of Dicer to bind with AGO2, thereby inhibits processing of precursor miRNAs into mature miRNAs [32]. Under hypoxia, phosphorylation of Tyr393 by EGFR enhances cell survival and invasiveness and this was associated with poor prognosis of breast cancer patients [32]. TGF-β and bone morphogenic protein (BMP) signaling increases miR-21 abundance; specific SMAD signal transducers are recruited to the Drosha microprocessor complex and thus promote processing of primary miR-21 (pri-miR-21) into precursor miR-21 (pre-miR-21) [33]. Global effects of growth factors on miRNA biogenesis are associated in tumors with genomic rearrangements, which cause deletions or amplification of specific miRNAs loci. Conceivably, cancer cells make use of both growth factors and genetic aberrations to change miRNAs abundance, and consequently harness cellular machineries in favor of better adaptation to their changing environments.

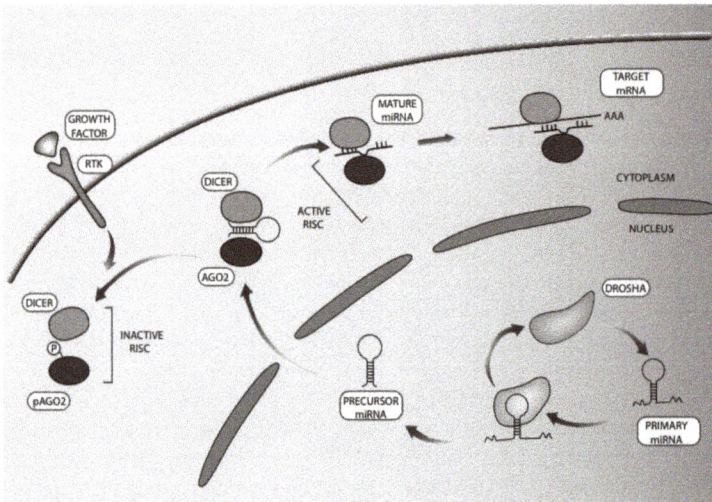

**Figure 2.** Schematic representation of microRNA biosynthesis and regulation by RTK signaling. microRNA biogenesis starts with transcription of the respective gene by RNA polymerase II. The formed long primary microRNA (pri-miRNA) consists of a hairpin stem, terminal loop and two single stranded regions. The RNase III endonuclease called Drosha processes pri-miRNAs into 70-nucleotide imperfect stem loop structures (pre-miRNAs). The latter are exported to the cytoplasm, to undergo processing by another RNase III endonuclease, Dicer, which removes the loop and joins the two arms. The resulting RNA duplex of 19–24 nucleotides allows one strand to be loaded into the RISC, while the other strand undergoes degradation. Mature microRNAs lead to translational repression or to mRNA degradation. Note that the RISC includes members of the Argonaute family, such as AGO2. It has been reported that phosphorylation of AGO2, at tyrosine 393, by EGFR is enhanced under hypoxia [32]. This is associated with dissociation of the AGO2-Drosha complex and with inhibition of processing of precursor microRNA molecules.

## 3. Networks of Growth Factors and microRNAs

### 3.1. Growth Factors Regulating miRNAs

Regulation of miRNA abundance might be induced, or otherwise influenced, by growth factors. Several studies analyzed changes in expression profiles of miRNAs following stimulation of cultured cells with specific growth factors. For instance, dynamic and coordinated changes in expression of groups of miRNAs were identified in normal mammary epithelial cells following stimulation with EGF. In less than 60 min post stimulation we observed both up- and down-regulation of distinct groups of miRNAs [34,35]. Interestingly the immediately down-regulated miRNAs we reported, a group consisting of 23 members, were over-represented among miRNAs that showed lower expression in breast cancer tumors compared to the surrounding normal tissue (peri-tumor) from the same patient [34]. Reciprocally, the up-regulated miRNAs were enriched among miRNAs with higher expression in the tumors [35]. Importantly, the mammary cells we tested, MCF10A, migrate in response to EGF stimulation [13,36]. Accordingly, we found that the migratory response of these cells is controlled by both up- and down-regulated miRNAs. For example, miR-15b, which was immediately up-regulated following EGF stimulation, significantly decelerated migration and invasion rates when silenced. In line with this observation, miR-15b expression was significantly higher in different breast cancer subtypes compared to control. MiR-15b's novel target, metastasis suppressor 1 (*MTSS1*), a lipid-binder cytoskeletal protein, which is lost in some advanced tumors, was down-regulated following EGF treatment and mediated the effects on migration and invasion of normal and cancerous cells [35] (Figure 3A). Manipulation of the immediately down-regulated miRNAs following EGF stimulation also affected migration. Thus, silencing miR-191, which targets the immediate early gene called *EGR1*, elevated cell migration. Like miR-191, a significant number of the targets of immediately down-regulated miRNAs are IEGs, such as *FOS* and *JUN*. Under steady state, when EGF is not introduced to cells, the immediately down-regulated miRNAs (ID-miRs) inhibit the expression of the IEGs, some of which are proto-oncogenes. Correspondingly, upon EGF stimulation the expression levels of these miRNAs are decreased and a rapid up-regulation of the IEGs is achieved. For example, one of the ID-miRs, miR-155, directly targets *FOS* (Figure 3B). Interestingly, the oncogenic viral form of c-*FOS*, v-*FOS*, harbors a shorter 3′UTR than the c-*FOS* 3′UTR, which does not include miR-155's target sequence. Hence, the transcript of v-*FOS* is not inhibited by miR-155, which allows v-*FOS* to exert its oncogenic ability [34]. In another comprehensive study, HeLa cells were stimulated with EGF for short times (15 min to 6 h) and miRNA expression levels were measured using microarray or deep-sequencing [37]. Dynamic changes in miRNA expression level were detected and the miRNA's predicted targets were found to be involved in molecular functions that relate to EGF signaling, such as cellular development, proliferation, cell morphology, cell death, and cell-to-cell signaling and interaction [37].

Up regulation of three miRNAs, miR-31, miR-181b, and miR-222, was detected in oral cancer cells following treatment with EGF, and this was mediated by AKT and C/EBPβ signaling, at least in the case of miR-31 [38]. Increased expression of miR-31 was also observed in EGF-stimulated mammary cells [35]. MiR-31 directly targets synaptojanin 2 (SYNJ2), a lipid phosphatase transiently up-regulated following EGF treatment (Figure 3C). Hence, it is possible that miR-31 fine-tunes the expression of *SYNJ2*, meaning that it induces down-regulation of SYNJ2 back to baseline expression level. In patients with breast and brain cancer, *SYNJ2*'s high abundance was negatively correlated with miR-31 expression and associated with poor prognosis [39]. Congruently, forced expression of *SYNJ2* enhanced tumor growth and metastasis in mice, and increased formation of invadopodia and lamellipodia, actin-filled cellular extensions involved in invasion and migration, respectively [39].

The delayed response to EGF stimulation (3–12 h post stimulation) involves miRNAs targeting both apoptotic and anti-apoptotic genes. Specifically, miR-134, miR-145, miR-146b, miR-432, and miR-494 had the largest number of apoptotic and anti-apoptotic targets, including targets that are part of the interferon pathway [40]. Other miRNAs that were identified as regulators of apoptosis and are induced by growth factor receptors, such as EGFR and MET, are miR-221/222 and miR-30b/30c. It was further suggested that in response to treatment of lung cancer cells with tyrosine kinase inhibitors these miRNAs repress the pro-apoptotic genes *APAF1* and *BIM*, making cells less susceptible to apoptosis (reviewed by [41]). The miR-30 family has a tumor suppressive role. These family members were induced by SRC inhibitors and down-regulated by oncogenic growth factors signals such as EGF and the hepatocyte growth factor (HGF). Additionally, several of miR-30's predicted targets, such as the MAPK-regulated transcription factor, ERG, are associated with epithelial-to-mesenchymal transition (EMT) [42]. In conclusion, several growth factor inducible miRNAs seem to act cooperatively to support survival, proliferation and motility, cellular functions vital for tumor progression.

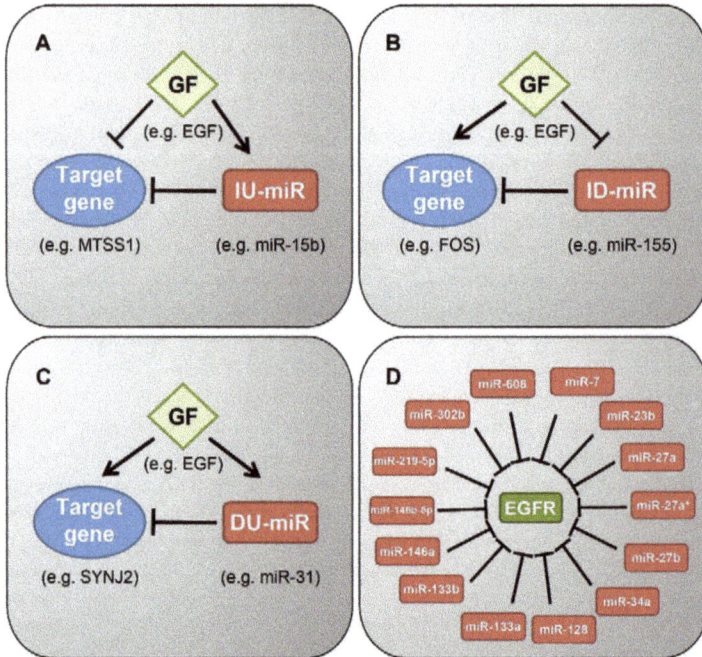

**Figure 3.** Network modules incorporating microRNAs and growth factor signaling pathways. (**A**) A feed-forward loop (FFL), whereby EGFR signaling down-regulates the expression of MTSS1, an inhibitor of metastasis. Inhibition of MTSS1 is strengthened by the induction of its targeting IU-miR, miR-15b; (**B**) A feed-forward loop whereby EGFR signaling up-regulates expression of the transcription factor FOS and, in parallel, down-regulates an ID-miR, miR-155, which inhibits *FOS*; (**C**) An incoherent FFL, whereby up-regulation of *SYNJ2*, a lipid phosphatase gene, by EGFR signaling is fine-tuned through the induction of the delayed up-regulated microRNA (DU-miR), miR-31, which inhibits *SYNJ2* expression; (**D**) Listed are miRNAs that directly target EGFR in different cancer cells. (ID-miR, immediately down-regulated miRNA; IU-miR, immediately up-regulated miRNA; DU-miR, delayed up-regulated miRNA).

## 3.2. Specific microRNAs Regulating Growth Factor Signaling

The other side of the miRNAs-growth factor networks is miRNAs that regulate the expression of growth factors, growth factor receptors, and their intracellular effectors. Specifically, we focus here on miRNAs that regulate EGFR, the EGFR pathway, and EGFR's family members. EGFR itself can be regulated by multiple miRNAs. MiR-7 was one of the first miRNA identified as directly regulating EGFR. In glioblastoma, lung and breast cancer cells miR-7 blocked EGFR expression by means of accelerating mRNA decay. Potentially, miR-7 induces tumor suppressive actions by regulating not only EGFR but also the downstream signaling pathway at multiple sites. For example, this miRNA can inhibit AKT and ERK1/2 in several human cancer cell lines and it might decrease invasiveness and arrest the cell cycle [43,44]. Similarly, miR-128 was among the first miRNAs identified as an upstream regulator of EGFR. Interestingly, miR-128 loss of heterozygosity was frequently detected in lung cancer samples, in correlation with patient survival following treatment with an EGFR-specific TKI [45]. Other miRNAs that directly target EGFR include miR-23b/27b [46], miR-133a [47,48], miR-133b [49], miR-146a [50], miR-146b-5p [51], miR-219-5p [52], miR-302b [53] and miR-608 [54] (Figure 3D).

As initially exemplified by miR-7, other miRNAs can also target more than one component of the EGFR pathway. These include miR-124, miR-147, and miR-193a-3p, which inhibit G1/S transition and cell proliferation by targeting EGFR-driven cell cycle proteins [55]. MiR-143 and miR-145 target *KRAS, BRAF* [56] and *MEK2* [57] in colorectal cancer and also in other types of cancer such as prostate tumors [58]. MiR-27a (miR-27a-3p) and the complementary miR-27a* (miR-27a-5p), both targeting EGFR, were found to be significantly down-regulated in multiple head and neck squamous cell carcinoma cell lines. Interestingly, miR-27a* targets also AKT and mTOR (mammalian target of rapamycin) within the EGFR signaling pathway [59].

Other members of the EGFR/ERBB family are also regulated by miRNAs in cancer. Using miRNA gain-of-function screens and two HER2-amplified cell lines enabled identification of the following direct regulators of HER2: miR-552, miR-541, miR-193a-5p, miR-453, miR-134, miR-498, and miR-331-3p [60]. MiR-331-3p was found to target HER2 also in glioblastoma and prostate cancer cell lines [61,62]. In a similar way, miR-148b, miR-149, miR-326, and miR-520a-3p simultaneously down-regulated HER3/ERBB3 and components of the downstream signaling pathway in response to the direct ligand of HER3, neuregulin [63]. Interestingly, miR-125a and miR-125b target both HER2 and HER3 in breast cancer cells, and consequently inhibit phosphorylation of ERK and AKT [64]. miR-193a-3p directly targets HER4/ERBB4. Repression of HER4 by overexpression of miR-193a-3p resulted in decreased proliferation, migration, invasion and EMT, as well as increased apoptosis of lung cancer cells. Moreover, miR-193a-3p, which negatively regulates HER4 in xenograft tumor models, bears anti-tumor effects [65,66]. In esophageal squamous cell carcinoma, miR-302 targeted HER4, inhibited proliferation and invasion and induced apoptosis [67]. Taken together, it is conceivable that other subgroups of receptors for growth factors are regulated by multiple miRNAs, and the latter might coordinately control components of the downstream signaling pathway.

### 3.3. Feedback Loops Linking microRNAs and Growth Factors

The plot thickens. Bilateral regulation of growth factors and miRNAs in tumors generates high order complexity that is increasingly emerging now. Specifically, feedback regulatory loops in which a miRNA is both targeting a specific pathway and, at the same time, is regulated by the same pathway, likely confer module versatility and dynamicity. For example, several miRNAs that directly target EGFR are also regulated by EGFR signaling. Thus, miR-34a is up-regulated immediately following EGF stimulation [35], but it is also directly regulating EGFR. Possibly, through this complex regulation, miR-34a acts as a tumor suppressor in the development of chordoma [54]. As discussed above, miR-7 is a well-established regulator of EGFR, however it was also shown that miR-7 might be regulated by EGFR signaling: EGFR activation in lung cancer cells can stimulate miR-7 expression in an ERK-dependent manner, suggesting that EGFR induces miR-7 expression via the RAS-ERK pathway [68]. Feedback loops that involve specific miRNAs and different components of the EGFR pathway also exist: miR-143 and miR-145 regulate the EGFR pathway genes *KRAS, BRAF*, and *MEK2* [56,57], but EGFR signals down-regulated these tumor suppressor miRNAs in a murine model of colon cancer [69]. In addition, in lung cancer cells, EGFR down-regulated miR-145 expression through ERK1/2 [70]. Other, less direct feedback loops, were also identified, in which EGFR regulated the expression of miRNAs that in turn targeted other partners of the same pathway. For example, miR-21 expression levels are regulated by EGFR via the activation of beta-catenin and AP-1 [71], and miR-21 is suppressed by the EGFR inhibitor, AG1478, suggesting that the EGFR can regulate miR-21 expression [72]. On the other hand, miR-21 regulates EGFR and AKT signaling through VHL/beta-catenin and the PPARα/AP-1axis [71]. These networks of miRNAs and growth factors have roles to play in cells motility, proliferation, and other processes that involved in cancer pathogenesis and metastasis. It is therefore important to resolve these networks in a global and systemic way.

### 4. Potential Clinical Applications of miRNAs Relevant to Growth Factors and Signal Transduction

Because growth factor signaling is pivotal to tumor progression and it is often targeted by anti-cancer drugs, major efforts are being made with the aim of better classifying malignancies and improving diagnosis and personalized therapy [73]. Since the first identification of miRNA dysregulation in cancer [74], profiling the abundance of miRNAs in tumor samples [75,76], as well as in patient fluids [77,78], is increasingly implicated as a tool enabling improved diagnosis, prognosis, and assessment of therapeutic responses. For example, in the pioneering case of let-7, reduced expression of this miRNA in human lung tumors is associated with shortened postoperative survival [79]. The use of let-7 and other miRNAs as biomarkers has been facilitated by their high stability in patient samples [77,80]. Furthermore, expression of miRNAs has been shown to be highly tissue specific [81], such that miRNA profiling might be able to infer developmental origins of specific tumors [76,82].

In the last few years, measuring global patterns of miRNAs is becoming an established method for classifying individual tumors of breast [83–86], lung [87,88], and other organs [89]. Some of these classifications will likely reach clinical application. For example, a microRNA-based test that identifies the primary origin of 42 different types of tumors (denoted miRview-mets2) has been established [90]. The panel involves testing 64 miRNAs, previously validated in 489 specimens, including 146 metastatic tumors from 42 tissues of origin. The panel is based on a tree-classifier, originally developed by Rosenfeld and co-workers, who profiled 205 primary *versus* 131 metastatic tumors from 22 different tumor origins [82]. Another comprehensive study by Nair and co-workers reported meta-analysis of 43 miRNA profiling studies across 20 types of malignancies [91]. These authors argue that stringent standardization must be introduced into the process of miRNA profiling. In addition, they found that for all classifier miRNAs in studies that evaluated overall survival across diverse malignancies, the miRNAs most frequently associated with poor outcome were let-7 (decreased expression in patients with cancer) and miR-21 (increased expression). In the context of growth factor signaling, relative abundance of subsets of EGF-regulated miRNAs in breast cancer models have been shown to correlate with the abundance of miRNAs in breast cancer patients [34,35]. Thus, miRNA classifiers, especially those based on molecular mechanisms of disease, will likely evolve into major diagnostic and prognostic tools of cancer pathologists.

## 5. MicroRNAs as Molecular Targets of Future Cancer Therapeutics

Apart from their increasing role in classification and prognosis of cancer, miRNAs are emerging as potential targets of novel drugs. Since miRNAs can function both as oncogenes and tumor suppressors, two complementary therapeutic approaches relate to miRNA-mediated therapy: silencing the action of a specific miRNA or re-introducing a specific miRNA into patients (reviewed in [92,93]). Initial efforts concentrated on silencing expression of specific miRNAs. For example, Krutzfeldt and co-workers conducted intravenous administration of "antagomirs" to mice. Injection of antagomirs resulted in significant reduction in abundance of several miRNAs in various tissues (*i.e.*, miR-16, miR-122, miR-192, and miR-194) [94]. Since then, many delivery methods have been developed to systemically administer miRNA antisense oligonucleotides, which directly silence oncogenic miRNAs in tumors [95,96] or in the surrounding microenvironment [97]. Attenuation of miRNA action has also been achieved using miRNA sponges [98] and miR-masks [99], which contain sequences complementary to the miRNA target site or to the miRNA itself, respectively. On the other hand, replacement therapy focuses on re-expression of tumor suppressor miRNAs. Overcoming the loss of miRNA expression might be achieved either through introduction of synthetic miRNA mimics in the form of small double stranded and chemically modified oligonucleotides [100], or by using adenovirus-associated vectors (AAV), which do not stably integrate into the host genome [101].

Currently there are only three miRNA-targeting therapeutics in clinical trials, two of them in oncology. The first, miR-122, is an abundant liver-specific miRNA involved in the pathology of liver diseases, such as replication of hepatitis C virus (HCV) [102]. Since HCV infection depends on functional interactions between miR-122 and the HCV genome [103], miravirsen, a LNA-modified DNA phosphorothioate antisense oligonucleotide against miR-122, was developed as a potential drug [104]. Currently, miravirsen is applied in seven clinical trials, some are already in phase II. Another therapeutic endeavor employs MRX34, a liposome-formulated mimic of miR-34a, which is administered to patients with primary liver cancer or to those with liver metastasis from other cancers. Notably, miR-34a is embedded in the p53 transcriptional network [105]. Overexpression of miR-34a was found to inhibit tumor growth and to prolong survival of tumor-bearing mice [100,106,107]. A similar endeavor, which reached phase I trials, involves the tumor suppressor miR-16. Mice injected with miR-16 mimics showed dose-dependent inhibition of Malignant Pleural Mesothelioma (MPM) tumors [108]. This led to the development of TargomiRs, nanoparticles containing miR-16 mimics, which are administered to patients with MPM or with non-small cell lung cancer (NSCLC). Importantly, the nanoparticles are conjugated to anti-EGFR bi-specific antibodies that facilitate their targeted delivery to EGFR-expressing cells. Targeting microRNA-based therapeutics to cancer cells represents only one of many pharmacological challenges. These relate not only to drug efficacy, but also to potential toxicity due to the biology of miRNAs and their multiple targets.

## 6. MicroRNAs as Modulators of Patient Response to Drugs Targeting Growth Factor Signaling

Anti-cancer drugs able to intercept growth factor signaling currently outnumber other classes of therapies available to medical oncologists [109]. These drugs are effective on a broad range of carcinomas, and some drugs are active in more than one clinical indication, which is a rare situation in oncology. So far, only two classes of drugs have been approved: (i) monoclonal antibodies (mAbs), either naked or conjugated to a cytotoxic compound; and (ii) tyrosine kinase inhibitors (TKIs), which are either mono-specific or designed to inhibit several receptors. Along with weak efficacy, development of patient resistance to therapy hinders the effectiveness of both TKIs and mAbs. Mechanisms leading to resistance are only partially understood, and they include activation of surrogate pathways, acquired structural modifications of the drug target, and histological transformation, such as epithelial to mesenchymal transition (EMT) and small cell transformation [110]. Several studies point to potential roles of miRNAs in emergence of resistance to various cancer treatments, including chemotherapy [111], radiotherapy [112], and targeted therapy [113]. Below we discuss resistance to targeted therapy, as well as summarize experimental data relevant to clinical applications of mAbs against oncogenic receptors (Table 1) and small molecule TKIs (Table 2).

Overexpression of miR-7, a well-known regulator of EGFR expression [43], was shown to enhance the effect of an EGFR TKI, erlotinib, in a head and neck cancer model system [114]. Another receptor-targeting miRNA, miR-375, was shown to target the receptor for the insulin-like growth factor 1 (IGF1R) [115]. Importantly, miR-375 abundance negatively correlates to the expression of IGF1R in breast cancer specimens. Moreover, overexpression of miR-375 restored sensitivity to trastuzumab, an anti-HER2 mAb, and increased efficacy of trastuzumab in a xenograft model [115]. Sensitivity of breast cancer cells to trastuzumab was increased also by overexpression of miR-200c, a well-known miRNA regulating various cellular processes, including EMT [116]. Adam and co-workers reported that miR-200c is also associated with modulation of sensitivity of bladder carcinoma cell lines to an EGFR mAb, cetuximab [117]. Efficiency of cetuximab treatment was found to benefit also from concomitant overexpression of miR-146a: exposing hepatocellular carcinoma (HCC) cell lines to both cetuximab and miR-146a mimics elicited synergistic effects leading to increased apoptosis and decreased cell growth [118]. Like cetuximab, nimotuzumab binds to EGFR, and its inhibitory effects were enhanced by reducing abundance of miR-566 in glioblastoma cells [119]. The case of miR-221 is especially interesting as it was shown in two independent studies to facilitate the therapeutic effect of both trastuzumab [120] and gefitinib [121], in breast and lung cancer models, respectively. While miR-221 (along with miR-222) was shown to target APAF-1 in the lung model, its main target in the mammary model was the tumor suppressor PTEN. PTEN was also shown to be targeted by miR-21 [122]. This later report showed that overexpression of miR-21 decreases sensitivity of lung cells to gefitinib. Additionally, knock-down of miR-21 restored gefitinib sensitivity to a gefitinib-resistant lung cell line and caused a dramatic reduction in tumor size [122].

Interestingly, many studies relating to TKI-resistance focus on lung cancer models, and particularly on resistance to the EGFR-specific TKI called gefitinib. Accordingly, overexpression of miR-138-5p [123], miR-34a [124], miR-103 [121], or miR-203 [121] all resulted in increased sensitivity to gefitinib in lung cancer models, albeit by targeting different effectors. Conversely, in the case of miR-30b and miR-30c, inhibition of miRNA expression, rather than overexpression, increased drug sensitivity of gefitinib-resistant cells [121]. Likewise, overexpression of miR-203 was shown to enhance the effect of another EGFR-targeting TKI, CI-1033, and to reduce tumor size in a xenograft model of RAS-driven cells [125]. Collectively, the results we reviewed underscore potential roles for specific miRNAs in the acquisition of resistance to cancer drugs, and support the ability of yet other miRNAs to restore drug sensitivity. Therefore, targeting miRNAs in combination with conventional treatments may improve therapeutic efficacy of personalized cancer therapy.

**Table 1.** miRNAs modulating the efficacy of monoclonal antibodies targeting receptor tyrosine kinases.

| miRNA | Target Gene(s) | Effect | Drug & Tumor | Reference |
|---|---|---|---|---|
| miR-566 | VHL | Knockdown of miR-566 inhibited cell proliferation and invasion and led to cell cycle arrest in glioma cells. It further sensitized glioblastoma cells to Nimotuzumab | Nimotuzumab (glioblastoma) | [119] |
| miR-200c | ZNF217, ZEB1 | Overexpression of miR-200c increased sensitivity to trastuzumab and suppressed invasiveness of breast cancer cell lines | Trastuzumab (breast) | [116] |
| miR-375 | IGF1R | Overexpression of miR-375 restored sensitivity to trastuzumab resistant cell lines and increased the efficacy of trastuzumab in a xenogarft model. | Trastuzumab (breast) | [115] |
| miR-221 | PTEN | Overexpression of miR-221 inhibited apoptosis, promoted metastasis and induced trastuzumab resistance in HER-2 positive breast cancer cells. | Trastuzumab (breast) | [120] |
| miR-200c | ERRFI-1 | Overexpression of miR-200c regains sensitivity of the resistant cell lines to cetuximab treatment resulting in reduced cell growth *in vitro* | Cetuximab (bladder) | [117] |
| miR-146a | EGFR signaling | Overexpression of miR-146a suppressed cell growth and increased cellular apoptosis in HCC cell lines and displayed synergistic effects with cetuximab | Cetuximab (hepatocellular) | [118] |
| miR-7 | EGFR | Overexpression of miR-7 enhanced the effect of erlotinib on growth inhibition of FaDu cells | Erlotinib (head&neck) | [114] |

**Table 2.** miRNAs modulating efficacy of TKIs.

| miRNA | Target Gene(s) | Effect | Drug & Tumor | Reference |
|---|---|---|---|---|
| miR-30b/30c and miR-221/222 | BIM, APAF-1 (respectively) | Knockdown of miR-30b, -30c, -221 and -222 in gefitinib-resistant cells induces increased sensitivity gefitinib | Gefitinib (lung) | [121] |
| miR-21 | PTEN | Overexpression of miR-21 decreased sensitivity of lung cells to gefitinib. Knock-down of miR-21 restored gefitinib sensitivity of the corresponding gefitinib-resistant cell line and caused a dramatic reduction in tumor size | Gefitinib (lung) | [122] |
| miR-34a | MET | Overexpression of miR-34a in EGFR mutant NSCLC increased sensitivity to gefitinib, resulting in increased inhibition of cell growth and to induced apoptosis, which resulted in tumor regression | Gefitinib (lung) | [124] |
| miR-138-5p | GPR124 | Overexpression of miR-138-5p in NSCLC cells increased sensitivity to gefitinib *in vitro* | Gefitinib (lung) | [123] |
| miR-103 and miR-203 | PKC-e, SRC (respectively) | Overexpression of miR-103 and miR-203 increased sensitivity to gefitinib in lung cells resistant to the drug | Gefitinib (lung) | [121] |
| miR-203 | EREG, TGFA, API5, BIRC2, TRIAP1 | Overexpression of miR-203 synergistically enhanced the effect of CI-1033 on reduction of tumor size in a xenograft model of nude mice injected with Ras-activated cells | CI-1033 (prostate) | [125] |

## 7. Concluding Remarks

MicroRNAs can target growth factor pathways and, vice versa, growth factor pathways can regulate miRNA biogenesis. This bilateral crosstalk creates complex networks that are involved in multiple sub-programs of tumor progression, such as cell cycle regulation, EMT, and metastasis. Moreover, as we discussed herein, the complexity and robustness of these networks are enhanced by recurring feedback regulatory modules. As expected, miRNAs and growth factor signals are embedded in larger regulatory networks that control patient response to therapeutic interventions, such as monoclonal antibodies. It is therefore essential to resolve miRNA networks at high granularity and understand their functional logic. Thus, comprehensive mapping and understanding of the miRNA and growth factor alliance holds promise in terms of more effective cancer treatments that avoid emergence of patient resistance. Other future applications might include utilization of the miRNAs-growth factor networks as classifiers of cancer subtypes and markers for cancer diagnostics and prognosis.

**Acknowledgments:** Our team is located at the Marvin Tanner Laboratory for Cancer Research. We thank Orit Bechar for artwork. Our research is supported by the National Cancer Institute, the European Research Council, the Seventh Framework Program of the European Commission, the German-Israeli Project Cooperation (DIP), the Israel Cancer Research Fund and the Dr. Miriam and Sheldon G. Adelson Medical Research Foundation. Yosef YardenY.Y. is the incumbent of the Harold and Zelda Goldenberg Professorial Chair.

**Conflicts of Interest:** The authors declare no conflict of interest.

**Author Contributions:** Merav Kedmi, Aldema Sas-Chen and Yosef Yarden conceived the review, wrote the text and designed the figures.

## References

1. Solomon, E.; Borrow, J.; Goddard, A.D. Chromosome aberrations and cancer. *Science* **1991**, *254*, 1153–1160. [CrossRef] [PubMed]

2. Fearon, E.R.; Vogelstein, B. A genetic model for colorectal tumorigenesis. *Cell* **1990**, *61*, 759–767. [CrossRef]
3. Tomasetti, C.; Vogelstein, B. Cancer etiology. Variation in cancer risk among tissues can be explained by the number of stem cell divisions. *Science* **2015**, *347*, 78–81. [CrossRef] [PubMed]
4. Chaffer, C.L.; Weinberg, R.A. How does multistep tumorigenesis really proceed? *Cancer Discov.* **2015**, *5*, 22–24. [CrossRef] [PubMed]
5. Beerenwinkel, N.; Antal, T.; Dingli, D.; Traulsen, A.; Kinzler, K.W.; Velculescu, V.E.; Vogelstein, B.; Nowak, M.A. Genetic progression and the waiting time to cancer. *PLoS Comput. Biol.* **2007**, *3*, e225. [CrossRef] [PubMed]
6. Witsch, E.; Sela, M.; Yarden, Y. Roles for growth factors in cancer progression. *Physiology (Bethesda)* **2010**, *25*, 85–101. [CrossRef] [PubMed]
7. Futreal, P.A.; Coin, L.; Marshall, M.; Down, T.; Hubbard, T.; Wooster, R.; Rahman, N.; Stratton, M.R. A census of human cancer genes. *Nat. Rev. Cancer* **2004**, *4*, 177–183. [CrossRef] [PubMed]
8. Sporn, M.B.; Todaro, G.J. Autocrine secretion and malignant transformation of cells. *N. Engl. J. Med.* **1980**, *303*, 878–880. [CrossRef] [PubMed]
9. Greco, A.; Fusetti, L.; Villa, R.; Sozzi, G.; Minoletti, F.; Mauri, P.; Pierotti, M.A. Transforming activity of the chimeric sequence formed by the fusion of collagen gene col1a1 and the platelet derived growth factor b-chain gene in dermatofibrosarcoma protuberans. *Oncogene* **1998**, *17*, 1313–1319. [CrossRef] [PubMed]
10. Shimizu, A.; O'Brien, K.P.; Sjoblom, T.; Pietras, K.; Buchdunger, E.; Collins, V.P.; Heldin, C.H.; Dumanski, J.P.; Ostman, A. The dermatofibrosarcoma protuberans-associated collagen type ialpha1/platelet-derived growth factor (pdgf) b-chain fusion gene generates a transforming protein that is processed to functional pdgf-bb. *Cancer Res.* **1999**, *59*, 3719–3723. [PubMed]
11. Hynes, N.E.; Watson, C.J. Mammary gland growth factors: Roles in normal development and in cancer. *Cold Spring Harb. Perspect. Biol.* **2010**, *2*, a003186. [CrossRef] [PubMed]
12. Kovacs, E.; Zorn, J.A.; Huang, Y.; Barros, T.; Kuriyan, J. A structural perspective on the regulation of the epidermal growth factor receptor. *Annu. Rev. Biochem.* **2015**, *84*, 739–764. [CrossRef] [PubMed]
13. Tarcic, G.; Avraham, R.; Pines, G.; Amit, I.; Shay, T.; Lu, Y.; Zwang, Y.; Katz, M.; Ben-Chetrit, N.; Jacob-Hirsch, J.; *et al.* Egr1 and the erk-erf axis drive mammary cell migration in response to egf. *FASEB J.* **2012**, *26*, 1582–1592. [CrossRef] [PubMed]
14. Huang, H.; Tindall, D.J. Dynamic foxo transcription factors. *J. Cell Sci.* **2007**, *120*, 2479–2487. [CrossRef] [PubMed]
15. Amit, I.; Citri, A.; Shay, T.; Lu, Y.; Katz, M.; Zhang, F.; Tarcic, G.; Siwak, D.; Lahad, J.; Jacob-Hirsch, J.; *et al.* A module of negative feedback regulators defines growth factor signaling. *Nat. Genet.* **2007**, *39*, 503–512. [CrossRef] [PubMed]
16. Tullai, J.W.; Schaffer, M.E.; Mullenbrock, S.; Sholder, G.; Kasif, S.; Cooper, G.M. Immediate-early and delayed primary response genes are distinct in function and genomic architecture. *J. Biol. Chem.* **2007**, *282*, 23981–23995. [CrossRef] [PubMed]
17. Avraham, R.; Yarden, Y. Feedback regulation of egfr signalling: Decision making by early and delayed loops. *Nat. Rev. Mol. Cell Biol.* **2011**, *12*, 104–117. [CrossRef] [PubMed]
18. Han, J.; Lee, Y.; Yeom, K.H.; Kim, Y.K.; Jin, H.; Kim, V.N. The drosha-dgcr8 complex in primary microrna processing. *Genes Dev.* **2004**, *18*, 3016–3027. [CrossRef] [PubMed]
19. Grishok, A.; Pasquinelli, A.E.; Conte, D.; Li, N.; Parrish, S.; Ha, I.; Baillie, D.L.; Fire, A.; Ruvkun, G.; Mello, C.C. Genes and mechanisms related to rna interference regulate expression of the small temporal rnas that control c. Elegans developmental timing. *Cell* **2001**, *106*, 23–34. [CrossRef]
20. Song, J.J.; Smith, S.K.; Hannon, G.J.; Joshua-Tor, L. Crystal structure of argonaute and its implications for risc slicer activity. *Science* **2004**, *305*, 1434–1437. [CrossRef] [PubMed]
21. Chendrimada, T.P.; Finn, K.J.; Ji, X.; Baillat, D.; Gregory, R.I.; Liebhaber, S.A.; Pasquinelli, A.E.; Shiekhattar, R. Microrna silencing through risc recruitment of eif6. *Nature* **2007**, *447*, 823–828. [CrossRef] [PubMed]
22. Tijsterman, M.; Plasterk, R.H. Dicers at risc; the mechanism of rnai. *Cell* **2004**, *117*, 1–3. [CrossRef]
23. Lewis, B.P.; Burge, C.B.; Bartel, D.P. Conserved seed pairing, often flanked by adenosines, indicates that thousands of human genes are microrna targets. *Cell* **2005**, *120*, 15–20. [CrossRef] [PubMed]
24. Zamore, P.D.; Haley, B. Ribo-gnome: The big world of small rnas. *Science* **2005**, *309*, 1519–1524. [CrossRef] [PubMed]

25. Baek, D.; Villen, J.; Shin, C.; Camargo, F.D.; Gygi, S.P.; Bartel, D.P. The impact of micrornas on protein output. *Nature* **2008**, *455*, 64–71. [CrossRef] [PubMed]

26. Croce, C.M.; Calin, G.A. Mirnas, cancer, and stem cell division. *Cell* **2005**, *122*, 6–7. [CrossRef] [PubMed]

27. Lin, S.; Gregory, R.I. Microrna biogenesis pathways in cancer. *Nat. Rev. Cancer* **2015**, *15*, 321–333. [CrossRef] [PubMed]

28. Hata, A.; Lieberman, J. Dysregulation of microrna biogenesis and gene silencing in cancer. *Sci. Signal.* **2015**, *8*, re3. [CrossRef] [PubMed]

29. Avery-Kiejda, K.A.; Braye, S.G.; Forbes, J.F.; Scott, R.J. The expression of dicer and drosha in matched normal tissues, tumours and lymph node metastases in triple negative breast cancer. *BMC Cancer* **2014**, *14*, 253. [CrossRef] [PubMed]

30. Poursadegh Zonouzi, A.A.; Nejatizadeh, A.; Rahmati-Yamchi, M.; Fardmanesh, H.; Shakerizadeh, S.; Poursadegh Zonouzi, A.; Nejati-Koshki, K.; Shekari, M. Dysregulated expression of dicer in invasive ductal breast carcinoma. *Med. Oncol.* **2015**, *32*, 643. [CrossRef] [PubMed]

31. Vincenzi, B.; Iuliani, M.; Zoccoli, A.; Pantano, F.; Fioramonti, M.; de Lisi, D.; Frezza, A.M.; Rabitti, C.; Perrone, G.; Onetti Muda, A.; *et al.* Deregulation of dicer and mir-155 expression in liposarcoma. *Oncotarget* **2015**, *6*, 10586–10591. [PubMed]

32. Shen, J.; Xia, W.; Khotskaya, Y.B.; Huo, L.; Nakanishi, K.; Lim, S.O.; Du, Y.; Wang, Y.; Chang, W.C.; Chen, C.H.; *et al.* Egfr modulates microrna maturation in response to hypoxia through phosphorylation of ago2. *Nature* **2013**, *497*, 383–387. [CrossRef] [PubMed]

33. Davis, B.N.; Hilyard, A.C.; Lagna, G.; Hata, A. Smad proteins control drosha-mediated microrna maturation. *Nature* **2008**, *454*, 56–61. [CrossRef] [PubMed]

34. Avraham, R.; Sas-Chen, A.; Manor, O.; Steinfeld, I.; Shalgi, R.; Tarcic, G.; Bossel, N.; Zeisel, A.; Amit, I.; Zwang, Y.; *et al.* Egf decreases the abundance of micrornas that restrain oncogenic transcription factors. *Sci. Signal.* **2010**, *3*, ra43. [CrossRef] [PubMed]

35. Kedmi, M.; Ben-Chetrit, N.; Korner, C.; Mancini, M.; Ben-Moshe, N.B.; Lauriola, M.; Lavi, S.; Biagioni, F.; Carvalho, S.; Cohen-Dvashi, H.; *et al.* Egf induces micrornas that target suppressors of cell migration: Mir-15b targets mtss1 in breast cancer. *Sci. Signal.* **2015**, *8*, ra29. [CrossRef] [PubMed]

36. Katz, M.; Amit, I.; Citri, A.; Shay, T.; Carvalho, S.; Lavi, S.; Milanezi, F.; Lyass, L.; Amariglio, N.; Jacob-Hirsch, J.; *et al.* A reciprocal tensin-3-cten switch mediates egf-driven mammary cell migration. *Nat. Cell Biol.* **2007**, *9*, 961–969. [CrossRef] [PubMed]

37. Llorens, F.; Hummel, M.; Pantano, L.; Pastor, X.; Vivancos, A.; Castillo, E.; Mattlin, H.; Ferrer, A.; Ingham, M.; Noguera, M.; *et al.* Microarray and deep sequencing cross-platform analysis of the mirrnome and isomir variation in response to epidermal growth factor. *BMC Genomics* **2013**, *14*, 371. [CrossRef] [PubMed]

38. Lu, W.C.; Kao, S.Y.; Yang, C.C.; Tu, H.F.; Wu, C.H.; Chang, K.W.; Lin, S.C. Egf up-regulates mir-31 through the c/ebpbeta signal cascade in oral carcinoma. *PLoS ONE* **2014**, *9*, e108049. [CrossRef] [PubMed]

39. Ben-Chetrit, N.; Chetrit, D.; Russell, R.; Korner, C.; Mancini, M.; Abdul-Hai, A.; Itkin, T.; Carvalho, S.; Cohen-Dvashi, H.; Koestler, W.J.; *et al.* Synaptojanin 2 is a druggable mediator of metastasis and the gene is overexpressed and amplified in breast cancer. *Sci. Signal.* **2015**, *8*, ra7. [CrossRef] [PubMed]

40. Alanazi, I.; Hoffmann, P.; Adelson, D.L. Micrornas are part of the regulatory network that controls egf induced apoptosis, including elements of the jak/stat pathway, in a431 cells. *PLoS ONE* **2015**, *10*, e0120337. [CrossRef] [PubMed]

41. Gomez, G.G.; Volinia, S.; Croce, C.M.; Zanca, C.; Li, M.; Emnett, R.; Gutmann, D.H.; Brennan, C.W.; Furnari, F.B.; Cavenee, W.K. Suppression of microrna-9 by mutant egfr signaling upregulates foxp1 to enhance glioblastoma tumorigenicity. *Cancer Res.* **2014**, *74*, 1429–1439. [CrossRef] [PubMed]

42. Kao, C.J.; Martiniez, A.; Shi, X.B.; Yang, J.; Evans, C.P.; Dobi, A.; deVere White, R.W.; Kung, H.J. Mir-30 as a tumor suppressor connects egf/src signal to erg and emt. *Oncogene* **2014**, *33*, 2495–2503. [CrossRef] [PubMed]

43. Kefas, B.; Godlewski, J.; Comeau, L.; Li, Y.; Abounader, R.; Hawkinson, M.; Lee, J.; Fine, H.; Chiocca, E.A.; Lawler, S.; *et al.* Microrna-7 inhibits the epidermal growth factor receptor and the akt pathway and is down-regulated in glioblastoma. *Cancer Res.* **2008**, *68*, 3566–3572. [CrossRef] [PubMed]

44. Webster, R.J.; Giles, K.M.; Price, K.J.; Zhang, P.M.; Mattick, J.S.; Leedman, P.J. Regulation of epidermal growth factor receptor signaling in human cancer cells by microrna-7. *J. Biol. Chem.* **2009**, *284*, 5731–5741. [CrossRef] [PubMed]

45. Weiss, G.J.; Bemis, L.T.; Nakajima, E.; Sugita, M.; Birks, D.K.; Robinson, W.A.; Varella-Garcia, M.; Bunn, P.A., Jr.; Haney, J.; Helfrich, B.A.; *et al.* Egfr regulation by microrna in lung cancer: Correlation with clinical response and survival to gefitinib and egfr expression in cell lines. *Ann. Oncol.: Off. J. Eur. Soc. Med. Oncol./ESMO* **2008**, *19*, 1053–1059. [CrossRef] [PubMed]

46. Chiyomaru, T.; Seki, N.; Inoguchi, S.; Ishihara, T.; Mataki, H.; Matsushita, R.; Goto, Y.; Nishikawa, R.; Tatarano, S.; Itesako, T.; *et al.* Dual regulation of receptor tyrosine kinase genes egfr and c-met by the tumor-suppressive microrna-23b/27b cluster in bladder cancer. *Int. J. Oncol.* **2015**, *46*, 487–496. [CrossRef] [PubMed]

47. Wang, L.K.; Hsiao, T.H.; Hong, T.M.; Chen, H.Y.; Kao, S.H.; Wang, W.L.; Yu, S.L.; Lin, C.W.; Yang, P.C. Microrna-133a suppresses multiple oncogenic membrane receptors and cell invasion in non-small cell lung carcinoma. *PLoS ONE* **2014**, *9*, e96765. [CrossRef] [PubMed]

48. Cui, W.; Zhang, S.; Shan, C.; Zhou, L.; Zhou, Z. Microrna-133a regulates the cell cycle and proliferation of breast cancer cells by targeting epidermal growth factor receptor through the egfr/akt signaling pathway. *FEBS J.* **2013**, *280*, 3962–3974. [CrossRef] [PubMed]

49. Liu, L.; Shao, X.; Gao, W.; Zhang, Z.; Liu, P.; Wang, R.; Huang, P.; Yin, Y.; Shu, Y. Microrna-133b inhibits the growth of non-small-cell lung cancer by targeting the epidermal growth factor receptor. *FEBS J.* **2012**, *279*, 3800–3812. [CrossRef] [PubMed]

50. Kumaraswamy, E.; Wendt, K.L.; Augustine, L.A.; Stecklein, S.R.; Sibala, E.C.; Li, D.; Gunewardena, S.; Jensen, R.A. Brca1 regulation of epidermal growth factor receptor (egfr) expression in human breast cancer cells involves microrna-146a and is critical for its tumor suppressor function. *Oncogene* **2014**. [CrossRef] [PubMed]

51. Katakowski, M.; Zheng, X.; Jiang, F.; Rogers, T.; Szalad, A.; Chopp, M. Mir-146b-5p suppresses egfr expression and reduces *in vitro* migration and invasion of glioma. *Cancer Investig.* **2010**, *28*, 1024–1030. [CrossRef] [PubMed]

52. Rao, S.A.; Arimappamagan, A.; Pandey, P.; Santosh, V.; Hegde, A.S.; Chandramouli, B.A.; Somasundaram, K. Mir-219-5p inhibits receptor tyrosine kinase pathway by targeting egfr in glioblastoma. *PLoS ONE* **2013**, *8*, e63164. [CrossRef] [PubMed]

53. Wang, L.; Yao, J.; Shi, X.; Hu, L.; Li, Z.; Song, T.; Huang, C. Microrna-302b suppresses cell proliferation by targeting egfr in human hepatocellular carcinoma smmc-7721 cells. *BMC Cancer* **2013**, *13*, 448. [CrossRef] [PubMed]

54. Zhang, Y.; Schiff, D.; Park, D.; Abounader, R. Microrna-608 and microrna-34a regulate chordoma malignancy by targeting egfr, bcl-xl and met. *PLoS ONE* **2014**, *9*, e91546. [CrossRef] [PubMed]

55. Uhlmann, S.; Mannsperger, H.; Zhang, J.D.; Horvat, E.A.; Schmidt, C.; Kublbeck, M.; Henjes, F.; Ward, A.; Tschulena, U.; Zweig, K.; *et al.* Global microrna level regulation of egfr-driven cell-cycle protein network in breast cancer. *Mol. Syst. Biol.* **2012**, *8*, 570. [CrossRef] [PubMed]

56. Pagliuca, A.; Valvo, C.; Fabrizi, E.; di Martino, S.; Biffoni, M.; Runci, D.; Forte, S.; de Maria, R.; Ricci-Vitiani, L. Analysis of the combined action of mir-143 and mir-145 on oncogenic pathways in colorectal cancer cells reveals a coordinate program of gene repression. *Oncogene* **2013**, *32*, 4806–4813. [CrossRef] [PubMed]

57. Pekow, J.R.; Dougherty, U.; Mustafi, R.; Zhu, H.; Kocherginsky, M.; Rubin, D.T.; Hanauer, S.B.; Hart, J.; Chang, E.B.; Fichera, A.; *et al.* Mir-143 and mir-145 are downregulated in ulcerative colitis: Putative regulators of inflammation and protooncogenes. *Inflamm. Bowel Dis.* **2012**, *18*, 94–100. [CrossRef] [PubMed]

58. Xu, B.; Niu, X.; Zhang, X.; Tao, J.; Wu, D.; Wang, Z.; Li, P.; Zhang, W.; Wu, H.; Feng, N.; *et al.* Mir-143 decreases prostate cancer cells proliferation and migration and enhances their sensitivity to docetaxel through suppression of kras. *Mol. Cell. Biochem.* **2011**, *350*, 207–213. [CrossRef] [PubMed]

59. Wu, X.; Bhayani, M.K.; Dodge, C.T.; Nicoloso, M.S.; Chen, Y.; Yan, X.; Adachi, M.; Thomas, L.; Galer, C.E.; Jiffar, T.; *et al.* Coordinated targeting of the egfr signaling axis by microrna-27a*. *Oncotarget* **2013**, *4*, 1388–1398. [PubMed]

60. Leivonen, S.K.; Sahlberg, K.K.; Makela, R.; Due, E.U.; Kallioniemi, O.; Borresen-Dale, A.L.; Perala, M. High-throughput screens identify micrornas essential for her2 positive breast cancer cell growth. *Mol. Oncol.* **2014**, *8*, 93–104. [CrossRef] [PubMed]

61. Giles, K.M.; Barker, A.; Zhang, P.M.; Epis, M.R.; Leedman, P.J. Microrna regulation of growth factor receptor signaling in human cancer cells. *Methods Mol. Biol.* **2011**, *676*, 147–163. [PubMed]

62. Epis, M.R.; Giles, K.M.; Barker, A.; Kendrick, T.S.; Leedman, P.J. Mir-331-3p regulates erbb-2 expression and androgen receptor signaling in prostate cancer. *J. Biol. Chem.* **2009**, *284*, 24696–24704. [CrossRef] [PubMed]

63. Bischoff, A.; Bayerlova, M.; Strotbek, M.; Schmid, S.; Beissbarth, T.; Olayioye, M.A. A global microrna screen identifies regulators of the erbb receptor signaling network. *Cell Commun. Signal.* **2015**, *13*, 5. [CrossRef] [PubMed]

64. Scott, G.K.; Goga, A.; Bhaumik, D.; Berger, C.E.; Sullivan, C.S.; Benz, C.C. Coordinate suppression of erbb2 and erbb3 by enforced expression of micro-rna mir-125a or mir-125b. *J. Biol. Chem.* **2007**, *282*, 1479–1486. [CrossRef] [PubMed]

65. Liang, H.; Liu, M.; Yan, X.; Zhou, Y.; Wang, W.; Wang, X.; Fu, Z.; Wang, N.; Zhang, S.; Wang, Y.; *et al.* Mir-193a-3p functions as a tumor suppressor in lung cancer by down-regulating erbb4. *J. Biol. Chem.* **2015**, *290*, 926–940. [CrossRef] [PubMed]

66. Yu, T.; Li, J.; Yan, M.; Liu, L.; Lin, H.; Zhao, F.; Sun, L.; Zhang, Y.; Cui, Y.; Zhang, F.; *et al.* Microrna-193a-3p and -5p suppress the metastasis of human non-small-cell lung cancer by downregulating the erbb4/pik3r3/mtor/s6k2 signaling pathway. *Oncogene* **2015**, *34*, 413–423. [CrossRef] [PubMed]

67. Zhang, M.; Yang, Q.; Zhang, L.; Zhou, S.; Ye, W.; Yao, Q.; Li, Z.; Huang, C.; Wen, Q.; Wang, J. Mir-302b is a potential molecular marker of esophageal squamous cell carcinoma and functions as a tumor suppressor by targeting erbb4. *J. Exp. Clin. Cancer Res.* **2014**, *33*, 10. [CrossRef] [PubMed]

68. Cho, W.C.; Chow, A.S.; Au, J.S. Mir-145 inhibits cell proliferation of human lung adenocarcinoma by targeting egfr and nudt1. *RNA Biol.* **2011**, *8*, 125–131. [CrossRef] [PubMed]

69. Zhu, H.; Dougherty, U.; Robinson, V.; Mustafi, R.; Pekow, J.; Kupfer, S.; Li, Y.C.; Hart, J.; Goss, K.; Fichera, A.; *et al.* Egfr signals downregulate tumor suppressors mir-143 and mir-145 in western diet-promoted murine colon cancer: Role of g1 regulators. *Mol. Cancer Res.* **2011**, *9*, 960–975. [CrossRef] [PubMed]

70. Guo, Y.H.; Zhang, C.; Shi, J.; Xu, M.H.; Liu, F.; Yuan, H.H.; Wang, J.Y.; Jiang, B.; Gao, F.H. Abnormal activation of the egfr signaling pathway mediates the downregulation of mir145 through the erk1/2 in non-small cell lung cancer. *Oncol. Rep.* **2014**, *31*, 1940–1946. [PubMed]

71. Zhang, K.L.; Han, L.; Chen, L.Y.; Shi, Z.D.; Yang, M.; Ren, Y.; Chen, L.C.; Zhang, J.X.; Pu, P.Y.; Kang, C.S. Blockage of a mir-21/egfr regulatory feedback loop augments anti-egfr therapy in glioblastomas. *Cancer Lett.* **2014**, *342*, 139–149. [CrossRef] [PubMed]

72. Seike, M.; Goto, A.; Okano, T.; Bowman, E.D.; Schetter, A.J.; Horikawa, I.; Mathe, E.A.; Jen, J.; Yang, P.; Sugimura, H.; *et al.* Mir-21 is an egfr-regulated anti-apoptotic factor in lung cancer in never-smokers. *Proc. Natl. Acad. Sci. USA* **2009**, *106*, 12085–12090. [CrossRef] [PubMed]

73. Perou, C.M.; Sorlie, T.; Eisen, M.B.; van de Rijn, M.; Jeffrey, S.S.; Rees, C.A.; Pollack, J.R.; Ross, D.T.; Johnsen, H.; Akslen, L.A.; *et al.* Molecular portraits of human breast tumours. *Nature* **2000**, *406*, 747–752. [CrossRef] [PubMed]

74. Calin, G.A.; Dumitru, C.D.; Shimizu, M.; Bichi, R.; Zupo, S.; Noch, E.; Aldler, H.; Rattan, S.; Keating, M.; Rai, K.; *et al.* Frequent deletions and down-regulation of micro- rna genes mir15 and mir16 at 13q14 in chronic lymphocytic leukemia. *Proc. Natl. Acad. Sci. USA* **2002**, *99*, 15524–15529. [CrossRef] [PubMed]

75. Volinia, S.; Calin, G.A.; Liu, C.G.; Ambs, S.; Cimmino, A.; Petrocca, F.; Visone, R.; Iorio, M.; Roldo, C.; Ferracin, M.; *et al.* A microrna expression signature of human solid tumors defines cancer gene targets. *Proc. Natl. Acad. Sci. USA* **2006**, *103*, 2257–2261. [CrossRef] [PubMed]

76. Lu, J.; Getz, G.; Miska, E.A.; Alvarez-Saavedra, E.; Lamb, J.; Peck, D.; Sweet-Cordero, A.; Ebert, B.L.; Mak, R.H.; Ferrando, A.A.; *et al.* Microrna expression profiles classify human cancers. *Nature* **2005**, *435*, 834–838. [CrossRef] [PubMed]

77. Mitchell, P.S.; Parkin, R.K.; Kroh, E.M.; Fritz, B.R.; Wyman, S.K.; Pogosova-Agadjanyan, E.L.; Peterson, A.; Noteboom, J.; O'Briant, K.C.; Allen, A.; *et al.* Circulating micrornas as stable blood-based markers for cancer detection. *Proc. Natl. Acad. Sci. USA* **2008**, *105*, 10513–10518. [CrossRef] [PubMed]

78. Chen, X.; Ba, Y.; Ma, L.; Cai, X.; Yin, Y.; Wang, K.; Guo, J.; Zhang, Y.; Chen, J.; Guo, X.; *et al.* Characterization of micrornas in serum: A novel class of biomarkers for diagnosis of cancer and other diseases. *Cell Res.* **2008**, *18*, 997–1006. [CrossRef] [PubMed]

79. Takamizawa, J.; Konishi, H.; Yanagisawa, K.; Tomida, S.; Osada, H.; Endoh, H.; Harano, T.; Yatabe, Y.; Nagino, M.; Nimura, Y.; *et al.* Reduced expression of the let-7 micrornas in human lung cancers in association with shortened postoperative survival. *Cancer Res.* **2004**, *64*, 3753–3756. [CrossRef] [PubMed]

80. Nelson, P.T.; Baldwin, D.A.; Scearce, L.M.; Oberholtzer, J.C.; Tobias, J.W.; Mourelatos, Z. Microarray-based, high-throughput gene expression profiling of micrornas. *Nat. Methods* **2004**, *1*, 155–161. [CrossRef] [PubMed]

81. Lagos-Quintana, M.; Rauhut, R.; Yalcin, A.; Meyer, J.; Lendeckel, W.; Tuschl, T. Identification of tissue-specific micrornas from mouse. *Curr. Biol.: CB* **2002**, *12*, 735–739. [CrossRef]

82. Rosenfeld, N.; Aharonov, R.; Meiri, E.; Rosenwald, S.; Spector, Y.; Zepeniuk, M.; Benjamin, H.; Shabes, N.; Tabak, S.; Levy, A.; *et al.* Micrornas accurately identify cancer tissue origin. *Nat. Biotechnol.* **2008**, *26*, 462–469. [CrossRef] [PubMed]

83. Dvinge, H.; Git, A.; Graf, S.; Salmon-Divon, M.; Curtis, C.; Sottoriva, A.; Zhao, Y.; Hirst, M.; Armisen, J.; Miska, E.A.; *et al.* The shaping and functional consequences of the microrna landscape in breast cancer. *Nature* **2013**, *497*, 378–382. [CrossRef] [PubMed]

84. Blenkiron, C.; Goldstein, L.D.; Thorne, N.P.; Spiteri, I.; Chin, S.F.; Dunning, M.J.; Barbosa-Morais, N.L.; Teschendorff, A.E.; Green, A.R.; Ellis, I.O.; *et al.* Microrna expression profiling of human breast cancer identifies new markers of tumor subtype. *Genome Biol.* **2007**, *8*, R214. [CrossRef] [PubMed]

85. Andorfer, C.A.; Necela, B.M.; Thompson, E.A.; Perez, E.A. Microrna signatures: Clinical biomarkers for the diagnosis and treatment of breast cancer. *Trends Mol. Med.* **2011**, *17*, 313–319. [CrossRef] [PubMed]

86. Enerly, E.; Steinfeld, I.; Kleivi, K.; Leivonen, S.K.; Aure, M.R.; Russnes, H.G.; Ronneberg, J.A.; Johnsen, H.; Navon, R.; Rodland, E.; *et al.* Mirna-mrna integrated analysis reveals roles for mirnas in primary breast tumors. *PLoS ONE* **2011**, *6*, e16915. [CrossRef] [PubMed]

87. Yanaihara, N.; Caplen, N.; Bowman, E.; Seike, M.; Kumamoto, K.; Yi, M.; Stephens, R.M.; Okamoto, A.; Yokota, J.; Tanaka, T.; *et al.* Unique microrna molecular profiles in lung cancer diagnosis and prognosis. *Cancer Cell* **2006**, *9*, 189–198. [CrossRef] [PubMed]

88. Hu, Z.; Chen, X.; Zhao, Y.; Tian, T.; Jin, G.; Shu, Y.; Chen, Y.; Xu, L.; Zen, K.; Zhang, C.; *et al.* Serum microrna signatures identified in a genome-wide serum microrna expression profiling predict survival of non-small-cell lung cancer. *J. Clin. Oncol.: Off. J. Am. Soc. Clin. Oncol.* **2010**, *28*, 1721–1726. [CrossRef] [PubMed]

89. Cho, W.C. Micrornas: Potential biomarkers for cancer diagnosis, prognosis and targets for therapy. *Int. J. Biochem. Cell Biol.* **2010**, *42*, 1273–1281. [CrossRef] [PubMed]

90. Meiri, E.; Mueller, W.C.; Rosenwald, S.; Zepeniuk, M.; Klinke, E.; Edmonston, T.B.; Werner, M.; Lass, U.; Barshack, I.; Feinmesser, M.; *et al.* A second-generation microrna-based assay for diagnosing tumor tissue origin. *Oncologist* **2012**, *17*, 801–812. [CrossRef] [PubMed]

91. Nair, V.S.; Maeda, L.S.; Ioannidis, J.P. Clinical outcome prediction by micrornas in human cancer: A systematic review. *J. Natl. Cancer Inst.* **2012**, *104*, 528–540. [CrossRef] [PubMed]

92. Garzon, R.; Marcucci, G.; Croce, C.M. Targeting micrornas in cancer: Rationale, strategies and challenges. *Nat. Rev. Drug Discov.* **2010**, *9*, 775–789. [CrossRef] [PubMed]

93. Shibata, C.; Otsuka, M.; Kishikawa, T.; Yoshikawa, T.; Ohno, M.; Takata, A.; Koike, K. Current status of mirna-targeting therapeutics and preclinical studies against gastroenterological carcinoma. *Mol. Cell. Ther.* **2013**, *1*, 5. [CrossRef] [PubMed]

94. Krutzfeldt, J.; Rajewsky, N.; Braich, R.; Rajeev, K.G.; Tuschl, T.; Manoharan, M.; Stoffel, M. Silencing of micrornas *in vivo* with "antagomirs". *Nature* **2005**, *438*, 685–689. [CrossRef] [PubMed]

95. Elmen, J.; Lindow, M.; Schutz, S.; Lawrence, M.; Petri, A.; Obad, S.; Lindholm, M.; Hedtjarn, M.; Hansen, H.F.; Berger, U.; *et al.* Lna-mediated microrna silencing in non-human primates. *Nature* **2008**, *452*, 896–899. [CrossRef] [PubMed]

96. Xie, J.; Ameres, S.L.; Friedline, R.; Hung, J.H.; Zhang, Y.; Xie, Q.; Zhong, L.; Su, Q.; He, R.; Li, M.; *et al.* Long-term, efficient inhibition of microrna function in mice using raav vectors. *Nat. Methods* **2012**, *9*, 403–409. [CrossRef] [PubMed]

97. Cheng, C.J.; Bahal, R.; Babar, I.A.; Pincus, Z.; Barrera, F.; Liu, C.; Svoronos, A.; Braddock, D.T.; Glazer, P.M.; Engelman, D.M.; *et al.* Microrna silencing for cancer therapy targeted to the tumour microenvironment. *Nature* **2015**, *518*, 107–110. [CrossRef] [PubMed]

98. Ebert, M.S.; Neilson, J.R.; Sharp, P.A. Microrna sponges: Competitive inhibitors of small rnas in mammalian cells. *Nat. Methods* **2007**, *4*, 721–726. [CrossRef] [PubMed]

99. Choi, W.Y.; Giraldez, A.J.; Schier, A.F. Target protectors reveal dampening and balancing of nodal agonist and antagonist by mir-430. *Science* **2007**, *318*, 271–274. [CrossRef] [PubMed]

100. Trang, P.; Wiggins, J.F.; Daige, C.L.; Cho, C.; Omotola, M.; Brown, D.; Weidhaas, J.B.; Bader, A.G.; Slack, F.J. Systemic delivery of tumor suppressor microrna mimics using a neutral lipid emulsion inhibits lung tumors in mice. *Mol. Ther.: J. Am. Soc. Gene Ther.* **2011**, *19*, 1116–1122. [CrossRef] [PubMed]

101. Kota, J.; Chivukula, R.R.; O'Donnell, K.A.; Wentzel, E.A.; Montgomery, C.L.; Hwang, H.W.; Chang, T.C.; Vivekanandan, P.; Torbenson, M.; Clark, K.R.; *et al.* Therapeutic microrna delivery suppresses tumorigenesis in a murine liver cancer model. *Cell* **2009**, *137*, 1005–1017. [CrossRef] [PubMed]

102. Zeisel, M.B.; Pfeffer, S.; Baumert, T.F. Mir-122 acts as a tumor suppressor in hepatocarcinogenesis *in vivo*. *J. Hepatol.* **2013**, *58*, 821–823. [CrossRef] [PubMed]

103. Jopling, C.L.; Yi, M.; Lancaster, A.M.; Lemon, S.M.; Sarnow, P. Modulation of hepatitis c virus rna abundance by a liver-specific microrna. *Science* **2005**, *309*, 1577–1581. [CrossRef] [PubMed]

104. Janssen, H.L.; Reesink, H.W.; Lawitz, E.J.; Zeuzem, S.; Rodriguez-Torres, M.; Patel, K.; van der Meer, A.J.; Patick, A.K.; Chen, A.; Zhou, Y.; *et al.* Treatment of hcv infection by targeting microrna. *N. Engl. J. Med.* **2013**, *368*, 1685–1694. [CrossRef] [PubMed]

105. He, L.; He, X.; Lim, L.P.; de Stanchina, E.; Xuan, Z.; Liang, Y.; Xue, W.; Zender, L.; Magnus, J.; Ridzon, D.; *et al.* A microrna component of the p53 tumour suppressor network. *Nature* **2007**, *447*, 1130–1134. [CrossRef] [PubMed]

106. Liu, C.; Kelnar, K.; Liu, B.; Chen, X.; Calhoun-Davis, T.; Li, H.; Patrawala, L.; Yan, H.; Jeter, C.; Honorio, S.; *et al.* The microrna mir-34a inhibits prostate cancer stem cells and metastasis by directly repressing cd44. *Nat. Med.* **2011**, *17*, 211–215. [CrossRef] [PubMed]

107. Hu, Q.L.; Jiang, Q.Y.; Jin, X.; Shen, J.; Wang, K.; Li, Y.B.; Xu, F.J.; Tang, G.P.; Li, Z.H. Cationic microrna-delivering nanovectors with bifunctional peptides for efficient treatment of panc-1 xenograft model. *Biomaterials* **2013**, *34*, 2265–2276. [CrossRef] [PubMed]

108. Reid, G.; Pel, M.E.; Kirschner, M.B.; Cheng, Y.Y.; Mugridge, N.; Weiss, J.; Williams, M.; Wright, C.; Edelman, J.J.; Vallely, M.P.; *et al.* Restoring expression of mir-16: A novel approach to therapy for malignant pleural mesothelioma. *Ann. Oncol.: Off. J. Eur. Soc. Med. Oncol./ESMO* **2013**, *24*, 3128–3135. [CrossRef] [PubMed]

109. Yarden, Y.; Pines, G. The erbb network: At last, cancer therapy meets systems biology. *Nat. Rev. Cancer* **2012**, *12*, 553–563. [CrossRef] [PubMed]

110. Lovly, C.M.; Shaw, A.T. Molecular pathways: Resistance to kinase inhibitors and implications for therapeutic strategies. *Clin. Cancer Res.: Off. J. Am. Assoc. Cancer Res.* **2014**, *20*, 2249–2256. [CrossRef] [PubMed]

111. Donzelli, S.; Mori, F.; Biagioni, F.; Bellissimo, T.; Pulito, C.; Muti, P.; Strano, S.; Blandino, G. Micrornas: Short non-coding players in cancer chemoresistance. *Mol. Cell. Ther.* **2014**, *2*, 16. [CrossRef] [PubMed]

112. Hummel, R.; Hussey, D.J.; Haier, J. Micrornas: Predictors and modifiers of chemo- and radiotherapy in different tumour types. *Eur. J. Cancer* **2010**, *46*, 298–311. [CrossRef] [PubMed]

113. MacDonagh, L.; Gray, S.G.; Finn, S.P.; Cuffe, S.; O'Byrne, K.J.; Barr, M.P. The emerging role of micrornas in resistance to lung cancer treatments. *Cancer Treat. Rev.* **2015**, *41*, 160–169. [CrossRef] [PubMed]

114. Kalinowski, F.C.; Giles, K.M.; Candy, P.A.; Ali, A.; Ganda, C.; Epis, M.R.; Webster, R.J.; Leedman, P.J. Regulation of epidermal growth factor receptor signaling and erlotinib sensitivity in head and neck cancer cells by mir-7. *PLoS ONE* **2012**, *7*, e47067. [CrossRef] [PubMed]

115. Ye, X.M.; Zhu, H.Y.; Bai, W.D.; Wang, T.; Wang, L.; Chen, Y.; Yang, A.G.; Jia, L.T. Epigenetic silencing of mir-375 induces trastuzumab resistance in her2-positive breast cancer by targeting igf1r. *BMC Cancer* **2014**, *14*, 134. [CrossRef] [PubMed]

116. Bai, W.D.; Ye, X.M.; Zhang, M.Y.; Zhu, H.Y.; Xi, W.J.; Huang, X.; Zhao, J.; Gu, B.; Zheng, G.X.; Yang, A.G.; *et al.* Mir-200c suppresses tgf-beta signaling and counteracts trastuzumab resistance and metastasis by targeting znf217 and zeb1 in breast cancer. *Int. J. Cancer. J. Int. Cancer* **2014**, *135*, 1356–1368. [CrossRef] [PubMed]

117. Adam, L.; Zhong, M.; Choi, W.; Qi, W.; Nicoloso, M.; Arora, A.; Calin, G.; Wang, H.; Siefker-Radtke, A.; McConkey, D.; *et al.* Mir-200 expression regulates epithelial-to-mesenchymal transition in bladder cancer cells and reverses resistance to epidermal growth factor receptor therapy. *Clin. Cancer Res.: Off. J. Am. Assoc. Cancer Res.* **2009**, *15*, 5060–5072. [CrossRef] [PubMed]

118. Huang, S.; He, R.; Rong, M.; Dang, Y.; Chen, G. Synergistic effect of mir-146a mimic and cetuximab on hepatocellular carcinoma cells. *BioMed Res. Int.* **2014**, *2014*, 384121. [CrossRef] [PubMed]

119. Zhang, K.L.; Zhou, X.; Han, L.; Chen, L.Y.; Chen, L.C.; Shi, Z.D.; Yang, M.; Ren, Y.; Yang, J.X.; Frank, T.S.; *et al.* Microrna-566 activates egfr signaling and its inhibition sensitizes glioblastoma cells to nimotuzumab. *Mol. Cancer* **2014**, *13*, 63. [CrossRef] [PubMed]

120. Ye, X.; Bai, W.; Zhu, H.; Zhang, X.; Chen, Y.; Wang, L.; Yang, A.; Zhao, J.; Jia, L. Mir-221 promotes trastuzumab-resistance and metastasis in her2-positive breast cancers by targeting pten. *BMB Rep.* **2014**, *47*, 268–273. [CrossRef] [PubMed]

121. Garofalo, M.; Romano, G.; di Leva, G.; Nuovo, G.; Jeon, Y.J.; Ngankeu, A.; Sun, J.; Lovat, F.; Alder, H.; Condorelli, G.; *et al.* Egfr and met receptor tyrosine kinase-altered microrna expression induces tumorigenesis and gefitinib resistance in lung cancers. *Nat. Med.* **2012**, *18*, 74–82. [CrossRef] [PubMed]

122. Shen, H.; Zhu, F.; Liu, J.; Xu, T.; Pei, D.; Wang, R.; Qian, Y.; Li, Q.; Wang, L.; Shi, Z.; *et al.* Alteration in mir-21/pten expression modulates gefitinib resistance in non-small cell lung cancer. *PLoS ONE* **2014**, *9*, e103305. [CrossRef] [PubMed]

123. Gao, Y.; Fan, X.; Li, W.; Ping, W.; Deng, Y.; Fu, X. Mir-138-5p reverses gefitinib resistance in non-small cell lung cancer cells via negatively regulating g protein-coupled receptor 124. *Biochem. Biophys. Res. Commun.* **2014**, *446*, 179–186. [CrossRef] [PubMed]

124. Zhou, J.Y.; Chen, X.; Zhao, J.; Bao, Z.; Chen, X.; Zhang, P.; Liu, Z.F.; Zhou, J.Y. Microrna-34a overcomes hgf-mediated gefitinib resistance in egfr mutant lung cancer cells partly by targeting met. *Cancer Lett.* **2014**, *351*, 265–271. [CrossRef] [PubMed]

125. Siu, M.K.; Abou-Kheir, W.; Yin, J.J.; Chang, Y.S.; Barrett, B.; Suau, F.; Casey, O.; Chen, W.Y.; Fang, L.; Hynes, P.; *et al.* Loss of egfr signaling regulated mir-203 promotes prostate cancer bone metastasis and tyrosine kinase inhibitors resistance. *Oncotarget* **2014**, *5*, 3770–3784. [PubMed]

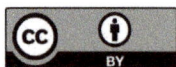

Journal of
*Clinical Medicine*

MDPI

*Review*

# Role of *MicroRNAs-221/222* in Digestive Systems

**Juntaro Matsuzaki [1] and Hidekazu Suzuki [2],***

[1]   Center for Preventive Medicine, Keio University Hospital, Tokyo 160-0016, Japan;
      juntaro.matsuzaki@gmail.com
[2]   Division of Gastroenterology and Hepatology, Department of Internal Medicine, Keio University School of
      Medicine, 35 Shinanomachi, Shinjuku-ku, Tokyo 160-8582, Japan
*    Author to whom correspondence should be addressed; hsuzuki.a6@keio.jp;
      Tel.: +81-3-5363-3914; Fax: +81-3-5363-3967.

Academic Editors: Takahiro Ochiya and Ryou-u Takahashi
Received: 29 June 2015; Accepted: 22 July 2015; Published: 6 August 2015

**Abstract:** *MiR-221* and *miR-222* (*miR-221/222*) are well-studied oncogenic microRNAs that are frequently upregulated in several types of human tumors, such as esophageal adenocarcinoma, gastric adenocarcinoma, colorectal adenocarcinoma, hepatocellular carcinoma, and pancreatic ductal adenocarcinoma. In these cancers, silencing *miR-221/222* could represent a novel anti-tumor approach to inhibit tumor growth and metastasis. On the other hand, *miR-221/222* also play onco-suppressive roles in cholangiocarcinoma and gastrointestinal stromal tumors (GISTs). Here we will review the roles of *miR-221/222* in digestive systems and their possibility as prognostic and therapeutic tools.

**Keywords:** microRNA; colorectal cancer; hepatocellular carcinoma; pancreatic cancer

## 1. Introduction

MicroRNAs (miRs) are ~22 nucleotide noncoding RNAs that can downregulate various gene products by translational repression when partially complementary sequences are present in the $3'$ untranslated regions ($3'$ UTR) of the target mRNAs or by directing mRNA degradation. Increasing evidence has demonstrated that miRs are involved in cancer initiation, progression, and metastasis, and may serve as diagnostic and prognostic biomarkers for cancers. Among the many miRNAs already identified as regulators of neoplastic transformation, invasion, and metastasis, *miR-221* and *miR-222* (*miR-221/222*) have emerged as key miRNAs deregulated in many cancers, such as gastrointestinal cancers, breast cancer, prostate cancer, thyroid cancer, and glioma [1–5]. *MiR-221* and *miR-222* are encoded in tandem from a gene cluster located on chromosome Xp11.3. Several reports indicated that *miR-221/222* could be used as a therapeutic tool to decrease cell proliferation or modulate sensitivity to anti-cancer agents [6–8]. Here we review the current knowledge about the role of *miR-221/222* in digestive systems, including hepatobiliary and pancreatic cancers.

## 2. Direct Targets of *miR-221/222*

The identification of target mRNAs is a key step for assessing the role of aberrantly expressed microRNAs in human cancer. To date, various direct targets of *miR-221/222* have been reported, even in the digestive system, as shown in Table 1. Among them, regulation of p27Kip1 by *miR-221/222* is well studied. Downregulation of p27Kip1 is required for cell cycle entry after growth factor stimulation. *MiR-221/222* are underactive towards p27Kip1-$3'$ UTRs in quiescent cells, as a result of target site hindrance. Pumilio-1 (PUM1) is a ubiquitously expressed RNA-binding protein (RBP) that interacts with p27Kip1-$3'$ UTR. In response to growth factor stimulation, PUM1 is upregulated and phosphorylated for optimal induction of its RNA-binding activity towards the p27Kip1-$3'$ UTR [9].

PUM1 binding induces a local change in RNA structure that favors association with *miR-221/222*, efficient suppression of p27Kip1 expression, and rapid entry to the cell cycle.

**Table 1.** Direct targets of *miR-221/222*.

| Target | Cancer Type | Reference |
| --- | --- | --- |
| p27Kip1 | Esophageal adenocarcinoma | Matsuzaki *et al.* (2013) |
| | Hepatocellular carcinoma | Pineau *et al.* (2010), Fu *et al.* (2011), Callegari *et al.* (2012) |
| | Pancreatic ductal adenocarcinoma | Park *et al.* (2009), Sarkar *et al.* (2013), Tanaka *et al.* (2015) |
| p57Kip2 | Colorectal adenocarcinoma | Sun *et al.* (2011) |
| | Pancreatic ductal adenocarcinoma | Sarkar *et al.* (2013) |
| PTEN | Gastric adenocarcinoma | Chun-Zhi *et al.* (2010) |
| | Hepatocellular carcinoma | Fornari *et al.* (2008), Callegari *et al.* (2012), Garofalo *et al.* (2009) |
| | Colorectal adenocarcinoma | Tsunoda *et al.* (2011), Xue *et al.* (2013) |
| | Pancreatic ductal adenocarcinoma | Sarkar *et al.* (2013) |
| RelA | Colorectal adenocarcinoma | Liu *et al.* (2014) |
| PDLIM2 | Colorectal adenocarcinoma | Liu *et al.* (2014) |
| RECK | Colorectal adenocarcinoma | Qin *et al.* (2014) |
| BMF | Hepatocellular carcinoma | Gramantieri *et al.* (2009), Callegari *et al.* (2012), He *et al.* (2014) |
| BBC3 | Hepatocellular carcinoma | He *et al.* (2014) |
| ANGPTL2 | Hepatocellular carcinoma | He *et al.* (2014) |
| HDAC6 | Hepatocellular carcinoma | Bae *et al.* (2015) |
| ERα | Hepatocellular carcinoma | Chen *et al.* (2015) |
| SOCS1 | Hepatocellular carcinoma | Xu *et al.* (2014) |
| SOCS3 | Hepatocellular carcinoma | Xu *et al.* (2014) |
| MDM2 | Hepatocellular carcinoma | Fornari *et al.* (2014) |
| DDIT4 | Hepatocellular carcinoma | Pineau *et al.* (2010) |
| TIMP3 | Hepatocellular carcinoma | Garofalo *et al.* (2009) |
| TIMP2 | Pancreatic ductal adenocarcinoma | Xu *et al.* (2015) |
| PIK3R1 | Colangiocarcinoma | Okamoto *et al.* (2013) |
| PUMA | Pancreatic ductal adenocarcinoma | Sarkar *et al.* (2013) |
| TRPS1 | Pancreatic ductal adenocarcinoma | Su *et al.* (2013) |
| KIT | Gastrointestinal stromal tumor | Koelz *et al.* (2011), Gits *et al.* (2013), Ihle *et al.* (2015) |

## 3. Esophageal Cancer

Duodeno-gastro-esophageal bile reflux contributes to development of esophageal adenocarcinoma. We recently reported that expression levels of *miR-221/222* increased, along with the activity of nuclear bile acid receptor/farnesoid X receptor (FXR), when cultured esophageal epithelial cells were exposed to bile acids [10]. Furthermore, *miR-221/222* expression was higher in esophageal adenocarcinoma than in the surrounding Barrett's esophagus, a precursor lesion of esophageal adenocarcinoma. p27Kip1 is known to inhibit the proteasomal protein degradation of the transcription factor CDX2. We also confirmed that the levels of p27Kip1 and CDX2 were lower in areas of esophageal adenocarcinoma than in those of Barrett's esophagus. Incubation of cells with bile acids increased degradation of CDX2; this process was reduced when cells were also incubated with proteasome inhibitors. Overexpression of *miR-221/222* reduced levels of p27Kip1 and CDX2, and knockdown of *miR-221/222* increased levels of these proteins in cultured cells. In addition, inhibitors of *miR-221/222* reduced growth of xenograft tumors in immunodeficient mice.

## 4. Gastric Cancer

Liu *et al.* reported that *miR-221* was upregulated in 88% of gastric cancer tissue samples compared with their paired adjacent non-tumor tissue samples [11]. High expression of *miR-221* showed a significant correlation with advanced tumor-node-metastasis stage, local invasion, and lymphatic metastasis. *MiR-221* overexpression was an unfavorable prognostic factor for overall survival in patients with gastric cancer.

In gastric cancer cells, upregulation of *miR-221/222* induced the malignant phenotype, whereas knockdown of *miR-221/222* reversed this phenotype via induction of PTEN, a direct target of *miR-221/222* [12]. In addition, knockdown of *miR-221/222* inhibited cell growth and invasion and increased the radiosensitivity.

## 5. Colorectal Cancer

*MiR-221* was upregulated in 90% of colorectal cancer (CRC) tissue samples compared to that in the adjacent non-tumorous tissue, and the expression level was positively correlated to an advanced TNM stage and local invasion [13–18]. A survival analysis indicated that high expression of *miR-221* was closely associated with a shorter survival time [14,19]. In CRC cells, *miR-221* overexpression enhances, whereas *miR-221* depletion reduces CRC cell proliferation, migration, invasion, and colony formation [16,17]. In mice with colitis, injection of lentiviruses expressing *miR-221/222* sponges led to formation of fewer tumors than injection of control lentiviruses [16]. Protein expressions of p57Kip2 and RECK, direct targets of *miR-221*, were decreased in the CRC tissues, and promoted CRC occurrence and progress [15,17].

Liu *et al.* reported that mimics of *miR-221/222* activated NF-κB and STAT3 in CRC cells [16]. *MiR-221/222* also reduced the ubiquitination and degradation of the RelA and STAT3 proteins by binding to the 3′ untranslated region of PDLIM2 mRNA (PDLIM2 is a nuclear ubiquitin E3 ligase for RelA and STAT3). In human CRC tissues, levels of *miR-221/222* positively correlated with levels of RelA and STAT3 mRNAs. Levels of PDLIM2 mRNA were lower than non-tumor tissues.

Xue *et al.* investigated the regulative effect of *miR-221* on CRC cell radiosensitivity [20]. X-ray radiation had an effect on the expression of *miR-221* in CRC cells in a dose-dependent manner. The protein levels of PTEN, a direct target of *miR-221*, reduced gradually during exposure to X-rays. Inhibition of *miR-221* upregulated expression of PTEN protein and enhanced the radiosensitivity. Moreover, the inhibitory effect was dramatically abolished by pretreatment with anti-PTEN-siRNA, suggesting that the enhancement of radiosensitivity was mediated by PTEN.

Tsunoda *et al.* reported that the increased expression of *miR-221/222* was observed in 3D culture as compared with 2D culture [18]. They showed that *miR-221/222* was regulated by oncogenic KRAS, which plays several key roles in 3D culture. The protein expression level of PTEN was reduced under the control of KRAS in a 3D-specific manner.

The plasma concentration of *miR-221* is a potential biomarker for differentiating CRC patients from controls [21]. Kaplan–Meier curve assessment shows that the elevated plasma *miR-221* level is a significant prognostic factor for poor overall survival in CRC patients. The immunohistochemistry analysis demonstrates a significant correlation between plasma *miR-221* level and p53 expression.

Stool-based *miR-221* can also be used as a non-invasive biomarker for the detection of CRC [13]. In stool samples, *miR-221* showed a significant increasing trend from normal controls to late stages of CRC. The AUC of stool *miR-221* was 0.73 for CRC patients as compared with normal controls. No significant differences in stool *miR-221* levels were found between patients with proximal and distal CRCs. The use of antibiotics did not influence stool *miR-221* levels.

## 6. Hepatocellular Carcinoma

*MiR-221/222* is a critical modulator in the hepatocellular carcinoma (HCC) signaling pathway [22]. *MiR-221/222* was upregulated in the human liver in a fibrosis progression-dependent manner with upregulation of α1 (I) collagen (COL1A1) and α-smooth muscle actin (αSMA) [23–25]. Upregulation of *miR-221* and downregulation of p27Kip1 and p57Kip2 were associated with tumor stages, local recurrence, metastasis, and poor prognosis [24–29]. In a mouse model of liver cancer, *miR-221* overexpression stimulated growth of tumorigenic murine hepatic progenitor cells [30,31]. Inhibition of *miR-221* decreased liver cancer cell proliferation, clonogenicity, migration, and invasion and also induced G1 arrest and apoptosis *in vitro* and *in vivo* [22,27,32].

In HCC cells or hepatocyte, various functions of *miR-221/222* have been investigated (Figure 1). In addition to p27Kip1 and p57Kip2, several direct targets of *miR-221/222* were identified, such as estrogen receptor-alpha (ERα) and a proapoptotic BH3-only protein (BMF) [33,34]. DNA damage-inducible transcript 4 (DDIT4), a modulator of mTOR pathway, was also a direct target of *miR-221* [30]. Garofalo *et al.* showed that *miR-221/222*, by targeting PTEN and TIMP3 tumor suppressors, induce TRAIL resistance and enhance cellular migration through the activation of the AKT pathway and metallopeptidases. Xu *et al.* reported that *miR-221* was upregulated by HCV infection [35]. In addition, an *miR-221* mimic could accentuate the anti-HCV effect of IFN-α in an HCV model, through the inhibition of two members of the suppressor of cytokine signaling (SOCS) family, SOCS1 and SOCS3.

In HCC cells, regulation systems of *miR-221/222* have also been investigated (Figure 1). JNK/c-Jun activation and NF-κB nuclear translocation were reported to be essential for the transcription of *miR-221/222* [23,36,37]. Hepatitis B virus X protein (HBx) leads to the promotion of cell proliferation and cell growth viability with overexpression of *miR-221* [33]. HCV infection could also upregulate the expression of *miR-221* in an NF-κB dependent manner [35,38]. Staphylococcal nuclease domain-containing 1 (SND1) is a multifunctional protein that is overexpressed in multiple cancers, including hepatocellular carcinoma (HCC). Santheladur *et al.* reported that SND1-induced activation of NF-κB resulted in induction of *miR-221* and subsequent induction of angiogenic factors Angiogenin and CXCL16 [39].

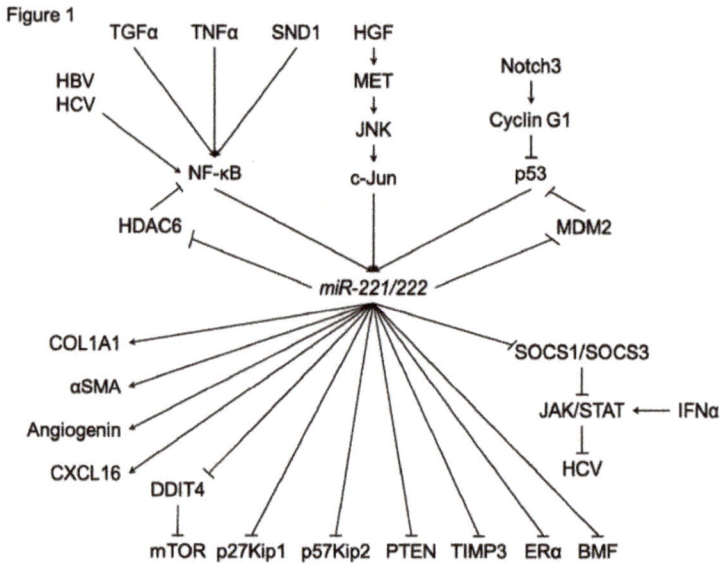

**Figure 1.** A schematic of the regulatory mechanisms of *miR-221/222* in hepatocarcinogenesis.

Bae *et al.* showed that the direct suppression of HDAC6 (histone deacetylase 6) by *miR-221* was induced by JNK/c-Jun signaling in liver cancer cells but not in normal hepatic cells [36]. In addition, NF-κB could be activated by *miR-221*, since HDAC6 suppressed the translocation of NF-κB.

Fornari *et al.* reported that MDM2 (E3 ubiquitin-protein ligase homolog), a known p53 (TP53) modulator, is identified as a direct target of *miR-221* [40]. *MiR-221* can activate the p53/mdm2 axis by inhibiting MDM2 and, in turn, p53 activation contributes to *miR-221* enhanced expression. Giovannini *et al.* reported that Notch3 silencing in HCC resulted in p53 upregulation [41]. They found that Notch3 regulated p53 at post-transcriptional level controlling both Cyclin G1 expression and the feed-forward circuit involving p53, *miR-221*, and MDM2.

## 7. Pancreatic Cancer

Expression of *miR-221/222* is upregulated in pancreatic cancer as compared with normal pancreatic duct epithelial cells or normal pancreas tissues [42–44]. Pancreatic cancer patients with high *miR-221* expression had a relatively shorter survival compared to those with lower expression [42]. Antisense to *miR-221* suppressed the proliferative capacity, increased the amount of apoptosis, and sensitized the effects of gemcitabine in pancreatic cancer cells with concomitant up-regulation of PTEN, p27Kip1, p57Kip2, and PUMA, which are the tumor suppressors and the predicted targets of *miR-221* [42,45,46].

Tanaka *et al.* reported that metformin suppressed the expression of *miR-221* in human pancreatic cancer cells, leading to G1-phase arrest via the upregulation of p27Kip1 [47]. In addition, Sarker *et al.* reported that the treatment of pancreatic cancer cells with isoflavone mixture (G2535), formulated 3,3′-diindolylmethane (BR-DIM), or synthetic curcumin analogue (CDF) could downregulate the expression of *miR-221* and consequently upregulate the expression of PTEN, p27Kip1, p57Kip2, and PUMA, leading to the inhibition of proliferation and migration of pancreatic cancer cells [42]. Therefore, these agents combined with conventional chemotherapeutics could be useful in designing novel targeted therapeutic strategy for the treatment of pancreatic cancer.

Matrix metalloproteinases (MMPs) are closely related to cell migration and invasion. Among the MMPs, MMP-2 and MMP-9 have been implicated in human cancer invasion. Xu *et al.* reported that the tissue inhibitor of metalloproteinase (TIMP)-2 was directly regulated by *miR-221/222* [43]. They also showed that *miR-221/222* mimic directly inhibited TIMP-2 expression, leading to the upregulation of MMP-2 and MMP-9.

The platelet-derived growth factor (PDGF) signaling pathway has been found to play important roles in the development and progression of human cancers by regulating the processes of cell proliferation, apoptosis, migration, invasion, metastasis, and the acquisition of the epithelial-mesenchymal transition (EMT) phenotype. Su *et al.* reported that *miR-221* expression was activated by PDGF signaling [48]. After the inhibition of *miR-221*, PDGF did not alter the levels of cell migration, proliferation, and acquisition of the EMT phenotype. These results showed that *miR-221* is essential for the PDGF-mediated EMT phenotype, migration, and growth of pancreatic cancer cells. Downregulation of TRPS1 by *miR-221* is critical for PDGF-mediated acquisition of the EMT phenotype.

Plasma *miR-221* concentration could be a useful biomarker for cancer detection, monitoring tumor dynamics, and predicting malignant outcomes in pancreatic cancer patients [44]. Plasma *miR-221* levels were higher in pancreatic cancer patients than in benign pancreatic tumors and controls, and were correlated with distant metastasis. In addition, plasma *miR-221* levels were reduced in postoperative samples.

Pancreatic cysts are a group of lesions with heterogeneous malignant potential. *MiR-221* concentration in the endoscopically acquired pancreatic cyst fluid samples could be useful for the diagnosis of pancreatic cysts. *MiR-221* was expressed at higher levels in malignant cysts compared with benign or premalignant cysts [49].

## 8. Cholangiocarcinoma

In contrast to the other epithelial cancers, *miR-221/222* was downregulated in intrahepatic cholangiocarcinoma tissues, suggesting that *miR-221/222* would play onco-suppressive roles [25]. Okamoto *et al.* reported a relationship between *miR-221* expression and the sensitivity of cholangiocarcinoma (CCA) cells to gemcitabine [50]. Microarray analysis was used to determine the miRNA expression profiles of two CCA cell lines, HuCCT1 and HuH28. HuCCT1 cells were more sensitive to gemcitabine than were HuH28 cells, and 18 miRNAs were differentially expressed between HuH28 and HuCCT1. To determine the effect of candidate miRNAs on gemcitabine sensitivity, expression of each candidate miRNA was modified via either transfection of a miRNA mimic or transfection of an anti-oligonucleotide. Among these 18 miRNAs, ectopic overexpression of each of three downregulated miRNAs in HuH28 (*miR-29b*, *miR-205*, and *miR-221*) restored gemcitabine sensitivity to HuH28. Selective siRNA-mediated downregulation of either of two software-predicted targets, PIK3R1 (target of *miR-29b* and *miR-221*) or MMP-2 (target of *miR-29b*), also conferred gemcitabine sensitivity to HuH28.

## 9. Gastrointestinal Stromal Tumor (GIST)

Gastrointestinal stromal tumors (GISTs) are characterized by high expression of the KIT receptor tyrosine kinase protein, resulting from oncogenic mutations in the extracellular, juxtamembrane, or kinase domains. KIT is known to be directly regulated by *miR-221/222*, suggesting that *miR-221/222* would also play onco-suppressive roles in GISTs [51]. In fact, expression of *miR-221/222* is reduced in GISTs compared to control tissue and other sarcomas [51–53]. Overexpression of *miR-221/222* in GIST cells inhibited cell proliferation, affected cell cycle progression, and induced apoptosis [51,52].

Ihle *et al.* analyzed expression of *miR-221/222* in six KIT exon 9, three KIT exon 11 mutated, and nine wild-type GISTs [52]. MiRNA expression was lower for the wild-type compared to mutated GISTs. Transient transfection of *miR-221/222* reduced viability and induced apoptosis by inhibition of KIT expression and its phosphorylation and activation of caspases 3 and 7 in GIST cells. p-AKT, AKT, and BCL2 expression were also reduced after *miR-221/222* transfection.

## 10. Conclusions and Prospects

The discovery of the important role of miRNAs in cancer has opened up a new era of cancer investigations that take into account new and emerging knowledge regarding the RNA signaling systems. The unraveling of *miR-221/222* signaling pathways and networks will be key to understanding the role that deregulated miRNA functioning can play in oncogenic or onco-suppressive processes and may be important for defining novel therapeutic molecules.

Recently miRNAs contained in exosomes have been shown to be released and to act as a signal transducer. However, the function of secretory *miR-221/222* has never been reported. Previous reports showed that *miR-221/222* play various roles not only in cancer but also in vascular smooth muscle cells, vascular endothelial cells, and adipose tissue [54,55]. These suggest that interactions between cancers and blood vessels or adipose tissue would be mediated by secretory *miR-221/222*. Revealing the inter-organic functions of miRNAs will also help us to better understand cancer biology.

**Acknowledgments:** This study was funded by a Grant-in-Aid for Young Scientists (B) (26860527, to Juntaro Matsuzaki), a Grant-in-Aid for Scientific Research (B) (25293178, to Hidekazu Suzuki), Grant-in-aid for Challenging Exploratory Research (26670065, to Hidekazu Suzuki) from the Japan Society for the Promotion of Science (JSPS), the Translational Research Network Program from Ministry of Education, Culture, Sports, Science and Technology of Japan (to Hidekazu Suzuki), Princess Takamatsu Cancer Research grants (to Hidekazu Suzuki), a grant from Takeda Science Foundation (to Juntaro Matsuzaki) and the Keio Gijuku Academic Development Fund (to Hidekazu Suzuki).

**Author Contributions:** Juntaro Matsuzaki wrote and Hidekazu Suzuki supervised and revised the manuscript.

**Conflicts of Interest:** The authors declare no conflict of interest.

## References

1.   Galardi, S.; Mercatelli, N.; Giorda, E.; Massalini, S.; Frajese, G.V.; Ciafre, S.A.; Farace, M.G. *MiR-221* and *miR-222* expression affects the proliferation potential of human prostate carcinoma cell lines by targeting p27kip1. *J. Biol. Chem.* **2007**, *282*, 23716–23724. [CrossRef] [PubMed]

2.   Kneitz, B.; Krebs, M.; Kalogirou, C.; Schubert, M.; Joniau, S.; van Poppel, H.; Lerut, E.; Kneitz, S.; Scholz, C.J.; Strobel, P.; *et al.* Survival in patients with high-risk prostate cancer is predicted by *miR-221*, which regulates proliferation, apoptosis, and invasion of prostate cancer cells by inhibiting IRF2 and SOCS3. *Cancer Res.* **2014**, *74*, 2591–2603. [CrossRef] [PubMed]

3. Falkenberg, N.; Anastasov, N.; Rappl, K.; Braselmann, H.; Auer, G.; Walch, A.; Huber, M.; Hofig, I.; Schmitt, M.; Hofler, H.; *et al. MiR-221/-222* differentiate prognostic groups in advanced breast cancers and influence cell invasion. *Br. J. Cancer* **2013**, *109*, 2714–2723. [PubMed]

4. Quintavalle, C.; Garofalo, M.; Zanca, C.; Romano, G.; Iaboni, M.; del Basso De Caro, M.; Martinez-Montero, J.C.; Incoronato, M.; Nuovo, G.; Croce, C.M.; *et al. MiR-221/222* overexpression in human glioblastoma increases invasiveness by targeting the protein phosphate ptpmu. *Oncogene* **2012**, *31*, 858–868. [PubMed]

5. He, H.; Jazdzewski, K.; Li, W.; Liyanarachchi, S.; Nagy, R.; Volinia, S.; Calin, G.A.; Liu, C.G.; Franssila, K.; Suster, S.; *et al.* The role of microRNA genes in papillary thyroid carcinoma. *Proc. Natl. Acad. Sci. USA* **2005**, *102*, 19075–19080. [CrossRef] [PubMed]

6. Moshiri, F.; Callegari, E.; D'Abundo, L.; Corra, F.; Lupini, L.; Sabbioni, S.; Negrini, M. Inhibiting the oncogenic *miR-221* by microRNA sponge: Toward microrna-based therapeutics for hepatocellular carcinoma. *Gastroenterol. Hepatol. Bed Bench* **2014**, *7*, 43–54. [PubMed]

7. Liu, Y.; Cui, H.; Wang, W.; Li, L.; Wang, Z.; Yang, S.; Zhang, X. Construction of circular miRNA sponges targeting miR-21 or *miR-221* and demonstration of their excellent anticancer effects on malignant melanoma cells. *Int. J. Biochem. Cell Biol.* **2013**, *45*, 2643–2650. [CrossRef] [PubMed]

8. Wang, X.; Han, L.; Zhang, A.; Wang, G.; Jia, Z.; Yang, Y.; Yue, X.; Pu, P.; Shen, C.; Kang, C. Adenovirus-mediated shrnas for co-repression of *miR-221* and *miR-222* expression and function in glioblastoma cells. *Oncol. Rep.* **2011**, *25*, 97–105. [PubMed]

9. Kedde, M.; van Kouwenhove, M.; Zwart, W.; Oude Vrielink, J.A.; Elkon, R.; Agami, R. A pumilio-induced RNA structure switch in p27-3' UTR controls *miR-221* and *miR-222* accessibility. *Nat. Cell Biol.* **2010**, *12*, 1014–1020. [CrossRef] [PubMed]

10. Matsuzaki, J.; Suzuki, H.; Tsugawa, H.; Watanabe, M.; Hossain, S.; Arai, E.; Saito, Y.; Sekine, S.; Akaike, T.; Kanai, Y.; *et al.* Bile acids increase levels of microRNAs 221 and 222, leading to degradation of CDX2 during esophageal carcinogenesis. *Gastroenterology* **2013**, *145*, 1300–1311. [CrossRef] [PubMed]

11. Liu, K.; Li, G.; Fan, C.; Diao, Y.; Wu, B.; Li, J. Increased expression of *microRNA-221* in gastric cancer and its clinical significance. *J. Int. Med. Res.* **2012**, *40*, 467–474. [CrossRef] [PubMed]

12. Chun-Zhi, Z.; Lei, H.; An-Ling, Z.; Yan-Chao, F.; Xiao, Y.; Guang-Xiu, W.; Zhi-Fan, J.; Pei-Yu, P.; Qing-Yu, Z.; Chun-Sheng, K. MicroRNA-221 and *microRNA-222* regulate gastric carcinoma cell proliferation and radioresistance by targeting pten. *BMC Cancer* **2010**, *10*, 367. [PubMed]

13. Yau, T.O.; Wu, C.W.; Dong, Y.; Tang, C.M.; Ng, S.S.; Chan, F.K.; Sung, J.J.; Yu, J. MicroRNA-221 and microRNA-18a identification in stool as potential biomarkers for the non-invasive diagnosis of colorectal carcinoma. *Br. J. Cancer* **2014**, *111*, 1765–1771. [CrossRef] [PubMed]

14. Tao, K.; Yang, J.; Guo, Z.; Hu, Y.; Sheng, H.; Gao, H.; Yu, H. Prognostic value of *miR-221*–3p, miR-342–3p and miR-491–5p expression in colon cancer. *Am. J. Transl. Res.* **2014**, *6*, 391–401. [PubMed]

15. Sun, K.; Wang, W.; Zeng, J.J.; Wu, C.T.; Lei, S.T.; Li, G.X. MicroRNA-221 inhibits cdkn1c/p57 expression in human colorectal carcinoma. *Acta Pharmacol. Sin.* **2011**, *32*, 375–384. [CrossRef] [PubMed]

16. Liu, S.; Sun, X.; Wang, M.; Hou, Y.; Zhan, Y.; Jiang, Y.; Liu, Z.; Cao, X.; Chen, P.; Chen, X.; *et al.* A *microRNA-221*- and 222-mediated feedback loop maintains constitutive activation of nfkappab and STAT3 in colorectal cancer cells. *Gastroenterology* **2014**, *147*, 847–859.e11. [CrossRef] [PubMed]

17. Qin, J.; Luo, M. MicroRNA-221 promotes colorectal cancer cell invasion and metastasis by targeting RECK. *FEBS Lett* **2014**, *588*, 99–104. [CrossRef] [PubMed]

18. Tsunoda, T.; Takashima, Y.; Yoshida, Y.; Doi, K.; Tanaka, Y.; Fujimoto, T.; Machida, T.; Ota, T.; Koyanagi, M.; Kuroki, M.; *et al.* Oncogenic KRAS regulates miR-200c and *miR-221/222* in a 3D-specific manner in colorectal cancer cells. *Anticancer Res.* **2011**, *31*, 2453–2459. [PubMed]

19. Cai, K.; Shen, F.; Cui, J.H.; Yu, Y.; Pan, H.Q. Expression of *miR-221* in colon cancer correlates with prognosis. *Int. J. Clin. Exp. Med.* **2015**, *8*, 2794–2798. [PubMed]

20. Xue, Q.; Sun, K.; Deng, H.J.; Lei, S.T.; Dong, J.Q.; Li, G.X. Anti-mirna-221 sensitizes human colorectal carcinoma cells to radiation by upregulating pten. *World J. Gastroenterol.* **2013**, *19*, 9307–9317. [CrossRef] [PubMed]

21. Pu, X.X.; Huang, G.L.; Guo, H.Q.; Guo, C.C.; Li, H.; Ye, S.; Ling, S.; Jiang, L.; Tian, Y.; Lin, T.Y. Circulating *miR-221* directly amplified from plasma is a potential diagnostic and prognostic marker of colorectal cancer and is correlated with p53 expression. *J. Gastroenterol. Hepatol.* **2010**, *25*, 1674–1680. [CrossRef] [PubMed]

22. He, X.X.; Guo, A.Y.; Xu, C.R.; Chang, Y.; Xiang, G.Y.; Gong, J.; Dan, Z.L.; Tian, D.A.; Liao, J.Z.; Lin, J.S. Bioinformatics analysis identifies *miR-221* as a core regulator in hepatocellular carcinoma and its silencing suppresses tumor properties. *Oncol. Rep.* **2014**, *32*, 1200–1210. [CrossRef] [PubMed]

23. Ogawa, T.; Enomoto, M.; Fujii, H.; Sekiya, Y.; Yoshizato, K.; Ikeda, K.; Kawada, N. *MicroRNA-221/222* upregulation indicates the activation of stellate cells and the progression of liver fibrosis. *Gut* **2012**, *61*, 1600–1609. [CrossRef] [PubMed]

24. Yoon, S.O.; Chun, S.M.; Han, E.H.; Choi, J.; Jang, S.J.; Koh, S.A.; Hwang, S.; Yu, E. Deregulated expression of *microRNA-221* with the potential for prognostic biomarkers in surgically resected hepatocellular carcinoma. *Hum. Pathol.* **2011**, *42*, 1391–1400. [CrossRef] [PubMed]

25. Karakatsanis, A.; Papaconstantinou, I.; Gazouli, M.; Lyberopoulou, A.; Polymeneas, G.; Voros, D. Expression of microRNAs, miR-21, miR-31, miR-122, miR-145, miR-146a, miR-200c, *miR-221, miR-222*, and miR-223 in patients with hepatocellular carcinoma or intrahepatic cholangiocarcinoma and its prognostic significance. *Mol. Carcinog* **2013**, *52*, 297–303. [CrossRef] [PubMed]

26. Fu, X.; Wang, Q.; Chen, J.; Huang, X.; Chen, X.; Cao, L.; Tan, H.; Li, W.; Zhang, L.; Bi, J.; *et al.* Clinical significance of *miR-221* and its inverse correlation with p27kip(1) in hepatocellular carcinoma. *Mol. Biol. Rep.* **2011**, *38*, 3029–3035. [CrossRef] [PubMed]

27. Rong, M.; Chen, G.; Dang, Y. Increased *miR-221* expression in hepatocellular carcinoma tissues and its role in enhancing cell growth and inhibiting apoptosis *in vitro*. *BMC Cancer* **2013**, *13*, 21. [CrossRef] [PubMed]

28. Fornari, F.; Gramantieri, L.; Ferracin, M.; Veronese, A.; Sabbioni, S.; Calin, G.A.; Grazi, G.L.; Giovannini, C.; Croce, C.M.; Bolondi, L.; *et al.* *MiR-221* controls CDKN1C/p57 and CDKN1B/p27 expression in human hepatocellular carcinoma. *Oncogene* **2008**, *27*, 5651–5661. [PubMed]

29. Li, J.; Wang, Y.; Yu, W.; Chen, J.; Luo, J. Expression of serum *miR-221* in human hepatocellular carcinoma and its prognostic significance. *Biochem. Biophys. Res. Commun.* **2011**, *406*, 70–73. [CrossRef] [PubMed]

30. Pineau, P.; Volinia, S.; McJunkin, K.; Marchio, A.; Battiston, C.; Terris, B.; Mazzaferro, V.; Lowe, S.W.; Croce, C.M.; Dejean, A. *MiR-221* overexpression contributes to liver tumorigenesis. *Proc. Natl. Acad. Sci. USA* **2010**, *107*, 264–269. [CrossRef] [PubMed]

31. Callegari, E.; Elamin, B.K.; Giannone, F.; Milazzo, M.; Altavilla, G.; Fornari, F.; Giacomelli, L.; D'Abundo, L.; Ferracin, M.; Bassi, C.; *et al.* Liver tumorigenicity promoted by *microRNA-221* in a mouse transgenic model. *Hepatology* **2012**, *56*, 1025–1033. [CrossRef] [PubMed]

32. Park, J.K.; Kogure, T.; Nuovo, G.J.; Jiang, J.; He, L.; Kim, J.H.; Phelps, M.A.; Papenfuss, T.L.; Croce, C.M.; Patel, T.; *et al.* *MiR-221* silencing blocks hepatocellular carcinoma and promotes survival. *Cancer Res.* **2011**, *71*, 7608–7616. [CrossRef] [PubMed]

33. Chen, J.J.; Tang, Y.S.; Huang, S.F.; Ai, J.G.; Wang, H.X.; Zhang, L.P. HBx protein-induced upregulation of *microRNA-221* promotes aberrant proliferation in HBV-related hepatocellular carcinoma by targeting estrogen receptor-alpha. *Oncol. Rep.* **2015**, *33*, 792–798. [PubMed]

34. Gramantieri, L.; Fornari, F.; Ferracin, M.; Veronese, A.; Sabbioni, S.; Calin, G.A.; Grazi, G.L.; Croce, C.M.; Bolondi, L.; Negrini, M. *MicroRNA-221* targets Bmf in hepatocellular carcinoma and correlates with tumor multifocality. *Clin. Cancer Res.* **2009**, *15*, 5073–5081. [CrossRef] [PubMed]

35. Xu, G.; Yang, F.; Ding, C.L.; Wang, J.; Zhao, P.; Wang, W.; Ren, H. *MiR-221* accentuates IFNs anti-HCV effect by downregulating SOCS1 and SOCS3. *Virology* **2014**, *462–463*, 343–350. [CrossRef] [PubMed]

36. Bae, H.J.; Jung, K.H.; Eun, J.W.; Shen, Q.; Kim, H.S.; Park, S.J.; Shin, W.C.; Yang, H.D.; Park, W.S.; Lee, J.Y.; *et al. MicroRNA-221* governs tumor suppressor HDAC6 to potentiate malignant progression of liver cancer. *J. Hepatol.* **2015**, *63*, 408–419. [PubMed]

37. Garofalo, M.; di Leva, G.; Romano, G.; Nuovo, G.; Suh, S.S.; Ngankeu, A.; Taccioli, C.; Pichiorri, F.; Alder, H.; Secchiero, P.; *et al. MiR-221&222* regulate TRAIL resistance and enhance tumorigenicity through PTEN and TIMP3 downregulation. *Cancer Cell* **2009**, *16*, 498–509. [PubMed]

38. Ding, C.L.; Xu, G.; Ren, H.; Zhao, L.J.; Zhao, P.; Qi, Z.T.; Wang, W. HCV infection induces the upregulation of *miR-221* in nf-kappab dependent manner. *Virus Res.* **2015**, *196*, 135–139. [CrossRef] [PubMed]

39. Santhekadur, P.K.; Das, S.K.; Gredler, R.; Chen, D.; Srivastava, J.; Robertson, C.; Baldwin, A.S., Jr.; Fisher, P.B.; Sarkar, D. Multifunction protein staphylococcal nuclease domain containing 1 (SND1) promotes tumor angiogenesis in human hepatocellular carcinoma through novel pathway that involves nuclear factor kappab and *miR-221*. *J. Biol. Chem.* **2012**, *287*, 13952–13958. [CrossRef] [PubMed]

40. Fornari, F.; Milazzo, M.; Galassi, M.; Callegari, E.; Veronese, A.; Miyaaki, H.; Sabbioni, S.; Mantovani, V.; Marasco, E.; Chieco, P.; *et al.* P53/mdm2 feedback loop sustains *miR-221* expression and dictates the response to anticancer treatments in hepatocellular carcinoma. *Mol. Cancer Res.* **2014**, *12*, 203–216. [CrossRef] [PubMed]

41. Giovannini, C.; Minguzzi, M.; Baglioni, M.; Fornari, F.; Giannone, F.; Ravaioli, M.; Cescon, M.; Chieco, P.; Bolondi, L.; Gramantieri, L. Suppression of p53 by Notch3 is mediated by Cyclin G1 and sustained by MDM2 and *miR-221* axis in hepatocellular carcinoma. *Oncotarget* **2014**, *5*, 10607–10620. [PubMed]

42. Sarkar, S.; Dubaybo, H.; Ali, S.; Goncalves, P.; Kollepara, S.L.; Sethi, S.; Philip, P.A.; Li, Y. Down-regulation of *miR-221* inhibits proliferation of pancreatic cancer cells through up-regulation of PTEN, p27(kip1), p57(kip2), and PUMA. *Am. J. Cancer Res.* **2013**, *3*, 465–477. [PubMed]

43. Xu, Q.; Li, P.; Chen, X.; Zong, L.; Jiang, Z.; Nan, L.; Lei, J.; Duan, W.; Zhang, D.; Li, X.; *et al. MiR-221/222* induces pancreatic cancer progression through the regulation of matrix metalloproteinases. *Oncotarget* **2015**, *6*, 14153–14164. [PubMed]

44. Kawaguchi, T.; Komatsu, S.; Ichikawa, D.; Morimura, R.; Tsujiura, M.; Konishi, H.; Takeshita, H.; Nagata, H.; Arita, T.; Hirajima, S.; *et al.* Clinical impact of circulating *miR-221* in plasma of patients with pancreatic cancer. *Br. J. Cancer* **2013**, *108*, 361–369. [CrossRef] [PubMed]

45. Park, J.K.; Lee, E.J.; Esau, C.; Schmittgen, T.D. Antisense inhibition of *microRNA-21* or -221 arrests cell cycle, induces apoptosis, and sensitizes the effects of gemcitabine in pancreatic adenocarcinoma. *Pancreas* **2009**, *38*, e190–e199. [CrossRef] [PubMed]

46. Basu, A.; Alder, H.; Khiyami, A.; Leahy, P.; Croce, C.M.; Haldar, S. *MicroRNA-375* and *microRNA-221*: Potential noncoding RNAs associated with antiproliferative activity of benzyl isothiocyanate in pancreatic cancer. *Genes Cancer* **2011**, *2*, 108–119. [CrossRef] [PubMed]

47. Tanaka, R.; Tomosugi, M.; Horinaka, M.; Sowa, Y.; Sakai, T. Metformin causes G1-phase arrest via down-regulation of *miR-221* and enhances trail sensitivity through DR5 up-regulation in pancreatic cancer cells. *PLoS ONE* **2015**, *10*, e0125779. [CrossRef] [PubMed]

48. Su, A.; He, S.; Tian, B.; Hu, W.; Zhang, Z. *MicroRNA-221* mediates the effects of pdgf-bb on migration, proliferation, and the epithelial-mesenchymal transition in pancreatic cancer cells. *PLoS ONE* **2013**, *8*, e71309. [CrossRef] [PubMed]

49. Farrell, J.J.; Toste, P.; Wu, N.; Li, L.; Wong, J.; Malkhassian, D.; Tran, L.M.; Wu, X.; Li, X.; Dawson, D.; *et al.* Endoscopically acquired pancreatic cyst fluid *microRNA 21* and *221* are associated with invasive cancer. *Am. J. Gastroenterol.* **2013**, *108*, 1352–1359. [CrossRef] [PubMed]

50. Okamoto, K.; Miyoshi, K.; Murawaki, Y. *MiR-29b, miR-205* and *miR-221* enhance chemosensitivity to gemcitabine in HuH28 human cholangiocarcinoma cells. *PLoS ONE* **2013**, *8*, e77623. [CrossRef] [PubMed]

51. Gits, C.M.; van Kuijk, P.F.; Jonkers, M.B.; Boersma, A.W.; van Ijcken, W.F.; Wozniak, A.; Sciot, R.; Rutkowski, P.; Schoffski, P.; Taguchi, T.; *et al.* MiR-17-92 and *miR-221/222* cluster members target KIT and ETV1 in human gastrointestinal stromal tumours. *Br. J. Cancer* **2013**, *109*, 1625–1635. [PubMed]

52. Ihle, M.A.; Trautmann, M.; Kuenstlinger, H.; Huss, S.; Heydt, C.; Fassunke, J.; Wardelmann, E.; Bauer, S.; Schildhaus, H.U.; Buettner, R.; *et al.* MiRNA-221 and *miRNA-222* induce apoptosis via the kit/akt signalling pathway in gastrointestinal stromal tumours. *Mol. Oncol.* **2015**. [CrossRef]

53. Koelz, M.; Lense, J.; Wrba, F.; Scheffler, M.; Dienes, H.P.; Odenthal, M. Down-regulation of *miR-221* and *miR-222* correlates with pronounced Kit expression in gastrointestinal stromal tumors. *Int. J. Oncol.* **2011**, *38*, 503–511. [CrossRef] [PubMed]

54. Meerson, A.; Traurig, M.; Ossowski, V.; Fleming, J.M.; Mullins, M.; Baier, L.J. Human adipose *microRNA-221* is upregulated in obesity and affects fat metabolism downstream of leptin and TNF-alpha. *Diabetologia* **2013**, *56*, 1971–1979. [CrossRef] [PubMed]

55. Liu, X.; Cheng, Y.; Yang, J.; Xu, L.; Zhang, C. Cell-specific effects of *miR-221/222* in vessels: Molecular mechanism and therapeutic application. *J. Mol. Cell. Cardiol.* **2012**, *52*, 245–255. [CrossRef] [PubMed]

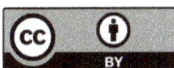

MDPI

St. Alban-Anlage 66

4052 Basel

Switzerland

Tel. +41 61 683 77 34

Fax +41 61 302 89 18

www.mdpi.com

*Journal of Clinical Medicine* Editorial Office

E-mail: jcm@mdpi.com

www.mdpi.com/journal/jcm